Molecular Testing in Cancer

George M. Yousef • Serge Jothy

Editors

Molecular Testing in Cancer

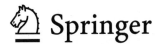 Springer

Editors

George M. Yousef
Department of Laboratory Medicine
and Pathobiology
University of Toronto
Toronto, ON, Canada

Serge Jothy
Department of Laboratory Medicine
and Pathobiology
University of Toronto
Toronto, ON, Canada

ISBN 978-1-4899-8049-6   ISBN 978-1-4899-8050-2 (eBook)
DOI 10.1007/978-1-4899-8050-2
Springer New York Heidelberg Dordrecht London

Library of Congress Control Number: 2014935231

Printed on acid-free paper

Springer is part of Springer Science+Business Media (www.springer.com)

Contents

Part II   Molecular Applications in Various Malignancies

Contributors

Nathanael G. Bailey, M.D. Department of Pathology, University of Michigan Medical School, Ann Arbor, MI, USA

Jyotsna Batra, Ph.D. Translational Research Institute, Queensland University of Technology, Woolloongabba, QLD, Australia

Amir Behdad, M.D. Department of Pathology, University of Michigan Medical School, Ann Arbor, MI, USA

Diana Bell, M.D. Department of Pathology, The University of Texas MD Anderson Cancer Center, Houston, TX, USA

Bryan L. Betz, Ph.D. Department of Pathology, University of Michigan Medical School, Ann Arbor, MI, USA

Paul C. Boutros, Ph.D. Ontario Institute for Cancer Research, Toronto, ON, Canada

Department of Medical Biophysics, University of Toronto, Toronto, ON, Canada

Department Pharmacology and Toxicology, University of Toronto, Toronto, ON, Canada

Judith Clements, Ph.D. Translational Research Institute, Queensland University of Technology, Woolloongabba, QLD, Australia

Kevin P. Conlon, B.Sc. Department of Pathology, University of Michigan Medical School, Ann Arbor, MI, USA

Elisabeth Dequeker, Ph.D. Department of Public Health, Research Unit, University of Leuven, Leuven, Belgium

Brendan C. Dickson, M.D. Department of Pathology and Laboratory Medicine, Mount Sinai Hospital, University of Toronto, Toronto, ON, Canada

Department of Laboratory Medicine and Pathobiology, University of Toronto, Toronto, ON, Canada

Michelle Dolan, M.D. Department of Laboratory Medicine and Pathology, University of Minnesota, Minneapolis, MN, USA

Louis Dubeau, M.D., Ph.D. USC/Norris Comprehensive Cancer Center, Keck School of Medicine of University of Southern California, Los Angeles, CA, USA

Kojo S. J. Elenitoba-Johnson, M.D. Department of Pathology, University of Michigan Medical School, Ann Arbor, MI, USA

Debora Fumagalli, M.D. Institut Jules Bordet, Université Libre de Bruxelles, Brussels, Belgium

Manal Y. Gabril, M.D. Department of Pathology and Laboratory Medicine, University Hospital, London, ON, Canada

Andrea Grin, M.D. Department of Laboratory Medicine, St. Michael's Hospital, University of Toronto, Toronto, ON, Canada

Department of Laboratory Medicine and Pathobiology, University of Toronto, Toronto, ON, Canada

Syed Haider, M.D. Ontario Institute for Cancer Research, Toronto, ON, Canada

Ehab Y. Hanna, M.D. Department of Head and Neck Surgery, The University of Texas MD Anderson Cancer Center, Houston, TX, USA

Carlo Hojilla, M.D., Ph.D. Department of Laboratory Medicine and Pathobiology, University of Toronto, Toronto, ON, Canada

Roland Hubaux, Ph.D. Department of Integrative Oncology, BC Cancer Agency, University of British Columbia, Vancouver, BC, Canada

Department of Pathology and Laboratory Medicine, University of British Columbia, Vancouver, BC, Canada

David M. Hwang, M.D., Ph.D. Department of Pathology, University Health Network, Toronto General Hospital, University of Toronto, Toronto, ON, Canada

Department of Laboratory Medicine and Pathobiology, University of Toronto, Toronto, ON, Canada

Serge Jothy, M.D., Ph.D. Department of Laboratory Medicine, St. Michael's Hospital, University of Toronto, Toronto, ON, Canada

Department of Laboratory Medicine and Pathobiology, University of Toronto, Toronto, ON, Canada

Rita A. Kandel, M.D. Department of Pathology and Laboratory Medicine, Mount Sinai Hospital, University of Toronto, Toronto, ON, Canada

Department of Laboratory Medicine and Pathobiology, University of Toronto, Toronto, ON, Canada

Jason Karamchandani, M.D. Department of Laboratory Medicine, St. Michael's Hospital, University of Toronto, Toronto, ON, Canada

Department of Laboratory Medicine and Pathobiology, University of Toronto, Toronto, ON, Canada

Shirin Karimi, M.D. Department of Pathology, University Health Network, Toronto General Hospital, University of Toronto, Toronto, ON, Canada

Department of Laboratory Medicine and Pathobiology, University of Toronto, Toronto, ON, Canada

Leon van Kempen, Ph.D. Department of Pathology, McGill University, Montreal, QC, Canada

Lady Davis Institute, Jewish General Hospital, Montreal, QC, Canada

Wan L. Lam, Ph.D. Department of Integrative Oncology, BC Cancer Agency, University of British Columbia, Vancouver, BC, Canada

Department of Pathology and Laboratory Medicine, University of British Columbia, Vancouver, BC, Canada

Philippe Lambin, M.D., Ph.D. Department of Radiation Oncology, Maastricht University Medical Center, Maastricht, The Netherlands

Evi S. Lianidou, Ph.D. Laboratory of Analytical Chemistry, Department of Chemistry, University of Athens, Athens, Greece

Megan S. Lim, M.D., Ph.D. Department of Pathology, University of Michigan Medical School, Ann Arbor, MI, USA

Victor D. Martinez, Ph.D. Department of Integrative Oncology, BC Cancer Agency, University of British Columbia, Vancouver, BC, Canada

Department of Pathology and Laboratory Medicine, University of British Columbia, Vancouver, BC, Canada

John D. McPherson, Ph.D. Ontario Institute for Cancer Research, Toronto, ON, Canada

Matthew T. Olson, M.D. Department of Pathology, Johns Hopkins University School of Medicine, Baltimore, MD, USA

Maria Pasic, Ph.D. Department of Laboratory Medicine and Pathobiology, University of Toronto, Toronto, ON, Canada

Jason D. Prescott, M.D., Ph.D. Department of Surgery, Johns Hopkins University School of Medicine, Baltimore, MD, USA

Margaret Redpath, M.D. Department of Pathology, McGill University, Montreal, QC, Canada

Caroline Robert, M.D. Dermatology Unit, Gustave Roussy Institute, Villejuif, France

Delphine Rolland, Ph.D. Department of Pathology, University of Michigan Medical School, Ann Arbor, MI, USA

Etienne Rouleau, Ph.D. Department of Genetics, Institut Curie, Paris, France

David Rowbotham, B.Sc. Department of Integrative Oncology, BC Cancer Agency, University of British Columbia, Vancouver, BC, Canada

Department of Pathology and Laboratory Medicine, University of British Columbia, Vancouver, BC, Canada

Soya S. Sam, Ph.D. Dartmouth Hitchcock Medical Center, Lebanon, NH, USA

Iris Schrijver, M.D. Department of Pathology, Stanford University School of Medicine, Stanford, CA, USA

Simon Patton, Ph.D. European Molecular Genetics Quality Network (EMQN) Genetic Medicine, St. Mary's Hospital, Manchester, UK

Gino R. Somers, M.D., Ph.D. Department of Paediatric Laboratory Medicine, Hospital for Sick Children, University of Toronto, Toronto, ON, Canada

Department of Laboratory Medicine and Pathobiology, University of Toronto, Toronto, ON, Canada

Christos Sotiriou, M.D., Ph.D. Institut Jules Bordet, Université Libre de Bruxelles, Brussels, Belgium

Alan Spatz, M.D. Departments of Pathology and Oncology, McGill University, Montreal, QC, Canada

Lady Davis Institute, Jewish General Hospital, Montreal, QC, Canada

Srilakshmi Srinivasan, Ph.D. Translational Research Institute, Queensland University of Technology, Woolloongabba, QLD, Australia

Maud H. W. Starmans, Ph.D. Informatics and Biocomputing Program, Ontario Institute for Cancer Research, Toronto, ON, Canada

Department of Radiation Oncology, Maastricht University Medical Center, Maastricht, The Netherlands

Sylviane Olschwang, Ph.D. UMR_S910, INSERM, Marseille, France

Department of Gastroenterology, Ambroise Paré Hospital, Marseille, France

Jeffrey J. Tanguay, M.D. Department of Pathology, University Health Network, Toronto General Hospital, University of Toronto, Toronto, ON, Canada

Department of Laboratory Medicine and Pathobiology, University of Toronto, Toronto, ON, Canada

Paul S. Thorner, M.D., Ph.D. Department of Paediatric Laboratory Medicine, Hospital for Sick Children, University of Toronto, Toronto, ON, Canada

Department of Laboratory Medicine and Pathobiology, University of Toronto, Toronto, ON, Canada

Ming-Sound Tsao, M.D. Department of Pathology, University Health Network, Toronto General Hospital, University of Toronto, Toronto, ON, Canada

Department of Laboratory Medicine and Pathobiology, University of Toronto, Toronto, ON, Canada

Gregory J. Tsongalis, Ph.D. Department of Pathology, Geisel School of Medicine at Dartmouth, Lebanon, NH, USA

Dartmouth Hitchcock Medical Center, One Medical Center Drive, Lebanon, NH, USA

Pamela M. Ward, Ph.D. USC/Norris Comprehensive Cancer Center, Keck School of Medicine of University of Southern California, Los Angeles, CA, USA

Kitchener D. Wilson, M.D., Ph.D. Department of Pathology, Stanford University School of Medicine, Stanford, CA, USA

Cindy Yao, M.Sc. Informatics and Biocomputing Program, Ontario Institute for Cancer Research, University of Toronto, Toronto, ON, Canada

Department of Medical Biophysics, University of Toronto, Toronto, ON, Canada

George M. Yousef, M.D., Ph.D. Department of Laboratory Medicine, St. Michael's Hospital, University of Toronto, Toronto, ON, Canada

Department of Laboratory Medicine and Pathobiology, University of Toronto, Toronto, ON, Canada

Dimitrios Zardavas, M.D. Institut Jules Bordet, Université Libre de Bruxelles, Brussels, Belgium

Martha A. Zeiger, M.D. Department of Surgery, Johns Hopkins University School of Medicine, Baltimore, MD, USA

Part I

Molecular Approaches and Techniques

Transitioning Diagnostic Molecular Pathology to the Genomic Era: Cancer Somatic Mutation Panel Testing

Kitchener D. Wilson and Iris Schrijver

Introduction

Treatment protocols for cancer patients are rapidly evolving as molecular genetic information is increasingly used to guide disease management decisions. Cancer diagnosis has traditionally been made according to histology, anatomic origin, cytogenetics as well as protein-based assays such as immunohistochemistry, and, more recently, high-dimension cell surface marker flow cytometry. Clinical oncologists still, in part, select the most appropriate treatment regiment based on these parameters and the extent of spread of the tumor. However, the integration of molecular testing with these conventional methods has ushered in an era of "precision" medicine in clinical oncology [1]. This new direction takes advantage of the data-intensive efforts over the past decades that have revealed large numbers of previously unknown genetic aberrations, many of which are likely to be fundamental molecular drivers of cancer. Although the majority of these molecular aberrations are, as yet, poorly understood, a limited subset has been found to occur across multiple cancer types and appears to be critical for oncogenesis and tumor progression. These are the molecular targets that are transforming clinical cancer care.

A direct result of this expanding catalogue of common molecular defects is the development of therapies that specifically target oncogenic pathways [2]. As a result, treatment decisions are now increasingly informed by genetic biomarkers, ultimately leading to targeted therapies that can augment, or even entirely replace, previously established chemotherapies. These successes have caused many to adopt a genomic view of cancer in which the myriad genetic events that occur during oncogenesis and tumor progression can be used to stratify patients for targeted therapies. For clinical molecular laboratories, next-generation sequencing (NGS) is obviously the key promising technology for tumor genomic profiling. Certainly in the coming decades, NGS instruments will become ubiquitous in clinical laboratories. This powerful technology has already revolutionized the basic research realm by enabling whole-genome, exome, and transcriptome sequencing at rates that are dramatically faster and cheaper than traditional Sanger-based methods. Major multinational efforts have been initiated with the goal of using NGS to understand a wide variety of cancers at the genome and epigenome level, including The Cancer Genome Atlas (TCGA) and the International Cancer Genome Consortium (ICGC) [3]. It is hoped that these molecular data will engender significant research by academia and industry that will result in many new drug targets

K.D. Wilson, M.D., Ph.D. • I. Schrijver, M.D. (✉)
Department of Pathology, Stanford University School of Medicine, 300 Pasteur Drive, Stanford, CA 94305, USA
e-mail: ischrijver@stanfordmed.org

and clinically useful biomarkers [4]. For clinical oncology, the goal of profiling every cancer for clinically actionable molecular targets using NGS underlies the ultimate ambition of precision cancer medicine [5].

Although NGS holds great promise for the field of oncology, both its cost and information-dense complexity require significant expertise and computational infrastructure that currently make it impractical for most clinical laboratories. Fortunately, over the long term, the cost of whole-genome sequencing will decrease to the point that it will be economically viable in the clinical setting, though the exact time frame for this is difficult to predict. Even with "thousand-dollar" whole-genome sequencing, however, it may not be the cost of sequencing that will impede the adoption of cancer genotyping but rather the complex data analysis that is required downstream. Here too there is some good news: techniques have been developed that can reduce the complexity of NGS by enriching only exonic DNA prior to sequencing ("exome sequencing"), thus avoiding the large inter-gene and intronic regions that remain poorly understood. Additional advancements such as DNA barcodes and pooling of samples may also increase NGS throughput while reducing cost [5]. And clearly there is an ongoing major attempt by academia and industry to streamline the bioinformatic pipeline so that non-computational laboratory personnel can align sequencing reads to the human genome for mutation discovery.

Regardless of these technical refinements, it will be several years before the NGS technology and computational infrastructure are affordable and mature enough for validation and generalized clinical use in cancer diagnostics. Furthermore, although NGS approaches may reveal biomarkers that are associated with disease progression or drug response in human patients, the information does not necessarily guarantee that they are the mechanisms and pathways that are at the root of the tumor phenotype and should therefore be considered therapeutic targets [6]. Thus, more sophisticated technical and analytical methods are needed that can define, and enrich for, the mutations that contribute directly to cancer progression and therapy response. This remains a formidable challenge that will dictate the pace of routine use of NGS for clinical cancer testing in the immediate future.

Despite these limitations, the successes with conventional methods of cancer genotyping (e.g., cytogenetics, FISH, PCR, Sanger sequencing, fragment analysis) have already forced oncologists and pathologists to reassess their reliance on anatomic origin and clinical progression for diagnosing cancer subtypes and then choosing treatments regardless of the underlying genetic change(s) [5]. While well established, these methods are frequently laborious and provide only limited information regarding the cancer genome status in clinical samples. To bridge this divide between traditional assays and the coming NGS era, relatively simple multiplexed diagnostic assays have been developed that use existing molecular techniques to provide high-content molecular information in an efficient and cost-effective manner. These newer assays exhibit high sensitivity and specificity for mutation detection, interrogate a large panel (on the order of hundreds) of mutations within oncogenes and tumor suppressor genes, and perform robust mutation detection in DNA from both frozen and formalin-fixed, paraffin-embedded (FFPE) tumor material. Importantly, these technologies allow molecular pathology laboratories to begin offering high-content oncologic molecular assays to treating physicians without the need for significant resource investment as would be required with NGS.

One example of such an approach is SNaPshot, a robust and highly sensitive tumor genotyping technique first developed at the Massachusetts General Hospital [2]. This high-throughput genetic profiling platform, whose only major instrumentation requirement is a capillary electrophoresis-automated DNA sequencer, can be multiplexed to assay hundreds of individual genomic positions at which known clinically actionable nucleotide changes frequently occur. Moreover, SNaPshot is rapid, sensitive, specific, cost-effective, and flexible enough to allow molecular targets to be added to the platform. When combined with other technologies such as Sanger sequencing and fragment size analysis, a comprehensive cancer assay is within reach for clinical molecular laboratories in terms of overall resource expenditure and technical expertise. An assay using this approach has been developed and offered at Stanford for high-content cancer genotyping since 2011. In this chapter, we will use our assay as an example of current methods for high-throughput clinical genotyping during the transition of diagnostic molecular pathology to the genomic era.

Multiplexed Mutation Testing with SNaPshot

The SNaPshot method consists of multiplexed PCR and a single-base extension sequencing reaction in which allele-specific probes that are fluorescently labeled with dideoxynucleotides (ddNTPs) interrogate genomic positions of interest (Figs. 1.1 and 1.2). The variable-length extension primers on each probe then enable resolution by electrophoresis and an automated DNA sequencer. Once size-resolved, the probes' molecular weight and color of the fluorescently

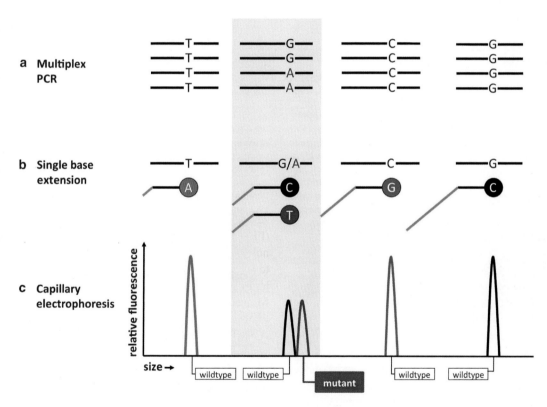

Fig. 1.1 Schematic of SNaPshot technology. After isolation of genomic DNA from tumor specimens, three basic steps are performed that together constitute the SNaPshot methodology. (**a**) Multiplexed PCR of genomic DNA. (**b**) Single-base extension in which allele-specific probes anneal with the target position. Each probe is fluorescently labeled according to nucleotide, using chain-terminating dideoxynucleotides. The four probes (for A, G, T, C) that target each position are barcoded using different length extension primers (*orange*) that allow for size reso-lution in Step 3. (**c**) Capillary electrophoresis of probe-target pairs reveals the relative nucleotide abundance at each target position based on probe size and the color and molecular weight of fluorescently labeled ddNTPs. For example, a mutation (G>A) is depicted in the schematic at one target position. Note that the red peak (mutation) is slightly shifted to the right of the wild-type peak (*black*) due to differences in molecular weight between the two fluorophores

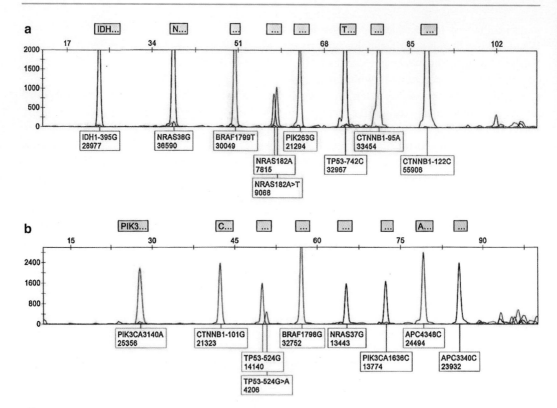

Fig. 1.2 Examples of multiplexed SNaPshot panels. (a) A positive control cell line with an *NRAS* c.182A>T (p.Q61L) mutation. The *gray boxes* above each peak demarcate regions where wild-type and mutant peaks are expected. Note the presence of low-level fluorescent background in each panel, emphasizing the importance of including positive, negative, and no-template controls in each run. (b) A specimen from a patient with non-small-cell lung cancer demonstrates a *TP53* c.524G>A (p.R175H) mutation. Fluorescent peak intensities may vary between targeted genomic regions, and so each laboratory must establish its own threshold criteria for accepting or rejecting these intensities, based on validation studies

labeled ddNTPs are used to identify the particular nucleotide(s) at each position. Overall, there are several obvious advantages of this relatively simple method to today's molecular pathology laboratory: (a) the required expertise and infrastructure are already present in most modern clinical laboratories, thus negating the need for investment in high-tech instrumentation, which can cost several hundreds of thousands of dollars; (b) the method is highly sensitive and (c) performs well with nucleic acid extracted from FFPE tissue; (d) due to the multiplexing features of the SNaPshot technique, the tissue requirements as well as cost are low; and (e) the system is modular and is able to incorporate more molecular predictors of response as they are identified.

In its current configuration, the Stanford Molecular Pathology Laboratory's genotyping platform "cancer somatic mutation panel" (CSMP) consists of a combination of SNaPshot, fragment sizing, and Sanger sequencing methods to query over 140 commonly mutated positions within 16 key cancer genes (Table 1.1). CSMP includes nine SNaPshot panels, each with six to eight multiplexed assays that target single-nucleotide changes. Because one limitation of SNaPshot technology is that it interrogates single-nucleotide changes and not larger genomic insertions/deletions, we have also added a separate capillary electrophoresis fragment sizing assay for several common size length mutations within *EGFR* and *ERRB2/HER2*. A second limi-

Table 1.1 The Stanford cancer somatic mutation panel (March 2013)

Gene	Known somatic mutations at each targeted location
APC	<u>Exon 16</u>: c.3340C>T (p.R1114X), c.4012C>T (p.Q1338X), c.4348C>T (p.R1450X), c.4660-4667insA (p.T1556fs)
BRAF	<u>Exons 11, 15</u>: c.1406G>C (p.G469A), c.1798G>A (p.V600M), c.1799T>C (p.V600A), c.1799T>A (p.V600E), c.1799T>G (p.V600G)
CTNNB1	<u>Exon 3</u>: c.95 A>C (p.D32A), c.95A>G (p.D32G), c.95 A>T (p.D32V), c.94G>T (p.D32Y), c.98C>G (p.S33C), c.98C>T (p.S33F), c.98C>A (p.S33Y), c.101G>A (p.G34E), c.101G>T (p.G34V), c.109T>G (p.S37A), c.109T>C (p.S37P), c.109T>A (p.S37T), c.110C>G (p.S37C), c.110C>T (p.S37F), c.110C>A (p.S37Y), c.121A>G (p.T41A), c.121A>C (p.T41P), c.121A>T (p.T41S), c.122C>T (p.T41I), c.122C>G (p.T41S), c.122C>A (p.T41N), c.133T>G (p.S45A), c.133T>C (p.S45P), c.133T>A (p.S45T), c.134C>G (p.S45C), c.134C>T (p.S45F), c.134C>A (p.S45Y)
DNMT3A	<u>Exon 23</u>: c.2644C>T (p.R882C), c.2644C>A (p.R882S), c.2645G>A (p.R882H), c.2645G>C (p.R882P)
EGFR	<u>Exons 18, 19, 20, 21</u>: c.2155G>T (p.G719C), c.2155G>A (p.G719S), c.2156G>C (p.G719A), c.2369C>T (p.T790M), c.2573T>A (p.L858Q), c.2573T>G (p.L858R), c.2582T>A (p.L861Q); *fragment sizing* for exon 19 deletions and exon 20 insertions
ERBB2/HER2	*Fragment sizing* for exon 20 insertions
IDH1	<u>Exon 4</u>: c.394C>T (p.R132C), c.394C>A (p.R132S), c.394C>G (p.R132G), c.395G>A (p.R132H), c.395G>T (p.R132L), c.395G>C (p.R132P)
IDH2	<u>Exon 4</u>: c.419G>A (p.R140Q), c.419G>T (p.R140L), c.514A>G (p.R172G), c.515G>T (p.R172M), c.515G>A (p.R172K), c.515G>A (p.R172K)
KRAS	<u>Exon 2</u>: c.34G>C (p.G12R), c.34G>A (p.G12S), c.34G>T (p.G12C), c.35G>C (p.G12A), c.35G>A (p.G12D), c.35G>T (p.G12V), c.37G>C (p.G13A), c.37G>A (p.G13S), c.37G>T (p.G13C), c.38G>C (p.G13A), c.38G>A (p.G13D), c.38G>T (p.G13V)
MYD88	<u>Exon 5</u>: c.794T>C (p.L265P)
NOTCH1	<u>Exon 26</u>: c.4724T>C (p.L1575P), c.4802T>C (p.L1601P)
NRAS	<u>Exon 2</u>: c.34G>T (p.G12C), c.34G>A (p.G12S), c.34G>C (p.G12R), c.35G>T (p.G12C), c.35G>A (p.G12D), c.35G>C (p.G12A), c.37G>T (p.G13C), c.37G>C (p.G13R), c.37G>A (p.G13S), c.38G>T (p.G13V), c.38G>C (p.G13A), c.38G>A (p.G13D), c.181C>A (p.Q61K), c.181C>G (p.Q61E), c.183 A>T (p.Q61H), c.183A>G (p.Q61Q), c.183A>C (p.Q61H),
PIK3CA	<u>Exons 10, 21</u>: c.263G>A (p.R88Q), c.1624G>A (p.E542K), c.1624G>C (p.E542Q), c.1633G>A (p.E545K), c.1633G>C (p.E545Q), c.1636C>G (p.Q546E), c.1636C>A (p.Q546K), c.1637A>T (p.Q546L), c.1637A>C (p.Q546P), c.1637A>G (p.Q546R), c.3139C>T (p.H1047Y), c.3140A>T (p.H1047L), c.3140A>G (p.H1047R), c.3145C>G (p.G1049R), c.3145G>A (p.G1049S)
PTEN	<u>Exons 5, 6, 7</u>: c.388C>T (p.R130X), c.388C>G (p.R130G), c.388C>A (p.R130R), c.517C>T (p.R173C), c.697C>T (p.R233X), c.697C>A (p.R233R), c.799delA (p.K267fs*9), c.800delA (p.K267fs*9)
TP53	<u>Exons 7, 8</u>: c.524G>A (p.R175H), c.524G>T (p.R175L), c.733G>T (p.G245C), c.733G>C (p.G245R), c.733G>A (p.G245S), c.742C>G (p.R248G), c.742C>T (p.R248W), c.743G>T (p.R248L), c.743G>C (p.R248P), c.743G>A (p.R248Q), c.817C>T (p.R273C), c.818G>A (p.R273H), c.818G>T (p.R273L), c.916C>T (p.R306X)
SF3B1	*Sanger sequencing* of exon 15 for the following targets: c.1866G>C (p.E622D), c.1873C>T (p.R625C), c.1874G>T (p.R625L), c.1986C>G (p.H662Q), c.1996A>C (p.K666Q), c.1997A>C (p.K666T), c.1997A>G (p.K666R), c.1998G>T (p.K666N); *SNaPshot* for c.2098A>G (p.K700E)

tation of SNaPshot may occur when a target gene contains a high number of clinically relevant nucleotide changes that render the single-base extension targeting of SNaPshot impractical for routine cancer diagnostics. One such example is the RNA-splicing subunit *SF3B1* [7] that has multiple mutation "hot spots" within exon 15. We therefore developed a Sanger DNA sequencing assay that targets exon 15 and is performed as part of CSMP on all specimens.

The Stanford CSMP initially consisted of genes targeted by FDA-approved therapies or by therapies in clinical trials. However, we have taken advantage of the platform's flexibility and have been able to add new gene mutations to our panels, when clinically warranted, within months of reports in the medical literature. One such example is the *MYD88* gene [8]. Importantly, although the mutations included in our CSMP test can be used to guide clinical decision making, the complete clinical implications of the mutations are still evolving. Thus, engaging with treating oncologists to discuss the many targets within a cancer genotyping assay and their clinical importance is an ongoing and required responsibility for the laboratory.

Although biomarker discovery and clinical molecular assay development will continue to advance the customization of cancer treatments, the pace of acceptance of molecular information has not been consistent across medical subspecialties. In our experience with CSMP testing, it has become clear that some clinical services (e.g., thoracic oncology, hematology/oncology) have been rapid adopters of high-content testing. Other services are incorporating such testing much more slowly, and from conversations with these physicians, we have found hesitancy related to the more complex interpretation and the immediate added value of large panels of mutations. Whereas it can easily be appreciated that high-content testing presents a shift in the traditional paradigm of "one disease, one marker," the coming wave of clinical NGS will bring with it even more challenges in the interpretation of complex molecular data. Familiarizing clinicians and clinical laboratories with a high-content but targeted genotyping approach such as CSMP will undoubtedly diminish some of these challenges and will help pave the way to an understanding of a new, genome-based reality.

Selecting Clinically Actionable Molecular Targets

Staying informed of the most recent developments in the fast-paced field of cancer biomarker discovery is a constant challenge for the clinical molecular laboratory. This chapter is not intended as a comprehensive review of biomarkers of cancer, which can be found elsewhere [4–6, 9].

However, the importance of understanding and selecting actionable molecular targets for clinical tumor genotyping is critical for maximizing their usefulness to treating physicians, and therefore knowledge of the cancer mutation field is essential. One of the most frequent questions regarding clinical genotyping assays is "which targets should be tested?". In practical terms, assaying for the most mutations possible is not always the best option because the resulting data complexity would likely be overwhelming. However, despite the difficulties in analyzing such high-dimension data, a comprehensive genotyping assay should, in theory, provide more information for each patient's tumor and therefore be more effective in guiding targeted treatments. A strategic balance must be made between offering as many cancer mutations as possible and acknowledging the limits of the technical and financial resources of the clinical laboratory to generate and interpret the resulting data. Finding the right balance is, of course, not necessarily straightforward.

Cancer mutations, sometimes referred to as biomarkers, are extremely diverse and may be prognostic, predictive, pharmacodynamic, or diagnostic [6]. Prognostic biomarkers provide information about overall cancer outcome, regardless of therapy, whereas predictive biomarkers give information about the potential effect of a therapeutic intervention. Pharmacodynamic biomarkers indicate the outcome of the interaction between a drug and a target, and diagnostic biomarkers are used to establish the presence of a specific disease [6]. Specific examples of mutations include single-base changes, deletions and amplifications, alternative splicing mutations, and translocations. Cumulatively, these molecular aberrations can be highly abundant in cancer cells [10, 11], although most are merely "passengers" that are a consequence of the high mutation rate in cancer [12]. A small subset is the molecular "drivers" that control cancer development and progression and may therefore have important therapeutic implications [4]. Differentiating driver from passenger mutations is a major challenge, made more difficult by the selective pressures of therapy that can lead to intra-tumor, inter-tumor, and between person clonal subpopulations [4, 13]. Clearly, the discovery and validation of clinically actionable biomarkers that consistently occur in a large proportion of cancers requires significant effort and expertise.

Whereas there is enormous diversity in the mutations and variants associated with cancer, which can make the clinical interpretation exceedingly difficult, in some cases the mutation is readily apparent from the data and clinical assays can be quickly developed. For example, a recent study applied whole-genome sequencing to patients with Waldenström's macroglobulinemia, an incurable lymphoplasmacytic lymphoma, and discovered a novel mutation, c.794T>C (p.L265P), in exon 5 of the *MYD88* gene [8]. Because of its immediate clinical applicability as a diagnostic biomarker, a SNaPshot assay for *MYD88* could be incorporated into CSMP within 6 months of publication of the original study. Similarly, a second study performed exome sequencing of patients with myelodysplastic syndrome (MDS), a precancerous lesion of blood forming cells, and identified a variety of mutations in *SF3B1* in 65 % of patients with a subtype of MDS, refractory anemia with ring sideroblasts (MDS-RARS) [7]. Soon after, Sanger sequencing of exon 15—the region where the majority of mutations occur—could be offered as part of CSMP. These experiences illustrate the overall flexibility of this approach to cancer genotyping, as well as the need to stay abreast of the latest discoveries in the cancer biomarker field.

In terms of predictive biomarkers, the clinical benefit observed with some targeted drugs is promising, but the ability to screen cancer patients in a cost-effective manner for clinically actionable targets remains challenging. For example, some kinase domain mutations in *EGFR* are associated with sensitivity to the tyrosine kinase inhibitors (TKI) gefitinib and erlotinib in non-small-cell lung cancer (NSCLC) [2, 14]. However, because only a small number of NSCLC tumors will have *EGFR* mutations, genotyping assays that are expensive and/or time-consuming are highly impractical for routine laboratory testing. Other examples include mutations in *BRAF* and *KRAS* in colorectal cancer [2, 4, 6, 15] that predict resistance to panitumumab and cetuximab and *KRAS* mutations that predict resistance to gefitinib and erlotinib in lung cancer [16]. In general, the advantage of utilizing high-content but low-cost tumor-genotyping assays such as SNaPshot that allow for selection of appropriate targeted therapies is underscored by the current enormous healthcare expenditure on cancer drugs. Inexpensive genotyping assays that lead to targeted therapies will reduce unnecessary treatments and associated costs, while also reducing patient morbidity due to the well-known toxic effects of standard chemotherapies.

Comprehensive- Versus Disease-Focused Tumor Genotyping

Deregulation of common signaling pathways is one of the major underlying causes driving human carcinogenesis. However, there is an ongoing debate in clinical molecular cancer testing regarding the need for large, comprehensive panels of gene mutations that are agnostic to the specific disease and/or tissue of origin of the tumor, in contrast to more targeted mutation panels that take into account the type of cancer. For example, should acute myelogenous leukemia (AML) and lung cancer be subjected to the same tumor-genotyping panel even if *DNMT3A* mutations are rarely detected in lung cancer and *EGFR* mutations in AML? Would it be more effective to offer targeted panels for lung cancer, for AML, for gastrointestinal tumors, etc.? With disease- or organ-specific mutation panels, some argue that those rare tumors that harbor unusual mutations and that might benefit from different classes of drugs will be missed. In contrast, others argue that it can be impractical and even wasteful to spend time and resources testing for mutations that are highly unusual in a particular cancer type. For the benefit of patient care, the right choice is not always "the more, the better," especially given that larger assays might increase turnaround time due to increased technical and analytical complexity.

As oncology and molecular diagnostics gradually continue to integrate, many physicians will undoubtedly prefer a more traditional approach to cancer treatment that focuses on well-characterized genetic hallmarks of cancer that have been verified in clinical trials. The disadvantage of this approach to cancer genotyping is that if we think of cancer as fundamentally a genetic disease, then cancer histology and tissue of origin should be de-emphasized as more drugs are developed that target specific genetic mutations, and smaller genotyping panels will thus lead to fewer opportunities for novel therapies. This discussion will only increase as NGS technologies are incorporated into tumor genotyping. In the future, it may be the case that genome sequencing will be performed on every specimen, but only data for genomic regions of interest will be released, while other regions are "masked" from the molecular pathologist and oncologist. This scenario, while perhaps preferable because of its reduction of complexity, does not take advantage of the power of NGS testing, especially if we expect that NGS should usher in an era of agnostic, unbiased analysis of the cancer genome. Regardless, this debate will continue in earnest as our knowledge, as well as the information content and throughput of mutation testing, increase.

Specimen Considerations

In addition to the challenges in selecting clinically actionable molecular targets, processing of the tissue samples themselves requires significant optimization and validation. Many specimens are derived from core biopsies that have relatively little material; nucleic acid is often fragmented or degraded due to the cross-linking caused by formalin fixation required for histology; and samples may be predominantly normal tissue with very little cancerous tissue, resulting in dilution of the mutant alleles of interest [2]. For heterogeneous specimens, FFPE does allow for assessment of tumor cellularity and demarcation of regions for macrodissection, though this is not always practical given limited time and resources.

Compounding these difficulties is the necessity for maintaining reasonable turnaround times that ensure maximum impact on patient care.

In general, the quality and quantity of tumor DNA are the critical criteria for performing a successful tumor-genotyping assay, and these criteria are ultimately dependent on the quality of the tissue specimen sent to the laboratory. Although the sensitivity of the assay for each mutation depends on the quality of the material and involvement of the block by tumor, our clinical laboratory's experience has found that specimens with >10 % cellularity are required for CSMP. Assays such as NGS with increased genomic coverage compared to targeted assays will obviously require greater quantities of tumor DNA. In the future, successful application of higher content NGS assays will thus require methods that enable genotyping from very small quantities of DNA.

There is an ongoing debate over the advantages of genotyping tissue from the primary tumor or metastatic lesion in advanced cancer patients [4]. Due to cancer's genomic instability and potential acquisition of new mutations that may arise during metastasis, as well as treatments that can select for drug-resistant clonal subpopulations [17, 18], genotyping a single biopsy from a patient may be inadequate for capturing the true genomic diversity of an evolving cancer. In fact, acquired mutations in different tumor sites may differ within the same patient [19] and even within the same tumor [13]. Some studies of *KRAS* mutations in colorectal cancer suggest that the differences are only marginal and the mutations are similar, if not identical, between primary and metastatic lesions [20, 21], while others have found discordant *PIK3CA* mutations between breast cancer primary and metastatic sites [22]. In many circumstances, the decision to choose a primary or metastatic biopsy for genotyping is often influenced by cost, convenience, and hospital practices rather than by evidence-based data [4]. Further studies are needed to determine whether mutation differences between primary and metastatic lesions will lead to different clinical treatment decisions and thus different patient outcomes.

Limitations of SNaPshot and CSMP

SNaPshot is limited by the number of reactions that can be multiplexed, which is ideally below ten per reaction [2]. The number of assays that can be performed on small biopsies is also limited. Furthermore, SNaPshot's single-base extension methodology allows testing only for point mutations in a few hot spots per reaction. To expand the repertoire of mutation targets and achieve a more comprehensive view of the cancer genome, clinical genotyping assays are greatly improved when other methods are incorporated that complement SNaPshot, for example, Sanger sequencing and fragment sizing by capillary electrophoresis. A relatively comprehensive molecular approach such as Stanford's CSMP can then be interpreted by oncologists in conjunction with conventional cytogenetic assays for alterations in gene copy number, as well as karyotyping and detection of large chromosomal rearrangements.

Clinical laboratories should also consider the overall size of their tumor genomic profiling assay, as the resulting complexity may pose challenges to the laboratory's personnel and resources. When introducing new mutation panels into cancer genotyping assays, it is important to realize that this added complexity may also lead to increased turnaround time and a greater possibility of repeat testing of select markers in order to achieve optimal results. Thus, added complexity does not necessarily translate into improved patient care. The number of molecular targets included in the assay, therefore, is limited by the ability of the laboratory to ensure precise, accurate results with good turnaround time for each assay run. Depending on laboratory resources and personnel, the typical maximum number of targets is on the order of hundreds. As mentioned earlier, the sensitivity of the assay is also dependent on the quality of the material and involvement of the block by tumor, and so the chances of a successful assay are easily compromised by samples of suboptimal quality. Communication with surgical pathologists is critical to ensure that high-quality blocks with high tumor percentage are sent for cancer genotyping.

With high-content assays also comes the potential for confusion and misunderstanding when reporting results to treating physicians. Therefore, reports must reflect the current state of knowledge, be as clear as possible, and emphasize that the molecular diagnostic test results should be interpreted in the context of histopathological and clinical findings. False negative results may be due to sampling error, sample handling, or clonal density below the level of detection with reagents and techniques used. Genotyping errors can also result, for example, from deletions or rare genetic variants that interfere with analysis, including polymorphisms in primer binding sites that prevent allele amplification. In such cases, alternative approaches may be helpful to investigate the underlying cause. In general, high-content testing requires excellent communication. Every attempt should be made to educate medical personnel and patients about the clinical implications of reported mutations, particularly with regard to prognostic or predictive biomarkers that are identified in a tumor. Up-to-date knowledge of the medical literature is central to effectively transmitting this knowledge among clinical pathologists, oncologists, and patients.

Conclusion

Targeted cancer therapy is revolutionizing clinical oncology by driving efforts to integrate tumor molecular analysis with clinical decision making. The continuing discovery of salient molecular biomarkers, as well as their use in the design of targeted therapies, is shifting oncology from tissue- and disease-based treatments to molecular target-based protocols. With the inclusion of clinical molecular diagnostics into standard cancer care, precision medicine is expected to progress rapidly as cancer biomarkers guide both therapy and monitoring of disease progression towards a future of individualized and customized therapies. Additionally, drugs that target specific mutations will potentially result in fewer side effects and will also be more efficacious against cancers in which conventional chemotherapy has failed.

The availability of ever-increasing molecular data sets will no doubt hasten all of these significant advancements.

With this revolution in genomic technologies, the age of precision medicine has not only defined how oncology is evolving today but also portends how it will be practiced in the future. These incredible advancements will greatly impact many established disciplines, bringing with them significant new challenges. For example, most institutions are not yet prepared for the associated infrastructure requirements, which include expansion in patient-informed consent and substantial laboratory information database hardware and software [5]. Educating physicians regarding the appropriate interpretation of this information is important and practice guidelines for its use must be established as well. Lastly, reimbursement for genomic diagnostics will continue to be a source of much discussion. Confronting these diverse challenges will require the careful organization of clinicians across multiple disciplines, laboratories, genetic counselors, bioethicists, information technology and informatics specialists, basic and translational researchers, health policy experts, and patient advocacy groups [5].

Although not without their own challenges, multiplexed platforms such as CSMP can serve as invaluable bridges between conventional cancer genotyping and the coming genomic era. The spectrum of mutations detected with the Stanford CSMP configuration are all potentially clinically actionable, typically involving signal pathway-activating mutations which have targeted therapies available or are under clinical investigation. Furthermore, due to its inherent modular design, CSMP (within limits) allows for rapid and efficient adoption of new targets as they are discovered. This is important because the list of actionable mutations continues to grow. Lastly, relatively straightforward high-content cancer genotyping platforms such as CSMP are giving oncologists and pathologists a glimpse of what precision cancer care will look like in the near future. In many respects, CSMP is a dry run for comprehensive testing by NGS, allowing clinical laboratories time to adapt to the increasing ana-lytic complexity and logistical challenges that are the defining characteristic of clinical NGS.

With this explosion in oncologic molecular data, the understanding of oncogenesis is becoming increasingly complex and it is critical that pathologists and oncologists stay abreast of the latest discoveries. Overall, these data have revealed that specific mutations are often observed across a range of cancers, albeit at different frequencies. It is therefore not unreasonable to ask whether cancer treatment itself will be transformed in the genomic era. One obvious question is whether tumors that have different histologies and/or tissues of origin, and which would traditionally be treated differently based on these parameters, should instead be treated the same if they carry identical genetic profiles. More specifically, if vemurafenib is effective in treating *BRAF* p.V600E positive melanoma, then would it be unreasonable to assume it might also be effective in *BRAF* p.V600E positive ovarian cancer [23]? Recent evidence appears to refute, at least in part, this hypothesis that a specific mutation is generalizable across cancers. For example, trastuzumab, which is effective in patients with *HER2*-positive breast and gastric cancer, is less effective in those with *HER2*-positive ovarian or endometrial cancer [24, 25]. However, if the sensitivity of a specific mutation to a targeted drug is even slightly similar across different cancers, then interrogating the cancer genome for all actionable mutations *regardless* of traditional taxonomy would be an ideal method to help guide treatment decisions.

Although there currently exist numerous examples of the successful integration of cancer genetic information with clinical oncologic treatments, particularly as high-content mutation panel testing such as SNaPshot gains in popularity, the future is likely to be less straightforward as NGS is implemented. Regardless of the challenges, genetic profiling strategies will be essential to dissecting the intricate connections between genotype and phenotype and will play an increasingly important role in cancer management decisions. While the basic and translational research contributions rapidly add to the medical knowledge base, application of CSMP and other high-content genotyping platforms will better prepare healthcare providers for the new genomic era, in which genomic testing of cancers becomes routine medical care.

References

1. Toward precision medicine: building a knowledge network for biomedical research and a new taxonomy of disease. National Research Council of the National Academies. 2011.
2. Dias Santagata D, Akhavanfard S, David S, Vernovsky K, Kuhlmann G, Boisvert S, et al. Rapid targeted mutational analysis of human tumours: a clinical platform to guide personalized cancer medicine. EMBO Mol Med. 2010;2:146–58.
3. Hudson TJ, Anderson W, Artez A, Barker A, Bell C, Bernabé R, et al. International network of cancer genome projects. Nature. 2010;464:993–8.
4. Dancey JE, Bedard PL, Onetto N, Hudson TJ. The genetic basis for cancer treatment decisions. Cell. 2012;148:409–20.
5. MacConaill L, Garraway L. Clinical implications of the cancer genome. J Clin Oncol. 2010;28:5219–28.
6. Ong F, Das K, Wang J, Vakil H, Kuo J, Blackwell W-L, et al. Personalized medicine and pharmacogenetic biomarkers: progress in molecular oncology testing. Expert Rev Mol Diagn. 2012;12:593–602.
7. Papaemmanuil E, Cazzola M, Boultwood J, Malcovati L, Vyas P, Bowen D, et al. Somatic SF3B1 mutation in myelodysplasia with ring sideroblasts. N Engl J Med. 2011;365:1384–95.
8. Treon S, Xu L, Yang G, Zhou Y, Liu X, Cao Y, et al. MYD88 L265P somatic mutation in Waldenström's macroglobulinemia. N Engl J Med. 2012;367:826–33.
9. Arteaga CL, Baselga J. Impact of genomics on personalized cancer medicine. Clin Cancer Res. 2012;18:612–8.
10. Stratton MR. Exploring the genomes of cancer cells: progress and promise. Science. 2011;331:1553–8.
11. Wong K, Hudson T, McPherson J. Unraveling the genetics of cancer: genome sequencing and beyond. Annu Rev Genomics Hum Genet. 2011;12:407–30.
12. Pleasance E, Cheetham RK, Stephens P, McBride D, Humphray S, Greenman C, et al. A comprehensive catalogue of somatic mutations from a human cancer genome. Nature. 2010;463:191–6.
13. Gerlinger M, Rowan A, Horswell S, Larkin J, Endesfelder D, Gronroos E, et al. Intratumor heterogeneity and branched evolution revealed by multiregion sequencing. N Engl J Med. 2012;366:883–92.
14. Maemondo M, Inoue A, Kobayashi K, Sugawara S, Oizumi S, Isobe H, et al. Gefitinib or chemotherapy for non-small-cell lung cancer with mutated EGFR. N Engl J Med. 2010;362:2380–8.
15. Di Nicolantonio F, Martini M, Molinari F, Sartore Bianchi A, Arena S, Saletti P, et al. Wild-type BRAF is required for response to panitumumab or cetuximab in metastatic colorectal cancer. J Clin Oncol. 2008;26:5705–12.
16. Pao W, Wang T, Riely G, Miller V, Pan Q, Ladanyi M, et al. KRAS mutations and primary resistance of lung adenocarcinomas to gefitinib or erlotinib. PLoS Med. 2005;2:e17-e.
17. Campbell P, Yachida S, Mudie L, Stephens P, Pleasance E, Stebbings L, et al. The patterns and dynamics of genomic instability in metastatic pancreatic cancer. Nature. 2010;467:1109–13.
18. Jones S, Laskin J, Li Y, Griffith O, An J, Bilenky M, et al. Evolution of an adenocarcinoma in response to selection by targeted kinase inhibitors. Genome Biol. 2010;11:R82-R.
19. Yachida S, Jones S, Bozic I, Antal T, Leary R, Fu B, et al. Distant metastasis occurs late during the genetic evolution of pancreatic cancer. Nature. 2010;467:1114–7.
20. Knijn N, Mekenkamp LJM, Klomp M, Vink-Börger ME, Tol J, Teerenstra S, et al. KRAS mutation analysis: a comparison between primary tumours and matched liver metastases in 305 colorectal cancer patients. Br J Cancer. 2011;104:1020–6.
21. Santini D, Loupakis F, Vincenzi B, Floriani I, Stasi I, Canestrari E, et al. High concordance of KRAS status between primary colorectal tumors and related metastatic sites: Implications for clinical practice. Oncologist. 2008;13:1270–5.
22. Jensen JD, Laenkholm A-V, Knoop A, Ewertz M, Bandaru R, Liu W, et al. PIK3CA mutations may be discordant between primary and corresponding metastatic disease in breast cancer. Clin Cancer Res. 2011;17:667–77.
23. Estep A, Palmer C, McCormick F, Rauen K. Mutation analysis of BRAF, MEK1 and MEK2 in 15 ovarian cancer cell lines: implications for therapy. PLoS One. 2007;2:e1279.
24. Bang Y-J, Van Cutsem E, Feyereislova A, Chung H, Shen L, Sawaki A, et al. Trastuzumab in combination with chemotherapy versus chemotherapy alone for treatment of HER2-positive advanced gastric or gastro-oesophageal junction cancer (ToGA): a phase 3, open-label, randomised controlled trial. Lancet. 2010;376:687–97.
25. Fleming G, Sill M, Darcy K, McMeekin DS, Thigpen JT, Adler L, et al. Phase II trial of trastuzumab in women with advanced or recurrent, HER2-positive endometrial carcinoma: a Gynecologic Oncology Group study. Gynecol Oncol. 2010;116:15–20.

Conventional and Molecular Cytogenetics in Cancer

Michelle Dolan

Introduction

Chromosomes were first identified in the mid-nineteenth century, but it took almost 75 years to count them accurately—it was not until 1956 that Tjio and Levan [1] reported their seminal observation that the human chromosome number was 46, not 48, as previously believed; Ford and Hamerton confirmed this finding later that year [2]. This serendipitous discovery (due to a laboratory error, hypotonic rather than isotonic solution was used during cell harvesting, which improved chromosome spreading) laid the foundation for further advances in cytogenetics (for reviews of the history of cytogenetics, see [3–7]). Continued improvements in cell culture and harvesting techniques permitted the identification of numerical abnormalities (e.g., Turner and Klinefelter syndromes and trisomies 13, 18, and 21) and major structural chromosomal abnormalities. Despite being able to identify chromosomes at that time only by size and centromere position, Peter Nowell and David Hungerford in 1960 noted that patients with chronic myelogenous leukemia (CML) had a small acrocentric chromosome that appeared deleted; this abnormal chromosome became known as the Philadelphia chromosome

after the city of its discovery [8, 9]. With the advent of banding techniques, however, Janet Rowley was able to recognize that the Philadelphia chromosome arose not from a deletion but rather from a reciprocal translocation between the long arms of a chromosome 9 and a chromosome 22 [10]. Later advances in molecular techniques enabled researchers to discover that the 9;22 translocation fused the *ABL1* gene in 9q34 to the *BCR* gene in 22q11.2 [11–14].

Such gene discoveries led to the next major advance in cytogenetic technology: molecular cytogenetics, specifically fluorescence in situ hybridization (FISH). Whereas conventional G-banded chromosomal analysis allows the entire genome to be analyzed, FISH evaluates specific genes and thus is a technique of much greater resolution and sensitivity. Although chromosomal banding and FISH may have been overshadowed in recent years by the tremendous advances made by highly complex technologies such as array-based comparative genomic hybridization and next-generation sequencing, still, the clinical utility of these two reliable techniques is undeniable. Not only is the demonstration by G-banding or FISH of specific chromosomal abnormalities and gene rearrangements a necessary component in the diagnosis of numerous malignancies, this information can often be obtained in less than 24 h and even, in some cases, the same day.

Since the discovery of the Philadelphia chromosome ushered in the era of genomic medicine, there has been extremely rapid growth in the

M. Dolan M.D. (✉)
Department of Laboratory Medicine and Pathology,
University of Minnesota, MMC 609,
420 Delaware St. SE, Minneapolis, MN 55455, USA
e-mail: dolan009@umn.edu

understanding of the genetic basis of neoplasia—there are now almost 63,000 cases of chromosome abnormalities and over 1,500 gene fusions that have been reported in cancer [15]. Further advances in technology, and in the bioinformatics needed to analyze the massive amounts of data these technologies yield, will no doubt transform the field of cytogenomics as profoundly as did the discovery of the number of human chromosomes.

Conventional Cytogenetics

Conventional cytogenetic analysis is performed on metaphase (dividing) cells and provides information about the entire chromosome complement. A variety of tissue types can be cultured to yield metaphase cells for analysis, including peripheral blood, chorionic villi, amniotic fluid, bone marrow, lymph nodes, and solid tumors. Analyses of peripheral blood, chorionic villi, and amniotic fluid are typically performed to identify and characterize constitutional abnormalities (i.e., those present at birth and, barring mosaicism, found in every cell). These specimen types involve somewhat different culture conditions than do those for neoplastic conditions and thus lie outside the scope of this chapter. At a basic level, however, culture procedures have the same goal, namely, optimizing the conditions of cell culture media, temperature, pH, and sterility to stimulate cells to proceed through the cell cycle to mitosis (various culture protocols are described in [3, 16–18]). Cells from the submitted specimens are first isolated, either through centrifugation (for liquid specimens) or disaggregation (for solid tissue specimens), and then placed in tissue culture media. Culture conditions are typically optimized in each laboratory for particular specimen types and include the type of culture (suspension vs. in situ), variations on the length of time in culture, additives such as mitogens, and exposure time to a spindle fiber poison such as colcemid. The cultured cells are then harvested after exposure to a hypotonic solution and placed in fixative, typically a 3:1 methanol to acetic acid mixture (Carnoy's fixative). The resulting cell

suspension is "dropped" via pipette onto glass slides, an often idiosyncratic process driven by ambient conditions (e.g., temperature and humidity) and specimen cellularity as well as technologist experience.

As noted above, different studies (constitutional or neoplastic) and different tissues require culture modifications to increase the likelihood of obtaining metaphases from the cells of interest. This is critical in cancer studies because, unlike constitutional abnormalities that are present in every cell of the body, chromosome aberrations associated with malignancies are present only in the involved tissue or even, in the case of leukemias, only one particular cell line. Thus, in neoplasms of mature cells (e.g., mature B cells and plasma cells), the malignant cells may not be actively dividing and may require the addition of a mitogen to stimulate those cells to enter the cell cycle. Studies have shown that the addition of CpG motif-containing oligonucleotides such as DSP30 together with interleukin-2 increases the yield of chromosomal aberrations in mature B-cell neoplasms by G-banding analysis [19, 20]. After the slides have been dropped and aged by heating them in an oven for several hours, they are treated with a proteolytic enzyme such as trypsin or pancreatin and stained with a Giemsa/buffer solution, resulting in the series of alternating light and dark bands (G-bands) characteristic of each of the 22 pairs of autosomes and two sex chromosomes.

The cytogenetic technologist then analyzes (by comparing the two homologues of a chromosome pair band-for-band along their entire lengths) at least 20 metaphase cells, taking care not to skip cells with poor chromosome morphology, because these may be the malignant cells. G-banding enables detection of both numerical (gain or loss of a chromosome) and structural (e.g., translocation, deletion, inversion, etc.) abnormalities throughout the entire genome. These cells are photographed with a digital camera affixed to the microscope, and the technologist interacts with the resulting images via specialized image analysis software. At least two karyograms, images in which the chromosome pairs have been aligned and placed in order, are prepared. G-banding analysis at diagnosis provides critical information about the types of abnormalities present, and whether or not they can be evaluated by FISH (see below); follow-up studies are compared with the diagnostic study to document therapeutic response. Periodic monitoring can detect cytogenetic evolution, which may even precede morphologic evidence of disease progression.

Even in the early days of cytogenetics, it was recognized that a uniform nomenclature was needed to describe and communicate findings accurately. In 1960, a group of cytogeneticists collaborated on a project to develop a system by which even complex numerical and/or structural abnormalities could be succinctly described. The resulting book would eventually come to be known as the International System for Human Cytogenetic Nomenclature (ISCN). Since its initial publication, the ISCN has been updated and revised several times (most recently in 2013) [21] to keep pace with the findings resulting from FISH and genomic microarray testing. The ISCN provides diagrammatic representations (ideograms) of each chromosome and its banding pattern at various levels of resolution; these ideograms permit cytogeneticists to identify breakpoints, the bands involved in structural rearrangements. The ISCN can be considered both a dictionary and a grammar book: the former, because it describes the abbreviations used for the various types of chromosomal abnormalities and defines basic concepts such as clones, and the latter, because it provides the rules for organizing nomenclature strings to describe the chromosomal complement. Below is an example of a nomenclature string that might be found in a case of CML (see also Fig. 2.1):

Because G-banding analysis can be performed on such a wide range of specimen types, it has been the principal means by which numerical and structural abnormalities have been identified in numerous neoplastic conditions. Because it provides a whole-genome view of these conditions, genome complexity can also be identified and investigated, which might otherwise be missed by more targeted approaches such as FISH. As will be described in a subsequent chapter, other whole-genome approaches such as array-based comparative genomic hybridization are now being commonly used, particularly in the evaluation of constitutional abnormalities and also in neoplastic conditions. Still, G-banding analysis has proved its utility since the discovery of the Philadelphia chromosome and for the foreseeable future will retain its important role in the diagnosis and treatment of malignant disorders.

Molecular Cytogenetics

As exemplified by the advances in the diagnosis and treatment of CML, conventional G-banding analyses often provide the initial clues as to which genes are involved in malignancies. Even if well-documented translocations are identified by G-banding, however, resolution is insufficient (each band can have 5–10 Mb of DNA) to determine if the characteristic gene rearrangement is present. Fluorescently labeled probes, typically several hundred Kb long and complementary to known genomic sequences, can be used to enumerate specific loci and to identify various structural rearrangements such as translocations and inversions. Such probes can also detect

46,XY,t(9;22)(q34;q11.2)[3/20]/48,sl,+8,+19[5/20]/49,sdl1,i(17)(q10),+der(22)t(9;22)[2/20]//46,XX[10/20]

| Clone 1 (stemline, sl): 15% of metaphases have a male karyotype with a reciprocal 9;22 translocation with breakpoints at 9q34 and 22q11.2 | Clone 2 (sideline [sdl] 1): In addition to the t(9;22) found in Clone 1(stemline), 25% of metaphases have gain of one extra copy each of chromosomes 8 and 19 | Clone 3 (sideline [sdl] 2): In addition to the abnormalities found in Clone 2 (sideline 1), 10% of metaphases have an isochromosome for the long arm of a chromosome 17 and gain of a second Philadelphia chromosome | This specimen shows chimerism for recipient (XY) and donor (XX) cells; 50% of metaphases are karyotypically normal female donor cells (listed after "//") |

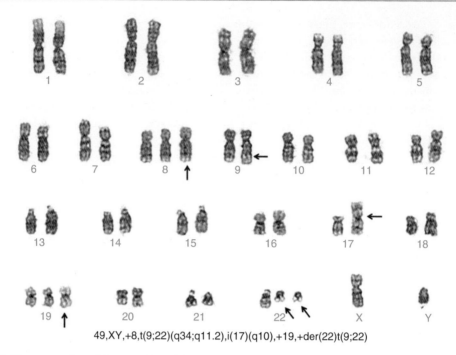

49,XY,+8,t(9;22)(q34;q11.2),i(17)(q10),+19,+der(22)t(9;22)

Fig. 2.1 Karyogram of a cell from a patient with chronic myelogenous leukemia. In addition to the t(9;22) resulting in the formation of the Philadelphia chromosome (the derivative chromosome 22), there are gains of one extra copy each of chromosomes 8 and 19, an isochromosome composed of the long arms of a chromosome 17 joined in mirror image at the centromere (resulting in net loss of 17p and net gain of 17q), and gain of an extra copy of the Philadelphia chromosome

abnormalities that are cryptic (i.e., undetectable by G-banding) due either to the lower resolution of G-banding or to the exchange of regions with similar banding characteristics. Although FISH can be performed on metaphase cells, in cancer cases it is most frequently performed on interphase (nondividing) cells, allowing a large number of cells to be examined quickly, resulting in greater sensitivity and a more rapid turnaround time than G-banding analysis. Interphase cells are often obtained after culturing specimens for concomitant G-banding analysis, but as FISH does not require dividing cells, it can also be performed on a variety of other substrates, including smears prepared from peripheral blood or bone marrow; touch imprints; cytologic preparations; formalin-fixed, paraffin-embedded (FFPE) tissues; or enriched cell populations (e.g., after processing by flow cytometry or magnetic bead separation based on surface antigens). The benefits and limitations of each are outlined in Table 2.1.

Probes to clinically relevant genes are readily available from commercial vendors and can also be developed in-house. With the exception of some probes that have been approved by the US Food and Drug Administration (FDA), most are sold as analyte-specific reagents, which require laboratory validation and verification of test performance before clinical use; guidelines for validation procedures have been published [22–24].

Procedures for setting up FISH are less time- and labor-intensive than those for G-banding analyses and, with some modifications depending on the type of substrate (suspension, smears, touch imprints, FFPE tissues), are essentially the same for all tissue types [16, 18, 25–27]. Briefly, an aliquot of the appropriate probe/buffer mixture is placed on a glass slide that has been etched to delimit an area with an appropriate concentration of nuclei. Cell concentration is important in that only nonoverlapping nuclei should be evaluated; thus, when making touch imprints, a gentle

Table 2.1 Suitability of various specimen types for FISH analysis

Substrate	Advantages	Disadvantages
Harvested cell suspensions	• Ability to correlate with G-banding findings • Typically yields uniform results	• Lineage of mononuclear cells cannot be readily identified • Need to wait until after harvest to obtain cells
Smears (blood, bone marrow)	• Readily available • Can be set up same day (no need to wait for cell culture)	• Red blood cells can sometimes obscure signals
Touch imprints	• Easy to prepare and store • FISH can be set up same day • Typically yield strong signals with little artifact	• Tissue architecture not preserved • If too thick, cell clumping precludes analysis
FFPE tissues	• Readily available • Tissue architecture preserved • Can be performed on archived specimens	• Signal strength can be affected by multiple factors (e.g., fixation time, type of fixative, decalcification) • Nuclear truncation due to cutting block during slide preparation results in artifactual loss of signals • Longer preparation time, same-day turnaround not possible
Isolated/separated cell populations	• Cell enrichment increases assay sensitivity	• Isolation process time- and labor-intensive • May yield weaker signal intensity

touch typically yields better results. A coverslip is placed over the probe and its edges sealed with rubber cement. Both the probe and the specimen DNA are heat denatured, typically using an automated instrument analogous to a thermocycler. After denaturation (2–5 min depending on the specimen type), the instrument cools to 37 °C, where the slide remains for approximately 6–14 h; this hybridization process permits binding of the probe to the target sequence. After a wash step to remove residual probe and the addition of a nuclear counterstain such as 4′,6-diamidino-2-phenylindole (DAPI), the cells can be evaluated under a fluorescence microscope. Interphase cells are evaluated according to criteria validated by each laboratory and according to manufacturer's recommendations and published criteria [22, 23]. It is important to have defined normal control ranges (cutoff values) to avoid false-positive results; laboratories also should have established criteria for how many cells are evaluated at diagnosis and for monitoring to rule out residual disease. Among the criteria evaluated when scoring are the sizes, intensity, and relative positions of

the signals as well as their number. Scoring at least some of the cells on single-pass filters (which allow only one color to be visualized and thus yield brighter signals) permits the detection of very small signals that may, in situations such as gene insertions, overlap but be masked by the signal of the partner gene. Unusual or unexpected patterns must also be evaluated (e.g., gain instead of rearrangement of a locus).

Several of the commonly used probe types are described below (see Fig. 2.2). As for conventional cytogenetics, ISCN designations allow the signal patterns identified to be conveyed succinctly. Examples of ISCN nomenclature for these FISH findings are provided in the legends accompanying these images.

Enumeration Probes (Fig. 2.2a)

• Directed against the centromeric or pericentromeric regions of each chromosome; these repetitive-sequence probes yield large, bright signals.

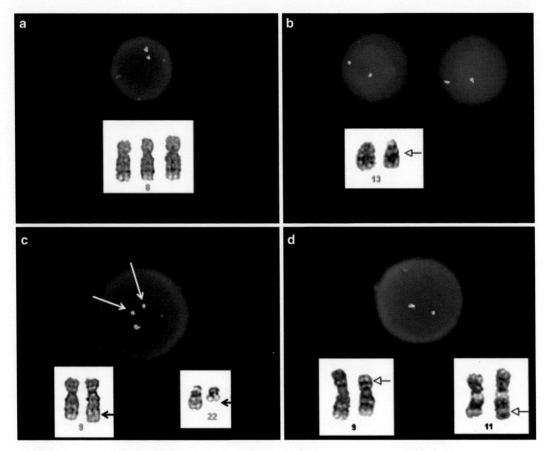

Fig. 2.2 (**a**) Three D8Z2 (centromere 8, *red*) signals and two D6Z1 (centromere 6, *green*) signals. ISCN designation: nuc ish(D8Z2x3,D6Z1x2). *Inset*: three copies of chromosome 8 by G-banding. (**b**) Left cell: one D13S319 (13q14, *red*) signal and two LAMP1 (13q34, *green*) signals, representing monoallelic loss of D13S319. ISCN designation: nuc ish(D13S319x1,LAMP1x2). *Inset*: G-banded chromosome 13 pair, one of which has an interstitial deletion involving 13q12-q14 (*arrow*). Right cell: no D13S319 (13q14, *red*) signal and two LAMP1 (13q34, *green*) signals, representing biallelic loss of D13S319. ISCN designation: nuc ish(D13S319x0,LAMP1x2). (**c**)

Three signals each for *ABL1* (*red*) and *BCR* (*green*), two of which are juxtaposed ("con") to form yellow fusion signals (*arrows*). ISCN designation: nuc ish(ABL1,BCR)x3(ABL1 con BCRx2). *Inset*: derivative chromosome 9 and derivative chromosome 22 resulting from a t(9;22) (q34;q11.2) (*arrows*). (**d**) Two *MLL* signals are present, one of which is intact (yellow fusion signal) and the other of which is separated ("sep") into its component 5′ (*green*) and 3′ (*red*) signals. ISCN designation: nuc ish(MLLx2) (5′MLL sep 3′MLLx1). *Inset*: derivative chromosome 9 and derivative chromosome 11 resulting from a t(9;11) (p22;q23) (*arrows*)

- One signal per chromosome; used to count the number of copies of the chromosome in each cell.
- Clinical uses include evaluation of monosomies or trisomies, often seen in hematologic malignancies such as myeloid neoplasms (monosomy 7, trisomy 8) and chronic lymphocytic leukemia (trisomy 12).

Locus Specific (Unique Sequence) (Fig. 2.2b)

- Directed against specific genes or loci.
- One signal per chromosome; used primarily to evaluate gain or loss of the gene/locus.
- Clinical uses include evaluation of losses of genes/loci such as *ATM* and 13q14 (chronic

lymphocytic leukemia) and loci on 5q and 7q (myeloid neoplasms).

Dual Fusion (Fig. 2.2c)

- Each gene involved in the translocation is labeled in a different color.
- Juxtaposition of the genes due to the translocation results in a fusion signal on each of the chromosome partners (derivative chromosomes).
- Clinical uses include evaluation of recurring translocations seen in leukemias and lymphomas (e.g., *BCR-ABL1* in CML, *IGH-CCND1* in mantle cell lymphoma and plasma cell dyscrasias, *IGH-BCL2* in follicular and diffuse large B-cell lymphoma, *IGH-MYC* in Burkitt and double-hit lymphomas).

Break Apart (Fig. 2.2d)

- 5′ and 3′ portions of a gene are labeled in different colors.
- Separation of fusion signal into separate red and green signals represents gene rearrangement.
- Clinical uses include evaluation of rearrangements involving promiscuous genes such as *MLL* that have multiple translocation partners or involving loci (e.g., *CBFB*, *MECOM*) associated with different types of rearrangements such as inversions and translocations.
- Easier to evaluate than dual-fusion probes in FFPE tissues in which nuclear overlap can cause false-positive fusion signals, thus, often used for solid tumors such as sarcomas (e.g., *EWSR1* in Ewing sarcoma, *SS18* in synovial sarcoma) for which only FFPE tissue may be available.

Paint (Fig. 2.3)

- Probe mixture hybridizes to the chromosome of interest along its entire length.
- Used on metaphase cells to further characterize complex rearrangements and chromosomes of unknown origin (e.g., marker chromosomes).

Because of its flexibility, FISH can be adapted to situations other than those mentioned above. For example, because it does not require dividing cells, it can be performed on uncultured cells to evaluate for the presence of diagnostic abnormalities (e.g., *PML-RARA* in acute promyelocytic leukemia) for which rapid turnaround time is crucial. FISH can also be performed on previously G-banded slides to further characterize G-banding findings in specific cells. Although these require a longer hybridization time (typically 36–48 h), abnormal metaphases can be located on the fluorescence microscope and the signal pattern evaluated. Many of the types of aberrations detectable by the FISH probes described above will be discussed in the relevant chapters on specific disease processes. However, several important findings that can be readily detected by FISH warrant mention here.

Gene amplification has important prognostic and therapeutic consequences in a variety of diseases, one of the most common of which is neuroblastoma. Although it can be suspected by G-banding, gene amplification requires confirmation by locus-specific (unique sequence) probes. Amplification of the *MYCN* locus in neuroblastoma is associated with aggressive disease and is a critical component in risk stratification and therapeutic regimens [28–31]. Although *MYCN* amplification can be evaluated in FFPE tissue, touch imprints are the preferred substrate due to ease of preparation, strength of signals, and more rapid turnaround time. Just as the American Society of Clinical Oncology/College of American Pathology (ASCO/CAP) Guidelines define the criteria for *HER2* amplification (see below), the International Neuroblastoma Risk Group Biology Committee has also issued criteria for *MYCN* amplification [28, 29]. Cases with *MYCN* amplification are often very highly amplified, precluding accurate enumeration of the signals (Fig. 2.4a). These signals are frequently scattered throughout the cell and reflect gene amplification on double minute chromosomes. In contrast, cases of acute lymphoblastic leukemia with *RUNX1* amplification often show much lower levels of amplification, with as few as 5–6 *RUNX1* signals per cell. These signals are often clustered together in interphase cells, representing amplification occurring within an abnormal chromosome 21 (Fig. 2.4b, c).

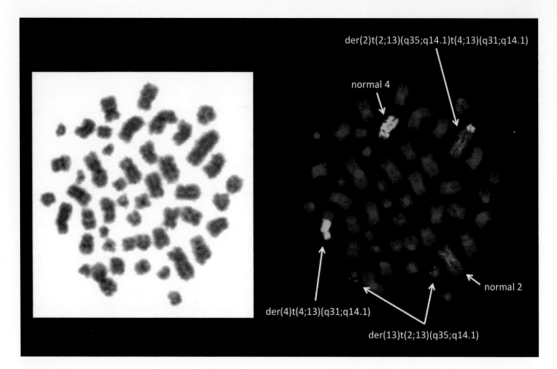

Fig. 2.3 Sequential FISH after G-banding using whole chromosome paint probes to chromosome 2 (*red*) and chromosome 4 (*green*). FISH confirmed that the complex rearrangements seen by G-banding resulted from a 2;13 translocation and a subsequent translocation of the derivative chromosome 2 and a chromosome 4. Two copies of the derivative chromosome 13 are present

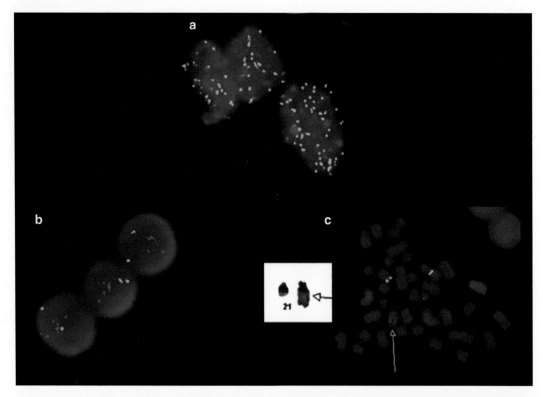

Fig. 2.4 (**a**) *MYCN* amplification: multiple *MYCN* (*green*) signals in the setting of three chromosome 2 centromere signals (*red*). (**b**) *RUNX1* amplification, interphase: multiple *RUNX1* (21q22, *red*) signals clustered; two normal *ETV6* (12p13, *green*) signals. (**c**) *RUNX1* amplification, metaphase: multiple *RUNX1* (*red*) signals clustered along the length of one copy of chromosome 21 (*arrow*), seen by both FISH and G-banding (*inset*)

Gene amplification is also well documented in breast cancer. *HER2* (*ERBB2*) amplification, found in approximately 10–30 % of cases of invasive breast cancer, has been associated with aggressive disease and also with response to particular chemotherapeutic regimens (reviewed in [32]). Patients with *HER2* amplification may also benefit from targeted therapy with trastuzumab, a monoclonal antibody directed against *HER2*. Although *HER2* amplification can also be seen in in situ carcinoma, its prognostic significance is limited to cases in which it is found in invasive carcinoma. Because it is critical to evaluate only invasive carcinoma, it is necessary to perform this assay on FFPE specimens to preserve tissue architecture. Before evaluating, a pathologist marks the areas of invasive carcinoma on a hematoxylin- and eosin-stained slide, and the technologist uses that marked slide to identify the corresponding area of invasive carcinoma on the FISH slide.

Because of its importance clinically and also as a criterion for entry onto various clinical trials, it is critical to perform, analyze, and interpret *HER2* cases according to uniform criteria. With the goal of ensuring accuracy and uniformity among laboratories performing *HER2* testing, the ASCO/CAP Guidelines [33] and the subsequent Update [34] defined specific preanalytic, analytic, and postanalytic criteria that each laboratory performing *HER2* testing must follow. In cases in which a dual-color probe set is used (*HER2* and the chromosome 17 centromere as a control), *HER2* amplification is defined as a *HER2*/centromere 17 ratio per cell of ≥ 2.0 or ≥ 6.0 copies of *HER2* per cell. The Guidelines also define an equivocal category (*HER2*/centromere 17 ratio of <2.0 and ≥ 4.0 and <6.0 *HER2* signals per cell). These scoring criteria are specifically for breast cancer; *HER2* analyses performed on other tissue types (e.g., esophageal or gastric tissue) use slightly different criteria [35, 36]. Subsequent to the publication of the first ASCO/CAP document, an expert panel published guidelines for evaluating cases with intratumoral heterogeneity, a well-documented challenge when performing *HER2* and other FFPE FISH [37]. In situ hybridization techniques other than FISH have also been used to detect *HER2* amplification [38–40].

A number of disease processes have several commonly occurring genetic abnormalities that may occur individually or together. Because probes can be readily multiplexed, mixtures of FISH probes ("panels") are often used to detect several of these abnormalities in a single assay. FISH panels to detect the most common abnormalities in voided urine [41, 42] and chronic lymphocytic leukemia [43] are commercially available (e.g., Abbott Molecular, Abbott Park, IL, USA; Cytocell, Cambridge, UK). These probe sets can also be used in other clinical situations; for example, the bladder cancer probe set (Abbott Molecular, Abbot Park, IL, USA) has also been used in cytologic specimens obtained from biliary tract brushings [42]. FISH is also playing an important role in therapy as well as diagnosis. As the documentation of genetic abnormalities is becoming increasingly important in determining responsiveness to therapeutic regimens, some guidelines mandate the use of FISH for the detection of certain abnormalities (e.g., *ALK* rearrangement in lung cancer) [44–47].

Although most clinical laboratories use commercially available probes for the more frequently occurring abnormalities, the ready availability of sequence data makes it possible for laboratories to design and label their own FISH probes. Reasons for doing this include but are not limited to lack of a commercially available probe for the region of interest or the need for smaller probes to detect abnormalities of very small genes. For example, the *TP53* gene is approximately 20 Kb, but commercially available probes may be severalfold larger; losses involving only the gene or with small flanking regions would be undetectable, as very small differences in signal size cannot be resolved at the microscope. Additionally, copy number abnormalities that are detected by other methods such as array-comparative genomic hybridization can be validated by FISH and used as a means to monitor the disease.

Conclusions

A number of new genomic techniques, such as array-based comparative genomic hybridization and next-generation sequencing, are entering widespread clinical use and have enabled researchers to make significant contributions to elucidating the genetic basis of both constitutional and acquired disorders. However, reliable and less complex methods such as G-banding and FISH still play an important role in the diagnosis, prognosis, and therapy of many diseases. Not only can they be used in concert to provide a whole-genome view with the capability of targeting specific loci, they also are able to detect low-level mosaicism and balanced rearrangements that might be missed by other techniques. In light of the rapid progress that is being made both clinically and in the laboratory, it is imperative that clinicians and pathologists educate each other and collaborate to incorporate these advances into routine practice and to determine the most informative combination of testing methods to diagnose, treat, and monitor patients.

References

1. Tjio JH, Levan A. The chromosome number of man. Hereditas. 1956;42:1–6.
2. Ford CE, Hamerton JL. The chromosomes of man. Nature. 1956;178:1020–3.
3. Gersen SL, Keagle MB, editors. The principles of clinical cytogenetics. 3rd ed. New York: Springer Science+Business Media; 2013.
4. Harper PS. First years of human chromosomes. Bloxham: Scion Publishing Ltd; 2006.
5. Smeets DF. Historical prospective of human cytogenetics: from microscope to microarray. Clin Biochem. 2004;37:439–46.
6. Sumner AT. Chromosome banding. London: Unwin Hyman; 1990.
7. Trask BJ. Human cytogenetics: 46 chromosomes, 46 years and counting. Nat Rev Genet. 2002;3:769–78.
8. Nowell PC, Hungerford DA. A minute chromosome in human chronic granulocytic leukemia. Science. 1960;132:1497.
9. Chandra HS, Heisterkamp NC, Hungerford A, Morrissette JJ, Nowell PC, Rowley JD, et al. Philadelphia Chromosome Symposium: commemoration of the 50th anniversary of the discovery of the Ph chromosome. Cancer Genet. 2011;204:171–9.
10. Rowley JD. A new consistent chromosomal abnormality in chronic myelogenous leukaemia identified by quinacrine fluorescence and Giemsa staining. Nature. 1973;243:290–3.
11. de Klein A, van Kessel AG, Grosveld G, Bartram CR, Hagemeijer A, Bootsma D, et al. A cellular oncogene is translocated to the Philadelphia chromosome in chronic myelocytic leukaemia. Nature. 1982;300:765–7.
12. Groffen J, Stephenson JR, Heisterkamp N, de Klein A, Bartram CR, Grosveld G. Philadelphia chromosomal breakpoints are clustered with a limited region, bcr, on chromosome 22. Cell. 1984;36:93–9.
13. Heisterkamp N, Stephenson JR, Groffen J, Hansen PF, de Klein A, Bartram CR, et al. Localization of the c-abl oncogene adjacent to a translocation break point in chronic myelocytic leukaemia. Nature. 1983;306:239–42.
14. Heisterkamp N, Stam K, Groffen J, de Klein A, Grosveld G. Structural organization of the bcr gene and its role in the Ph' translocation. Nature. 1985;315:758–61.
15. Mitelman F, Johansson B, Mertens F, editors. Mitelman database of chromosome aberrations and gene fusions in cancer. 2013. http://cgap.nci.nih.gov/Chromosomes/Mitelman
16. Barch MJ, Knutsen T, Spurbeck JL, editors. The AGT cytogenetics laboratory manual. 3rd ed. Philadelphia: Lippincott-Raven; 1997.
17. Swansbury J, editor. Cancer cytogenetics—methods and protocols. Totowa: Humana Press; 2003.
18. Wegner R-D, editor. Diagnostic cytogenetics. Berlin: Springer; 1999.
19. Heerema NA, Byrd JC, Cin PSD, Dell' Aquila ML, Koduru PRK, Aviram A, et al. Stimulation of chronic lymphocytic leukemia cells with CpG oligodeoxynucleotide gives consistent karyotypic results among laboratories: a CLL Research Consortium (CRC) Study. Cancer Genet Cytogenet. 2010;203:134–40.
20. Dicker F, Schnittger S, Haferlach T, Kern W, Schoch C. Immunostimulatory oligonucleotide-induced metaphase cytogenetics detect chromosomal aberrations in 80% of CLL patients: a study of 132 CLL cases with correlation to FISH, IgVH status, and CD38 expression. Blood. 2006;108:3152–60.
21. Shaffer LG, McGowan-Jordan J, Schmid M, editors. ISCN (2013): an international system for human cytogenetic nomenclature. Basel: S. Karger; 2013.
22. Mascarello JT, Hirsch B, Kearney HM, Ketterling RP, Olson SB, Quigley DI, et al. Section E9 of the American College of Medical Genetics technical standards and guidelines: fluorescence in situ hybridization. Genet Med. 2011;13:667–75.
23. Wolff DJ, Bagg A, Cooley LD, Dewald GW, Hirsch BA, Jacky PB, et al. Guidance for fluorescence in situ hybridization testing in hematologic disorders. J Mol Diagn. 2007;9:134–43.
24. Wiktor AE, van Dyke DL, Stupca PJ, Ketterling RP, Thorland EC, Shearer BM, et al. Preclinical validation of fluorescence in situ hybridization assays for clinical practice. Genet Med. 2006;8:16–23.
25. Liehr T, editor. Fluorescence in situ hybridization (FISH). Berlin: Springer; 2009.
26. Bridger JM, Volpi EV, editors. Fluorescence in situ hybridization (FISH)—protocols and applications. New York: Springer Science+Business Media; 2010.

27. Al-Mulla F, editor. Formalin-fixed paraffin-embedded tissues—methods and protocols. New York: Springer Science + Business Media; 2011.
28. Ambros PF, Ambros IM, Brodeur GM, Haber M, Khan J, Nakagawara A, et al. International consensus for neuroblastoma molecular diagnostics: report from the International Neuroblastoma Risk Group (INRG) Biology Committee. Br J Cancer. 2009;100:1471–82.
29. Cohn SL, Pearson ADJ, London WB, Monclair T, Ambros PF, Brodeur GM, et al. The International Neuroblastoma Risk Group (INRG) classification system: an INRG task force report. J Clin Oncol. 2009;27:289–97.
30. Schneiderman J, London WB, Brodeur GM, Castleberry RP, Look AT, Cohn SL. Clinical significance of MYCN amplification and ploidy in favorable-stage neuroblastoma: a report from the Children's Oncology Group. J Clin Oncol. 2008;26:913–8.
31. Mueller S, Matthay KK. Neuroblastoma: biology and staging. Curr Oncol Rep. 2009;11:431–8.
32. Ross JS, Slodkowska EA, Symmans WF, Pusztai L, Ravdin PM, Hortobagyi GN. The HER-2 receptor and breast cancer: ten years of targeted anti-HER-2 therapy and personalized medicine. Oncologist. 2009;14:320–68.
33. Wolff AC, Hammond MEH, Schwartz JN, Hagerty KL, Allred DC, Cote RJ, et al. American Society of Clinical Oncology/College of American Pathologists guideline recommendations for human epidermal growth factor receptor 2 testing in breast cancer. J Clin Oncol. 2006;25:118–45.
34. Wolff AC, Hammond MEH, Hicks DG, Dowsett M, McShane LM, Allison KH, et al. Recommendations for human epidermal growth factor receptor 2 testing in breast cancer. American Society of Clinical Oncology/College of American Pathologists clinical practice guideline update. Arch Pathol Lab Med. doi:10.5858/arpa.2013-0953-SA.
35. Bang Y-J, Van Cutsem E, Feyereislova A, Chung HC, Shen L, Sawaki A, et al. Trastuzumab in combination with chemotherapy versus chemotherapy alone for treatment of HER2-positive advanced gastric or gastro-oesophageal junction cancer (ToGA): a phase 3, open-label, randomised controlled trial. Lancet. 2010;376:687–97.
36. Yoon HH, Shi Q, Sukov WR, Wiktor AE, Khan M, Sattler CA, et al. Association of HER2/ErbB2 expression and gene amplification with pathologic features and prognosis in esophageal adenocarcinomas. Clin Cancer Res. 2012;18:546–54.
37. Vance GH, Barry TS, Bloom KJ, Fitzgibbons PL, Hicks DG, Jenkins RB, et al. Genetic heterogeneity in HER2 testing. Arch Pathol Lab Med. 2009;133:611–2.
38. Laudadio J, Quigley DI, Tubbs R, Wolff DJ. HER2 testing: a review of detection methodologies and their clinical performance. Expert Rev Mol Diagn. 2007;7:53–62.
39. Gruver AM, Peerwani Z, Tubbs RR. Out of the darkness and into the light: bright field in situ hybridisation for delineation of ERBB2 (HER2) status in breast carcinoma. J Clin Pathol. 2010;63:210–9.
40. Mansfield AS, Sukov WR, Eckel-Passow JE, Sakai Y, Walsh FJ, Lonzo M, et al. Comparison of fluorescence in situ hybridization (FISH) and dual-ISH (DISH) in the determination of HER2 status in breast cancer. Am J Clin Pathol. 2013;139:144–50.
41. Sokolova IA, Halling KC, Jenkins RB, Burkhardt HM, Meyer RG, Seelig SA, et al. The development of a multitarget, multicolor fluorescence in situ hybridization assay for the detection of urothelial carcinoma in urine. J Mol Diagn. 2010;2:116–23.
42. Halling KC, Kipp BR. Fluorescence in situ hybridization in diagnostic cytology. Hum Pathol. 2007;38:1137–44.
43. Haferlach C, Dicker F, Schnittger S, Kern W, Haferlach T. Comprehensive genetic characterization of CLL: a study on 506 cases analysed with chromosome banding analysis, interphase FISH, IgVH status and immunophenotyping. Leukemia. 2007;21:2442–51.
44. Lindeman NI, Cagle PT, Beasley MB, Chitale DA, Dacic S, Giaccone G, et al. Molecular testing guideline for selection of lung cancer patients for EGFR and ALK tyrosine kinase inhibitors: guideline from the College of American Pathologists, International Association for the Study of Lung Cancer, and Association for Molecular Pathology. Arch Pathol Lab Med. 2013;137:828–60.
45. Yi ES, Chung J-H, Kulig K, Kerr KM. Detection of anaplastic lymphoma kinase (ALK) gene rearrangement in non-small cell lung cancer and related issues in ALK inhibitor therapy. Mol Diagn Ther. 2012;16:143–50.
46. Camidge DR, Theodoro M, Maxson DA, Skokan M, O'Brien T, Lu X, et al. Correlations between the percentage of tumor cells showing an anaplastic lymphoma kinase (ALK) gene rearrangement, ALK signal copy number, and response to crizotinib therapy in ALK fluorescence in situ hybridization-positive nonsmall cell lung cancer. Cancer. 2012;118:4486–94.
47. Gerber DE, Minna JD. ALK inhibition for non-small cell lung cancer: from discovery to therapy in record time. Cancer Cell. 2010;18:548–51.

Comparative Genomic Hybridization and Array Based CGH in Cancer

Roland Hubaux *, Victor D. Martinez *,
David Rowbotham, and Wan L. Lam

Chromosomal Rearrangements and Cancer

Genomic instability is a hallmark of cancer [1]. Genetic alterations accumulate during tumor development and progression, and genomic instability is an indicator of poor prognosis [2]. Chromosomal instability (CIN), a prevalent form of genome instability, involves the deletion and duplication of whole or a portion of a chromosome, known as dosage alterations [2–4]. Focal DNA dosage alterations, such as small *in*sertions or *del*etions (indels) up to 10 Kb in length, are commonly detected in tumor genomes [5–7].

Somatic DNA dosage alterations and rearrangements resulting in gain or loss of genetic material are classified as unbalanced, as opposed to balanced alterations, for example, translocation events where no net gain or loss occurs (Fig. 3.1). While gain or amplification of DNA segments containing oncogenes, such as *HER-2/neu* and *MYC*, and deletion of chromosomal regions containing tumor suppressor genes, such as *TP53*, are common events across a broad spectrum of cancers, many genetic alterations are characteristic to specific tumor types and subtypes [8–11]. Array comparative genomic hybridization (aCGH) is a molecular cytogenetic technology commonly used in both research and clinical laboratory settings for the identification of DNA dosage alterations in tumor genomes.

Principles of aCGH Technology

Prior to the invention of comparative genomic hybridization technology, karyotyping techniques and fluorescence *in situ* hybridization (FISH) methods were commonly used for the detection of chromosome-wide and locus-specific alterations, respectively. The staining of chromosomes in metaphase nuclei with Giemsa dye allows visual analysis of chromosomal rearrangements by tracking G-band patterns characteristic of individual chromosomes [12]. FISH methods utilize locus-specific probes to identify deletions, duplications, and translocations of specific DNA segments [13]. Chromosome painting and spectral karyotyping methods extend FISH analysis to simultaneously interrogating multiple human chromosomes or chromosomal segments [14–16] (Table 3.1).

The principles behind aCGH that distinguish it from other methods are (1) "reverse FISH," where the probes are immobilized and the sample is labeled, and (2) "competitive hybridization,"

*Author contributed equally with all other contributors.

R. Hubaux, Ph.D. • V.D. Martinez, Ph.D. (✉)
D. Rowbotham, B.SC. • W.L. Lam, Ph.D.
Department of Integrative Oncology, BC Cancer
Agency and Department of Pathology and Laboratory
Medicine, University of British Columbia,
Vancouver, BC, Canada
e-mail: vmartinez@bccrc.ca

G.M. Yousef and S. Jothy (eds.), *Molecular Testing in Cancer*,
DOI 10.1007/978-1-4899-8050-2_3, © Springer Science+Business Media New York 2014

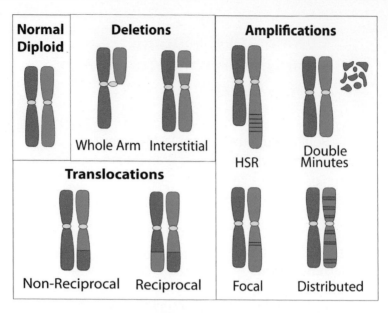

Fig. 3.1 Chromosomal rearrangements. Normal diploid chromosome with a 2n DNA dosage. An abnormal number of chromosomes (chromosomal aneuploidy) or segments (segmental aneuploidy) are common events in tumorigenesis and have a significant impact on patient prognosis. Deletions result in loss of genetic material. A deletion event can affect a whole chromosomal arm or specific segments (interstitial deletion, not involving chromosome ends). Translocations: In nonreciprocal translocations, genetic material is gained or lost, while reciprocal translocations result in no net change in the amount of genetic material. Amplifications: Homologous stained regions (HSR) are chromosomal structures where a segment of the chromosome is duplicated or amplified but remains on the same chromosome. Double minutes are the manifestation of gene amplification events in small extrachromosomal fragments. Focal amplification involves an increased number of copies of a specific DNA segment—frequently encompassing one or a few genes that can be selected for in clonal expansion. Distributed insertion events occur when a chromosomal fragment is amplified and inserted into different locations in another chromosome

Table 3.1 Platforms for clinical detection of chromosomal rearrangements and their applications

Technique	Resolution	Scale	Detection	Sample type	Limitations
G-banding	Chromosome band	Karyotyping	Translocations, duplications, deletions	Metaphase nuclei	Requires dividing cells; low resolution
FISH	10 Kb	Locus specific	Translocation, duplication, deletion	Fresh or fixed cells, FFPE, FNA	Detect known alterations
Multicolor FISH (SKY, M-FISH, CCK)	10 Mb	Karyotyping	Translocation, duplication, deletion	Cultured cells from specimen	Requires dividing cells; low resolution
Chromosomal CGH	2 Mb	Karyotyping	Segmental gains and loss	Fresh or fixed cells	Low resolution
BAC aCGH	0.1–1 Mb	Regional and whole genome	Segmental gains and losses	Fresh or fixed cells, FFPE	Moderate resolution
SNP oligonucleotide microarray	<30 Kb	Regional and whole genome	Segmental gains and losses, allelic imbalance	Fresh or fixed cells, FFPE	Limited utility for FFPE samples

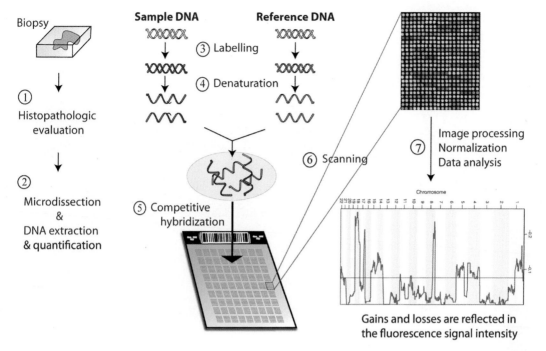

Fig. 3.2 Analysis of tumor samples using aCGH. (*1*) Depending on the type of platform, aCGH technology is capable of analyzing samples derived from fresh frozen tumors and formalin-fixed, paraffin-embedded (FFPE) tissue. (*2*) FFPE or a fresh frozen tumor is microdissected to enrich for tumoral cells. (*3*) DNA is then extracted from both tumor and matched normal or a reference sample and differentially labeled with fluorescent dyes. (*4*) Sample DNA is denatured. (*5*) Tumor and normal (reference) DNA are deposited onto the array where both samples competitively co-hybridize with probes on the array surface. (*6*) Sequences that have undergone DNA amplification in the tumor will have a skewed signal. Likewise, sites of DNA losses in tumor will allow increased hybridization of normal DNA. (*7*) Fluorescence intensity ratios on the array are captured by a scanner, and output data from the array is normalized and plotted using different available visualization and analysis software

where the tumor sample DNA and a diploid genomic DNA reference (differentially labeled) compete for binding to immobilized probe targets [17–19] (Fig. 3.2). Before the development of genomic microarrays, normal metaphase nuclei were fixed onto a glass slide so that spreaded chromosomes were used as targets for competitive hybridization [20].

Development of CGH Array Platforms

The first generations of genome-wide aCGH platforms employed cloned DNA fragments spotted in microarray format to investigate selected targets distributed throughout the genome [18, 19]. For example, Pollack and colleagues assembled a CGH array using 3,360 unique complementary (cDNA) clones [21]. Snijders et al. used bacterial artificial chromosome (BAC) and other clones, containing human DNA fragments of ~0.1 Mb, to survey 2,460 loci for copy-number alteration [22].

The development of tiling path arrays enabled complete genome coverage based on the physical map of the human genome. The submegabase resolution tiling set (SMRT) array, developed in 2004, was first to offer whole-genome coverage, with 32,433 overlapping BAC clones spotted in triplicate [23]. The overlapping arrangement of these BAC clones abrogated the need to infer genetic events between marker clones. The SMRT array technology is capable of detecting DNA copy-number alterations of >80 Kb in size (Fig. 3.3) [23].

High-density arrays increased the resolution of CGH arrays [24]. Oligonucleotide probes, rep-

a

Array CGH

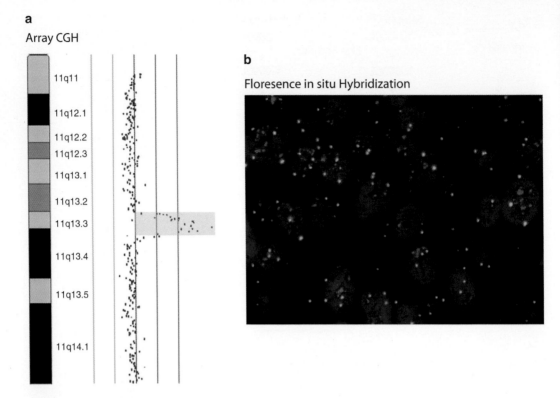

b

Floresence in situ Hybridization

Fig. 3.3 FISH validation of DNA amplification detected by aCGH. (**a**) DNA copy-number alteration for each probe is aligned with their chromosomal position and displayed by SeeGH software. Region of gene amplification detected by aCGH on 11q13 is highlighted in *red* and contains the gene encoding for *Cyclin D1* (*CCND1*). (**b**) Gene amplification is validated by fluorescence in situ hybridization (FISH), by using a sequence-specific probe for *CCND1* (*red*), and by a probe specifically hybridizing for chromosome 11 (*green*). Multiple signals observed from the *CCDN1* probe confirm the high-level amplification affecting this gene

resenting targets of 25–80 nucleotides in length, were densely arranged to produce CGH array platforms that contain hundreds of thousands to millions of oligonucleotide probes. The inclusion of single-nucleotide polymorphism (SNP) probes provides allelic data, yielding information on copy-neutral loss of heterozygosity (LOH), and allelic imbalances, where only one allele is duplicated or amplified [25].

Contemporary Array CGH Platforms

As genomic array technology evolves, contemporary aCGH platforms mainly employ high-density arrays, for example, the Agilent SurePrint G3 Human CGH Microarray, which contains ~1 million probes. For applications where both copy number and allelic information are desirable, platforms such as the Affymetrix Genome-Wide Human SNP Array 6.0 (containing 906,600 SNP markers and 946,000 CGH markers) and the Illumina HumanOmni5-Quad BeadChip (featuring ~4.3 million probes per array, including 2.3 million SNP probes) are commercially available (Table 3.2). Each platform uses a proprietary array production technology: Agilent's SurePrint technology produces 60-mer oligonucleotide probes, Affymetrix combines chemistry and photolithography to synthesize 25-mer oligonucleotide probes, while Illumina's BeadChip technology utilizes beads covered with immobilized oligonucleotide probes. The length of the oligonucleotide probes is optimal for the technical requirement of individual platforms. Affymetrix designed paired 25-mer probes to distinguish

Table 3.2 Example of contemporary array CGH platforms

Platform	Source	Array type (probe size)	No. markers	Median spacing	Sample amount	Use FFPE samples
Genome-Wide Human SNP Array 6.0	Affymetrix	SNP and CNV (25 mer)	1.8 M	<0.7 kb	0.5 µg	
HumanOmni5-Quad BeadChip	Illumina	SNP and CNV (50 mer)	4.3 M	0.36 kb	0.4 µg	
SurePrint G3 Human CGH Microarray 1 × 1M	Agilent	CNV (60 mer)	963,029	2.1 kb	1–2 µg	
SMRT array v.2	BCCRC	CNV (BAC, 100–150 Kb)	32,433	Tiling	0.2 µg	Yes
Human Genome CGH 244A	Agilent	SNP (60 mer)	~236,000	8.9 kb	0.5–1 µg	
Illumina HumanExon510s-duo	Illumina	CNV (25 mer)	511,354	3.2 kb	0.75 µg	
Infinium CytoSNP-850K BeadChip	Illumina	SNP (50 mer)	~850,000	6.2 kb	1–2 µg	Requires restoration
CGX array	PerkinElmer	Oligonucleotide	~164,000			
CytoChip Cancer 4 × 180K	BlueGnome	Oligonucleotide	153,442	20 kb		
CytoSure Consortium Cancer + SNP	Oxford Gene Technology	Oligonucleotide	~180,000			
OncoScan™ FFPE Assay	Affymetrix	Oligonucleotide	334,183 (~900 cancer genes)	9 kb	80 ng	Yes

perfect match and mismatch to the DNA sample being analyzed, while Agilent and Illumina use 50–60-mer oligonucleotides to maximize sensitivity [26, 27]. It is important to note that the resolution of an array is not defined by the length of the array elements (i.e., an array consisting of 25-mer elements will not offer a resolution of 25 bp) but rather by probe density and distribution. Smaller probe size will increase the ability to detect smaller alterations [24].

Application of aCGH to Identify Genetic Alterations in Cancer

In hematological cancers, the ability of genome scanning at a high resolution, provided by array-based CGH, has enabled the identification of cryptic recurrent genomic imbalances not detected by conventional cytogenetic techniques. Such findings have proven relevant to patient prognosis and understanding disease mechanisms. Copy-number alterations identified in myelodysplastic syndromes (MDS) are a case in

point [28]. The localization of deletion breakpoints on chromosome arm 5q facilitated the identification of MDS patients with shorter overall survival, as well as microRNA gene deletions as mediators of the 5q-syndrome phenotype potentially through haploinsufficency [28–32]. The use of aCGH to track DNA alterations in longitudinal cohorts of chronic lymphocytic leukemia (CLL) patients showed complex clonal evolution during disease progression and the development of chemotherapy resistance [33, 34]. Likewise, aCGH has enabled genomic comparison of clonal cell populations within the same patient. Recent studies revealed that multiple subclones in the lymph nodes originate from a common clone, suggesting clonal evolution of adult T-cell leukemia/lymphoma taking place in lymph nodes [35]. These findings were also observed in mantle cell lymphoma [36].

In sarcomas, mutation and DNA copy-number profilings have led to the identification of subtype-specific genomic alterations and promising therapeutic targets [37]. Array-based CGH yielded genomic signatures that predict poor outcome in

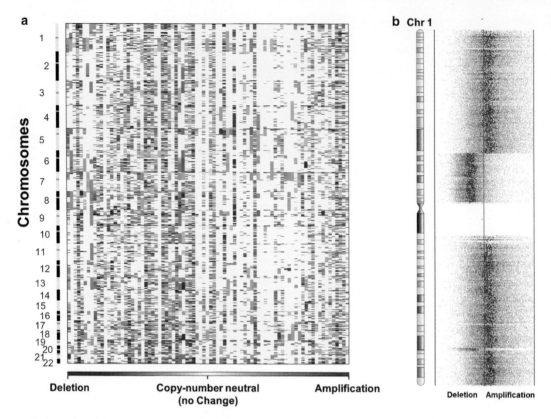

Fig. 3.4 Analysis of array comparative genomic hybridization data in tumor genomes. (**a**) Heatmap representing somatic copy-number alterations across a panel of 83 lung adenocarcinomas (*columns*). Analysis was performed with the GISTIC bioinformatic package. DNA gains (in *red*) and losses (*blue*) for each chromosome are shown. (**b**) Copy-number analysis performed with the Partek® Genomics Suite™ (version 6). Data derived from Affymetrix Genome-Wide Human SNP Array 6.0. Copy-number status for probes mapping to chromosome 1 is shown. Central *blue line* indicates diploid status. DNA copy-number losses are shown to the *left*, while DNA gains are plotted to the *right*

undifferentiated pleomorphic sarcomas and leiomyosarcomas [38]. Similarly, a combined aCGH and expression profiling approach has yielded prognostic signatures able to predict metastatic outcome in soft tissue sarcomas on the basis of a gene expression signature related to genome complexity [39].

In solid tumors, aCGH has been instrumental in identifying disease-specific genetic alterations (Fig. 3.4). For example, in non-small cell lung cancer, aCGH comparison of squamous cell carcinoma and adenocarcinoma subtypes revealed lineage-specific genetic alterations [10, 40]. For example, the *NK2 homeobox 1* (*NKX2-1*) gene at 14q13, also known as *thyroid transcription factor 1* (*TTF-1* or *TITF1*), is amplified in adenocarcinoma, while *SRY-BOX 2* (*SOX2*) at 3q26.33 and

the *BRF2 subunit of RNA polymerase III transcription initiation factor* (*BRF2*) gene at 8p11.23 are primarily amplified in squamous cell carcinomas. These genes are prime examples of cell lineage-survival oncogenes [40–46].

The biological effect of DNA copy-number alteration is not limited to a single gene. In a multiple-component system such as a signaling pathway or a protein complex, alteration of a single-component gene can disrupt the entire complex. Individual component genes may be altered at a low frequency, but when different components are altered in different patients, the disruption of the protein complex can become a common event [47]. For example, gene dosage alteration is found to be a low-frequency event but a prominent genetic mechanism in disrupting each component of the KEAP1-CUL3-RBX1 complex and its NF-κB stimulating substrate, IKBKB. Remarkably when all components are considered, more than half of the tumors analyzed showed genetic alteration in one or more complex components in a recent non-small cell lung cancer study [47]. Multiple-component disruption of this complex represents a novel mechanism of NF-κB activation in lung cancer.

Gene dosage alteration also impacts response to therapy. For example, the amplification of the *HER-2/neu* gene and *EGFR* (*epidermal growth factor receptor*) copy-number status can predict the likelihood of response to EGFR-targeted therapies. Lung cancer patients that have *EGFR* amplification show significantly better response rates to gefitinib (an EGFR inhibitor) compared to patients with normal gene or protein levels [48]. Furthermore, combination of aCGH and next-generation sequencing (NGS) has been useful in determining complex genomic rearrangements in circulating tumor cells, which provides new options for monitoring tumor progression, treatment, and relapse [49].

Technical Considerations

Clinical specimens are often confounded by limited DNA quality and quantity and by the heterogeneity of cell populations. Fresh frozen tumors provide high-quality genomic DNA; however, typical specimens from hospital archives, especially historic samples with clinical outcome, exist as formalin-fixed, paraffin-embedded (FFPE) material. Formalin fixation has been found to cause DNA degradation. Much effort has been made to develop strategies for restoring DNA isolated from FFPE samples, and protocols for DNA extraction and sample amplification have been developed and applied to aCGH analysis of a variety of cancers [50–55]. BAC-based array platforms have proven effective in producing aCGH profiles from microdissected (low-quantity) and FFPE (low-quality) specimens, due to the large size of hybridization targets (~0.1 Mb) capturing ample signals from the fluorescently labeled samples [19, 56]. However, the limited resolution of BAC arrays has prompted development of labeling and hybridization strategies for FFPE samples that are compatible with high-density oligonucleotide array alternatives (Table 3.2). The Agilent arrays utilize a protocol based on Kreatech's Universal Linkage System (ULS™) technology, a nonenzymatic direct labeling methodology [57]. The Illumina Infinium CytoSNP-850K BeadChip is also able to process FFPE samples, although an initial sample DNA restoration process is required [50]. The Affymetrix OncoScan™ express array provides data on copy-number changes and copy-neutral LOH on FFPE samples at ~900 cancer gene loci, through the use of molecular inversion probe (MIP) DNA amplification technology [58].

Sample DNA amplification can drastically reduce the amount of primary material required; however, noise and bias are introduced by nonlinear amplification of sequences, limiting utility in the analysis of low-yield clinical specimens, such as microdissected samples, sorted cell populations, and preneoplastic lesions [59]. Current aCGH platforms have very different primary material quantity requirements. BAC-based arrays have the lowest input sample DNA requirements (~200 ng), while oligonucleotide- and SNP-based platforms require higher amounts in the microgram range (Table 3.2).

Use of Next-Generation Sequencing to Identify Dosage Alterations

A common limitation of the aCGH technology is that it is unable to detect sequence mutations and balanced chromosomal rearrangements, such as balanced translocation and inversion events. With lowering cost for whole-genome sequencing and advancing bioinformatics capability for NGS, this approach is an emerging technology for profiling tumor genomes. The detection of structural variations through NGS approaches takes advantage of the mapping of sequence reads to the human genome. The accuracy of calling alterations is influenced by the depth of sequencing (the number of times that each sequence is read) [60–62]. Sequence alignment maps the exact location of the alteration, while depth of coverage provides information on the magnitude of the alteration. NGS technology has been proven successful in identifying challenging alterations, such as small indels, balanced translocations, and inversions [63–65]. The most recent NGS-based approaches for copy-number analysis use targeted breakpoint capture followed by sequencing [66]. Overall, NGS offers an approach complementary to array CGH technologies to provide a comprehensive identification of structural chromosomal rearrangements in tumor genomes.

aCGH: From Bench to Bedside

Array CGH platforms are becoming a routine tool in clinical molecular diagnostics laboratories. For prenatal diagnosis, the International Standard Cytogenomic Array (ISCA) Consortium supports the use of aCGH as a first-line clinical diagnostic test for individuals with developmental disabilities or congenital anomalies [67]. For cancer molecular cytogenetics, the Cancer Cytogenomics Microarray Consortium (CCMC) is aiming to establish platform-neutral and cancer-specific microarray designs for diagnostic purposes. BlueGnome (Illumina) has developed *CytoChip Cancer* using standards set by ISCA and CCMC which covers 670 cancer genes with ~20,000 disease-targeted oligonucleotide probes.

Conclusions

The array-based CGH technology has greatly expanded the scope of molecular cytogenetics beyond karyotype analysis. This technology has experienced tremendous progress in the past decade with continual improvement in array resolution and genome coverage. These advancements are accompanied by a steady reduction in the cost of assays and increased reproducibility due to the establishment of robust protocols and the manufacturing of genomic arrays and quality controlled reagents by commercial vendors. The development of robust methods for sample amplification and labeling to reduce material

quantity and quality requirement of clinically relevant specimens and the increasing availability of user-friendly bioinformatic tools for processing and interpreting aCGH data contribute to the acceptance and implementation of aCGH as a tool for molecular cytogenetics in cancer research and clinical diagnostics.

References

1. Hanahan D, Weinberg RA. Hallmarks of cancer: the next generation. Cell. 2011;144(5):646–74. PubMed PMID: 21376230. Epub 2011/03/08. eng.
2. Pikor L, Thu K, Vucic E, Lam W. The detection and implication of genome instability in cancer. Cancer metastasis reviews. 2013;32(3-4):341-52. Epub 2013/05/02.
3. Aguilera A, Garcia-Muse T. Causes of genome instability. Annual review of genetics. 2013;47:1–32. Epub 2013/08/06.
4. Gordon DJ, Resio B, Pellman D. Causes and consequences of aneuploidy in cancer. Nat Rev Genet. 2012;13(3):189–203. PubMed PMID: 22269907. Epub 2012/01/25. eng.
5. Iskow RC, Gokcumen O, Lee C. Exploring the role of copy number variants in human adaptation. Trends Genet. 2012;28(6):245–57. PubMed PMID: 22483647. Pubmed Central PMCID: 3533238.
6. Quinlan AR, Hall IM. Characterizing complex structural variation in germline and somatic genomes. Trends Genet. 2012;28(1):43–53. PubMed PMID: 22094265. Pubmed Central PMCID: 3249479.
7. Greenman C, Stephens P, Smith R, Dalgliesh GL, Hunter C, Bignell G, et al. Patterns of somatic mutation in human cancer genomes. Nature. 2007;446(7132):153–8. PubMed PMID: 17344846. Pubmed Central PMCID: 2712719. Epub 2007/03/09. eng.
8. Kumar N, Cai H, von Mering C, Baudis M. Specific genomic regions are differentially affected by copy number alterations across distinct cancer types, in aggregated cytogenetic data. PLoS One. 2012;7(8): e43689. PubMed PMID: 22937079. Pubmed Central PMCID: 3427184. Epub 2012/09/01. eng.
9. Li Y, Zhang L, Ball RL, Liang X, Li J, Lin Z, et al. Comparative analysis of somatic copy-number alterations across different human cancer types reveals two distinct classes of breakpoint hotspots. Hum Mol Genet. 2012;21(22):4957–65. PubMed PMID: 22899649. Pubmed Central PMCID: 3607479. Epub 2012/08/18. eng.
10. Lockwood WW, Wilson IM, Coe BP, Chari R, Pikor LA, Thu KL, et al. Divergent genomic and epigenomic landscapes of lung cancer subtypes underscore the selection of different oncogenic pathways during tumor development. PLoS One. 2012;7(5):e37775.

PubMed PMID: 22629454. Pubmed Central PMCID: 3357406.

11. Mitelman F, Johansson B, Mertens F. Mitelman database of chromosome aberrations and gene fusions in cancer. 2013. http://cgap.nci.nih.gov/Chromosomes/Mitelman.

12. Seabright M. A rapid banding technique for human chromosomes. Lancet. 1971;2(7731):971–2. PubMed PMID: 4107917. Epub 1971/10/30. eng.

13. Van Prooijen-Knegt AC, Van Hoek JF, Bauman JG, Van Duijn P, Wool IG, Van der Ploeg M. In situ hybridization of DNA sequences in human metaphase chromosomes visualized by an indirect fluorescent immunocytochemical procedure. Exp Cell Res. 1982;141(2):397–407. PubMed PMID: 6754395. Epub 1982/10/01. eng.

14. Bayani J, Squire J. Multi-color FISH techniques. Curr Protoc Cell Biol. 2004;Chapter 22:Unit 22.5. PubMed PMID: 18228456.

15. Bayani JM, Squire JA. Applications of SKY in cancer cytogenetics. Cancer Invest. 2002;20(3):373–86. PubMed PMID: 12025233.

16. Schrock E, du Manoir S, Veldman T, Schoell B, Wienberg J, Ferguson-Smith MA, et al. Multicolor spectral karyotyping of human chromosomes. Science. 1996;273(5274):494–7. PubMed PMID: 8662537. Epub 1996/07/26. eng.

17. Albertson DG, Pinkel D. Genomic microarrays in human genetic disease and cancer. Hum Mol Genet. 2003;12 Spec No 2:R145–52. PubMed PMID: 12915456.

18. Pinkel D, Albertson DG. Array comparative genomic hybridization and its applications in cancer. Nat Genet. 2005;37(Suppl):S11–7. PubMed PMID: 15920524.

19. Lockwood WW, Chari R, Chi B, Lam WL. Recent advances in array comparative genomic hybridization technologies and their applications in human genetics. Eur J Hum Genet. 2006;14(2):139–48. PubMed PMID: 16288307.

20. Kallioniemi A, Kallioniemi OP, Sudar D, Rutovitz D, Gray JW, Waldman F, et al. Comparative genomic hybridization for molecular cytogenetic analysis of solid tumors. Science. 1992;258(5083):818–21. PubMed PMID: 1359641.

21. Pollack JR, Perou CM, Alizadeh AA, Eisen MB, Pergamenschikov A, Williams CF, et al. Genome-wide analysis of DNA copy-number changes using cDNA microarrays. Nat Genet. 1999;23(1):41–6. PubMed PMID: 10471496. Epub 1999/09/02. eng.

22. Snijders AM, Nowak N, Segraves R, Blackwood S, Brown N, Conroy J, et al. Assembly of microarrays for genome-wide measurement of DNA copy number. Nat Genet. 2001;29(3):263–4. PubMed PMID: 11687795. Epub 2001/11/01. eng.

23. Ishkanian AS, Malloff CA, Watson SK, DeLeeuw RJ, Chi B, Coe BP, et al. A tiling resolution DNA microarray with complete coverage of the human genome. Nat Genet. 2004;36(3):299–303. PubMed PMID: 14981516. Epub 2004/02/26. eng.

24. Coe BP, Ylstra B, Carvalho B, Meijer GA, Macaulay C, Lam WL. Resolving the resolution of array CGH. Genomics. 2007;89(5):647–53. PubMed PMID: 17276656. Epub 2007/02/06. eng.

25. Corver WE, Middeldorp A, ter Haar NT, Jordanova ES, van Puijenbroek M, van Eijk R, et al. Genome-wide allelic state analysis on flow-sorted tumor fractions provides an accurate measure of chromosomal aberrations. Cancer Res. 2008;68(24):10333–40. PubMed PMID: 19074902. Epub 2008/12/17. eng.

26. Shchepinov MS, Case-Green SC, Southern EM. Steric factors influencing hybridisation of nucleic acids to oligonucleotide arrays. Nucleic Acids Res. 1997;25(6):1155–61. PubMed PMID: 9092624. Pubmed Central PMCID: 146580. Epub 1997/03/15. eng.

27. Hughes TR, Mao M, Jones AR, Burchard J, Marton MJ, Shannon KW, et al. Expression profiling using microarrays fabricated by an ink-jet oligonucleotide synthesizer. Nat Biotechnol. 2001;19(4):342–7. PubMed PMID: 11283592. Epub 2001/04/03. eng.

28. Thiel A, Beier M, Ingenhag D, Servan K, Hein M, Moeller V, et al. Comprehensive array CGH of normal karyotype myelodysplastic syndromes reveals hidden recurrent and individual genomic copy number alterations with prognostic relevance. Leukemia. 2011;25(3):387–99. PubMed PMID: 21274003. Epub 2011/01/29. eng.

29. Starczynowski DT, Vercauteren S, Sung S, Brooks-Wilson A, Lam WL, Karsan A. Copy number alterations at polymorphic loci may be acquired somatically in patients with myelodysplastic syndromes. Leuk Res. 2011;35(4):444–7. PubMed PMID: 20801506. Epub 2010/08/31. eng.

30. Starczynowski DT, Kuchenbauer F, Argiropoulos B, Sung S, Morin R, Muranyi A, et al. Identification of miR-145 and miR-146a as mediators of the 5q- syndrome phenotype. Nat Med. 2010;16(1):49–58. PubMed PMID: 19898489. Epub 2009/11/10. eng.

31. Starczynowski DT, Vercauteren S, Telenius A, Sung S, Tohyama K, Brooks-Wilson A, et al. High-resolution whole genome tiling path array CGH analysis of CD34+ cells from patients with low-risk myelodysplastic syndromes reveals cryptic copy number alterations and predicts overall and leukemia-free survival. Blood. 2008;112(8):3412–24. PubMed PMID: 18663149. Epub 2008/07/30. eng.

32. Evers C, Beier M, Poelitz A, Hildebrandt B, Servan K, Drechsler M, et al. Molecular definition of chromosome arm 5q deletion end points and detection of hidden aberrations in patients with myelodysplastic syndromes and isolated del(5q) using oligonucleotide array CGH. Genes Chromosomes Cancer. 2007;46(12):1119–28. PubMed PMID: 17823930. Epub 2007/09/08. eng.

33. Braggio E, Kay NE, VanWier S, Tschumper RC, Smoley S, Eckel-Passow JE, et al. Longitudinal genome-wide analysis of patients with chronic lymphocytic leukemia reveals complex evolution of clonal architecture at disease progression and at the

time of relapse. Leukemia. 2012;26(7):1698–701. PubMed PMID: 22261920. Epub 2012/01/21. eng.

34. Knight SJ, Yau C, Clifford R, Timbs AT, Sadighi Akha E, Dreau HM, et al. Quantification of subclonal distributions of recurrent genomic aberrations in paired pre-treatment and relapse samples from patients with B-cell chronic lymphocytic leukemia. Leukemia. 2012;26(7):1564–75. PubMed PMID: 22258401. Pubmed Central PMCID: 3505832. Epub 2012/01/20. eng.

35. Umino A, Nakagawa M, Utsunomiya A, Tsukasaki K, Taira N, Katayama N, et al. Clonal evolution of adult T-cell leukemia/lymphoma takes place in the lymph nodes. Blood. 2011;117(20):5473–8. PubMed PMID: 21447829. Epub 2011/03/31. eng.

36. Liu F, Yoshida N, Suguro M, Kato H, Karube K, Arita K, et al. Clonal heterogeneity of mantle cell lymphoma revealed by array comparative genomic hybridization. Eur J Haematol. 2013;90(1):51–8. PubMed PMID: 23110670. Epub 2012/11/01. eng.

37. Barretina J, Taylor BS, Banerji S, Ramos AH, Lagos-Quintana M, Decarolis PL, et al. Subtype-specific genomic alterations define new targets for soft-tissue sarcoma therapy. Nat Genet. 2010;42(8):715–21. PubMed PMID: 20601955. Pubmed Central PMCID: 2911503. Epub 2010/07/06. eng.

38. Silveira SM, Villacis RA, Marchi FA, Barros Filho Mde C, Drigo SA, Neto CS, et al. Genomic signatures predict poor outcome in undifferentiated pleomorphic sarcomas and leiomyosarcomas. PLoS One. 2013;8(6):e67643. PubMed PMID: 23825676. Pubmed Central PMCID: 3692486. Epub 2013/07/05. Eng.

39. Chibon F, Lagarde P, Salas S, Perot G, Brouste V, Tirode F, et al. Validated prediction of clinical outcome in sarcomas and multiple types of cancer on the basis of a gene expression signature related to genome complexity. Nat Med. 2010;16(7):781–7. PubMed PMID: 20581836. Epub 2010/06/29. eng.

40. Kwei KA, Kim YH, Girard L, Kao J, Pacyna-Gengelbach M, Salari K, et al. Genomic profiling identifies TITF1 as a lineage-specific oncogene amplified in lung cancer. Oncogene. 2008;27(25):3635–40. PubMed PMID: 18212743. Pubmed Central PMCID: 2903002.

41. Cabarcas S, Schramm L. RNA polymerase III transcription in cancer: the BRF2 connection. Mol Cancer. 2011;10:47. PubMed PMID: 21518452. Pubmed Central PMCID: 3098206.

42. Winslow MM, Dayton TL, Verhaak RG, Kim-Kiselak C, Snyder EL, Feldser DM, et al. Suppression of lung adenocarcinoma progression by Nkx2-1. Nature. 2011;473(7345):101–4. PubMed PMID: 21471965. Pubmed Central PMCID: 3088778.

43. Wilbertz T, Wagner P, Petersen K, Stiedl AC, Scheble VJ, Maier S, et al. SOX2 gene amplification and protein overexpression are associated with better outcome in squamous cell lung cancer. Mod Pathol. 2011;24(7):944–53. PubMed PMID: 21460799.

44. Bass AJ, Watanabe H, Mermel CH, Yu S, Perner S, Verhaak RG, et al. SOX2 is an amplified lineage-survival oncogene in lung and esophageal squamous cell carcinomas. Nat Genet. 2009;41(11):1238–42. PubMed PMID: 19801978. Pubmed Central PMCID: 2783775.

45. Weir BA, Woo MS, Getz G, Perner S, Ding L, Beroukhim R, et al. Characterizing the cancer genome in lung adenocarcinoma. Nature. 2007;450(7171):893–8. PubMed PMID: 17982442. Pubmed Central PMCID: 2538683.

46. Lockwood WW, Chari R, Coe BP, Thu KL, Garnis C, Malloff CA, et al. Integrative genomic analyses identify BRF2 as a novel lineage-specific oncogene in lung squamous cell carcinoma. PLoS Med. 2010;7(7):e1000315. PubMed PMID: 20668658. Pubmed Central PMCID: 2910599. Epub 2010/07/30. eng.

47. Thu KL, Pikor LA, Chari R, Wilson IM, Macaulay CE, English JC, et al. Genetic disruption of KEAP1/CUL3 E3 ubiquitin ligase complex components is a key mechanism of NF-kappaB pathway activation in lung cancer. J Thorac Oncol. 2011;6(9):1521–9. PubMed PMID: 21795997. Pubmed Central PMCID: 3164321.

48. Cappuzzo F, Hirsch FR, Rossi E, Bartolini S, Ceresoli GL, Bemis L, et al. Epidermal growth factor receptor gene and protein and gefitinib sensitivity in non-small-cell lung cancer. J Natl Cancer Inst. 2005;97(9):643–55. PubMed PMID: 15870435. Epub 2005/05/05. eng.

49. Heitzer E, Auer M, Gasch C, Pichler M, Ulz P, Hoffmann EM, et al. Complex tumor genomes inferred from single circulating tumor cells by array-CGH and next-generation sequencing. Cancer Res. 2013;73(10):2965–75. PubMed PMID: 23471846. Epub 2013/03/09. eng.

50. Pokholok DK, Le JM, Steemers FJ, Ronaghi M, Gunderson KL. Analysis of restored FFPE samples on high-density SNP arrays. In: Proceedings of the 101st annual meeting of the American Association for cancer research, Apr 17–21. Washington, DC; 2010. Abstract nr LB-34.

51. Salawu A, Ul-Hassan A, Hammond D, Fernando M, Reed M, Sisley K. High quality genomic copy number data from archival formalin-fixed paraffin-embedded leiomyosarcoma: optimisation of universal linkage system labelling. PLoS One. 2012;7(11):e50415. PubMed PMID: 23209738. Pubmed Central PMCID: 3510175.

52. van Essen HF, Ylstra B. High-resolution copy number profiling by array CGH using DNA isolated from formalin-fixed, paraffin-embedded tissues. Methods Mol Biol. 2012;838:329–41. PubMed PMID: 22228020.

53. Krijgsman O, Israeli D, Haan JC, van Essen HF, Smeets SJ, Eijk PP, et al. CGH arrays compared for DNA isolated from formalin-fixed, paraffin-embedded material. Genes Chromosomes Cancer. 2012;51(4):344–52. PubMed PMID: 22162309.

54. Pikor LA, Enfield KS, Cameron H, Lam WL. DNA extraction from paraffin embedded material for

genetic and epigenetic analyses. J Vis Exp. 2011;(49). pii: 2763. PubMed PMID: 21490570. Pubmed Central PMCID: 3197328.

55. Hostetter G, Kim SY, Savage S, Gooden GC, Barrett M, Zhang J, et al. Random DNA fragmentation allows detection of single-copy, single-exon alterations of copy number by oligonucleotide array CGH in clinical FFPE samples. Nucleic Acids Res. 2010;38(2):e9. PubMed PMID: 19875416. Pubmed Central PMCID: 2811007.

56. Ylstra B, van den Ijssel P, Carvalho B, Brakenhoff RH, Meijer GA. BAC to the future! or oligonucleotides: a perspective for micro array comparative genomic hybridization (array CGH). Nucleic Acids Res. 2006;34(2):445–50. PubMed PMID: 16439806. Pubmed Central PMCID: 1356528. Epub 2006/01/28. eng.

57. Kreatech. ULS™ (Universal Linkage System) technology. 2013. http://www.kreatech.com/products/universal-linkage-systemtm-labeling-kits/the-ulstm-labeling-technology.html

58. Wang Y, Cottman M, Schiffman JD. Molecular inversion probes: a novel microarray technology and its application in cancer research. Cancer Genet. 2012;205(7–8):341–55. PubMed PMID: 22867995. Epub 2012/08/08. eng.

59. Gilbert I, Scantland S, Dufort I, Gordynska O, Labbe A, Sirard MA, et al. Real-time monitoring of aRNA production during T7 amplification to prevent the loss of sample representation during microarray hybridization sample preparation. Nucleic Acids Res. 2009;37(8):e65. PubMed PMID: 19336411. Pubmed Central PMCID: 2677895. Epub 2009/04/02. eng.

60. Hormozdiari F, Alkan C, Eichler EE, Sahinalp SC. Combinatorial algorithms for structural variation detection in high-throughput sequenced genomes. Genome Res. 2009;19(7):1270–8. PubMed PMID: 19447966. Pubmed Central PMCID: 2704429. Epub 2009/05/19. eng.

61. Korbel JO, Urban AE, Affourtit JP, Godwin B, Grubert F, Simons JF, et al. Paired-end mapping reveals extensive structural variation in the human genome. Science. 2007;318(5849):420–6. PubMed PMID: 17901297. Pubmed Central PMCID: 2674581. Epub 2007/09/29. eng.

62. Xie C, Tammi MT. CNV-seq, a new method to detect copy number variation using high-throughput sequencing. BMC Bioinformatics. 2009;10:80. PubMed PMID: 19267900. Pubmed Central PMCID: 2667514. Epub 2009/03/10. eng.

63. Grossmann V, Kohlmann A, Klein HU, Schindela S, Schnittger S, Dicker F, et al. Targeted next-generation sequencing detects point mutations, insertions, deletions and balanced chromosomal rearrangements as well as identifies novel leukemia-specific fusion genes in a single procedure. Leukemia. 2011;25(4):671–80. PubMed PMID: 21252984. Epub 2011/01/22. eng.

64. Grimm D, Hagmann J, Koenig D, Weigel D, Borgwardt K. Accurate indel prediction using paired-end short reads. BMC Genomics. 2013;14:132. PubMed PMID: 23442375. Pubmed Central PMCID: 3614465. Epub 2013/02/28. eng.

65. Mills RE, Luttig CT, Larkins CE, Beauchamp A, Tsui C, Pittard WS, et al. An initial map of insertion and deletion (INDEL) variation in the human genome. Genome Res. 2006;16(9):1182–90. PubMed PMID: 16902084. Pubmed Central PMCID: 1557762. Epub 2006/08/12. eng.

66. Sobreira NL, Gnanakkan V, Walsh M, Marosy B, Wohler E, Thomas G, et al. Characterization of complex chromosomal rearrangements by targeted capture and next-generation sequencing. Genome Res. 2011;21(10):1720–7. PubMed PMID: 21890680. Pubmed Central PMCID: 3202288. Epub 2011/09/06. eng.

67. Miller DT, Adam MP, Aradhya S, Biesecker LG, Brothman AR, Carter NP, et al. Consensus statement: chromosomal microarray is a first-tier clinical diagnostic test for individuals with developmental disabilities or congenital anomalies. Am J Hum Genet. 2010;86(5): 749–64. PubMed PMID: 20466091. Pubmed Central PMCID: 2869000. Epub 2010/05/15. eng.

Polymerase Chain Reaction

Maria Pasic, Carlo Hojilla, and George M. Yousef

Introduction

Nucleic acid amplification by polymerase chain reaction (PCR) is a molecular technique that is used to amplify the copy number of a specific DNA region of interest [1, 2]. It has revolutionized the field of molecular biology since its Nobel award-winning discovery by Mullis and colleagues in the mid-1980s [3]. Its relative simplicity, versatility, and high amenability for automation have allowed for the many impactful discoveries in the fields of microbiology, genetics, and oncology [4–6].

In this chapter, we will discuss the technical aspects of PCR as well as optimization and troubleshooting of the reaction. We will also elaborate on the variations and types of PCR. Finally, current and prospective clinical applications of PCR will be discussed.

Principle and Basic Steps of PCR

The principle of PCR has been extensively described in the literature [7–13]. At its simplest, the starting reagents in a PCR include a DNA template, a reaction buffer, a cocktail of deoxynucleotide triphosphates (dNTPs), a heat-stable DNA polymerase enzyme, magnesium ions (Mg^{2+}), and specific DNA primers that flank the region to be amplified (this region is also called the amplicon). A typical PCR cycle is divided into three basic steps, namely, thermal-induced separation (denaturation) of the double-stranded target DNA, annealing of synthetic oligonucleotide primers to the target sequence, and extension of the annealed primer-target sequence by a DNA polymerase (Fig. 4.1). This cycle is repeated 25–40 times. Some protocols supply the enzyme in an inactive form to prevent nonspecific binding of the primers, and this requires an additional initial enzyme activation step (usually by heat). PCR products are then analyzed and/or quantified by a variety of methods. Modifications to the reagents, the steps, and detection methods have improved on this basic concept to truly showcase the potential of this method for research and clinical applications.

The Denaturation Step

Thermal denaturation of the double-stranded DNA (dsDNA) target is the first step in the reaction. Often a failed reaction is due to inadequate denaturation of DNA. dsDNA is denatured into single-stranded DNA (ssDNA) that can hybridize to single-stranded primers. Initial denaturation of target DNA is typically set at 94 °C for 6–8 min, which in subsequent cycles can be reduced to 1–2 min. As genomic DNA targets decrease and amplified PCR targets increase during the progression

M. Pasic, Ph.D. • C. Hojilla, M.D., Ph.D.
G.M. Yousef, M.D., Ph.D. (✉)
Department of Laboratory Medicine and Pathobiology,
University of Toronto, Medical Sciences Building,
1 King's College Circle, Toronto, ON M5S 1A8, Canada
e-mail: yousefg@smh.ca

G.M. Yousef and S. Jothy (eds.), *Molecular Testing in Cancer*,
DOI 10.1007/978-1-4899-8050-2_4, © Springer Science+Business Media New York 2014

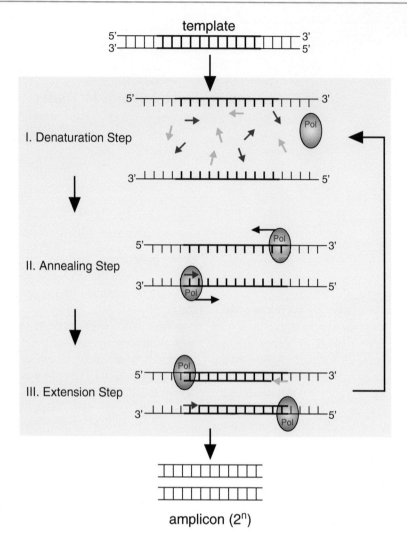

Fig. 4.1 A simplified schematic of the basic steps of a polymerase chain reaction. A typical PCR cycle consists of three steps: a denaturation step to separate the double-stranded DNA template into two single stands, annealing step where the primers hybridize to the template, and extension step where a complimentary copy is made by the polymerase enzyme (Pol) (*red arrow* = forward primer; *green arrow* = reverse primer). Theoretically, if you start with two stands of DNA, the exponential PCR amplicon production after n number of cycles will be 2^n

of the PCR, it has been suggested to use a lower denaturation temperature to minimize thermal denaturation of the Taq polymerase enzyme.

tion to the primer over target reannealing as the smaller primers move more rapidly in solution than larger ssDNA molecules.

The Annealing Step

The primer annealing step is largely determined by the composition of the primers and their melting temperature. Having primers in molar excess concentration promotes target hybridiza-

The Extension Step

The primer extension step requires adjusting the temperature and the extension time. Extension temperature is determined by the optimal functional temperature of the DNA polymerase used while the extension time is determined by the length of the target sequence. For example, using Taq polymerase, the typical extension temperature is 72 °C, with an extension time of 1 min for products up to 2 kb in length. Some protocols merge annealing and extension into one step.

Cycle Number

The number of cycles required is inversely dependent on the starting copy number of the target DNA. For example, a starting concentration of 10^5 template molecules requires 25 cycles for an ethidium bromide-visible signal on gel electrophoresis. Lower copy numbers of target DNA require more amplification cycles. Given that target DNA is doubled for every PCR cycle, if you start with two copies of DNA, the theoretical exponential PCR amplicon production after n number of cycles will be 2^n. However as the reaction progresses past 25 cycles, the PCR amplicon production begins to plateau as the reaction components (most often dNTPs) become rate limiting as they are consumed by the reaction. In addition, there is a steady decline in efficiency of the DNA polymerase due to thermal denaturation.

The PCR Reagents

Target-Specific Primers

One of the key advantages of PCR over other nucleic acid analysis methods is its high specificity, mediated by the use of target-specific primers. Two single-stranded primers are employed, which flank the 5′ and 3′ ends of the desired dsDNA sequence. The primers (commonly designated as the forward and reverse primers) are complementary to opposite ends of the denatured ssDNA of the sequence of choice (designated correspondingly, as the reverse or forward strands). Inherent in the design of primers is the knowledge of the DNA sequence of interest.

There are general concepts for ideal primer design. First, the primer sequence should be unique in the target DNA sequence to minimize the chance of nonspecific amplification. Second, primers should have minimal intra- and inter-sequence complementarity to mitigate the formation of primer-dimer sequences, which can negatively impact the yield of the reaction or, worse, lead to spurious results. Stretches with more than three or four of the same base, secondary structures such as hairpin loops, and palindromic sequences should be avoided. Third, primer concentration should be added in molar excess compared to the target DNA, as primers are incorporated and consumed at each cycle. Finally, optimizing the annealing temperature is essential to specificity as nonspecific binding occurs at lower annealing temperatures, whereas annealing might not happen if the temperature is too high. The annealing temperature is determined by the primer melting temperature. There are a number of free online tools that can help designing primers and also calculate the annealing temperature for each primer.

DNA Template

The robustness of PCR stems from its ability to amplify DNA from various sources such as tissues, peripheral blood, or other material such as hair or nail specimens. Tissues can be fresh, frozen, or formalin-fixed. Furthermore, the nucleic acid source can be RNA, genomic DNA, or mitochondrial DNA. Indeed, PCR is so remarkably robust that even fragmented DNA, such as archived material from formalin-fixed paraffin wax-embedded tissues, in nanogram quantities, can be sufficient for amplification [14]. A rate limiting step, therefore, is the DNA extraction procedure. In general, proteinase K digestion of fresh tissue yields the highest and best quality DNA. However, this process is laborious and involves multiple phenol-chloroform extraction steps. An alternative, faster extraction method, but one that produces a lower yield and quality, is achieved by boiling the fresh tissue in sterile water for 15 min. DNA can be extracted successfully from archival samples, stained sections, or cytological preparations using either approach described above. In all these methods, the use of EDTA- containing buffers should be avoided as it affects Mg^{2+} ion concentrations. Also, contamination with organic solvents should be minimized as this affects other PCR reagents.

dNTPs

dNTPs can be obtained either as freeze-dried or neutralized aqueous solutions. They are also available as labeled nucleotides (radioactive or fluorescent labeled) for use in subsequent hybridization or sequencing (as discussed below) reactions. Currently, they are commonly supplied by the manufacturers of a proprietary PCR kit as aqueous solutions at a stock concentration, with a final working concentration of 50–200 μM, which is sufficient to synthesize 6.5–25 μg of DNA.

PCR Buffer

Tris buffer at a concentration of 10 mM and pH of 8.5 or 9.0 at 25 °C is the buffer of choice for most PCRs. The pH of Tris is temperature dependent such that a buffer made to pH 8.8 at 25 °C will have a pH value of 7.4 at 72 °C. This is the optimal working temperature and pH for Taq polymerase. Primer annealing is further facilitated by 50 mM KCl or NaCl salts; however, concentrations in excess will inhibit Taq polymerase activity. Phosphate salts are generally avoided as they can precipitate Mg^{2+} at the high temperatures used in the PCR [15]. Another key ingredient to the reaction buffer is Mg^{2+} ions at a concentration that is specific and empirically determined per amplification reaction (as discussed in the optimization section below). Also, additives can be used to further optimize the PCR amplification. Most reaction buffers are bundled and supplied by manufacturers as a 10× proprietary stock, with or without Mg^{2+} and additives.

DNA Polymerase

The key reagent that revolutionized PCR is the heat-stable DNA polymerase found in microorganisms surviving in extreme environments. Whereas most proteins are denatured at the temperature required for DNA denaturation, these polymerases are still functional. Three commonly used DNA polymerases are Pfu (Pyrococcus furiosus), Vent or Tli (Thermococcus litoralis), and Taq polymerase (Thermus aquaticus), with the latter being the most common commercially available polymerase. These polymerases are functionally quite robust in that they can extend DNA at a wide range of temperatures as long as a primer-template hybrid is present. However, the optimal working temperature for these enzymes is 70 °C and a pH of 7.0–7.5. Nonetheless, the half-life of Taq DNA polymerase activity is >2 h at 92.5 °C, 40 min at 95 °C, and 5 min at 97.5 °C, which explains the decline in fidelity and the plateau effect towards cycles greater than 25. Notably, Taq polymerase lacks a $3'–5'$ proofreading exonuclease activity leading to an error rate of 1 in 9,000 bases [15]. Additionally, Taq polymerase is sensitive to Mg^{2+} concentration.

Detection, Characterization, and Quantification of PCR Products

At the completion of the PCR amplification, the DNA product can then be detected, quantified, and analyzed by various methods, as shown in Box 4.1. The most cost-efficient, widely used method is agarose gel electrophoresis of the PCR product that is visualized by ethidium bromide (EtBr) staining. This process allows for analysis of the PCR-generated product based on size. DNA fragments are visualized under UV illumination. A DNA ladder of known sizes is used to correlate with the size of the product. Primer dimers and other small products also appear as diffuse bands close to the leading edge of the gel. Other additional bands on the gel may be the result of single-stranded products or nonspecific priming [16].

Semiquantitative analysis of the PCR product after gel electrophoresis can be done by measuring the densitometry of the product compared to the densitometry values of a known housekeeping gene. Multiplex and mimic PCR offered a more accurate quantitative method where serial dilutions of a competitive DNA fragment (the mimic) are added to constant amounts of complementary DNA (cDNA). During PCR, competition occurs between template and the mimic for a given primer set, and because a known quantity of mimic is added, the concentrations of a particular cDNA and hence messenger RNA (mRNA) can be determined [15]. In quantitative real-time PCR (Q-PCR), the quantification is based on measuring the accumulated product after each cycle, as described below [17].

Gel electrophoresis can be also followed by Southern blot hybridization, which allows for confirmation of the amplicon through hybridization of a probe with denatured amplicon DNA fixed on a membrane. This method is quite laborious and involves use to radioactively labeled probes. Southern blotting is now supplanted by sequencing or fluorescence-based assays.

Optimization of PCR

Optimization is critical in obtaining a successful PCR [18]. A number of factors need to be optimized, as summarized in Box 4.2, and discussed below in more details. Negative results in the PCR can be due to a number of reasons, including lack of optimization, in addition to absence of the target in the examined specimen, as shown in Box 4.3. In general, a number of controls are included in a PCR: a negative control (usually no DNA template), a positive control (usually a cloned dsDNA copy of the target), and a second PCR control which is usually a housekeeping gene that is abundantly expressed in every tissue.

Melting and Annealing Temperatures

The melting temperature (T_m) is the temperature at which 50 % of the oligonucleotide primers are bound to their complementary sequence and the other 50 % are separated into single-stranded molecules. The T_m of the primer depends on both its length and its nucleotide sequence composition, specifically the ratio of the number of guanines and cytosines to the number of adenines and thymidines. For sequences less than 14 nucleotides, the formula is

$$T_m = (wA + xT) \times 2 + (yG + zC) \times 4$$

where w, x, y, and z are the numbers of the bases A, T, G, and C in the sequence, respectively.

For sequences longer than 13 nucleotides, the equation used is

$$T_m = 64.9 + 41 \times (yG + zC - 16.4) / (wA + xT + yG + zC)$$

Both above equations assume that the annealing occurs under the standard conditions of 50 nM of primer, 50 mM of Na$^+$, and pH 7.0 for the reaction. The melting temperature serves as a starting point for choosing the annealing temperature for the PCR. Optimal annealing temperature is determined experimentally by comparing a range of temperatures around the estimated degree. Additionally, melting curve analysis is a powerful post-amplification analysis that is used in real-time PCR to determine characterizations of mutations or single-nucleotide polymorphisms (SNPs) in the DNA sequence of interest (as discussed below) [19, 20].

Magnesium Ion Concentration

Magnesium ions are essential to DNA polymerase function as they associate with DNA, dNTPs, and the polymerase. Because of this, Mg^{2+} can affect the T_m of the primers and consequently the specificity of the PCR and the fidelity of the DNA polymerase. As a rule of thumb, the Mg^{2+} concentration in the reaction mixture is generally 0.5–2.5 mM greater than the concentration of dNTPs. The optimal concentration is specific and must be determined empirically per reaction.

Reaction Additives

To further optimize the reaction, organic additives can be used in some cases to improve the specificity and yield of the PCR amplification. Several organic additives, nonionic detergents,

and bovine serum albumin have been described. The mechanism of action for each of these additives may be multifactorial and varied. For example, dimethyl sulfoxide (DMSO) may play a role in altering the T_m that favors a more specific primer-target binding. On the other hand, bovine serum albumin may sequester protein inhibitors of the PCR amplification. Titration of the concentration of these additives in the reaction is usually required to determine the optimal concentration.

Thermal Cyclers

While each manufacturer's model may be slightly different, a good thermal cycler should have thermal uniformity, a cooling system, a heating block, and a programmable memory. Variations between thermal cyclers include the type and capacity of reaction vessels used (i.e., plates vs. tubes vs. glass slides; 48-well vs. 96-well plates). Some have smaller separate heating blocks that allow for multiple reactions to run simultaneously (which is especially useful when optimizing Mg^{2+} and annealing temperatures per reaction). Others also use heated covers to allow for the omission of mineral oil additives in the reaction. For real-time PCR, thermal cyclers are capable of exciting fluorophores and detecting emitted light wavelengths. Furthermore, they are equipped with post-amplification software that can analyze fluorescence values that can be used to track the PCR amplification curve, optimize the reaction, quantify PCR amplified products, and perform melting curve analyses.

Common PCR Variants and Modifications

There are different types and variants of the PCR, as outlined in Table 4.1. The common variants are discussed here in more details.

Reverse Transcription PCR

Gene expression studies have greatly benefited from a modification in the basic PCR with a preceding step of reverse transcription [21]. Using

Table 4.1 PCR types and variants

Type	Description
Reverse transcription PCR	See text for details
Multiplex PCR	Using two or more pairs of primer to target different DNA regions in the same reaction for the same specimen [39]
Nested PCR	The product of initial amplification is re-amplified with a new set of primers that are located within the first set to enhance sensitivity [40]
Quantitative (real time) PCR	See text for details
Restriction fragment length polymorphism	PCR followed by restriction digestion of the product. Mutations will alter the size of the fragment produced by restriction digestion
Single-stranded conformational polymorphism	See text for details
Cold PCR protocols	G/T to A/G mutations decrease the melting temperature of the targets and thus lower denaturation temperature can be used to preferentially amplify mutant DNA if it is present in a minority component [41]
Methylation-specific PCR	A method for analysis of DNA methylation patterns in CpG islands. DNA is modified by sodium bisulfite, converting all unmethylated, but not methylated, cytosines to uracil and PCR performed with two primer pairs for methylated and unmethylated DNA, respectively [42]
In situ PCR	Combines the extreme sensitivity of the PCR with the anatomical localization provided by in situ hybridization [43]

reverse transcriptase (RT) enzyme, mRNA sequences are transcribed into cDNA which can then serve as the DNA template for the subsequent PCR. Most RT enzymes are isolated from viruses, for example, the avian myeloblastosis virus (AMV) and the Moloney murine leukemia virus (MMLV). AMV reverse transcriptase has the advantage that the optimum temperature for reverse transcription is 42 °C, which is of benefit if the RNA template has a high degree of secondary structure [18].

Briefly, the method involves the initial conversion of mRNA to cDNA using a RT enzyme. This can be primed by various strategies including the use of a downstream antisense PCR primer that is specific to the RNA of interest, random hexamers, or an oligo d(T) primer targeted at the poly(A) tail of mRNA. Using antisense primers offers the advantage of specificity but limits subsequent PCR to testing a single product. Random hexamers and oligo d(T) primers offer the advantage of having cDNA template that can be used for a number of independent PCRs within the same tube. However, oligo d(T) primers suffer fidelity issues with long mRNA sequences or those with secondary RNA struc-tures. The single-stranded cDNA produced by the RT reaction is then amplified during the first cycle of the standard PCR by Taq polymerase to yield double-stranded cDNA, which is then amplified in further cycles.

Real-Time (Quantitative) PCR

An evolutionary improvement of PCR came with the introduction of quantitative (real-time) analysis [22, 23]. The powerful advantage of real-time PCR is its ability to quantify the amplified product in the reaction with extremely high analytic sensitivity. In real-time PCR, amplification is combined with simultaneous detection and analysis of PCR products as they are synthesized in real time rather than waiting until the end of the reaction when quantification can be misleading due to a plateau effect (Fig. 4.2). At the end of each cycle, the fluorescence intensity produced (which is proportional to the amount of accumulated product) is detected and plotted against the PCR cycle number. The cycle number at which a set fluorescence intensity threshold is attained is called the *crossing threshold* or *cycle threshold*

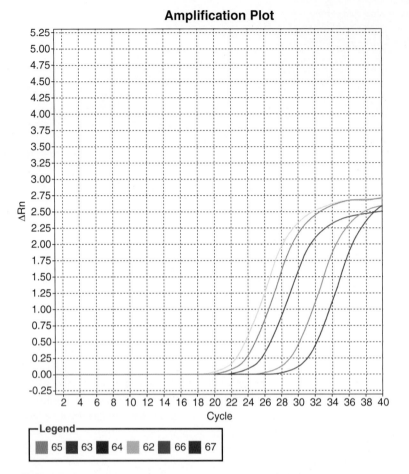

Fig. 4.2 A representative blot of a quantitative PCR. The cycle number is shown on the *X*-axis, and the florescent signal is displayed on the *Y*-axis. The intensity of the fluorescent signal is measured at the end of each cycle and is proportional to amount of the PCR product for each sample. The cycle number at which a set fluores- cence intensity threshold is attained is called the *crossing threshold* or *cycle threshold* (Ct) for the reaction, and it is inversely proportional to the initial concentration of the DNA target in the template. At the end of the reaction, all samples reached a plateau, and the PCR product of all samples will be the same

(Ct) for the reaction. This threshold is set early in the log-linear growth phase of the PCR amplification curve and roughly corresponds to the starting amount of the template DNA of the sample.

There are myriad applications of real-time PCR's ability to detect and analyze a particular target. At its most basic application, real-time PCR can be used to quantify the gene expression levels of a target cDNA. Moreover, depending on the chemistry and the analytic software used, post-amplification, real-time PCR can be also used for other purposes, like detection of SNPs using end point analysis or for gene mutation analysis through post-amplification melting curve analysis.

Real-Time PCR: Probe Design

Two broad fluorescence strategies are used: nonspecific and specific to a target DNA sequence. The nonspecific fluorescence makes use of an intercalating dye such as SYBR green or ethidium bromide, which binds to the minor groove of dsDNA. This allows for a low-cost and quick method of quantifying amplicons as

Fig. 4.3 Most common real-time (quantitative) PCR probe design strategies: (**a**) hybridization-based probes, (**b**) hydrolysis-based probes, and (**c**) molecular beacon-based probes. *FRET* fluorescence resonance energy transfer. Probes are denoted by *blue arrows*

a. Hybridization-based probe design

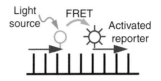

b. Hydrolysis-based probe design

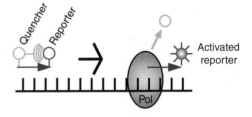

c. Molecular beacon-based probe design

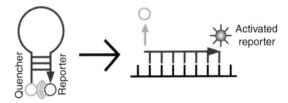

the fluorescence accumulates per PCR cycle. However, as the dye is nonspecific, other double-stranded sequences such as primer dimers will be also detected.

Specific methods for detection employ the use of fluorescent-labeled amplicon-specific oligonucleotide probes. Probes are designed to be complimentary to a DNA target region and have a fluorophore (with or without a nearby quencher moiety) that absorbs and emits light at specific wavelength that is detectable by the thermal cycler (Fig. 4.3). During the PCR amplification, the probes have either a change in their emission spectra only when bound to the target DNA in a specific orientation or they produce a fluorescence signal in proportion to the amount of amplicon generated. The most commonly employed probe designs include hybridization probes, hydrolysis or TaqMan® probes, minor groove-binding (MGB) probes, and molecular beacon probes.

Hybridization Probes

The hybridization probe method uses two oligonucleotide probes that are both fluorescently labeled (a donor and a reporter fluorophore) (Fig. 4.3a). These probes are designed to be complementary to two regions that are in close proximity to each other on the target DNA. This method depends on the physical property of fluorescence resonance energy transfer (FRET), wherein when two fluorophores are in close proximity to one another, the donor fluorophore is excited by the thermal cycler light source and emits light at a wavelength in the absorption range of the second reporter fluorophore. During a PCR cycle, binding of the two probes during the annealing step allows for FRET to occur, and the reporter absorbs the donor emission and emits light at a wavelength detected by the real-time PCR thermal cycler. The amount of product generated per cycle is proportional to the FRET fluorescence generated. Hybridization probes are also useful for detection of small deletion or insertion mutations.

Hydrolysis and Minor Groove-Binding Probes

As shown in Fig. 4.3b, the hydrolysis or *Taq*Man™ probe method requires an oligonucleotide probe that is labeled with a reporter fluorophore at the 5′ end and a fluorescence quencher at the 3′ end and a DNA polymerase with a 5′ exonuclease activity. At the beginning of the PCR, the probe does not fluoresce as the quencher dye absorbs the light emitted from the reporter. During the annealing and extension steps of each cycle, the probe is incorporated into the PCR product, and the 5′ exonuclease activity of the DNA polymerase cleaves the probe and releases the reporter dye from the effect of the quencher. The amount of free fluorescence is proportional to the amount of PCR product accumulating after each cycle.

MGB probes work in similar principle to the hydrolysis probes in that this method uses a dual-labeled probe and requires a 5′ exonuclease activity. The difference is the addition of a covalently linked molecule that can bind to the minor groove of dsDNA which further stabilizes the hybridization of the probe to target DNA which raises the melting temperature of the reaction.

Hydrolysis probes are useful for the identification of SNPs. A specific probe is designed to an allele of interest. A perfect match will allow for the release of the reporter dye, which is detected as fluorescence and any mismatch will not yield one at the end of the reaction. MGB probes are particularly useful for shorter probes due to the inherent stability of the minor groove-binding property of the probe.

Molecular Beacon Probes

The molecular beacon probe method shares a similar design to the hydrolysis probes, except that the 5′ and 3′ terminal sequences of the probe are complimentary to one another (Fig. 4.3c). As such, the fluorophore and quencher dyes are brought to close proximity during the unbound state, creating a loop secondary structure with a double-stranded terminal stem. During PCR amplification, the stem is melted, and the loop portion, which is complimentary to the target DNA, is allowed to anneal. This permits separation of the fluorophore and quencher and light emission. Another difference from the hydrolysis probe is that the DNA polymerase does not cleave the probe. It simply displaces it and makes it available for use in subsequent cycles.

SNPs and mutations can be detected after the PCR by performing melting curve analyses of the final PCR products. The melting point is the temperature at which 50 % of DNA is denatured. Different dsDNA molecules melt at different temperatures, dependent upon a number of factors including GC content, amplicon length, secondary and tertiary structure. The sequence with mutation will have a different melting curve compared to the wild-type sequence (Fig. 4.4). To perform a melting curve, the final PCR product is exposed to an increasing temperature gradient while fluorescence readouts are continually collected. Temperature will cause denaturation of dsDNA. The point at which the dsDNA melts into ssDNA is observed as a drop in fluorescence as the dye dissociates. This can be displayed as distinct melting peaks by plotting the first negative derivative of the fluorescence as a function of temperature.

Single-Stranded Conformation Polymorphism Analysis

Single-stranded conformation polymorphism (SSCP) analysis is based on the differential rate of migration of ssDNA depending on its ability to fold into a specific secondary structure based on its sequence [24–26]. Wild-type and mutant DNA are amplified by PCR and denatured. The products are analyzed by electrophoresis under non-denaturing conditions in a polyacrylamide matrix. Mutations affect the

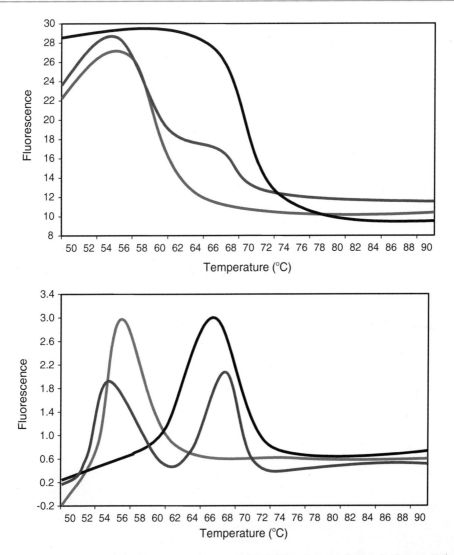

Fig. 4.4 Melting curve analysis is useful to detect SNPs and mutations in the amplified target region. The final PCR product is exposed to a temperature gradient while fluorescence readouts are continually collected. This causes denaturation of dsDNA. The point at which the dsDNA melts into ssDNA is observed as a drop in fluorescence as the dye dissociates (*upper*). The melt curves are converted to distinct melting peaks by plotting the first negative derivative of the fluorescence as a function of temperature (−dF/dT) (*lower*). In this example, we have three products: the *black* sample has the wild-type allele with a melting temperature of 68°, the *blue* sample has the mutant allele with a melting temperature of 56°, and the *red* sample is heterozygous with both the wild-type and mutant alleles

secondary structure and consequently the migration properties which can be visualized by radiography or ethidium bromide staining/ UV illumination. Mutant ssDNA bands will migrate to different positions compared to wild-type ssDNA. If a heterozygous mutation is present, both types of bands are generated. Current advancements in SSCP analysis allows for use with RNA samples, as RNA creates more stable conformations than ssDNA. One of the key advantages of this technique is its simplicity and sensitivity to screening for mutations, with up to 70–90 % sensitivity in sequences less than 200 bases [27, 28].

It should be noted that SSCP is a screening tool, which needs sequencing for confirmation [15]. Another limitation of SSCP analysis is its sensitivity to temperature, ionic environment, and pH which affects conformation. Hence these parameters must be tightly controlled during the process. SSCP is also less sensitive for G>C mutation detection. Contaminants such as excess primers or nonspecific PCR amplicons from low-fidelity reactions can bind ssDNA and alter its migration properties. The sensitivity of SSCP analysis decreases as fragment lengths increase beyond 200 bases, which can be improved by restriction enzyme digestion and multiplexing variably sized ssDNA fragments into one gel lane (a process known as restriction endonuclease fingerprinting SSCP) [29].

> **Box 4.4   Advantages and Limitations of PCR Technology**
>
> *Advantages*
> - High sensitivity (can be done on very small amounts of DNA material)
> - Fast
> - Reasonable cost
> - Can be automated
> - Can be quantified
>
> *Disadvantages and Limitations*
> - Specificity (mispriming can cause misleading results)
> - Easy contamination
> - Not suitable for mutation analysis of large DNA fragments
> - Limited ability to detect translocations and large deletions

---

Restriction Fragment Length Polymorphism Analysis

Restriction enzymes are bacterial enzymes capable of cleaving specific DNA sequences. Mutations, naturally occurring or user introduced, may create a new restriction site or disrupt one. The normal sequence can be differentiated from the mutation by the pattern of fragments following the restriction enzyme digestion, a process known as restriction mapping or restriction fragment length polymorphism (RFLP) analysis [30, 31].

RFLP analysis can be used to quickly characterize mutations of PCR products [32, 33]. PCR amplicons with known and predicted restriction maps are digested with specific restriction enzymes. The digestion products are then analyzed by gel electrophoresis and compared to size controls. RFLP analysis can be used to detect restriction site polymorphisms and mutations that are associated with the creation or destruction of restriction sites. The obliteration of a restriction site generates a longer DNA sequence, whereas the introduction of a restriction site will produce two shorter DNA fragments on gel electrophoresis.

Clinical Applications of PCR

The use of PCR techniques in molecular oncology has greatly expanded over the years, with a wide range of applications currently in use. Although PCR is a great technology that is widely used in molecular oncology due to its many advantages, it also has certain limitations, as outlined in Box 4.4. The ability of PCR to detect very small or even single-nucleotide mutations, as well as larger ones like deletions, rearrangements, or translocations, makes it a very economically feasible, easy, and rapid method for monitoring disease [34, 35]. The flexibility to quantify genomic material also makes PCR an ideal method for predicting the response to cancer treatments (example applications in [36, 37]). Additionally, genetic determinations can assist in the selection of appropriate treatment for a particular individual, which has led to evolution of the field of "personalized medicine" [6]. For example, p53 mutations in breast cancer can be indicative of poor response to tamoxifen [38], while mutations in KRAS can indicate if a person will benefit from the cancer drug panitumumab [37]. The spectrum of PCR applications in molecular oncology is outlined in Table 4.2.

Table 4.2 Spectrum of application of PCR in molecular oncology

	Application	Example
1	Detection of DNA mutations, deletions/insertions	BRCA1 and BRCA2 in breast/ovarian cancers [44]
		MSH2 and MLH1 in colon carcinoma and polyps [45]
		Rb1 mutations in retinoblastoma [46]
		P53 mutations in soft tissue sarcoma [47]
2	Oncogene or tumor suppressor gene expression	Increased erbB2 expression in breast cancer: associated with poor prognosis [48]
		Increased myc expression in lung cancer: associated with tumor progression and poor response to chemotherapy [49]
3	Single-nucleotide polymorphism analysis	SNPs in the microRNA miR-143/145 can predict increased or decreased risk for colorectal cancer [50]
4	Methylation analysis	Promoter methylation of E-cadherin results in reduced expression and aberrant nuclear localization in epithelial ovarian cancer [51]
5	Large-scale screening of mRNA expression	PCR-based expression arrays
6	miRNA expression	miR409-3p, miR-7, and miR93 panel can be used for early detection of colorectal cancer [52]
7	PCR-based miRNA global screening	Identification of differentially expressed miRNAs in non-small cell lung cancer as biomarkers for early cancer detection [53]
8	Genotyping of somatic mutations	JAK2 V617F in myeloproliferative disorders [54]
		KRAS mutations in codons 12 and 13 for colon cancer [55]
		BRAF V600E mutation in melanomas [56]
9	Detection of residual disease	BCR-ABL1 copy number in chronic myelogenous leukemia treated with Gleevec [57]
10	Detection of chromosomal rearrangements	T cell receptor gene and immunoglobulin heavy chain gene rearrangements, respectively, in T cell and B cell non-Hodgkin's lymphomas [58]
11	Amplification of microsatellite repeats	Identification of microsatellite instability in mismatch repair genes in Lynch syndrome [59]
12	Quantification of viral load for cancer patient management	EBV load in posttransplant lymphoproliferative disorder patients can predict likelihood of disease development, and thus, proper amount of suppression can be controlled [60]
13	Tumor commonality assay	Clonality detection in Hodgkin's lymphoma [61]
14	Detection of chromosomal translocations	2;5 translocation in anaplastic large cell non- Hodgkin's lymphoma [62]
		9;22 translocation in chronic myeloid leukemia [63]
		11;22 translocation in Ewing's sarcoma [64]
15	Loss of heterozygosity (LOH) for investigation of clonality in tumors	LOH on chromosome 16 in lobular carcinoma of the breast [65]
16	Detection of infectious agents (viruses) causing neoplasms	Human papillomavirus associated with cervical cancer [66]
		Epstein-Barr virus associated with Burkitt's lymphoma [67]
		Human herpesvirus 8 associated with Kaposi's sarcoma [68]

References

1. Bossler A, van Deerlin V. Conventional and real-time polymerase chain reaction. In: Tubbs RR, Stoler MH, editors. Cell and tissue based molecular pathology. Philadelphia, PA: Churchill Livingstone Elsevier Inc.; 2009. p. 33–49.

2. Rennert H, Leonard DGB. Molecular methods in the diagnostic laboratory. In: Leonard DGB, editor. Diagnostic molecular pathology. Philadelphia: Saunders; 2003. p. 25–52.

3. Mullis K, Faloona F, Scharf S, Saiki R, Horn G, Erlich H. Specific enzymatic amplification of DNA in vitro: the polymerase chain reaction. Cold Spring Harb Symp Quant Biol. 1986;51(Pt 1):263–73.

4. Gazdar AF. Personalized medicine and inhibition of EGFR signaling in lung cancer. N Engl J Med. 2009;361(10):1018–20.
5. Gonzalez-Angulo AM, Hennessy BT, Mills GB. Future of personalized medicine in oncology: a systems biology approach. J Clin Oncol. 2010;28(16):2777–83.
6. Pasic MD, Samaan S, Yousef GM. Genomic medicine: new frontiers and new challenges. Clin Chem. 2013;59(1):158–67.
7. Bej AK, Mahbubani MH, Atlas RM. Amplification of nucleic acids by polymerase chain reaction (PCR) and other methods and their applications. Crit Rev Biochem Mol Biol. 1991;26(3–4):301–34.
8. Coleman WG, Tsongalis GJ. Essential concepts in molecular pathology. San Diego, CA: Elsevier; 2010.
9. Gibbs RA. DNA amplification by the polymerase chain reaction. Anal Chem. 1990;62(13):1202–14.
10. Kubista M, Andrade JM, Bengtsson M, Forootan A, Jonak J, Lind K, et al. The real-time polymerase chain reaction. Mol Aspects Med. 2006;27(2–3):95–125.
11. Lo YM, Chan KC. Setting up a polymerase chain reaction laboratory. Methods Mol Biol. 2006; 336:11–8.
12. Remick DG, Kunkel SL, Holbrook EA, Hanson CA. Theory and applications of the polymerase chain reaction. Am J Clin Pathol. 1990;93(4 Suppl 1):S49–54.
13. Templeton NS. The polymerase chain reaction. History, methods, and applications. Diagn Mol Pathol. 1992;1(1):58–72.
14. Mies C. Molecular biological analysis of paraffin-embedded tissues. Hum Pathol. 1994;25(6):555–60.
15. Baumforth KR, Nelson PN, Digby JE, O'Neil JD, Murray PG. Demystified … the polymerase chain reaction. Mol Pathol. 1999;52(1):1–10.
16. Killeen AA. Principles of molecular pathology. New Jersey: Humana Press; 2004.
17. Crotty PL, Staggs RA, Porter PT, Killeen AA, McGlennen RC. Quantitative analysis in molecular diagnostics. Hum Pathol. 1994;25(6):572–9.
18. Oliver D. Polymerase chain reaction and reverse transcription-polymerase chain reaction. In: Cagle PT, Allen TC, editors. Basic concepts of molecular pathology. New York: Springer; 2009. p. 73–85.
19. Ririe KM, Rasmussen RP, Wittwer CT. Product differentiation by analysis of DNA melting curves during the polymerase chain reaction. Anal Biochem. 1997;245(2):154–60.
20. Wienken CJ, Baaske P, Duhr S, Braun D. Thermophoretic melting curves quantify the conformation and stability of RNA and DNA. Nucleic Acids Res. 2011;39(8):e52.
21. Joyce C. Quantitative RT-PCR. A review of current methodologies. Methods Mol Biol. 2002;193:83–92.
22. Deepak S, Kottapalli K, Rakwal R, Oros G, Rangappa K, Iwahashi H, et al. Real-time PCR: revolutionizing detection and expression analysis of genes. Curr Genomics. 2007;8(4):234–51.
23. Freeman WM, Walker SJ, Vrana KE. Quantitative RT-PCR: pitfalls and potential. Biotechniques. 1999;26(1):112–22, 24–5.

24. Hayashi K. PCR-SSCP: a simple and sensitive method for detection of mutations in the genomic DNA. PCR Methods Appl. 1991;1(1):34–8.
25. Liu Q, Feng J, Buzin C, Wen C, Nozari G, Mengos A, et al. Detection of virtually all mutations-SSCP (DOVAM-S): a rapid method for mutation scanning with virtually 100% sensitivity. Biotechniques. 1999;26(5):932, 6–8, 40–2.
26. Orita M, Iwahana H, Kanazawa H, Hayashi K, Sekiya T. Detection of polymorphisms of human DNA by gel electrophoresis as single-strand conformation polymorphisms. Proc Natl Acad Sci U S A. 1989;86(8):2766–70.
27. Noakes MA, Reimer T, Phillips RB. Genotypic characterization of an MHC class II locus in lake trout (Salvelinus namaycush) from Lake Superior by single-stranded conformational polymorphism analysis and reference strand-mediated conformational analysis. Mar Biotechnol (NY). 2003;5(3):270–8.
28. Pajak B, Stefanska I, Lepek K, Donevski S, Romanowska M, Szeliga M, et al. Rapid differentiation of mixed influenza A/H1N1 virus infections with seasonal and pandemic variants by multitemperature single-stranded conformational polymorphism analysis. J Clin Microbiol. 2011;49(6):2216–21.
29. Liu MS, Rampal S, Hsiang D, Chen FT. Automated DNA mutation analysis by single-strand conformation polymorphism using capillary electrophoresis with laser-induced fluorescence detection. Mol Biotechnol. 2000;15(1):21–7.
30. Farkas DH, Holland CA. Overview of molecular diagnostic techniques and instrumentation. In: Tubbs RR, Stoler MH, editors. Cell and tissue based molecular pathology. Philadelphia, PA: Churchill Livingstone Elsevier Inc; 2009. p. 19–35.
31. Lo YM, Chan KC. Introduction to the polymerase chain reaction. Methods Mol Biol. 2006;336:1–10.
32. Case C, Kandola K, Chui L, Li V, Nix N, Johnson R. Examining DNA fingerprinting as an epidemiology tool in the tuberculosis program in the Northwest Territories, Canada. Int J Circumpolar Health. 2013 May 8;72. doi: 10.3402/ijch.v72i0.20067. Print 2013. PubMed PMID: 23671837; PubMed Central PMCID: PMC3650219.
33. Priyadarshini A, Chakraborti A, Mandal AK, Singh SK. Asp299Gly and Thr399Ile polymorphism of TLR-4 gene in patients with prostate cancer from North India. Indian J Urol. 2013;29(1):37–41.
34. Bernard PS, Wittwer CT. Real-time PCR technology for cancer diagnostics. Clin Chem. 2002;48(8):1178–85.
35. Crocker J. Demystified… Molecular pathology in oncology. Mol Pathol. 2002;55(6):337–47.
36. Darb-Esfahani S, Kronenwett R, von Minckwitz G, Denkert C, Gehrmann M, Rody A, et al. Thymosin beta 15A (TMSB15A) is a predictor of chemotherapy response in triple-negative breast cancer. Br J Cancer. 2012;107(11):1892–900.
37. Kim ST, Sung JS, Jo UH, Park KH, Shin SW, Kim YH. Can mutations of EGFR and KRAS in serum be

predictive and prognostic markers in patients with advanced non-small cell lung cancer (NSCLC)? Med Oncol. 2013;30(1):328.

38. Berns EM, Foekens JA, Vossen R, Look MP, Devilee P, Henzen-Logmans SC, et al. Complete sequencing of TP53 predicts poor response to systemic therapy of advanced breast cancer. Cancer Res. 2000;60(8): 2155–62.

39. Chamberlain JS, Gibbs RA, Ranier JE, Nguyen PN, Caskey CT. Deletion screening of the Duchenne muscular dystrophy locus via multiplex DNA amplification. Nucleic Acids Res. 1988;16(23): 11141–56.

40. Llop P, Bonaterra A, Penalver J, Lopez MM. Development of a highly sensitive nested-PCR procedure using a single closed tube for detection of Erwinia amylovora in asymptomatic plant material. Appl Environ Microbiol. 2000;66(5):2071–8.

41. Milbury CA, Li J, Makrigiorgos GM. PCR-based methods for the enrichment of minority alleles and mutations. Clin Chem. 2009;55(4):632–40.

42. Ku JL, Jeon YK, Park JG. Methylation-specific PCR. Methods Mol Biol. 2011;791:23–32.

43. Komminoth P, Long AA. In-situ polymerase chain reaction. An overview of methods, applications and limitations of a new molecular technique. Virchows Arch B Cell Pathol Incl Mol Pathol. 1993;64(2): 67–73.

44. Hernan I, Borras E, de Sousa DM, Gamundi MJ, Mane B, Llort G, et al. Detection of genomic variations in BRCA1 and BRCA2 genes by long-range PCR and next-generation sequencing. J Mol Diagn. 2012;14(3):286–93.

45. Wang Y, Friedl W, Sengteller M, Jungck M, Filges I, Propping P, et al. A modified multiplex PCR assay for detection of large deletions in MSH2 and MLH1. Hum Mutat. 2002;19(3):279–86.

46. Shimizu T, Toguchida J, Kato MV, Kaneko A, Ishizaki K, Sasaki MS. Detection of mutations of the RB1 gene in retinoblastoma patients by using exon-by-exon PCR-SSCP analysis. Am J Hum Genet. 1994;54(5): 793–800.

47. Yin L, Liu CX, Nong WX, Chen YZ, Qi Y, Li HA, et al. Mutational analysis of p53 and PTEN in soft tissue sarcoma. Mol Med Rep. 2012;5(2):457–61.

48. O'Malley FP, Saad Z, Kerkvliet N, Doig G, Stitt L, Ainsworth P, et al. The predictive power of semiquantitative immunohistochemical assessment of p53 and c-erb B-2 in lymph node-negative breast cancer. Hum Pathol. 1996;27(9):955–63.

49. Iwakawa R, Kohno T, Kato M, Shiraishi K, Tsuta K, Noguchi M, et al. MYC amplification as a prognostic marker of early-stage lung adenocarcinoma identified by whole genome copy number analysis. Clin Cancer Res. 2011;17(6):1481–9.

50. Li L, Pan X, Li Z, Bai P, Jin H, Wang T, et al. Association between polymorphisms in the promoter region of miR-143/145 and risk of colorectal cancer. Hum Immunol. 2013;74(8):993–7.

51. Makarla PB, Saboorian MH, Ashfaq R, Toyooka KO, Toyooka S, Minna JD, et al. Promoter hypermethylation profile of ovarian epithelial neoplasms. Clin Cancer Res. 2005;11(15):5365–9.

52. Wang S, Xiang J, Li Z, Lu S, Hu J, Gao X, et al. A plasma microRNA panel for early detection of colorectal cancer. Int J Cancer. 2013 Mar 2. doi:10.1002/ijc.28136. [Epub ahead of print] PubMed PMID: 23456911.

53. Hennessey PT, Sanford T, Choudhary A, Mydlarz WW, Brown D, Adai AT, et al. Serum microRNA biomarkers for detection of non-small cell lung cancer. PLoS One. 2012;7(2):e32307.

54. Olsen RJ, Tang Z, Farkas DH, Bernard DW, Zu Y, Chang CC. Detection of the JAK2(V617F) mutation in myeloproliferative disorders by melting curve analysis using the LightCycler system. Arch Pathol Lab Med. 2006;130(7):997–1003.

55. Ma ES, Wong CL, Law FB, Chan WK, Siu D. Detection of KRAS mutations in colorectal cancer by high-resolution melting analysis. J Clin Pathol. 2009;62(10):886–91.

56. Kumar R, Angelini S, Czene K, Sauroja I, Hahka-Kemppinen M, Pyrhonen S, et al. BRAF mutations in metastatic melanoma: a possible association with clinical outcome. Clin Cancer Res. 2003;9(9):3362–8.

57. Kantarjian HM, Talpaz M, Cortes J, O'Brien S, Faderl S, Thomas D, et al. Quantitative polymerase chain reaction monitoring of BCR-ABL during therapy with imatinib mesylate (STI571; gleevec) in chronic-phase chronic myelogenous leukemia. Clin Cancer Res. 2003;9(1):160–6.

58. Rezuke WN, Abernathy EC, Tsongalis GJ. Molecular diagnosis of B- and T-cell lymphomas: fundamental principles and clinical applications. Clin Chem. 1997;43(10):1814–23.

59. Terdiman JP, Gum Jr JR, Conrad PG, Miller GA, Weinberg V, Crawley SC, et al. Efficient detection of hereditary nonpolyposis colorectal cancer gene carriers by screening for tumor microsatellite instability before germline genetic testing. Gastroenterology. 2001;120(1):21–30.

60. Tsai DE, Nearey M, Hardy CL, Tomaszewski JE, Kotloff RM, Grossman RA, et al. Use of EBV PCR for the diagnosis and monitoring of post-transplant lymphoproliferative disorder in adult solid organ transplant patients. Am J Transplant. 2002;2(10):946–54.

61. Tapia G, Sanz C, Mate JL, Munoz-Marmol AM, Ariza A. Improved clonality detection in Hodgkin lymphoma using the BIOMED-2-based heavy and kappa chain assay: a paraffin-embedded tissue study. Histopathology. 2012;60(5):768–73.

62. Downing JR, Shurtleff SA, Zielenska M, Curcio-Brint AM, Behm FG, Head DR, et al. Molecular detection of the (2;5) translocation of non-Hodgkin's lymphoma by reverse transcriptase-polymerase chain reaction. Blood. 1995;85(12):3416–22.

63. Chasseriau J, Rivet J, Bilan F, Chomel JC, Guilhot F, Bourmeyster N, et al. Characterization of the different

BCR-ABL transcripts with a single multiplex RT-PCR. J Mol Diagn. 2004;6(4):343–7.

64. Downing JR, Khandekar A, Shurtleff SA, Head DR, Parham DM, Webber BL, et al. Multiplex RT-PCR assay for the differential diagnosis of alveolar rhabdomyosarcoma and Ewing's sarcoma. Am J Pathol. 1995;146(3):626–34.

65. Cleton-Jansen AM. E-cadherin and loss of heterozygosity at chromosome 16 in breast carcinogenesis: different genetic pathways in ductal and lobular breast cancer? Breast Cancer Res. 2002;4(1):5–8.

66. Schlecht NF, Kulaga S, Robitaille J, Ferreira S, Santos M, Miyamura RA, et al. Persistent human papillomavirus infection as a predictor of cervical intraepithelial neoplasia. JAMA. 2001;286(24):3106–14.

67. Fan H, Gulley ML. Epstein-Barr viral load measurement as a marker of EBV-related disease. Mol Diagn. 2001;6(4):279–89.

68. Mancuso R, Biffi R, Valli M, Bellinvia M, Tourlaki A, Ferrucci S, et al. HHV8 a subtype is associated with rapidly evolving classic Kaposi's sarcoma. J Med Virol. 2008;80(12):2153–60.

Single Nucleotide Polymorphisms (SNPs)

5

Jyotsna Batra, Srilakshmi Srinivasan, and Judith Clements

Introduction

Human genomic DNA consists of three billion deoxyribonucleotide bases (A, C, G or T) distributed between 23 pairs of chromosomes, the pattern and sequence of which differs among individuals—these variations are called polymorphisms. It is estimated that up to 0.1 % of the human genome is polymorphic. It is thus estimated that a polymorphism is present every 300 nucleotide base pairs. Recent improvements in DNA sequencing technology ('next generation' sequencing platforms) have sharply reduced the cost of sequencing and allowed for large investigations into common genetic variations in the human population. The 1000 Genomes project [1, 2] is an international collaboration to sequence the genomes of a substantial number of people ($N = 2,500$) to provide a comprehensive resource on human genetic variations and their haplotype contexts. This project has identified up to 50 % more novel genetic variants in comparison to the existing most comprehensive single nucleotide polymorphism (SNP) database, HapMap [3–5], with an estimate of more than 5.9 million variant nucleotide positions in the human genome. The most common type of variation in the human genome is the SNP, representing approximately 90 %

of all sequence variations [6] among other variations such as insertion, deletion, structural variations (copy number variations) and short tandem repeats. SNPs are generally proposed to have originated as a result of copying errors of genetic material during the replication process and are inherited from generation to generation. SNPs are observed in coding (gene) and more frequently in the noncoding regions of the genome. Two-thirds of SNPs involve the replacement of cytosine (C) with thymine (T). Notably, a total of 68,300 non-synonymous SNPs were identified through the 1000 Genomes pilot project, 34,161 of which were found to be novel. A fraction of these variations have been associated with various diseases and assigned a biological role, while others have been proposed to be silent variations with no effect [2].

SNPs are conventionally defined as common variations at a single nucleotide position in the genome such that the least common allele is present in at least 1 % of a given population. However, some researchers distinguish between these 'polymorphic SNPs' and 'common SNPs' with a minor allele frequency of at least 5 % in the population [7–10]. Inherited genetic variants can be further segregated into two categories: rare, high-risk genetic variants (mutations) and common, low-risk genetic variants. High-risk variants have a large relative risk and many of these have been identified using family-based studies.

In the recent era, SNPs have been the major drivers of various disease-association studies, which test for a correlation between disease status and genetic variation to identify candidate

J. Batra, Ph.D. • S. Srinivasan, Ph.D.
J. Clements, Ph.D. (✉)
Translational Research Institute, Queensland University of Technology, 37 Kent Street, Woolloongabba, QLD 4102, Australia
e-mail: j.clements@qut.edu.au

G.M. Yousef and S. Jothy (eds.), *Molecular Testing in Cancer*,
DOI 10.1007/978-1-4899-8050-2_5, © Springer Science+Business Media New York 2014

genes or genomic regions that contribute to a specific disease. SNPs are the most widely used polymorphisms in association studies due to their mostly bi-allelic nature, low genotyping cost, ease of genotyping and due to the development of various statistical and bioinformatic tools for analysing the results of association studies involving SNPs [11–15]. The current chapter deals with these common low-risk variants detailing their clinical utility mostly in genetic association studies and the methods of SNP detection and genotyping.

Clinical Uses of SNPs and SNP Databases

Single SNPs but mainly a combination of SNPs on an array have been used classically in the research environment and recently shown to have many clinical applications.

Chromosome instability and copy number alterations (CNAs) including duplications, amplifications and long contiguous stretches of homozygosity (LCSH) are an important molecular signature in cancer initiation, development and progression and in many other diseases. When a deletion or other mutational event occurs within the normal allele at a particular locus (heterozygous for a deleterious mutant allele and a normal allele) rendering the cell either hemizygous (one deleterious allele and one deleted allele) or homozygous for the deleterious allele, it is defined as LOH [16]. Chromosomal abnormalities including LOH are further correlated with poor prognosis, disease classification, risk stratification and treatment selection. Recent SNP array studies have shown that solid tumours such as prostate, ovarian, breast, endometrial, gastric cancer and liver cancer show LOH, as do nonsolid malignancies such as hematologic malignancies [16–24]. Recently, the utility of SNPs has been extended to the clinical environment to provide detection of not only deletion and mosaics, chimerism and ploidy levels but also the copy-neutral LOH (also called uniparental disomy or gene conversion), where one allele or whole chromosome from a parent is missing. This prob-

lem leads to duplication of the other parental allele, which could be pathological. Mosaicism for structural and numerical chromosome abnormalities can be identified by conventional analysis; however, low level mosaics may go undetected by routine karyotyping. In addition, the culturing necessary for preparing metaphase chromosomes for karyotyping can alter the mosaic levels and lead to false negatives. For example, approximately 40–50 % of myelodysplastic syndrome patients do not have karyotypic abnormalities that are detectable using classical metaphase cytogenetic techniques. Microarray platforms that measure genomic DNA without the need for culturing offer a more accurate method of revealing the true mosaic state [25–28]. Previous studies involving dilution series of known chromosomal abnormalities using array comparative genomic hybridization (aCGH) platforms have determined the lower limit of detection for mosaicism to be approximately 20 %, while SNP-based arrays, for example, Illumina's Infinium-based microarrays, can accurately detect mosaicism down to 5 % [26, 27, 29]. The reason Illumina's SNP arrays offer increased detection sensitivity for low level mosaicism is due to the long 50-mer SNP probes, and at least 15× replication of each SNP bead on the array, and empirical selection of probes for a better performance. These arrays have limited ability to detect single-exon copy number variants (CNVs) due to the distribution of SNPs across the genome.

SNP array, combined with aCGH, is a useful technique allowing detection of CNAs and LOH including copy-neutral LOH together in a single experiment [30–34]. Bruno et al. reported SNP array data performed on 5,000 clinical samples and were able to emphasize the clinical utility of SNP genotyping data for the investigation of individuals with intellectual disability, developmental delay, abnormal growth, autism or congenital abnormalities [35]. In this study, 25 clinically significant aberrations were revealed by the SNP genotyping data alone. Their data suggests that the incidence of low level mosaics has previously been underestimated and that chromosome mosaics frequently occur in the absence of clinical features; thus, using the

SNP-based arrays can shed new insights into the disease. Van et al. recently developed ASCAT (allele-specific copy number analysis of tumours) suite of tools to analyse SNP array data to analyse the complex data due to intratumour heterogeneity (http://www.ifi.uio.no/forskning/grupper/bioinf/Projects/ASCAT/). The ASCAT algorithm determines the fraction of nonaberrant cells and the tumour ploidy (the average number of DNA copies), and calculates an ASCAT profile, which can be used to visualize both copy number aberrations and copy number-neutral events [36]. SNP genotyping is also especially suitable for use in the analysis of the genetic purity of model organisms such as the mouse and various cell lines used in laboratory settings [37].

In addition, genetic association studies using SNPs have been at the forefront of identifying novel genetic biomarkers for a plethora of disorders and for measuring the efficacy of drug therapies designed specifically for individuals (commonly known as pharmacogenomics). These studies have further identified the novel disease-associated genes and pathways with potential to be future drug targets. The most common method used for association studies is case–control analysis, apart from the family-based (mostly considered in trio samples of proband with mother and father) and sib-pair analysis. Genetic association studies have been mainly performed at a candidate gene level to date, but are increasingly being performed at the genome-wide level without an a priori hypothesis as detailed below.

Candidate gene association studies: Prior to 2007, the candidate gene approach was the predominant method to explore inherited low-risk genetic variants. This approach is based on previous knowledge of the gene(s) of interest in the pathogenesis of the phenotype and involves the examination of a relatively small number of genetic variants (between 1 and 100 SNPs) [38]. This approach has led to the identification of a number of alleles that may influence the risk of various cancers and immunological diseases [12, 39–49]. Notwithstanding the advantages of candidate gene association studies, this method has been criticized at various levels due to non-

replication of results. One of the major issues for non-replication of the results involves population stratification. Population stratification can easily be circumvented by considering a replication study using an independent and random cohort of test and control populations, which reduces the chance of occurrence of a similar admixture showing similar patterns of variations [50].

Most of the candidate gene studies are presented with an ambiguity in results which makes it unclear if the results portray disease susceptibility of a common variant, or are just due to certain ancestral differences existing by chance between the mixes of test or control populations. Further, many of the candidate gene association studies do not consider correction for multiple testing while reporting their results. The multiple comparisons issue can be addressed in two ways—first, by computing Bonferroni adjustments of the significance criterion (alpha) according to the number of genes/SNPs/haplotypes examined and second, by performing permutation analysis of the association with allelic variation in the associating haplotype block. Although some argue that candidate gene studies must still meet statistical criteria for genome-wide significance, such a conservative threshold seems overly stringent, particularly in the context of a disorder with no (known) major gene effects.

Another reason for non-replication and identifying a number of false positive findings could involve systemic genotyping errors, lack of statistical power due to smaller samples and, also, in some cases false negative findings (type II error) [51, 52]. False negative findings can be attributed to under-evaluation of gene–gene interactions and gene–environment interactions [51], failing to include all causative polymorphisms in linkage disequilibrium (LD) [53], which is equally valid for the genome-wide association studies (GWAS).

Considering these aspects along with cumulative effect of multiple loci, and also complex disease heterogeneity, a fine tuning of the candidate gene approach in the future has been highly recommended [52, 53].

Genome-wide association studies: GWAS are the studies wherein research subjects are typed for a large number of genetic variants, typically between

300,000 and 1,500,000 polymorphisms, and the allele or genotype frequencies are evaluated for differences between groups (e.g. disease versus non-disease groups). The advantage of GWAS is that they allow for a wide search of genetic variants associated with disease, without having to specify a particular gene of interest. However, due to the massive number of joint statistical tests performed, there is a higher level of type-1 error. Therefore, statistical corrections for multiple hypotheses testing are essential and a $p < 10^{-7}$ has been proposed as an appropriate significance level for evidence of a genome-wide association [54]. Because of this, large sample sizes are required for GWAS to ensure adequate statistical power to detect an association with small p-values.

To reduce the cost of GWAS and the redundancy in the information collected, an informative subset of the SNPs, termed tag SNPs, is genotyped in GWAS. Tag SNPs are selected by utilizing the correlation structure between the SNPs, referred to as linkage disequilibrium (LD). The non-random associations of alleles at different loci are called gametic phase disequilibrium or more simply linkage disequilibrium. The most widely recognized measure for LD is r^2, where r is the correlation coefficient between two loci with alleles (A, a, B, b) in association [55]. Taking PA, Pa, PB and Pb as frequency of alleles at the two loci, $r^2 = D2/(pApBpapb)$ where one measure of the magnitude of LD is $D = PAB - PAPB$. D is the measure of LD signifying the difference between frequency of distribution observed at a two locus haplotype and the frequency if the two alleles segregate at random as expected [56]. $0.8 < r^2 < 1$ shows a strong LD. The international HapMap Project (http://hapmap.ncbi.nlm.nih.gov/) took the initiative of genotyping sections of human populations worldwide to carry out a Haplotype Map, and accelerate the search for haplotypes and tag SNPs specifically to narrow down on statistically significant, reviewed disease-associated loci, while understanding the patterns of genetic distribution in humans [5]; and currently provides this data to refine further GWAS results and analysis. Most recently the 1000 Genomes project (http://www.1000genomes.org/), which aims to use 'next-gen' sequencing techniques to characterize common and low-frequency variants in a large and ethnically diverse population sets, is producing a better genetic map to be utilized in SNP selection processes [57].

The intrinsic design of the GWAS is such that the significantly associated SNPs are seldom those that are causally linked to the phenotype, and are instead in LD with a functionally important variant. Identification of the causal variant is important to understand the molecular mechanisms underlying the pathogenesis of disease. Consequently, additional intensive studies are required to complement GWAS to identify disease-causing alleles, such as fine-mapping and imputation studies. These involve examining the association of all known common sequence variants in the vicinity of the GWAS-identified SNP with the disease of interest. Appropriate common sequence variants may be identified by accessing SNP databases, using sequencing data from the 1000 Genomes project, or by performing re-sequencing studies of the region of interest. Another method to refine GWAS signals and identify causal SNPs is to perform imputation. Genotype imputation is the process of predicting (or imputing) genotypes for known variants that are not directly assayed in a sample of individuals. These non-genotyped variants can then be tested for association with the trait. Imputation involves the comparison of study samples genotyped for a relatively large number of genetic markers (100,000–1,000,000 SNPs) to a reference panel of haplotypes derived from a number of individuals genotyped at all markers of interest [58]. To date, the HapMap database has typically served as this reference panel, with Phase II of this project including over 3.1 million SNPs genotyped on four panels of individuals [10], but other reference panels such as the 1000 Genomes project can also be used (http://www.1000genomes.org).

Since the advent of GWAS technology, highly statistically significant and robust associations with SNPs in over 230 diseases and traits have been successfully identified [59]. The National Human Genome Research Institute (NHGRI) maintains a catalogue of published GWAS that can be accessed at http://www.genome.gov/gwastudies/. As of 08/01/13, the catalogue includes 1,664 publications and 11,039 SNPs (Fig. 5.1).

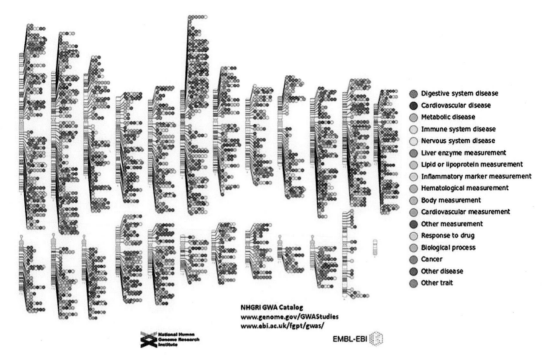

Digestive system disease
Cardiovascular disease
Metabolic disease
Immune system disease
Nervous system disease
Liver enzyme measurement
Lipid or lipoprotein measurement
Inflammatory marker measurement
Hematological measurement
Body measurement
Cardiovascular measurement
Other measurement
Response to drug
Biological process
Cancer
Other disease
Other trait

NHGRI GWA Catalog
www.genome.gov/GWAStudies
www.ebi.ac.uk/fgpt/gwas/

National Human
Genome Research
Institute

EMBL-EBI

Fig. 5.1 Published Genome-Wide Associations through 12/2012 at $p \leq 5 \times 10^{-8}$ for 17 trait categories (Hindorff LA, MacArthur J (European Bioinformatics Institute), Morales J (European Bioinformatics Institute), Junkins HA, Hall PN, Klemm AK, and Manolio TA. A Catalog of Published Genome-Wide Association Studies. Available at: http://www.genome.gov/gwastudies. Accessed on 15/08/2013)

Many of these SNPs are now part of the multiplex platforms starting to be used in the predictive and pre-symptomatic testing for many disease/trait-related, including certain cancers and pharmacogenetic tests, as well as for ophthalmologic, cardiac, renal and neurological disorders (among others). Several commercial companies now provide versions of clinical genotyping services to consumers, such as the Personal Genome Service from 23andMe (https://www.23andme.com/), Pathway Genomics (https://www.pathway.com/) and Navigenics (https://www.navigenics.com/), to name but a few. Although these SNP-based tests are easy to conduct and can easily be used in a clinical environment, the result output is probabilistic in nature rather than deterministic. For example, a single common SNP can predict an individual's risk of having a disease up to 1.5-fold. However, the combination of many SNPs has been proven useful especially when analysed in a high-risk group, e.g. individuals with family history. As the study of human genomics transitions into the next generation, our ability to identify genetic variants associated with complex traits and diseases will advance dramatically, due in large part to anticipated improvements in genotyping array technology and greater access to low-cost sequencing.

SNP Detection and Genotyping: Various Platforms

SNPs were originally used to be computationally detected by overlapping the sequences of various clones harbouring the genomic DNA. Shotgun sequencing and Sanger sequencing then took over as the common methods of SNP detection in larger populations to determine their allelic frequencies (Table 5.1). In the era of next generation sequencing (NGS), most of the SNPs in humans have been detected by sequencing and aligning the genomic DNAs

Table 5.1 Summary of the SNP genotyping and detection methods

Method	Advantages	Disadvantages	Reference	Comments
Low-throughput techniques				
RFLP	Powerful, but very laborious strategy	Limited throughput and is applicable to a limited number of SNPs	[102]	Traditional method
T-ARMS-PCR	Involves single-tube PCR and no additional sample manipulation	PCR primer design is restricted due to limitation of size discrimination between PCR products	[44]	Low assay time and low cost
Invader assay	High signal amplification and allows direct analysis of SNPs from zeptomolar quantities of genomic DNA without the need for PCR amplification	Requires independent reactions per SNP and sample and cannot be used for high-throughput genotyping projects	[48]	Normal FLAP endonuclease
PCR-SSCP	Simultaneous genotyping of multiple SNPs using strands of unknown SNPs in a sample of different sizes and four-colour labelling. PCR-SSCP can also be used for detection of unknown SNPs in a sample	Does not reveal the position of the SNP	[52]	Detection method based on conformation of DNA
Heteroduplex analysis (HA)	Genotype detection based on conformation of duplex DNA	Sensitivity is dependent on nucleotide base	[54]	Similar to SSCP
DHPLC	High sensitivity to distinguish homoduplexes from heteroduplexes and is an automated sequencing technique	Not useful for highly polymorphic species, optimum assay temperature for each of the target has to be determined	[55]	A priori knowledge of exact SNP site not needed
Pyrosequencing	Sequencing of up to 50 bases	Expensive, difficult to multiplex	[38]	Needs dedicated equipment
Oligonucleotide hybridization probes—molecular beacons	High target specificity	High cost of synthesis, and design of probes and requirement of expensive labelled oligos	[103]	Characteristic stem–loop structure
OLA—rolling circle amplification method	Amplifies a number of ligated circularized padlock probes to a level required for detecting single-copy sequences	Steric hindrance on solid phases	[59]	Homogenous, isothermal assay can be done in a microtiter plate
5'-Nuclease—TaqMan® assay	Discrimination of polymorphism is solely by hybridization and not by enzyme activity	Limited availability of reporter-quencher combination	[104]	Low multiplexing ability

Mid-high-throughput techniques

Technique	Description	Disadvantage	Ref	Note
iPLEX Sequenom	No labelling involved	Expensive instrument	[105]	Simple assay with modest multiplexing
SNaPshot	Multiplexing capacity	Size separation step required	[69]	Compatible with capillary DNA sequencers
Fluidigm assay	Highly reliable microfluidic assay	Uses nanoliter scale of sample	[68]	Simple assay with high accuracy
Illumina GoldenGate assay	Primer extension–ligation bead array with high specificity	Low flexibility	[79]	Medium to large throughput of SNPs
Illumina Infinium assay	Detection by hybridization	Requires thousands of samples to find a significant association	[107]	Large/small–large-scale throughput
SLAF-seq	De novo SNP discovery with reduced cost and high accuracy	Needs	[5]	Double barcode system ensures simultaneous genotyping of large populations
Affymetrix™ assay	High genomic coverage	Generates huge data and need complex algorithms for analysis	[93]	Whole-genome sequencing

SNP detection methods

Technique	Description	Disadvantage	Ref	Note
454 sequencing	Long read-lengths, relatively fast run times of instrument	Errors due to poor interpretation of the homopolymers (consecutive bases such as AAA and GGG)	[92]	First introduced NGS technique
Illumina (Solexa) Genome Analyzer	Most widely used, short read-length approach	Aberrant incorporation of incorrect dNTPs by polymerases	[106]	Low multiplexing ability
ABI SOLiD system	Reduction in error rates relative to Illumina NGS by using 2-base encoding	Long run times, complex analysis requirements	[74]	Two-base sequencing method
Heliscope™ sequencer	Nonbiased DNA sequence	High NTP incorporation error rates	[108]	Single-molecule sequencing
Ion Torrent sequencing	First platform to eliminate cost and complexity with 4-colour optical detection used by other NGS platforms	Low parallelism, focuses on short sequences	[98]	No need for modified dNTPs

from various human populations and have been submitted to various databases. These SNPs can be further genotyped in various populations or disease conditions to answer a specific research question. The extent and number of SNPs to be analysed determines the method of genotyping and the downstream statistical analysis. The SNP genotyping methods can be segregated into low, mid and high-throughput techniques according to the number of SNP genotypes that can be determined per reaction and sample. A combination of these methods has been further successful in genotyping large numbers of SNPs.

Low-Throughput Methods

Single SNP genotyping assays were performed classically and have a long history. Many methods based on polymerase chain reaction (PCR), enzyme-based and other approaches were used. Although these techniques are considered to be traditional methods and less used, they still are valuable and economical in small laboratories for a low-throughput genotyping and don't require sophisticated and expensive equipment. Some of these include the following.

Restriction fragment length polymorphisms (RFLP): Alteration in restriction sites in the genome in the presence of alternative alleles was used in the first attempts to identify SNPs in the human genome [60]. The technique utilizes distinct classes of enzymes to cleave DNA by recognition of a specific sequence and structure. DNA samples subjected to restriction digestion are then separated and transferred onto nylon membranes. These Southern blots are then probed with a labelled DNA probe to identify variations in the restriction fragment lengths. Alternatively, PCR can be conducted to amplify the region of interest, which after digestion with a suitable endonuclease can be separated by gel electrophoresis and stained using DNA intercalating dyes. The requirement for a specific endonuclease to identify the exact SNP and the slow nature of the gel assays make RFLP a poor choice for high-throughput analysis.

Pyrosequencing (PSQ): PSQ is a robust quantitative sequencing-by-synthesis method for determining an SNP genotype and can also be used for mutation screening, methylation analysis and viral/bacterial DNA typing [61]. Compared to other SNP genotyping methods, PSQ can also display the 50–100 bp sequence next to the SNP and help in evaluating other variations—such as bi-, tri- and tetra-allelic SNPs, insertions/deletions and point mutations, as well as quality of the PSQ template. About four to five closely located SNPs can be analysed in one reaction and up to 96 SNPs can be run on one plate within 1 h. The assay is based on detecting the real-time pyrophosphate (PPi) release during synthesis of the complementary strand to a PCR product [62]. The three primers used for the synthesis of the complementary PCR product are designed using PSQ™ Assay Design software to amplify a 100–200 bp DNA sequence surrounding the SNP. One of the primers is biotinylated at the 5′ end to allow capture of a single strand of PCR as template for the PSQ reaction. The sequencing primer is designed complementary to the PSQ template with its 3′ end annealing next to, or few bases upstream of, the SNP. This sequencing primer hybridizes to a single-stranded DNA (ssDNA) biotin-labelled template and mixed with the enzymes—DNA polymerase, ATP sulfurylase, luciferase and apyrase. Cycles of four dNTPs are separately added to the reaction mixture iteratively. The cycle starts with a polymerization reaction in which PPi is released as a result of nucleotide incorporation followed by release of inorganic pyrophosphate (PPi) in a quantity equimolar to the amount of incorporated nucleotide. The released PPi is converted to ATP by ATP sulfurylase in the presence of adenosine 5′ phosphate (APS). The generated ATP drives the luciferase-mediated conversion of luciferin to oxyluciferin producing light proportional to the amount of ATPs present (Fig. 5.2).

The light is captured by a charge-coupled device (CCD) camera or photomultiplier. The *pyrogram*™ can be converted automatically into a nucleotide sequence by dedicated software. However, a very low DNA concentration may generate peak heights close to the noise level;

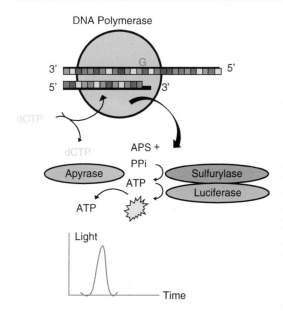

Fig. 5.2 Principle of pyrosequencing. Sequencing primer hybridizes to the single-stranded, amplified DNA template and incubated with enzymes DNA polymerase, ATP sulfurylase, luciferase and apyrase. Cycles of four dNTPs are separately added to the reaction mixture iteratively. DNA polymerase catalyses the incorporation of the nucleotide complementary to the template DNA (**C**). The incorporation of the nucleotide is accompanied by the release of the inorganic pyrophosphate (PPi) in a quantity equimolar to the amount of incorporated nucleotide. The released PPi is converted to ATP by ATP sulfurylase in the presence of adenosine 5′ phosphate (APS). The generated ATP drives the luciferase-mediated conversion of luciferin to oxyluciferin producing light proportional to the amount of ATPs present. The light is captured and monitored by a camera. The height of each peak is proportional to the number of incorporated nucleotides. Apyrase, a nucleotide degrading enzyme, degrades ATP and unincorporated dNTPs. This turns off the light generation and the next dNTP is then added

compilation of signals from Multiple Amplicon Sample (MAS—a sample with multiple target amplicons) by *pyrogram*™ and its inability to distinguish each amplicon-specific signal can lead to the interpretation of incorrect nucleotides. MAS signals are usually generated in numerous diagnostic applications by using multiplex pyrosequencing where several primers are simultaneously used. This can lead to overlapping of primer-specific pyrosequencing signals so recently mPSQed, MultiPSQ assays [63, 64] and virtual pyrogram generator (Pyromaker) [65]

software were developed to aid researchers in analysing multiplex pyrosequencing. These techniques have some drawbacks such as the requirement for a built-in formula, which is mutation specific and is not universal for all SNPs. Therefore, a novel approach based on reconstruction of sparse signal using a small number of measurements also known as Single Amplicon Sample (SAS) was developed called AdvISER-PYRO. This technique can convert SAS into correct single sequence and translate MAS signals into the correct sequence pair compared to the pyrosequencing software. The software can be implemented in an R package and used in broad range of clinical applications in heterogenous tumour cell samples [66]. This traditional sequencing method is not considered to be powerful enough for standard sequencing needs because of the short read-lengths it generates to detect SNPs.

ARMS-PCR: Allele-specific PCR-based methods offer inexpensive, flexible SNP genotyping methods with a reasonable throughput. Among the many PCR methods, tetra-primer amplification refractory mutation system PCR (T-ARMS-PCR) employs a combination of two allele-specific inner primers in a single PCR followed by electrophoresis separation [67]. The primers are designed such that the two allele-specific primers overlap at an SNP location but each matches perfectly to one of the possible SNP alleles. A PCR product will be obtained only if the given allele is present in the genomic DNA. The PCR products are of varying lengths allowing for easy discrimination by gel electrophoresis. For the first time, six SNPs in a single reaction using T-ARMS-PCR were developed recently and have been used to genotype 186 samples of breast cancer and cervical cancer patients. The results obtained were 100 % consistent with direct sequencing and have demonstrated their application for screening of multiple SNPs [68]. An advancement of the PCR-based methods includes chimeric-primer-based multiplex PCR which adds a universal 5′-tag to the sequence-specific primers for identifying multiple targets in a single reaction to improve

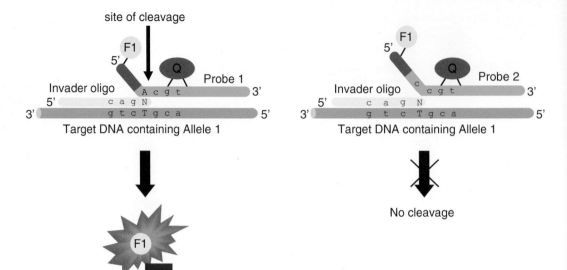

Fig. 5.3 Allele-specific cleavage in an Invader assay by FENs. Hybridization of the Invader oligo and the probe to the complementary oligo (shown on *left*) generates a three-dimensional invader structure over the SNP site that can be recognized by the cleavase, an FEN enzyme. The enzyme cleaves the probe 3′ of the base complementary to the SNP site. If probes are designed as a fluorescence resonance energy transfer (FRET) molecule containing a fluorophore at the 5′ end as an internal quencher molecule, the cleavage reaction separates the fluorophore from the quencher and generates a fluorescent signal and, employing data analysis tools, allows efficient automated computational assessment of genotypes. If the probe does not match the SNP allele in the target DNA (shown on *right*) no invader structure is formed and the probe is not cleaved (figure reproduced from Olivier et al. [72])

throughput and efficiency of PCRs [69]. However, improved detection of a large number of SNPs is still not possible given the limitations of the subsequent gel electrophoresis separation.

Invader Assay: The thermostable flap endonuclease (FEN) isolated from Archea catalyses structure-specific cleavage and is highly sensitive to sequence mismatches and thus can be used for sensitive detection of SNPs which is the basis of the Invader assay. This technique uses oligonucleotide probes hybridized to target DNA containing a polymorphic site, an allele-specific primary probe and an Invader® probe. The Invader® oligo is complementary to the target sequence 3′ of the polymorphic site and ends with a non-matching base overlapping the SNP nucleotide. The allele-specific primary probe contains the complementary base of the SNP allele and extends to the sequence 5′ of the polymorphic site. Once the two nucleotides are annealed to the target DNA, a three-dimensional invader structure over the SNP site is formed that can be recognized by the cleavase, an FEN enzyme. The enzyme cleaves the probe 3′ of the base complementary to the SNP site. If probes are designed as a fluorescence resonance energy transfer (FRET) molecule containing a fluorophore at the 5′ end as an internal quencher molecule, the cleavage reaction separates the fluorophore from the quencher and generates a fluorescent signal (Fig. 5.3) and, employing data analysis tools, allows efficient automated computational assessment of genotypes [70]. If the probe does not match the SNP allele in the target DNA no invader structure is formed and the probe is not cleaved. This signal amplification can also be used to quantify DNA targets, from both PCR product and genomic DNA, as well as mRNA targets for gene expression monitoring [71]. An improved version, to address the difficulties with the initial Invader® assay by reducing the long incubation times (3–4 h) and large amounts of genomic DNA required, is the biplex SISAR (serial invasive signal amplification reaction) Invader® assay. This assay is similar to the initial Invader® assay until the initial reaction format, but results in two separate distinct fluorescent signals for the two SNP alleles.

While these assays allow highly specific SNP genotyping, it requires a large amount of target molecules to generate a detectable fluorescent signal and requires initial PCR amplification of the target region followed by the Invader reaction. In addition, the assay requires two separate allele-specific probes labelled with a fluorophore and a quencher molecule. Hence the assay is considered to be relatively expensive making it unsuitable for large-scale genotyping techniques [72].

Single strand conformation polymorphism (SSCP): SSCP stands out as a fast and easy detection method of SNPs by detecting the alleles by altered mobility of single-stranded conformation. The gene of interest is amplified by PCR and then denatured using heat and formamide to produce ssDNA [73]. The fragments are then separated by denaturing electrophoresis during which the ssDNA folds into a nucleotide sequence-dependent conformation, which determines its mobility in the gel [74]. Recently this assay was used for identifying *SOD1* and *SOD2* gene polymorphisms in gastric cancer patients [75]. On the negative side, the size of the PCR products significantly affects sensitivity of the assay and can generate false positive results. Therefore, the assay needs empirical optimization of assay conditions, as it is not possible to predict the electrophoretic patterns expected during SSCP analysis [76].

Heteroduplex analysis (HA): HA depends on the conformation of duplex DNA resolved on a native gel. The PCR-amplified DNA with strands harbouring single-base pair mismatch may form heteroduplexes [77] and retards its mobility during electrophoresis compared to homoduplexes [73]. However the separation of heteroduplexes from homoduplexes varies with nucleotide base. For example, G:G/C:C mismatches can be more easily identified than A:A/T:T mismatches [78]. HA has a detection rate similar to SSCP and requires empirical optimization. In many cases SSCP and HA are combined to increase detection sensitivity.

Denaturing high-performance liquid chromatography (DHPLC): DHPLC uses heteroduplex formation between wild-type and the polymorphic DNA strands to identify SNPs. While SSCP and HA employ ssDNA, DHPLC utilizes dsDNA. Heteroduplexes are separated from homoduplexes by ion-pair, reverse-phase liquid chromatography on a special matrix with partial heat denaturation of DNA strands [79]. Under partial denaturing conditions, the heteroduplexes have lower affinity to the column than homoduplexes and are easier to elute. DHPLC is more efficient than conventional DNA sequencing methods, as the interpretation of the generated data by DHPLC is less subjective and labour-intensive. Also, it is more cost-effective to perform DNA sequencing just to confirm and analyse the SNPs initially detected by DHPLC. The sensitivity of the DHPLC is 100 % and can be used to analyse up to 200 samples a day [80].

Oligonucleotide ligation assay (OLA): This assay is based on the joining of two adjacent oligonucleotide probes (Capture and Reporter Oligos) using a DNA ligase while they are annealed to a complementary PCR product containing the SNP. The capture probes can be labelled (biotin, fluorescence or radioactive label) in a genotype-specific manner, and therefore for each allele there are two capture probes. These probes differ only at the last base at the 3′ end. The unlabelled reporter probe is a common probe complementary to the target DNA sequence immediately downstream (3′) of the SNP site and harbours a phosphate at the 5′ end. Allele discrimination is based on the specificity of the ligase to join perfectly matched probes; a 3′ mismatch in the capture probe prevents ligation. The ligated and unligated products can then be detected by gel electrophoresis, matrix-assisted laser desorption/ionization time-of-flight mass spectrometry (MALDI-TOF MS) and capillary electrophoresis. Colorimetric-based detection techniques using microtiter plates which utilize the principle of enzyme-linked immunosorbent assay (ELISA) for detection of wild-type and variant alleles in two different ligation reactions were earlier performed. As the sample throughput with detection in microplates is limited and is more suitable for smaller sample sizes, employing flow cytometers that can detect microspheres increases the throughput. The common probes

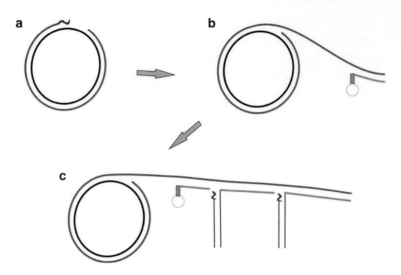

Fig. 5.4 Rolling circle amplification and FRET. A circular probe formed in the ligation serves as a target in the amplification. The first primer (orange spiral ~) hybridizes to the circularized probe and initiates the amplification (**a**). While strand-displacing DNA polymerase elongates the primer, a single-stranded concatamer of the ligated probe is formed. The second primer, small hairpin structure containing a complementary sequence for the amplification product and a hairpin structure, in which there is a fluorescent dye in both ends, hybridizes to each tandem repeat of the original probe (**b**). When the hairpin structure is present FRET is detected due to the close proximity of two fluorescent dyes. However, during the elongation of the second primer, a new recognition site for the first primer is exposed. While this primer is elongated, the hairpin loop is opened and only the fluorescence of the donor is detected in the reaction (**c**)

are labelled with fluorescein at the 3′-end and have a unique 5′ end with a tail that can hybridize to capture probes. Capture probes can be identified individually by their fluorescence and therefore can be used for the detection of alleles [81]. Ligation reactions performed on a biosensor chip surface into which the allele-specific probes are covalently attached have raised the OLA assay's throughput to a higher level [82] to detect several hundreds of SNPs on one single chip. FRET is detected when the oligonucleotide probes labelled with a donor dye (5′-Carboxyfluorescein) are in close proximity to the other probe labelled with acceptor dye (Rhodamine dyes—ROX and TAMARA). FRET was also utilized in the rolling circle amplification method, where only one probe containing an allele-specific sequence at one end and the unlabelled common sequence at the other is used for detection of each allele. Probe sequences of 80 nucleotides are designed so as to bring the 5′- and 3′-ends next to each other when they hybridize to the target sequence generating a closed loop or padlock probe. Primers annealing to this circle (Fig. 5.4) can be extended with a strand-displacing DNA polymerase, so that when the nascent strand completes the circle and encounters itself, it is continually displaced generating a long concatemer that is easy to detect using fluorescent methods [83].

SNP detection using oligonucleotide hybridization probes: Screening of SNPs in homogenous assays using PCR can be performed by using hybridization probes such as molecular beacons. These are single-stranded probes with a specific hairpin (stem-and-loop) conformation and undergo a conformational reorganization when bound to a perfect complementary sequence [84]. The loop is complementary to a predetermined sequence of the target DNA sequence and the stem is formed by annealing of arm sequences, complementary to each other, on either side of the probe sequence. One arm is linked to a fluorescent moiety and the other arm is bound to a quencher. The complementarity of the stem sequences keep the two moieties in close proximity and therefore the emission spectrum of the fluorophore need not be matched to the quencher. This provides the researcher the choice of many available fluorophores. Perfect complementary hybrids can be distinguished from mismatched targets by their higher fluorescence at a given temperature. The presence of hairpin stem enhances the specificity of molecular beacons to their complementary targets compared to the linear probes such as TaqMan probes [84]. Spectral genotyping can be performed by SNP detection with templates of various origins using up to four colours for molecular beacons [85]. Due to their high target specificity these oligonucleotide hybridization probes have wider applications besides being used in SNP detection such as quantification of RNA transcripts and as probes on microarrays [86].

5′-Nuclease assays: The PCR-based assays described above involve specific amplification of the mutant or the polymorphic allele using PCR (ARMS) or utilize fluorogenic changes of reporter molecules based on the presence of the specific allele (Invader assay). These assays have limited sensitivity, multiple time-consuming steps and are not amenable for rapid throughput for a large sample size. With the rapid progression of fluorescent-based technologies, using a fluorogenic 5′ nuclease PCR more high-throughput and precise assays have emerged (e.g. TaqMan® assay). The probes consist of an oligonucleotide labelled with a reporter dye linked at the 5′-end and a non-fluorescent quencher at the 3′-end of the probe. When the probe is intact, the quencher suppresses the fluorescence of the reporter. During PCR, the probe anneals to its specific complementary sequence. Cleavage liberates the reporter dye, resulting in increased fluorescence at every PCR cycle, and occurs only when the complementary sequence to the probe is amplified. For allelic discrimination of bi-allelic systems, probes specific to each allele are differently labelled with fluorescent reporter dyes (e.g. FAM, VIC) and both are added in the PCR [87]. Low fluorescence reflects low efficiency and mismatches between probe and target, and a high fluorescence is observed for heterozygotes (Fig. 5.5). Thus labelled probes are designed to hybridize to a specific SNP allele, with a different 5′ fluorophore colour for each allele. As a specific colour or both colours light up during amplification,

the genotype at a particular SNP can be easily determined. The TaqMan assay is hence a single-plex reaction, also termed 'one tube, one SNP reaction' although it can be multiplexed to three or four SNPs per reaction with additional fluorescent colours. TaqMan assays have been commonly used for post-GWAS to study a small number of SNPs in validation assays. For example, a panel of 31 SNPs from previous GWAS were genotyped by TaqMan assay in 2,230 prostate cancer cases of Ashkenazic descent and were able to identify 4 SNPs to be associated with aggressive prostate cancer [88].

Mid-High-Throughput Genotyping Techniques

Primer extension/single-base extension (SBE): The primer extension technique allows hybridization of a probe to the bases immediately upstream of the SNP nucleotide followed by a mini-sequencing reaction, in which a DNA polymerase extends the hybridized primer by adding a single nucleotide at the position of the SNP. Many approaches are available for primer extension product analysis and many of these monitor the differences in physical properties between starting reagents and primer extension products. Primer extension assays utilize either a common primer for detecting either alleles or specific primers to detect each allele. The former is predominantly used: an example is the common primer (CPE) reaction in which a primer is annealed to the 3′ end adjacent to an SNP site and extended by DNA polymerase. The identity of the extended base is determined by either fluorescence or mass to reveal the SNP genotype. Many commercial systems such as MassEXTEND™ and PinPoint assay utilize CPE methods that use MALDI-TOF MS for allele discrimination.

On a similar principle, Sequenom's iPLEX SNP genotyping method uses MassARRAY MS in which a locus-specific PCR takes place, followed by locus-specific primer extension reaction (iPLEX assay). In the first step the primer anneals upstream of the polymorphic site being genotyped and in the iPLEX assay, the primer and amplified target DNA are incubated with

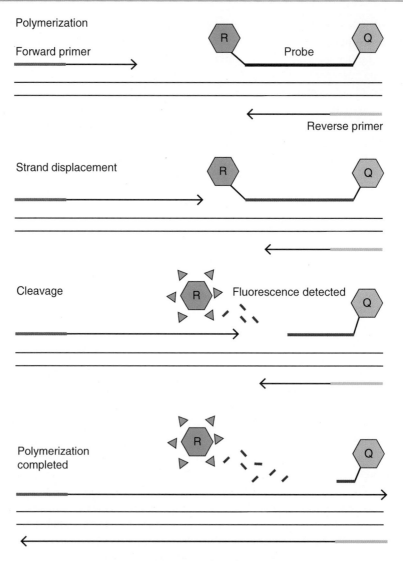

Fig. 5.5 5′ Nuclease assay. Two probes are used for SNP identification. Each probe is labelled with two dyes, a fluorescent reporter (R) specific to the allele and a fluorescent quencher (Q). A reporter dye is quenched by the quencher when bound to the probe. During polymeriza- tion, the matching probe hybridizes to the target, and DNA polymerase cleaves the reporter dye during extension. The non-matching probe does not bind well and no cleavage is observed. After cleavage, the reporter fluoresces and helps in discriminating the SNP allele

mass-modified nucleotides (difference in mass for each nucleotide by at least 12 Da). The MALDI-TOF MS determines the mass of the extended primer. The primer's mass indicates the sequence and, therefore, the allele present at the polymorphic site. The Sequenom software (SpectroTYPER) automatically translates the mass of the observed primers into a genotype for each reaction (Fig. 5.6). A typical iPLEX Gold assay can run a 36-plex format and would offer the best choice for second-tier applications as validating hits after (first-tier) GWAS. This is because the arrays are too expensive to run on a large number of samples whereas singleplex assays like TaqMan are too cumbersome to use for many SNPs.

CPE approaches using fluorescence-based detection involve single base extension (SBE) of a primer with fluorescently labelled dideoxynucleotides (ddNTPs). This leads to the generation

PCR amplification

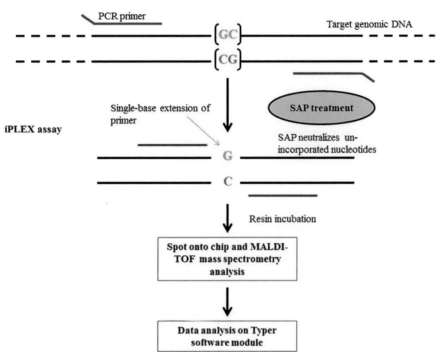

Fig. 5.6 Overview of the iPLEX assay. PCR primers designed to amplify ~100 bp region surrounding SNP of interest anneal to the target genomic DNA and make amplified copies in the first PCR step. The unincorporated nucleotides are dephosphorylated by Shrimp Alkaline Phosphatase (SAP) by cleaving the phosphate groups from the 5′ termini. Extension primers are designed immediately adjacent to the SNP which is extended by just one mass-modified nucleotide in the iPLEX assay. Resin incubation helps in removal of the salts that might result in background noise. The samples are spotted onto a SpectroCHIP and placed into the mass spectrometer and each spot is shot with a laser under vacuum by the MALDI method. MALDI-TOF mass spectrometry helps to determine the mass of the extended primer and the primer's mass indicates the nucleotide incorporated

of fluorescently labelled extension products that are detected by capillary electrophoresis and used for genotype determination [89]. A different approach uses tagged primers in a homogenous reaction followed by capture of extension products on a solid support using an array of complementary tags. The array is then washed and scanned for a fluorescent signal to determine the genotype for each SNP. SNPstream™ assay uses this approach for SBE of 12 tagged primers in each well of a 384-well plate to achieve genotyping throughput [90]. Specific primer extension (SPE) employs two allele-specific primers that are identical except for a mismatch at their 3′ end. The extension of these primers is possible only if the 3′ end is complementary to the SNP, allowing allele-specific discrimination.

Allele-specific primer extension (ASPE) uses extension of allele-specific primers with a PCR-amplified template, and the extended products are analysed by fluorescence to determine the SNP genotype [91].

Another important technique utilizing this primer extension principle is SNaPshot genotyping (Applied Biosystems) technique. SNaPshot incorporates PCR multiplexing for about 10 SNPs and each DNA sample is PCR-amplified and subjected to a symmetric PCR where each primer is annealed to target DNA either directly upstream or downstream to the SNP site. The primer is then extended by DNA polymerase by just one fluorescent-labelled di-deoxynucleotide (four nucleotides labelled with four different fluorescent dyes, each emitting fluorescence of varying wavelength) [92].

Multiplex PCR

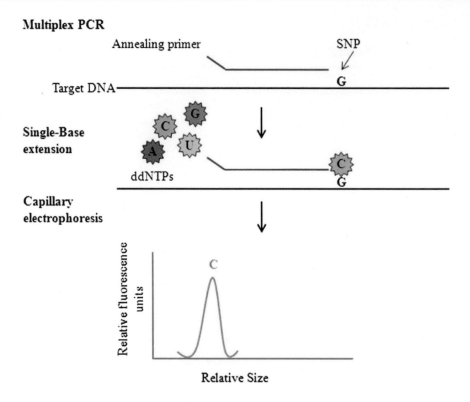

Fig. 5.7 SNaPshot technique principle. The primer anneals to the target sequence immediately upstream of the SNP site and is extended by just one base (**C**) in the presence of four fluorescently labelled dNTPs. Each fluorescent dNTP emits a different wavelength and is translated into a specific colour for each base

The extended product which is the initial probe plus one fluorescent base is then analysed by gel electrophoresis and genotypes are determined by the colour and location of the peak that is generated from the emitted fluorescence. Data can then be analysed with the ABI GeneScan™ or GeneMapper™ (Applied Biosystems, Foster City, CA) software using size standards for verification of the peaks (Fig. 5.7). Accuracy of genotyping depends on the primer design, DNA template purification and failure to remove unincorporated ddNTPs which can lead to extraneous fluorescence. SNaPshot has increased sensitivity (~10 %) compared with standard sequencing, allowing detection of a single-base pair difference in each test tube. A study comparing the performance of SNaPshot and Sequenom has found that the SNaPshot platform was useful to narrow down the mutations for highly prevalent genetic abnormalities in non-small lung cancer patients compared to Sequenom [93].

A separation-free technique based on SBE which utilizes two-photon fluorescence excitation technology, known as ArcDia™ TPX technology, to identify SNPs was introduced in 2004. In this method, template-directed SBE is carried out for primers immobilized on microparticles. Depending on the template DNA sequence, the primers are extended with either a labelled or unlabelled nucleotide. The genotype is then determined by the two-photon-excited fluorescence of individual microparticles. The reliability and sensitivity of this assay as evaluated by a statistical tool—'Z'-factor', a dimensionless simple statistical characteristic which accounts for both the signal response and the signal viability of a screening assay—suggested it to be comparable to the SNaPshot™ method [94]. This assay enables sensitive, separation-free and cost-effective genotyping with low to medium sample throughput yielding ±0.5 bp standard deviation up to 105 bp (Applied

Biosystems). The limitations include the need for sample pre-amplification and long detection time per sample.

Both SNaPShot and Sequenom panels are widely used in the cancer research community and show promise for clinical use [95]. It is noteworthy that these genomic tests only detect the expression of known variants and oncogenes and do not have the ability to discover new or additional drug targets [93].

Nanofluidics technique: Recent advances in nanofluidics utilize integrated fluidic circuits (IFCs) for high-throughput real-time PCR [96]. Nanoliter-scale of samples and reagents are channelled into thousands of nanoliter-scale chambers in which distinct real-time PCRs can be run. Recently, Fluidigm (South San Francisco, CA) introduced a nanofluidic chip, the Dynamic array chip, compatible with existing TaqMan genotyping assays [92]. Fluidigm was originally developed for real-time quantitative PCR and low-throughput SNP genotyping but recently Access Array was released, allowing retrieval of the PCR product for targeted sequencing applications. This Access Array system can perform parallel PCRs for 24–96 samples by 24–96 singleplex assays with the promise of low use of reagents and time but high accuracy. Proof-of-concept of this approach was demonstrated by genotyping human DNA samples from the prostate, lung, colon and ovarian (PLCO) cancer screening trial and HapMap samples of cell lines [92]. This study demonstrated 99.5 % call accuracy using this dynamic array genotyping system compared to the iPlex and Illumina GoldenGate assay with a comparatively lesser accuracy. Concordance rates of 99–100 % between TaqMan real-time PCR and Fluidigm platforms were achieved in a clinical setting [97].

Bead array-based genotyping: Genetic association studies indicate the requirement of genotyping several hundreds of thousands of SNPs per individual across hundreds to many thousands of samples to map a causal variant by LD analysis. Development of bead array-based techniques allows to genotype hundreds of thousands of SNPs efficiently in a single array experiment. The multiplexed assays can detect up to 1,536 SNPs in a single DNA sample. Illumina provides

the highest density array platform currently available. One of the assays is GoldenGate genotyping assay which allows a high degree of loci specific multiplexing in a single reaction through extension and amplification steps. The interesting aspect of this assay is that it genotypes directly on the genomic DNA and does not require prior PCR amplification of the target sequence. The DNA sample is activated for binding to paramagnetic particles and this activation step requires a minimum input of at least 250 ng. Assay oligonucleotides, hybridization buffer and paramagnetic particles are combined with activated DNA in the hybridization step. Three assay oligonucleotides are designed for each SNP locus. Two oligos are specific to each allele of the SNP site, called allele-specific oligos (ASOs). The third oligo hybridizes between 1 and 20 bases downstream from the ASO site and is called locus-specific oligo (LSO). The 1–20 bp distance allows probe design flexibility to avoid non-specific sequences flanking the SNP or neighbouring SNPs. All the three oligonucleotides include regions of complementarity and universal primer sites; the LSO contains unique address sequence complementary to a specific bead type. During hybridization, the assay nucleotides bind to the genomic DNA bound to the paramagnetic particles. As hybridization occurs prior to any amplification there is no chance of amplification bias during the assay. After hybridization, a polymerase extends the ASO(s) complementary to the SNP site. The polymerase lacking the strand displacement or exonuclease activity is employed and therefore just fills the gap between the ASO and LSO. The polymerase drops off the genomic DNA as it reaches the LSO and a DNA ligase seals the nick between the extended ASO and LSO to form template that can be amplified by universal PCR primers. The extended ASO ligated to LSO joins information about the genotype at the SNP site to the address sequence on LSO. These joined products are amplified by three fluorescently labelled universal primers P1, P2 and P3. P1 and P2 are labelled with different cytochrome dyes. Thermal cycling and processing of the single-stranded labelled DNA products of the GoldenGate assay are hybridized to their perfect complementary bead type through their address sequence. This hybridization of the products onto the Sentrix arrays allows readout of the SNP genotype and the BeadArray Reader analyses the fluorescence signal on the Array matrix or BeadChip. A scan of 96 hybridized samples in Sentrix Array Matrix represents data acquired from 4.5 million discrete beads. This assay represents the highest resolution of any scanning platform used for microarray-based genetic analysis applications [98].

More recently Illumina introduced the Infinium™ assay, a high-throughput whole-genome genotyping (WGG) approach that allows analysis of thousands of SNPs per sample. This method consists of four components—(1) a single-tube amplification step, (2) an array-based hybridization capture step using 50-mer probes, (3) an enzymatic ASPE step, and (4) an amplified-signal detection step [99]. The Infinium assay complements the fine-mapping capabilities of the GoldenGate custom genotyping assay and features single-tube sample preparation without the need of a prior PCR. Sample handling-errors and labour are minimal and the enzymatic discrimination provides high call rates and accuracy. It allows researcher the advantages of whole-genome approach combining the sophistication of unlimited multiplexing with unrestrained SNP selection. The number of SNP readout is only limited by the number of bead types on the array. This is particularly important in assaying custom sets of SNPs, including haplotype-tagging SNPs [5], coding SNPs and high-value SNPs. Ability to choose SNPs of interest increases the power of association studies relative to random SNPs, particularly with respect to maximizing LD with markers in genes and conserved regions [100]. This WGG method allows almost any SNP to be assayed and a study has used cell lines harbouring one to four X chromosomes, to detect single-copy changes in chromosomal copy number with low variability levels. The study has also demonstrated the utility of this technique to study the LOH in tumour samples at sub-100 kb effective resolution [101]. The data delivered is comparable to the GoldenGate assay with respect to call rate, reproducibility and accuracy [102].

SNP microarray: In high-density oligonucleotide SNP arrays, hundreds of thousands of probes are analysed on a chip. The high-density microarrays for genetic variation analysis such as Affymetrix Genome-wide SNP arrays have enabled studies in common diseases such as diabetes, heart disease and cancer. Affymetrix has been the first to commercially produce SNP arrays over a decade ago. The HuSNP assay was designed initially to genotype less than 1,500 SNPs on one chip and have currently increased to 946,000 for the new Genome-Wide Human SNP Array 6.0, which have probes for SNPs as well as copy number variations. Every SNP is interrogated by a set (two alleles for an SNP) of 25-mer probes unlike the 50-mer for Infinium assay. The alleles are conventionally referred to as allele A and allele B. The probe is designed to be a perfect match for allele A (PM_A) and to a perfect match for the allele B (PM_B). A mismatch probe is synthesized for each allele (MM_A and MM_B) to detect non-specific binding. This quartet (PM_A, MM_A, PM_B, MM_B) is the base for genotyping and the computational goal is to convert these 8–10 probe quartet intensity measures from raw data into a genotype interference—AA, AB or BB. With every new version by the manufacturer new algorithms developed and have influenced the array design. So the array should be chosen for which the algorithm works best. For example, for a 10K version [103], a partitioning around medoids (PAM)-based algorithm was chosen [104]. For the current Human SNP Array 6.0 only six or eight perfect match probes—three or four replicates of the same probe for each of the two alleles are being used [105]. The intensity data for each SNP therefore have two sets of repeated measurements. A study investigating the coverage of important pharmacogenes by comparing the performance of a range of Affymetrix's arrays and Illumina arrays has found the Affymetrix 6.0 array to have the highest coverage. These results help to understand the limitations of these arrays to detect the association of known functional variation with clinical drug response [106].

Specific-locus-amplified fragment sequencing (SLAF-seq): Whole-genome sequencing (described in the next section) for large populations is still cost-prohibitive and high population size greatly affects the accuracy of association studies. Therefore, low-cost but efficient high-throughput sequence-based SNP genotyping techniques have evolved recently such as SLAF-seq [107]. This technique reduces the complexity of high-quality reference genome library required for other NGS techniques and uses the strategy of reduced representation library (RRL) method. This method, therefore, does not require reference genome sequence and polymorphism information and uses barcode multiplexed sequencing for genotyping multiple loci simultaneously. It combines the locus-specific amplification and high-throughput sequencing for de novo SNP detection. A bioinformatics statistical model used by this technique improves the efficiency of DNA fragment selection for the subsequent amplification of specific locus based on the training data. The DNA fragments include randomly sequenced BAC sequences and genome draft sequences. The double barcode system distinguishes individuals in large populations of about 10,000 samples. A study testing the efficiency of the SLAF-seq on rice and soybean genome has observed the genotyping data to be accurate and the density of the genetic map to be high compared to all the genome data available by other methods so far. The same study genotyped 211 individual carp samples by just utilizing 55 double barcode system. The data generated by this study found the SLAF-seq to be highly efficient and accurate method with reduced repetitive regions compared to Affymetrix and GoldenGate techniques. Therefore, SLAF-seq represents a low-cost large-scale genotyping technique with an important role in genetic association studies.

SNP Detection: Next Generation Sequencing Techniques

Since the advent of Sanger sequencing in 1977, DNA sequencing has relied on this technique until the early 1990s. The technique is simple generating an amplified target using a 'cycle sequencing reaction' where cycles of template denaturation, primer annealing and primer exten-

sion are performed. Each round of primer extension is then terminated by fluorescently labelled ddNTPs which reveals the identity of the extended nucleotide. After 3 decades of improvement, the read-lengths by Sanger sequencing are up to ~1,000 bp with 99.99 % accuracy and a cost of $0.50 per kb. The evolution of the NGS techniques has dramatically accelerated biomedical and biological research by enabling a more comprehensive analysis of genomes to become inexpensive, routine and widespread with less production-scale efforts. Some of these NGS techniques are described below. These platforms are quite diverse in sequencing biochemistry and array generation but their workflow is conceptually similar. Libraries are usually made by random shearing of DNA followed by ligation with common adaptors.

(a) *Sequencing-by-synthesis technology*: The first NGS platform commercially available that was utilizing this technique was the Roche 454 GS20 which later was replaced by 454 GS FLX Titanium sequencer [108]. The 454 (454; Branford, CT, USA; now Roche, Basel) sequencing is a miniature of pyrosequencing technique which allows direct incorporation of natural nucleotides rather than repeated cycles of incorporation, detection and cleavage. The sheared DNA template strands attached to adapters are bound to capture streptavidin bead arrays and amplified *en masse* by emulsion PCR [109]. Each bead in emulsion acts as an independent amplification reactor producing ~10^7 clonal copies of a unique DNA template per bead. The individual beads are transferred into a well of a picotiter plate along with DNA polymerase, primers and enzymes for pyrosequencing [108]. The pyrophosphate released during this pyrosequencing can be traced by *pyrogram*™ or enzymatic luminometric inorganic pyrophosphate detection assay (ELLIDA) which corresponds to the order of correct nucleotides that have been incorporated (Fig. 5.8) [110]. Since the chemiluminescent signal intensity is proportional to the amount of pyrophosphate released and hence the number of bases incorporated, the pyrosequencing approach is prone to errors that result from

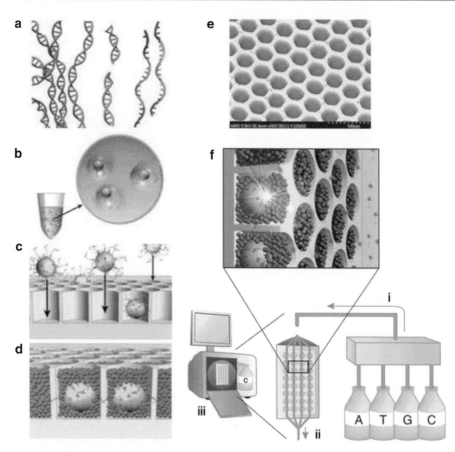

Fig. 5.8 454 sequencing. (**a**) Genomic DNA is isolated, fragmented, ligated to adapters and denatured into single strands. (**b**) DNA fragments are bound to streptavidin-coated magnetic beads under conditions that allow one fragment per bead; the beads are isolated and grouped in the droplets of a PCR-mixture-in-oil emulsion and PCR amplification occurs within each droplet. (**c**) The emulsion is broken, the DNA strands are denatured and beads carrying single-stranded DNA templates are enriched (not shown) and deposited into wells of a fiber-optic slide. (**d**) Smaller beads carrying enzymes required for a solid phase pyrophosphate sequencing reaction are deposited into each well. (**e**) Scanning electron micrograph of a portion of a fiber-optic slide, showing fiber-optic cladding and wells before bead deposition. (**f**) The 454 sequencing instrument consists of the following major subsystems: a fluidic assembly (object i), a flow cell that includes the well-containing fiber-optic slide (object ii), a CCD camera-based imaging assembly with its own fiber-optic bundle used to image the fiber-optic slide (part of object iii) and a computer that provides the necessary user interface and instrument control (part of object iii) (figure reproduced from Rothberg et al. with permission [84])

incorrectly estimating the length of homopolymeric sequence stretches (i.e. indels) [111]. A hidden Markov model (HMM) was proposed to statistically and explicitly formulate these sequencing errors called PyroHMMsnp. PyroHMMsnp is an SNP-calling program that realigns the read sequences according to the error model and infers the underlying genotype by a Bayesian approach [112]. The current state-of-the-art 454 platform marketed by Roche Applied Science with the GS FLX Titanium system is capable of generating 700 megabase (Mb) of sequence in 700 bp reads in a 23 h run with an accuracy of 99.9 % after filter. In late 2009, Roche combined the GS Junior, a bench top system, into the 454 sequencing system and the output was upgraded to 14 gigabases (G) per run [113].

Although the sequencing reads produced by these sequencers are thought to be proportional to the number of incorporated bases, in reality the signal generated varies substantially and can lead to misinterpretations as over-calls and under-calls. These over- or under-calls are often manifested as insertions and deletion errors [114] leading to inaccuracy of sequencing estimates.

The NGS technique next introduced was by Illumina combining the clonal amplification of a single DNA molecule with a cyclical sequencing-by-synthesis approach. Several instruments were commercialized by Illumina, ranging from bench top MiSeq sequencer to the high-throughput HiSeq 2500 sequencer. The first introduced instrument of these is the Illumina (Solexa) Genome Analyzer (GA), released by Solexa in 2007 after the release of Roche 454 in 2006 and is the current dominating sequencing technique in the market [115]. The library with fixed adaptors is denatured to single strands and grafted to the flow cell, followed by amplification to produce 100–200 million spatially separated template clusters. These templates with free ends can be hybridized to adjacent universal sequencing primers (isothermal bridging amplification) to form clusters and initiate the NGS reaction. Before sequencing, the library denatures into single strands with the help of a cleavage enzyme. From the four nucleotides (ddATP, ddGTP, ddCTP, ddTTP) with different cleavable fluorescent dyes and a terminating/inhibiting group, DNA polymerase bound to the primed template adds just one fluorescently labelled nucleotide which represents the complement of the template base [10]. The unbound nucleotides are washed away and imaging is performed to determine the identity of the incorporated nucleotide.

The first instrument, Solexa GA, had an output of 1 G/run and with improvement in the enzyme, buffer and flow cell conditions and with the upgraded Genome AnalyzerIIx series now attains 85 G/run. The latest HiSeq 2500/2000 which uses same sequencing technique of the genome analyser can give an output of 600 G in 2–11 days but with a low read-length of 200 bp compared to 700 bp by 454 sequencing system. The error rate is as low as 2 % on average after filtering [113]. The HiSeq 2000 is the cheapest sequencing method to date with \$0.02/million

bases and needs HiSeq control software for program control, real-time analyser software for base-calling and CASAVA for secondary analysis. High GC content of the DNA has always been associated with low efficiency of sequencing techniques and HiSeq 2000 is convenient for GC-rich DNA templates. Efficiently mapping the short reads generated by these sequencers to the reference genome is challenging and recently many alignment algorithms have emerged to help researchers in taking full advantage of the NGS technologies. These alignment algorithms must be able to efficiently align millions of sequence and be able to detect the true genomic polymorphisms [116]. Traditional algorithms, such as BLAST [117] and BLAT [118], are time-consuming and unaffordable. Recently the cancer genome atlas project (TCGA) compared many algorithms for efficient mapping of their sequencing reads generated from Illumina Genome Analyzer II and found two algorithms, BWA and Bowtie, to be efficient among others [119].

(b) *Sequencing by Oligo Ligation and Detection*: The ABI SOLiD system utilizing this method originated from the system described by Jay Shendure and colleagues in 2005 [120] and in-house work by Applied Biosystems since 2006. The sequencer utilizes the technique of two-base sequencing based on ligation sequencing. Libraries may be made by any method that gives rise to a mixture of short, adaptor-flanked fragments. These oligo adaptor-linked DNA fragments with 1-μm paramagnetic beads tethered to complementary oligos amplify each bead–DNA complex by emulsion PCR. The template for sequencing is generated by emulsion PCR with amplicons captured on paramagnetic beads. On the SOLiD flow cell, two slides are processed per run; one slide receives sequencing reactants as the second slide is imaged. A universal primer complementary to the adaptor sequence is hybridized to the array of amplicon-bearing beads. Each cycle of sequencing starts with annealing of this universal primer complementary to the SOLiD-specific adaptors on the library fragments. Sequencing by synthesis is driven by DNA ligase rather than a polymerase. An octamer oligonucleotide (8-mer) that is complementary to the adaptors is added and is ligated to the DNA fragment sequence adjacent to the 3′ end. Fluorescent readout identifies the fixed base of the octamer and corresponding position to second or fifth depending on the cycle number. A chemical cleavage step removes the sixth to eighth base by attacking the linkage between bases 5 and 6 removing the fluorescent group and enabling a subsequent round of ligation. Progressive steps of octamer ligation enable sequencing of every fifth base. After many cycles, the extended primer is denatured to reset the system.

Performance comparison of sequence mapping software in aligning reads from samples of TCGA project showed the overall best performance for the NovoalignC compared to other programs like ZOOM, SeqMap and RMAP [119].

(c) *HeliScope*: Helicos Heliscope™ Sequencer is also called a single-molecule sequencing system. The platform includes two flow cells to enable billions of DNA molecules captured on a surface. The template DNA prepared by random fragmentation and poly-A tailing is captured by hybridization to surface-tethered poly-T primers to yield an array of primed single-molecule sequencing templates. Fluorescently labelled single species of dNTPs and DNA polymerase are added to allow elongation in a template-dependent manner of these hybridized template strands. The unincorporated dNTPs are washed away followed by imaging, removal of fluorescent groups and subsequent cycles of extension and imaging. After several hundred cycles of single-base extension, average read-lengths of 25 bp or greater can be achieved [121]. Notable features of this system include its similarity to the 454 platform as asynchronous method of sequencing in a sequence-dependent manner (i.e. some templates may fall ahead or behind because of its failure to incorporate despite having the appropriate base at the next position). There is no terminating moiety on the labelled nucleotides therefore; homopolymer runs may be an issue, which can be mitigated by limiting the rate of incorporation events. Also, consecutive incorporation of labelled nucleotide on homopolymers produces a quenching interaction and may lead to difficulties in inferring the discreet number of incorporations (e.g. A versus AA versus AAA) [121].

(d) *Semiconductor chip technique*: Ion Torrent system harnesses the power of semiconductor technology by detecting the protons released as nucleotides which are incorporated during synthesis. A unique aspect making this system different from other sequencing techniques is its ability to detect the polymerization events by measuring pH rather than light. The preparation of the library is similar to the 454 sequencing system [122]. The fragmented DNA fragments are linked to specific adapter sequences, and a single DNA template is affixed to a bead (Ion Sphere Particle) and clonally amplified by using emulsion PCR. The beads are loaded onto the chip and the dNTPs are flowed over the surface of these beads in a predetermined sequence with zero or more dNTPs ligating during each flow. Whereas the 454 sequencing system can introduce 4 nucleotides sequentially, the Ion Torrent can include 32 nucleotides. This complex flow cycle referred to as *Samba* improves the synchronicity of clonal templates on the bead at the cost of a flow-sequence not optimized for read-length. The protons released for every nucleotide incorporated decrease the net pH in the surrounding solution that can be measured by an ionic sensor and then converted to a flow value. A base-caller corrects these flow-values for phase and signal loss, normalizes to the key and generates corrected base calls for each flow in each well to produce the sequencing reads. Each read is sequentially passed between two signal-based filters to exclude less accurate reads. Per-base quality values are predicted by the Phred method [123] that quantifies the similarity between the phasing model predictions and the observed signal.

Conclusion

Recent advances in high-throughput experimental technologies like whole-genome large-scale gene expression profiling, the GWAS and next generation DNA sequencing provide an advantage of scoping the genome for disease-associated genetic variants hypothesis-free, without detailing a specific gene of interest [124]. Moreover, GWAS have made feasible the discoverability of many intricate interactions in the genome spread apart across different regions [125]. In addition SNP-based methods are now being used in clinical environment to identify various structural anomalies including LOH and mosaicism. Further work in the future improving SNP discovery and genotyping platforms is bound to give rich dividends in terms of elucidation of complex disease mechanisms, better prognosis and diagnosis of patients in a short time, and in an efficient way.

References

1. Siva N. 1000 Genomes project. Nat Biotechnol. 2008;26(3):256.
2. Pennisi E. Genomics. 1000 Genomes Project gives new map of genetic diversity. Science. 2010;330(6004): 574–5.
3. Montpetit A, Chagnon F. The Haplotype Map of the human genome: a revolution in the genetics of complex diseases. Med Sci (Paris). 2006;22(12): 1061–7.
4. International HapMap Consortium. A haplotype map of the human genome. Nature. 2005;437(7063): 1299–320.
5. International HapMap Consortium. The International HapMap Project. Nature. 2003;426(6968):789–96.
6. Collins FS, Brooks LD, Chakravarti A. A DNA polymorphism discovery resource for research on human genetic variation. Genome Res. 1998;8(12): 1229–31.
7. Brookes AJ. The essence of SNPs. Gene. 1999;234(2): 177–86.
8. Kruglyak L, Nickerson DA. Variation is the spice of life. Nat Genet. 2001;27(3):234–6.
9. Ladiges W, et al. Human gene variation: from SNPs to phenotypes. Mutat Res. 2004;545(1–2):131–9.
10. Frazer KA, et al. A second generation human haplotype map of over 3.1 million SNPs. Nature. 2007;449(7164):851–61.
11. Hegele RA. SNP judgments and freedom of association. Arterioscler Thromb Vasc Biol. 2002;22(7): 1058–61.

12. Stram DO. Tag SNP selection for association studies. Genet Epidemiol. 2004;27(4):365–74.
13. Gu CC, Rao DC. Designing an optimum genetic association study using dense SNP markers and family-based sample. Front Biosci. 2003;8:s68–80.
14. Martino A, Mancuso T, Rossi AM. Application of high-resolution melting to large-scale, high-throughput SNP genotyping: a comparison with the TaqMan method. J Biomol Screen. 2010;15(6):623–9.
15. Mendisco F, et al. Application of the iPLEX Gold SNP genotyping method for the analysis of Amerindian ancient DNA samples: benefits for ancient population studies. Electrophoresis. 2011; 32(3–4):386–93.
16. Li X, et al. Direct inference of SNP heterozygosity rates and resolution of LOH detection. PLoS Comput Biol. 2007;3(11):e244.
17. Arzimanoglou II, et al. Frequent LOH at hMLH1, a highly variable SNP in hMSH3, and negligible coding instability in ovarian cancer. Anticancer Res. 2002;22(2A):969–75.
18. Dumur CI, et al. Genome-wide detection of LOH in prostate cancer using human SNP microarray technology. Genomics. 2003;81(3):260–9.
19. Goransson H, et al. Quantification of normal cell fraction and copy number neutral LOH in clinical lung cancer samples using SNP array data. PLoS One. 2009;4(6):e6057.
20. Huggins R, et al. Nonparametric estimation of LOH using Affymetrix SNP genotyping arrays for unpaired samples. J Hum Genet. 2008;53(11–12):983–90.
21. Huijsmans CJ, et al. Single nucleotide polymorphism (SNP)-based loss of heterozygosity (LOH) testing by real time PCR in patients suspect of myeloproliferative disease. PLoS One. 2012;7(7):e38362.
22. Pfeifer D, et al. Genome-wide analysis of DNA copy number changes and LOH in CLL using high-density SNP arrays. Blood. 2007;109(3):1202–10.
23. Pfeiffer J, et al. LOH-profiling by SNP-mapping in a case of multifocal head and neck cancer. World J Clin Oncol. 2012;3(2):24–8.
24. Zhou X, et al. Concurrent analysis of loss of heterozygosity (LOH) and copy number abnormality (CNA) for oral premalignancy progression using the Affymetrix 10K SNP mapping array. Hum Genet. 2004;115(4):327–30.
25. Izumi K, et al. Mosaic maternal uniparental disomy of chromosome 15 in Prader-Willi syndrome: utility of genome-wide SNP array. Am J Med Genet A. 2013;161A(1):166–71.
26. Conlin LK, et al. Utility of SNP arrays in detecting, quantifying, and determining meiotic origin of tetrasomy 12p in blood from individuals with Pallister-Killian syndrome. Am J Med Genet A. 2012; 158A(12):3046–53.
27. Zhang L, et al. Clonal diversity analysis using SNP microarray: a new prognostic tool for chronic lymphocytic leukemia. Cancer Genet. 2011;204(12): 654–65.
28. Cross J, et al. Resolution of trisomic mosaicism in prenatal diagnosis: estimated performance of a 50K

SNP microarray. Prenat Diagn. 2007;27(13): 1197–204.

29. Kearney HM, Kearney JB, Conlin LK. Diagnostic implications of excessive homozygosity detected by SNP-based microarrays: consanguinity, uniparental disomy, and recessive single-gene mutations. Clin Lab Med. 2011;31(4):595–613. ix.

30. Konecny M, et al. Identification of rare complete BRCA1 gene deletion using a combination of SNP haplotype analysis, MLPA and array-CGH techniques. Breast Cancer Res Treat. 2008;109(3):581–3.

31. Lai Y, Zhao H. A statistical method to detect chromosomal regions with DNA copy number alterations using SNP-array-based CGH data. Comput Biol Chem. 2005;29(1):47–54.

32. Mackinnon RN, et al. CGH and SNP array using DNA extracted from fixed cytogenetic preparations and long-term refrigerated bone marrow specimens. Mol Cytogenet. 2012;5:10.

33. Siggberg L, et al. High-resolution SNP array analysis of patients with developmental disorder and normal array CGH results. BMC Med Genet. 2012;13:84.

34. Wiszniewska J, et al. Combined array CGH plus SNP genome analyses in a single assay for optimized clinical testing. Eur J Hum Genet. 2013; 22(1):79–87.

35. Bruno DL, et al. Pathogenic aberrations revealed exclusively by single nucleotide polymorphism (SNP) genotyping data in 5000 samples tested by molecular karyotyping. J Med Genet. 2011;48(12): 831–9.

36. Van Loo P, et al. Analyzing cancer samples with SNP arrays. Methods Mol Biol. 2012;802:57–72.

37. Cui SF, Zhou Q, Qu XH. SNP genotyping for the genetic monitoring of laboratory mice by using a microarray-based method with dualcolour fluorescence hybridisation. Altern Lab Anim. 2012;40(3): 155–63.

38. Savage SA. Cancer genetic association studies in the genome-wide age. Per Med. 2008;5(6):589–97.

39. Anaya JM, et al. Evaluation of genetic association between an ITGAM non-synonymous SNP (rs1143679) and multiple autoimmune diseases. Autoimmun Rev. 2012;11(4):276–80.

40. Batra J, et al. Association between prostinogen (KLK15) genetic variants and prostate cancer risk and aggressiveness in Australia and a meta-analysis of GWAS data. PLoS One. 2011;6(11):e26527.

41. Batra J, et al. A Kallikrein 15 (KLK15) single nucleotide polymorphism located close to a novel exon shows evidence of association with poor ovarian cancer survival. BMC Cancer. 2011;11:119.

42. Batra J, et al. Kallikrein-related peptidase 10 (KLK10) expression and single nucleotide polymorphisms in ovarian cancer survival. Int J Gynecol Cancer. 2010;20(4):529–36.

43. Dhillon PK, et al. Common polymorphisms in the adiponectin and its receptor genes, adiponectin levels and the risk of prostate cancer. Cancer Epidemiol Biomarkers Prev. 2011;20(12):2618–27.

44. FitzGerald LM, et al. Association of FGFR4 genetic polymorphisms with prostate cancer risk and prognosis. Prostate Cancer Prostatic Dis. 2009;12(2): 192–7.

45. Iida R, et al. Multiplex single base extension method for simultaneous genotyping of non-synonymous SNP in the three human SOD genes. Electrophoresis. 2008;29(23):4788–94.

46. Lose F, et al. Common variation in Kallikrein genes KLK5, KLK6, KLK12, and KLK13 and risk of prostate cancer and tumor aggressiveness. Urol Oncol. 2013;31(5):635–43.

47. Shui IM, et al. Genetic variation in the toll-like receptor 4 and prostate cancer incidence and mortality. Prostate. 2012;72(2):209–16.

48. Stevens VL, et al. Genetic variation in the toll-like receptor gene cluster (TLR10-TLR1-TLR6) and prostate cancer risk. Int J Cancer. 2008;123(11):2644–50.

49. Yu Z, et al. Analysis of GABRB2 association with schizophrenia in German population with DNA sequencing and one-label extension method for SNP genotyping. Clin Biochem. 2006;39(3):210–8.

50. Burdick KE, et al. Genetic variation in the MET proto-oncogene is associated with schizophrenia and general cognitive ability. Am J Psychiatry. 2010; 167(4):436–43.

51. Pharoah PDP, et al. Association studies for finding cancer-susceptibility genetic variants. Nat Rev Cancer. 2004;4(11):850–60.

52. Braem MGM, et al. Genetic susceptibility to sporadic ovarian cancer: a systematic review. Biochim Biophys Acta. 2011;1816(2):132–46.

53. Tabor HK, Risch NJ, Myers RM. Candidate-gene approaches for studying complex genetic traits: practical considerations. Nat Rev Genet. 2002;3(5): 391–7.

54. Thomas DC, Haile RW, Duggan D. Recent developments in genomewide association scans: a workshop summary and review. Am J Hum Genet. 2005; 77(3):337–45.

55. Weiss KM, Clark AG. Linkage disequilibrium and the mapping of complex human traits. Trends Genet. 2002;18(1):19–24.

56. Ardlie KG, Kruglyak L, Seielstad M. Patterns of linkage disequilibrium in the human genome. Nat Rev Genet. 2002;3(4):299–309.

57. 1000 Genomes Project Consortium, Abecasis GR, Altshuler D, Auton A, Brooks LD, Durbin RM, Gibbs RA. A map of human genome variation from population-scale sequencing. Nature. 2010; 467(7319):1061–73.

58. Browning SR. Missing data imputation and haplotype phase inference for genome-wide association studies. Hum Genet. 2008;124(5):439–50.

59. Welter D et al. The NHGRI GWAS Catalog, a curated resource of SNP-trait associations. Nucleic Acids Res. 2013 Dec 6. [Epub ahead of print].

60. Botstein D, et al. Construction of a genetic linkage map in man using restriction fragment length polymorphisms. Am J Hum Genet. 1980;32(3):314–31.

61. Fakhrai-Rad H, Pourmand N, Ronaghi M. Pyrosequencing: an accurate detection platform for single nucleotide polymorphisms. Hum Mutat. 2002;19(5):479–85.

62. Alderborn A, Kristofferson A, Hammerling U. Determination of single-nucleotide polymorphisms by real-time pyrophosphate DNA sequencing. Genome Res. 2000;10(8):1249–58.

63. Dabrowski PW, Nitsche A. MPSQed: a software for the design of multiplex pyrosequencing assays. PLoS One. 2012;7(6):e38140.

64. Dabrowski PW, Schroder K, Nitsche A. MultiPSQ: a software solution for the analysis of diagnostic n-plexed pyrosequencing reactions. PLoS One. 2013;8(3):e60055.

65. Chen G, et al. A virtual pyrogram generator to resolve complex pyrosequencing results. J Mol Diagn. 2012;14(2):149–59.

66. Ambroise J, et al. AdvISER-PYRO: amplicon identification using SparsE representation of PYROsequencing signal. Bioinformatics. 2013; 29(16):1963–9.

67. Ye S, Humphries S, Green F. Allele specific amplification by tetra-primer PCR. Nucleic Acids Res. 1992;20(5):1152.

68. Zhang C, et al. A novel multiplex tetra-primer ARMS-PCR for the simultaneous genotyping of six single nucleotide polymorphisms associated with female cancers. PLoS One. 2013;8(4):e62126.

69. Shuber AP, Grondin VJ, Klinger KW. A simplified procedure for developing multiplex PCRs. Genome Res. 1995;5(5):488–93.

70. Olivier M, et al. High-throughput genotyping of single nucleotide polymorphisms using new biplex invader technology. Nucleic Acids Res. 2002;30(12): e53.

71. de Arruda M, et al. Invader technology for DNA and RNA analysis: principles and applications. Expert Rev Mol Diagn. 2002;2(5):487–96.

72. Olivier M. The Invader assay for SNP genotyping. Mutat Res. 2005;573(1–2):103–10.

73. Nataraj AJ, et al. Single-strand conformation polymorphism and heteroduplex analysis for gel-based mutation detection. Electrophoresis. 1999;20(6): 1177–85.

74. Humphries SE, et al. Single-strand conformation polymorphism analysis with high throughput modifications, and its use in mutation detection in familial hypercholesterolemia. International Federation of Clinical Chemistry Scientific Division: Committee on Molecular Biology Techniques. Clin Chem. 1997;43(3):427–35.

75. Han L, et al. Association of SOD1 and SOD2 single nucleotide polymorphisms with susceptibility to gastric cancer in a Korean population. APMIS. 2013;121(3):246–56.

76. Balogh K, et al. Genetic screening methods for the detection of mutations responsible for multiple endocrine neoplasia type 1. Mol Genet Metab. 2004;83(1–2):74–81.

77. Nagamine CM, Chan K, Lau YF. A PCR artifact: generation of heteroduplexes. Am J Hum Genet. 1989;45(2):337–9.

78. Highsmith Jr WE, et al. Use of a DNA toolbox for the characterization of mutation scanning methods. I: construction of the toolbox and evaluation of heteroduplex analysis. Electrophoresis. 1999;20(6): 1186–94.

79. O'Donovan MC, et al. Blind analysis of denaturing high-performance liquid chromatography as a tool for mutation detection. Genomics. 1998;52(1):44–9.

80. Kurzawski G, et al. Mutation analysis of MLH1 and MSH2 genes performed by denaturing high-performance liquid chromatography. J Biochem Biophys Methods. 2002;51(1):89–100.

81. Iannone MA, et al. Multiplexed single nucleotide polymorphism genotyping by oligonucleotide ligation and flow cytometry. Cytometry. 2000;39(2): 131–40.

82. Zhong XB, et al. Single-nucleotide polymorphism genotyping on optical thin-film biosensor chips. Proc Natl Acad Sci U S A. 2003;100(20):11559–64.

83. Lizardi PM, et al. Mutation detection and single-molecule counting using isothermal rolling-circle amplification. Nat Genet. 1998;19(3):225–32.

84. Tyagi S, Bratu DP, Kramer FR. Multicolor molecular beacons for allele discrimination. Nat Biotechnol. 1998;16(1):49–53.

85. Marras SA, Kramer FR, Tyagi S. Multiplex detection of single-nucleotide variations using molecular beacons. Genet Anal. 1999;14(5–6):151–6.

86. Mhlanga MM, Malmberg L. Using molecular beacons to detect single-nucleotide polymorphisms with real-time PCR. Methods. 2001;25(4):463–71.

87. Lee LG, Connell CR, Bloch W. Allelic discrimination by nick-translation PCR with fluorogenic probes. Nucleic Acids Res. 1993;21(16):3761–6.

88. Agalliu I, et al. Characterization of SNPs associated with prostate cancer in men of Ashkenazic descent from the set of GWAS identified SNPs: impact of cancer family history and cumulative SNP risk prediction. PLoS One. 2013;8(4):e60083.

89. Le Hellard S, et al. SNP genotyping on pooled DNAs: comparison of genotyping technologies and a semi automated method for data storage and analysis. Nucleic Acids Res. 2002;30(15):e74.

90. Bell PA, et al. SNPstream UHT: ultra-high throughput SNP genotyping for pharmacogenomics and drug discovery. BioTechniques 2002;Suppl:70–2, 74, 76–7.

91. Ugozzoli L, et al. Detection of specific alleles by using allele-specific primer extension followed by capture on solid support. Genet Anal Tech Appl. 1992;9(4):107–12.

92. Wang J, et al. High-throughput single nucleotide polymorphism genotyping using nanofluidic dynamic arrays. BMC Genomics. 2009;10:561.

93. Li T, et al. Genotyping and genomic profiling of non-small-cell lung cancer: implications for current and future therapies. J Clin Oncol. 2013;31(8):1039–49.

94. Vaarno J, et al. New separation-free assay technique for SNPs using two-photon excitation fluorometry. Nucleic Acids Res. 2004;32(13):e108.

95. MacConaill LE, et al. Profiling critical cancer gene mutations in clinical tumor samples. PLoS One. 2009;4(11):e7887.

96. Spurgeon SL, Jones RC, Ramakrishnan R. High throughput gene expression measurement with real time PCR in a microfluidic dynamic array. PLoS One. 2008;3(2):e1662.

97. Chan M, et al. Evaluation of nanofluidics technology for high-throughput SNP genotyping in a clinical setting. J Mol Diagn. 2011;13(3):305–12.

98. Shen R, et al. High-throughput SNP genotyping on universal bead arrays. Mutat Res. 2005;573(1–2): 70–82.

99. Steemers FJ, et al. Whole-genome genotyping with the single-base extension assay. Nat Methods. 2006; 3(1):31–3.

100. Simpson CL, et al. MaGIC: a program to generate targeted marker sets for genome-wide association studies. Biotechniques. 2004;37(6):996–9.

101. Peiffer DA, et al. High-resolution genomic profiling of chromosomal aberrations using Infinium whole-genome genotyping. Genome Res. 2006;16(9):1136–48.

102. Fan JB, et al. Highly parallel SNP genotyping. In: Cold Spring Harbor symposia on quantitative biology, vol 68; 2003. p. 69–78.

103. Matsuzaki H, et al. Parallel genotyping of over 10,000 SNPs using a one-primer assay on a high-density oligonucleotide array. Genome Res. 2004;14(3):414–25.

104. Liu WM, et al. Algorithms for large-scale genotyping microarrays. Bioinformatics. 2003;19(18):2397–403.

105. McCarroll SA, et al. Integrated detection and population-genetic analysis of SNPs and copy number variation. Nat Genet. 2008;40(10):1166–74.

106. Peters EJ, McLeod HL. Ability of whole-genome SNP arrays to capture 'must have' pharmacogenomic variants. Pharmacogenomics. 2008;9(11):1573–7.

107. Sun X, et al. SLAF-seq: an efficient method of large-scale de novo SNP discovery and genotyping using high-throughput sequencing. PLoS One. 2013;8(3): e58700.

108. Margulies M, et al. Genome sequencing in microfabricated high-density picolitre reactors. Nature. 2005;437(7057):376–80.

109. Dressman D, et al. Transforming single DNA molecules into fluorescent magnetic particles for detection and enumeration of genetic variations. Proc Natl Acad Sci U S A. 2003;100(15):8817–22.

110. Ronaghi M, et al. Real-time DNA sequencing using detection of pyrophosphate release. Anal Biochem. 1996;242(1):84–9.

111. Morozova O, Marra MA. Applications of next-generation sequencing technologies in functional genomics. Genomics. 2008;92(5):255–64.

112. Zeng F, Jiang R, Chen T. PyroHMMsnp: an SNP caller for Ion Torrent and 454 sequencing data. Nucleic Acids Res. 2013;41(13):e136.

113. Liu L, et al. Comparison of next-generation sequencing systems. J Biomed Biotechnol. 2012;2012: 251364.

114. Quinlan AR, et al. Pyrobayes: an improved base caller for SNP discovery in pyrosequences. Nat Methods. 2008;5(2):179–81.

115. Metzker ML. Sequencing technologies—the next generation. Nat Rev Genet. 2010;11(1):31–46.

116. Mardis ER. The impact of next-generation sequencing technology on genetics. Trends Genet. 2008;24(3): 133–41.

117. Altschul SF, et al. Basic local alignment search tool. J Mol Biol. 1990;215(3):403–10.

118. Kent WJ. BLAT—the BLAST-like alignment tool. Genome Res. 2002;12(4):656–64.

119. Cox DG, et al. Common variants of the BRCA1 wild-type allele modify the risk of breast cancer in BRCA1 mutation carriers. Hum Mol Genet. 2011;20(23):4732–47.

120. Shendure J, et al. Accurate multiplex polony sequencing of an evolved bacterial genome. Science. 2005;309(5741):1728–32.

121. Harris TD, et al. Single-molecule DNA sequencing of a viral genome. Science. 2008;320(5872):106–9.

122. Rothberg JM, et al. An integrated semiconductor device enabling non-optical genome sequencing. Nature. 2011;475(7356):348–52.

123. Ewing B, Green P. Base-calling of automated sequencer traces using phred. II. Error probabilities. Genome Res. 1998;8(3):186–94.

124. The Wellcome Trust Case Control Consortium. Genome-wide association study of 14,000 cases of seven common diseases and 3,000 shared controls. Nature. 2007;447(7145):661–78.

125. Manolio TA. Genomewide association studies and assessment of the risk of disease. N Engl J Med. 2010;363(2):166–76.

Clinical Application of DNA Sequencing: Sanger and Next-Generation Platforms

John D. McPherson

Cancer is a disease of the genome and all cancers arise due to alterations in DNA. An initial nucleotide aberration that is either inborn (germ line) or arises during cell replication (somatic) lays the foundation for further changes in the nucleotide sequence that ultimately confers a growth advantage to the altered cell [1]. These changes allow the cell to override the checks and balances that are essential for controlled growth and differentiation [2]. The clinical management of cancer has largely been guided by knowing the tissue of origin and histopathological appearance of the tumor. Additionally, many of the genomic alterations result in altered expression of proteins that can be measured by immunohistochemical methods and provide diagnostic and prognostic value (e.g., trastuzumab for HER2-overexpressing breast cancer; [3, 4]). In a growing number of cases, the direct measurement of the underlying nucleotide changes is providing specific treatment guidance (e.g., vemurafenib for BRAFmutated malignant melanoma; [7]). The clinical standard for the determination of DNA alterations has been to detect these few specific mutations by Sanger sequencing [5] of a polymerase chain reaction product [6] encompassing the locus of interest. This method provides a highly robust and accurate readout of the targeted nucleotide sequence. Sanger sequencing is however only able to detect variants that are present at greater than ~20 % of the DNA within a sample—an important limitation as discussed below.

Ten years ago Sanger sequencing chemistry and capillary-based sequencer technology was used to produce a highly accurate sequence of the first reference human genome [7]. This first human genome took thousands of individuals' efforts, 13 years and approximately one billion dollars. While suitable for analyzing a few key loci for guiding treatment decisions, the Sanger/capillary technologies do not scale to the timely analysis of many sites of interest or to rapid whole-genome analyses. Fortunately, DNA and RNA sequencing methods have advanced at an extraordinary rate in the past 8 years with current instruments capable of sequencing whole human genomes in only a couple of days with very few technical staff. These next-generation sequencing (NGS) platforms continue to evolve but have in common the ability to sequence templates in a massively parallel fashion generating millions of sequences simultaneously. Excellent reviews of the basic chemistry and technology behind these advances as well as the strategies for their implementation have recently been published [8–10]. Technical details of common NGS platforms are found in Chap. 5 of this book. A hallmark of the new NGS instruments compared to the traditional Sanger/capillary platforms is a much shorter achievable individual sequence read length, although the gap has closed significantly. In addition, the error rates observed for individual

J.D. McPherson, Ph.D. (✉)
Ontario Institute for Cancer Research, 101 College Street, Suite 800, Toronto, ON, Canada M5G 0A3
e-mail: john.mcpherson@oicr.on.ca

sequence reads are higher than previous platforms. Nonetheless, the sheer magnitude of quality sequence achievable provides consensus accuracy and heralds a new era of cancer genome investigation whereby the determination of the full spectrum of molecular changes in a tumor is now possible on a large scale. Projects such as The Cancer Genome Atlas (TCGA; cancergenome.nih.gov) and The International Cancer Genome Consortium (ICGC, http://www.icgc.org; [11]) are performing genome-wide sequencing of hundreds of tumors across many diverse tumor types and submitting these results to Internet-accessible public repositories. These are rich data sets that will reveal novel insights into the mechanisms of cancer with possible therapeutic potential. A recent study analyzed nearly five million mutations in greater than 7,000 primary tumors from 30 different tumor types [12]. DNA from normal-matched tissue was available to ensure that the variants analyzed were of somatic origin. The number of somatic mutations observed in these samples varied from 0.001 to 400 per megabase of genome with most tumors harboring 0.5–100 somatic mutations per megabase. Tumors associated with chronic exposure to mutagens such as tobacco smoke (lung cancer) or ultraviolet light (melanoma) exhibited the highest prevalence of mutation. This study identified 21 mutational signatures that are likely correlated with the different underlying mutational process that initiated the neoplastic events. It remains to be seen how these signatures may help guide treatment in the future. It is clear from these large-scale studies that there are many similarities among the genes and pathways that are altered in cancers of different anatomical origin and that significant mutational variation exists between tumors of the same type from different individuals. More precise targeting of the dominant altered pathway in an individual tumor has been proposed as an alternative to treatments based on tissue of tumor origin alone. Limited studies have been initiated that are using DNA analysis to derive a molecular profile of a tumor with respect to somatic mutations that can then be used to match specific drugs or treatments to the individual patient [13–16]. This personalized

medicine approach brings the hope that by understanding the specific underlying genetic alterations driving malignant growth of a tumor, treatment regimens specifically targeting the aberrant gene pathways can be deployed. These analyses are meant to augment histopathological and immunohistochemical analyses and not replace them. Therapeutic agents targeting the V660E *BRAF* mutation commonly observed in melanoma is ineffective in colorectal tumors with the same mutation without additionally inhibiting the *EGFR* signaling, as this pathway provides a cellular bypass of the *BRAF* inhibition not present in melanoma [17].

Unlike genome sequencing to determine the underlying cause of a de novo or Mendelian disorder where the variant allele is present in 50 % of the DNA sample generally derived from blood [18, 19], tumor sequencing presents many challenges. Few solid tumors exist as a uniform population of neoplastic cells but rather are a mixture of mutation-harboring cells and genotypically normal cells including immune cells, fibroblasts, and endothelial cells [20]. The tumor cellularity, the proportion of tumor cells present, can vary dramatically. For example, pancreatic ductal adenocarcinoma tumors typically have less than 20 % mutant cells [21]. In such cases, bulk processing of these tumors for DNA sequencing will result in only 10 % the sequence reads derived from a mutant locus present in all tumor cells. This falls below the reliable detection threshold of Sanger/capillary sequencing resulting in false-negative or ambiguous results. NGS platforms can achieve a lower detection threshold of a few percent through the generation of sufficient depth of sequence coverage (200- to 500-fold).

Further confounding the sequence analysis of tumors is the degree of heterogeneity observed within a tumor. Recent individual studies and the large-scale TCGA and ICGC data sets paint a clear picture that tumors are seldom a simple clonal population but rather are a complex mixture of cells evolving either independently or ancestrally from a precursor mutant cell [1]. This population is under selection for growth advantage with the early initiating mutational events often dominating but with many mutant derivatives spawning new clonal populations that may continue to evolve. This can even result in mutational profiles that vary between regions within the same tumor whereby some regions harbor somatic mutations not observed elsewhere within the tumor [22]. This latter property suggests that NGS analysis of a single biopsy in some tumors may be inadequate, potentially increasing the diagnostic burden. This heterogeneity within tumors also unfortunately means that therapies directed at a single dominant mutation often only have transient effects with recurrence frequent. In addition, recurrent tumors analyzed after initial clinical treatments often harbor a different mutation that on analysis has been shown to present at lower frequency in the initial tumor population [23, 24].

Lastly, the current clinical samples available for analysis are often not well suited for NGS. Formalin-fixed paraffin-embedded (FFPE) specimens are common clinical currency with the extracted DNA and RNA from these samples often of low quality and quantity. Nucleic acids are fragmented and harbor nucleotide damage that hinder sequencing steps limiting sequence yield and increasing error rates [25]. Older FFPE samples may yield no adequate analyte at all, but the situation has vastly improved with the adoption of standard operating procedures limiting the fixation times and using neutral-buffered formalin. Fresh-frozen samples are better for NGS but are not as suitable for pathological analyses. Sample collection practices should also be standardized limiting ischemic times as well as ensuring that non-necrotic tissue is provided for DNA and RNA extraction.

The proportion of the genome (a gene set; all genes—the exome or whole genome) that is to be sequenced is an important consideration for molecular testing. For research purposes, whole-genome sequencing affords the most comprehensive data set for discovery. The same cannot be said for clinical applications. If the goal is to provide a precise targeted therapy then the genes of interest are limited to those that have a therapeutic value. This is not limited to only genes that have a therapeutic agent that acts upon them but also members of the related pathway that can be impacted by targeting a node in the pathway. Genes on this list may also provide a prognostic value. With this definition of utility, the current actionable cancer gene list is likely limited to less than 300 genes. As discussed above, the depth of sequence coverage desired for detection of somatic mutations is 200- to 500-fold, so this limited gene list is advantageous as increasing sequence requirements come with increasing costs. Whole-genome sequencing is currently limited to ~50-fold coverage at any reasonable cost. Whether a limited gene set or all genes are targeted requires that these loci be isolated from the larger genome. The most robust method uses long complementary oligonucleotides directed towards the genes of interest [26–28]. The specificity for the captured target is through design of oligonucleotide sequences complementary to the target regions while excluding repetitive sequence. Genomic DNA is sheared, and adapters are added as in the first steps of preparing a whole-genome library. The prepared DNA is hybridized in solution to a pool of the long oligonucleotide baits, and the captured fragments are isolated using a biotin-streptavidin capture modality [27]. Unwanted DNA is removed by washing the captured fragments, and the targeted DNA is eluted, amplified, and used for sequencing. An alternative method uses highly multiplexed PCR combining thousands of PCR primers in a single reaction tube. This is an active area of development with new and more robust methods reaching the market regularly.

From a technical standpoint whole-genome sequencing is the easiest method as it avoids the steps above for isolating targeted regions. This simpler workflow may also require less input DNA. As previously mentioned, it does come with added costs due to the larger sequence target, but it also comes with another potential consequence for cancer diagnostics. With the actionable cancer gene list being somewhat limited, much of the genome is of little clinical value to the oncologist. Depth of sequence coverage is sacrificed for breadth of sequence coverage with the latter contributing little to treatment guidance. In addition, the analyzed genome may also harbor other variants of significance to a patient's health and possibly their relatives beyond the immediate cancer diagnostic need. The American College of Medical Genetics and Genomics recently released guidelines recommending that specific incidental findings be reported in a growing gene list with known or expected pathogenic variants [29].

DNA sequence data generation is only one part of the equation for using NGS as a molecular testing tool. The analysis of the data to derive somatic mutational profiles is very complex, and these concepts and challenges have been recently reviewed [30]. The complexity of the analyses is a hindrance to the adoption of NGS into widespread routine clinical practice. The NGS platform vendors and other independent companies are providing data analysis pipelines, but these are rapidly evolving and typically do not provide all necessary tools for comprehensive tumor analyses. Even the basics of the analyses involving aligning the sequence reads to a reference genome and determining single-nucleotide differences are fraught with complexities arising from multiple regions of the human genome with high sequence similarity. Once somatic mutations are identified, the task remains of determining the functional impact of the variant. Many mutations observed fall outside of the known annotated variants with verified functional consequences such as constitutive activation of a kinase. Mutations nearby may have no affect or even an opposite inactivating phenotype. The observed high frequency of any mutation within a tumor type may indicate its importance in the disease but is an indirect inference without supporting functional studies.

Discussions so far have been limited largely to single-nucleotide variants and small insertions and deletions (less than the length of a sequence read). Copy number alterations [31, 32] and structural rearrangements [33–35] can also be derived from NGS data. The latter is less robust with much work yet to be done to make the detection of large insertions and deletions and translocations routine analyses. Epigenetic alterations of tumor DNA can also be determined by NGS, but methods are not yet suitable for clinical appli-cation. All of these variant classes are important in cancer genomic diagnostics and will become part of the NGS repertoire in molecular testing of cancer.

Lastly, gene expression profiling is a robust NGS methodology (RNA-seq [36]). In general, much like the actionable gene list, the gene expression signatures involve a limited number of genes and are best assayed by other methods such as the MammaPrint and Oncotype DX prognostic biomarkers for aggressive breast cancer [37, 38]. RNA-seq is a tremendous research tool at present providing insight into differential expression and splicing, RNA editing, and allele-specific expression that may provide additional molecular testing potential in the future.

Conclusion

As the NGS technologies continue to evolve, costs will drop, read lengths and accuracy will increase, and analyses methods will improve. This will make whole-genome sequencing and RNA-seq more mainstream providing comprehensive cancer genome analyses. This will press the issue of reporting incidental findings but with improved diagnostic and prognostic capabilities providing the fuel for individualized treatments.

References

1. Stratton MR, Campbell PJ, Futreal PA. The cancer genome. Nature. 2009;458:719–24.
2. Hanahan D, Weinberg RA. Hallmarks of cancer: the next generation. Cell. 2011;144:646–74.
3. Slamon DJ, et al. Use of chemotherapy plus a monoclonal antibody against HER2 for metastatic breast cancer that overexpresses HER2. N Engl J Med. 2001;344:783–92.
4. Slamon D, et al. Adjuvant trastuzumab in HER2-positive breast cancer. N Engl J Med. 2011;365: 1273–83.
5. Sanger F, Nicklen S, Coulson AR. DNA sequencing with chain-terminating inhibitors. Proc Natl Acad Sci U S A. 1977;74:5463–7.
6. Saiki RK, et al. Primer-directed enzymatic amplification of DNA with a thermostable DNA polymerase. Science. 1988;239:487–91.

7. Lander ES, et al. Initial sequencing and analysis of the human genome. Nature. 2001;409:860–921.
8. Metzker ML. Sequencing technologies—the next generation. Nat Rev Genet. 2010;11:31–46.
9. Mardis ER. A decade's perspective on DNA sequencing technology. Nature. 2011;470:198–203.
10. Mardis ER. Genome sequencing and cancer. Curr Opin Genet Dev. 2012;22:245–50.
11. International Cancer Genome Consortium, et al. International network of cancer genome projects. Nature. 2010;464:993–8.
12. Alexandrov LB, et al. Signatures of mutational processes in human cancer. Nature. 2013;500:415–21.
13. von Hoff DD, et al. Pilot study using molecular profiling of patients' tumors to find potential targets and select treatments for their refractory cancers. J Clin Oncol. 2010;28:4877–83.
14. Roychowdhury S, et al. Personalized oncology through integrative high-throughput sequencing: a pilot study. Sci Transl Med. 2011;3:111ra121.
15. Welch JS, et al. Use of whole-genome sequencing to diagnose a cryptic fusion oncogene. JAMA. 2011;305:1577–84.
16. Tran B, et al. Feasibility of real time next generation sequencing of cancer genes linked to drug response: results from a clinical trial. Int J Cancer. 2013;132:1547–55.
17. Prahallad A, et al. Unresponsiveness of colon cancer to BRAF(V600E) inhibition through feedback activation of EGFR. Nature. 2012;483:100–3.
18. Ng SB, et al. Exome sequencing identifies MLL2 mutations as a cause of Kabuki syndrome. Nat Genet. 2010;42:790–3.
19. Bainbridge MN, et al. Whole-genome sequencing for optimized patient management. Sci Transl Med. 2011;3:87re3.
20. Bremnes RM, et al. The role of tumor-infiltrating immune cells and chronic inflammation at the tumor site on cancer development, progression, and prognosis: emphasis on non-small cell lung cancer. J Thorac Oncol. 2011;6:824–33.
21. Biankin AV, et al. Pancreatic cancer genomes reveal aberrations in axon guidance pathway genes. Nature. 2012;491:399–405.
22. Gerlinger M, et al. Intratumor heterogeneity and branched evolution revealed by multiregion sequencing. N Engl J Med. 2012;366:883–92.
23. Ding L, et al. Clonal evolution in relapsed acute myeloid leukaemia revealed by whole-genome sequencing. Nature. 2012;481:506–10.
24. Walter MJ, et al. Clonal architecture of secondary acute myeloid leukemia. N Engl J Med. 2012;366:1090–8.
25. Hadd AG, et al. Targeted, high-depth, next-generation sequencing of cancer genes in formalin-fixed. Paraffin-embedded and fine-needle aspiration tumor specimens. J Mol Diagn. 2013;15:234–47.
26. Albert TJ, et al. Direct selection of human genomic loci by microarray hybridization. Nat Methods. 2007;4:903–5.
27. Gnirke A, et al. Solution hybrid selection with ultra-long oligonucleotides for massively parallel targeted sequencing. Nat Biotechnol. 2009;27:182–9.
28. Hodges E, et al. Hybrid selection of discrete genomic intervals on custom-designed microarrays for massively parallel sequencing. Nat Protoc. 2009;4:960–74.
29. Green RC, et al. ACMG recommendations for reporting of incidental findings in clinical exome and genome sequencing. Genet Med. 2013;15:565–74.
30. International Cancer Genome Consortium Mutation Pathways and Consequences Subgroup of the Bioinformatics Analyses Working Group, et al. Computational approaches to identify functional genetic variants in cancer genomes. Nat Methods. 2013;10:723–9.
31. Xie C, Tammi MT. CNV-seq, a new method to detect copy number variation using high-throughput sequencing. BMC Bioinformatics. 2009;10:80.
32. Krumm N, et al. Copy number variation detection and genotyping from exome sequence data. Genome Res. 2012;22:1525–32.
33. Chen K, et al. BreakDancer: an algorithm for high-resolution mapping of genomic structural variation. Nat Methods. 2009;6:677–81.
34. Wang J, et al. CREST maps somatic structural variation in cancer genomes with base-pair resolution. Nat Methods. 2011;8:652–4.
35. Ye K, Schulz MH, Long Q, Apweiler R, Ning Z. Pindel: a pattern growth approach to detect break points of large deletions and medium sized insertions from paired-end short reads. Bioinformatics. 2009;25:2865–71.
36. Wang Z, Gerstein M, Snyder M. RNA-Seq: a revolutionary tool for transcriptomics. Nat Rev Genet. 2009;10:57–63.
37. Galanina N, Bossuyt V, Harris LN. Molecular predictors of response to therapy for breast cancer. Cancer J. 2011;17:96–103.
38. O'Toole SA, et al. Molecular assays in breast cancer pathology. Pathology. 2011;43:116–1127.

Microarray-Based Investigations in Cancer

7

Maud H.W. Starmans *, Syed Haider *, Cindy Yao *,
Philippe Lambin, and Paul C. Boutros

Introduction

A number of methods have been introduced since 1990 that have led to the application of microarray techniques to cancer investigations [1–4]. Although several different platforms exist, the basis for all microarrays is the same: it consists of a large panel of "probes" that are fixed on a solid substrate (the "slide" or "chip"). Each probe is designed to specifically recognize a single target molecule, making it possible to profile an enormous amount of target molecules simultaneously. Labeled target material is hybridized to the microarray and molecules will bind their respective probes. Because the location of each probe is annotated, scanning the intensities of each label gives a parallel measurement of target signal. This signal intensity is proportional to the abundance of the detected species in the range above the detection limit and below saturation (i.e., within the dynamic range of the system). The technology is inherently flexible, and changing the type of probes placed on the microarray allows the measurement of different molecular species. For example, a microarray with antibodies as probes can be constructed for proteomic analyses [5]. The most widely used type of microarray, however, is the DNA microarray, which uses DNA-based probes to quantitate DNA or RNA (often via cDNA). DNA microarray technology can be adopted for a large variety of applications, such as array-based comparative genomic hybridization (aCGH) [6], array-based genotyping [7], epigenetic profiling (e.g., DNA methylation) [8], and

*Author contributed equally with all other contributors.

M.H.W. Starmans, Ph.D.
Informatics and Biocomputing Program,
Ontario Institute for Cancer Research, 101 College
Street, Suite 800, Toronto, ON, Canada M5G 0A3

Department of Radiation Oncology (Maastro),
Maastricht University Medical Center, Maastricht,
The Netherlands

S. Haider, M.D.
Ontario Institute for Cancer Research, 101 College
Street, Suite 800, Toronto, ON, Canada M5G 0A3

C. Yao, M.Sc.
Informatics and Biocomputing Program,
Ontario Institute for Cancer Research, 101 College
Street, Suite 800, Toronto, ON, Canada M5G 0A3

Department of Medical Biophysics, University
of Toronto, Toronto, ON, Canada

P. Lambin, M.D., Ph.D.
Department of Radiation Oncology (Maastro),
Maastricht University Medical Center, Maastricht,
The Netherlands

P.C. Boutros, Ph.D. (✉)
Ontario Institute for Cancer Research, 101 College
Street, Suite 800, Toronto, ON, Canada M5G 0A3

Department of Medical Biophysics,
University of Toronto, Toronto, ON, Canada

Department of Pharmacology & Toxicology,
University of Toronto, Toronto, ON, Canada
e-mail: Paul.Boutros@oicr.on.ca

G.M. Yousef and S. Jothy (eds.), *Molecular Testing in Cancer*,
DOI 10.1007/978-1-4899-8050-2_7, © Springer Science+Business Media New York 2014

characterization of alternatively spliced transcript isoforms [9]. Perhaps most importantly, however, DNA-based microarrays remain the standard approach for transcriptome analysis. Because of their widespread and flexible use, this chapter will focus on DNA microarrays.

Types of Microarrays

A large variety of DNA microarrays exist, and these vary in both their construction and design, as well as in the techniques used for their analysis. Three general classifications can be made which illustrate the major differences. DNA microarrays can be categorized based on (1) the methodology used to create the microarray, (2) the type of probes used for the microarray, and (3) the number of samples that are hybridized to the microar-

ray slide. We first overview each of these in turn and then outline the benchmarking studies and software/databases that have emerged over the past decade to facilitate microarray data analysis.

Construction of Microarrays

Numerous technologies have been developed to produce microarrays, with the greatest difference being in the way probes are deposited onto the microarray slides. Two main concepts have been introduced to do this: spotting and in situ synthesis (Fig. 7.1). For the first technique, probes are pre-synthesized and subsequently attached to the microarray by spotting them on the slide. The probes are either deposited with a pin [2] or printed with a specialized inkjet-like printer onto the slide [10]. In the second

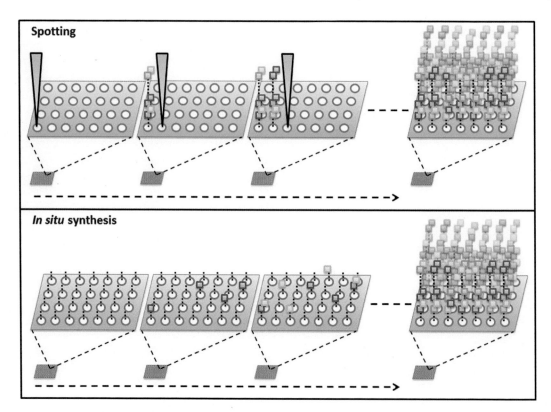

Fig. 7.1 Overview of the two main concepts for DNA microarray fabrication: spotting (*top*) and in situ synthesis (*bottom*). For spotting fabrication, probes are synthesized first and are then spotted onto a microarray slide. This can

be achieved through either pin deposit or inkjet printing. In contrast, in situ fabrication works by synthesizing probes directly on the slide and this is achieved using photolithography method, the probes are directly synthesized on the slide using photolithographic synthesis methodology [4]. The most widely used in situ-synthesized microarray is the GeneChip from Affymetrix (Affymetrix, Santa Clara, CA). Other companies producing them include Roche NimbleGen (Madison, WI).

In general, spotted microarrays have a lower density than their in situ-synthesized counterparts because of the relative difference in spot sizes. The technology to manufacture spotted microarrays does not require specific equipment or complex chemistry; therefore, it is possible to generate them in-house and multiple institutes have established core facilities to do this [11]. For in situ-synthesized microarrays, this is much more complex and these are in general manufactured commercially. This difference has several consequences. The use of spotting microarrays provides much more flexibility; it is easy to change the probe content of the microarray to the user's needs. However, in situ-synthesized microarrays have a better reproducibility due to commercial manufacturing and standardization of reagents and instrumentation [12].

Microarray Probes

There are two main types of probes used for DNA microarrays [13]. Double-stranded DNA (dsDNA), commonly obtained with polymerase chain reaction (PCR), is one of these. PCR amplicons, typically varying in length from approximately 200 to 800 base pairs (bp), are created using PCR primers. Primers can be designed from cDNA libraries, shotgun library clones, or known genomic sequence. These probes can only be used with spotting techniques, since they can only be synthesized prior to printing them on the microarray. The second type of probe is the oligonucleotide, a short chemical-synthesized sequence. The typical probe length for oligonucleotides ranges from 20 to 100 bp [14]. Unlike the dsDNA probe, this probe type can be used for both spotted and in situ-synthesized microarrays.

Since dsDNA probes are longer than oligonucleotides, in theory, they should have better sensitivity and specificity. However, longer probes

are more open to cross-hybridization (e.g., gene families) and may contain nonspecific elements, which would decrease specificity [15]. Further to increase sensitivity, the oligonucleotide-based microarray is designed to include multiple probes for the same target. The use of shorter fragments also makes it possible to increase resolution, for example, to examine specific exons or to interrogate polymorphisms [16].

Microarray Sample Hybridization

Another important distinction between types of microarrays involves the number of samples that are hybridized to a single microarray slide. Some microarrays can measure a single sample, while other types can measure two samples simultaneously (Fig. 7.2). Prior to hybridization, a sample is labeled with a fluorophore and target signal is measured by detection of fluorescence. When a single sample is hybridized to the array, one fluorophore is used (one-color microarray). However, in the case of two sample arrays, different fluorophores are used for each sample. These are subsequently mixed and hybridized together on a single microarray slide (two-color array), and they then competitively hybridize to the probes on the array. With the one-color microarray, absolute fluorescence is measured, whereas two-color arrays provide ratios. Notably, due to differences in hybridization affinity between probes, neither platform is effective at measuring absolute RNA/DNA abundances [17, 18]. A significant literature has been developed to describe the optimal ways to design multicolor microarray experiments [19].

Advances in Microarrays: Benchmarking Studies

Since the introduction of DNA microarrays, technology has evolved substantially. The first microarrays were limited to detect a few hundred targets; current arrays can measure millions of features. Technological advances besides probe density, both with respect to microarray design and production and DNA/RNA amplification methods,

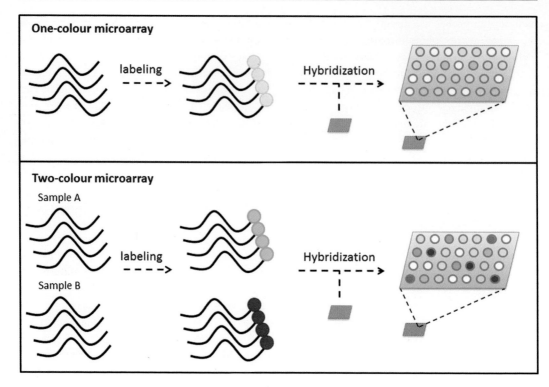

Fig. 7.2 Outline of a one-color (*top*) and a two-color (*bottom*) microarray. For one-color array, one fluorophore is used to label the sample prior to hybridization and direct fluorescence is measured. For two-color arrays, samples are labeled with different fluorophores; the two pools of samples are then mixed and hybridized to one microarray slide and a ratio of the two intensities is given

have resulted in a dramatic reduction in the amount of start material needed [20], making it recently possible to zoom onto the single cell level [21].

Since the first DNA microarrays, our understanding of the human genome and transcriptome has also evolved tremendously. Around the time DNA microarrays were first being developed and introduced, the Human Genome Project was initiated to sequence the complete human genome. In 2001 the first draft sequence of the human genome was published, with approximately a quarter of the sequence in its final form [22, 23]. Using this information showed that large proportions of probes were incorrectly assigned [24, 25]. Accordingly methods to update probe annotation and map microarray probes between platforms and species have been developed [26, 27], and these have resulted in better data reproducibility/comparability between different platforms [28, 29].

Other efforts to address DNA microarray data reproducibility and reliability have been undertaken. The MicroArray Quality Control (MAQC) studies I [30] and II [31] showed that with appropriate analyses, high consensus data could be generated. The specific analytical techniques for microarray data, standardization of manufacturing [32], sample preparation, and hybridization [33] as well as in analyses methods [34] have further increased repeatability and reliability.

Software and Databases

With the recognition that data quality and reproducibility was complex and multifaceted, a need for transparent reporting of data and computational methods became apparent [35, 36]. The importance of sharing data, especially with DNA microarray data, upon publishing is twofold. First, others can duplicate the analyses. Second, data can be explored by others providing additional insights. Further in the case of patient

Table 7.1   An overview of public microarray repositories

Repository	Web link
Gene Expression Omnibus (GEO)	http://www.ncbi.nlm.nih.gov/geo/
ArrayExpress	http://www.ebi.ac.uk/arrayexpress/
caArray	https://array.nci.nih.gov/caarray
Stanford Microarray Database (SMD)	http://smd.stanford.edu/
Princeton University MicroArray database (PUMAdb, will replace SMD)	http://puma.princeton.edu/

Table 7.2   An overview of microarray analysis tools

Software	Free	Open source	Website
Affymetrix Power Tools (APT)	Yes	Yes	http://www.affymetrix.com/partners_programs/programs/developer/tools/powertools.affx
Aroma.affymetrix	Yes	Yes	http://www.aroma-project.org/
ArrayStar	No	No	http://www.dnastar.com/
Babelomics	Yes	No	http://babelomics.bioinfo.cipf.es/
BioArray Software Environment (BASE)	Yes	Yes	http://base.thep.lu.se/
Bioconductor	Yes	Yes	http://www.bioconductor.org/
BRB Array Tools	Yes	Yes	http://linus.nci.nih.gov/BRB-ArrayTools.html
DNA Chip Analyzer (dChip)	Yes	Yes	http://www.hsph.harvard.edu/cli/complab/dchip/
GeneSifter	No	No	https://login.genesifter.net/
GeneSpring GX	No	No	http://genespring-support.com/
ImaGene	No	No	http://www.biodiscovery.com/software/imagene/
Partek Genomics Suite	No	No	http://www.partek.com/partekgs
Spotfire	No	No	http://spotfire.tibco.com/
TM4	Yes	Yes	http://www.tm4.org/
WebArray	Yes	Yes	http://www.webarray.org/

data, it offers the opportunity to perform meta-analyses, increasing the potential power of, e.g., biomarker studies. Public data repositories, such as the Gene Expression Omnibus (GEO) [37] and ArrayExpress [38], have been established to meet these needs. An overview of public repositories is presented in Table 7.1. Further a standard for reporting microarray experiments was introduced: Minimum Information About a Microarray Experiment (MIAME) [39]. MIAME describes the information that should be specified for microarray experiments; however, these are only recommendations regarding the content not regarding technical format. Therefore, despite the adoption of MIAME, it has often been difficult either to obtain the data or to reproduce results [40, 41]. Making high-throughput data available is often a condition of publication or funding as it is one of the MIAME criteria [42].

Comprehensive software packages for microarray data processing and analyses have been developed both commercially and as an open source. For example, the open-source software Bioconductor provides a wide array of tools for sophisticated microarray data analyses and provides researchers with the option to develop additional methods and make them easily available to others [43]. In Table 7.2 an overview of DNA microarray analysis tools is provided.

Applications of Microarrays

Measuring RNA Abundances

Several different types of RNA molecules can be profiled using microarrays; these include, but are not limited to, messenger RNA (mRNA), microRNA (miRNA), and RNA interference (RNAi). For studies of transcripts, mRNA is typically reverse-transcribed into cDNA and then hybridized to either one-color or two-color arrays (as detailed in section "Microarray Sample Hybridization"), although direct labeling of RNA can also be performed [44]. Similarly, miRNAs are reverse-transcribed, labeled with different fluorophore molecules [44, 45], and then hybridized onto a pre-spotted array [46–48]. Usually for one-channel mRNA expression data, robust multi-array average (RMA) algorithm is used to preprocess the data [45, 49]. RMA involves three key steps—background correction, quantile normalization (forcing intensity values from different arrays to have the same distribution), and summarization using a median polish. In contrast, there is no general consensus in a normalization method for two-color mRNA arrays. Different algorithms can be used [50–56] (e.g., empirical Bayes model [54], limma [56], and variance-stabilizing models [53]) and method selection is largely data dependent. Similarly, multiple normalization methods exist for miRNA data including median centering, quantile normalization, and variance-stabilizing normalization where inter-sample variation is calibrated so that it is independent of mean intensity [57, 58]. Lastly, microarray-based approaches have been developed to study short hairpin RNA (shRNA), molecules that are widely used to assess gain- or loss-of-function mutation in genes. A method termed Gene Modulation Array Platform (GMAP) is designed to allow for the study of genome-wide gene-dosage screens of >248,000 unique shRNAs simultaneously [59]. Cells are infected with lentiviral shRNA pools and genomic DNA are prepared and hybridized to GMAP array. GC-background correction for nonspecific binding probes and normalization using Cyclic Loess are applied to reduce inter-replicate variances.

Measuring Other Aspects of RNAs

Although measuring the abundance of different RNA species is likely the most common use of microarray technologies, they can also be used to study other aspects of RNA molecules. For example, ribonucleoprotein complexes (RNPs) are interesting assemblies comprised of both RNA and proteins, which play important roles in mRNA translation and maturation [60]. RNPs can be profiled using RNA immunoprecipitation (RIP). RIP starts with a cross-linking process, which preserves the interaction between RNA and protein [61], and is followed by incubation with an antibody. Extracted RNA is then reverse-transcribed to cDNA and hybridized to a microarray [62–64] (known as RIP-Chip). Different analysis methods are available for analyzing RIP-Chip data [62, 64–67]. For example, one method works by dividing individual probe intensity by the mean probe intensity across the array and then taking a sliding window approach to calculate the sum of all probe intensities that fall within the given window [66]. Those probes that fall below a prespecified adjusted p-value threshold are deemed significant.

mRNA turnover rate can also be studied using microarrays and is an important area because of its role in regulating gene expression. Time-series experiments of mRNA in combination with microarray-based technology can allow for the global characterization of mRNA decay [68]. Following stress induction, cells are harvested at various time points [68, 69], which are then metabolically labeled with [^{35}S]methionine, pulse-chased and immunoprecipitated [70, 71]. Isolated mRNA is hybridized onto a microarray for global profiling. RNA intensities are often normalized to internal controls and a nonlinear model is used to calculate the decay rate constant and half-life of each mRNA [72].

Similarly, mRNA translation, which is important for development, cell cycle, and drug resistance [73–77], can be profiled using a whole-genome approach [78–82]. During mRNA translation, multiple ribosomes are attached to RNA and this structure is called polysomes. mRNA translation can be profiled by capturing these polysome structures. This process starts by first arresting ribosome movement. Sucrose gradient centrifugation is then used to separate the complex into fractions [82]. Purified RNA from each of the fractions is reverse-transcribed, labeled with different dyes, and hybridized to a microarray. Normalization is done relative to a pool of normalization controls so that intensity signals from all normalization controls are equal to one on each array [78]. Fractions with the highest average values are defined as the peak fractions and differences in peak fractions show whether these RNA molecules are actively or inactively translating [78, 82].

Analyzing DNA Sequence and Structure

Microarrays can interrogate several aspects of DNA structure, including the presence or absence of specific base-pair-level sequence aberrations (also called resequencing or genotyping) and the copy number status of different regions of the genome.

Single nucleotide polymorphisms (SNPs) are DNA sequence variants of a single nucleotide in size that occur in a portion of the population. With the advancements of technologies, these single nucleotide alterations can be readily picked up by high-throughput assays such as microarray. Several fractionation-based SNP-enrichment approaches are available [68, 69, 83–85]. Briefly, the process starts by incubating DNA in a cocktail of restriction enzymes, which leaves short overhangs at the ends of the DNA fragments. Primers that recognize these overhangs are then ligated to the DNA fragments and are used for adaptor-mediated PCR amplification [86]. Sometimes a size-selection step is used prior to PCR amplification to reduce sample complexity. Amplified DNA is fragmented, labeled with fluorophores, and hybridized to an SNP array. Affymetrix offers various types of arrays, each with different resolutions, including the 10, 100, and 500 k arrays [87]. Prior to genotyping calling of AA, AB, or BB, SNP arrays need to be preprocessed. Various preprocessing methods exist for SNP arrays [88–91]. Some methods correct for probe sequence and fragment length prior to normalization. Array intensities are then quantile normalized to ensure that all samples have the same distribution [88–91]. Summarization of probes that correspond to the same allele of the same SNP is often done using median polish [88–90]. Multiple genotyping algorithms are available and the more successful ones involve initial training on known genotypes (e.g., BRLMM [88], CRLMM-1 [87], BRLMM-P [89], Birdseed [91], and CRLMM-2 [90]). In addition to genotyping, copy number status can also be inferred from SNP arrays through use of both hidden Markov models (HMM) [92–96] and non-HMM approaches which use hierarchical clustering or p-value threshold selection [91, 97–101].

More frequently, copy number variation analyses are achieved through comparative genomic hybridization (CGH), which allows for the simultaneous interrogation of four million oligonucleotides. Genomic DNA from one sample (e.g., tumor) and that of another (e.g., normal) are labeled with different fluorophores (Cy5 and Cy3, respectively). DNA from both samples is then hybridized onto a cDNA microarray [6] (Fig. 7.3). The ratio of Cy5/Cy3 fluorescence indicates copy number status where red (Cy5) represents copy number gain in the tumor samples, green (Cy3) represents a copy number loss in the tumor samples, and yellow represents no change in DNA copy number in comparison to the normal sample. Multiple segmentation methods are available for dividing data into sets of equal copy number; some of the methods include HMM approach (HMM) [102], circular binary segmentation (CBS) [103], and Gaussian model-based approach (GLAD) [99].

Epigenetic Applications

In addition to direct measures of RNA and DNA molecules, microarray-based techniques can also be applied to investigate the relationship between proteins and DNA. Chromatin immunoprecipitation (ChIP) can detect transcription factor binding sites through cross-linking of DNA and proteins by formaldehyde and sonication and breaking up of nonbinding DNA fragments. The protein of interest is then probed with the respective antibodies to complete the immunoprecipitation process. DNA bound to the protein

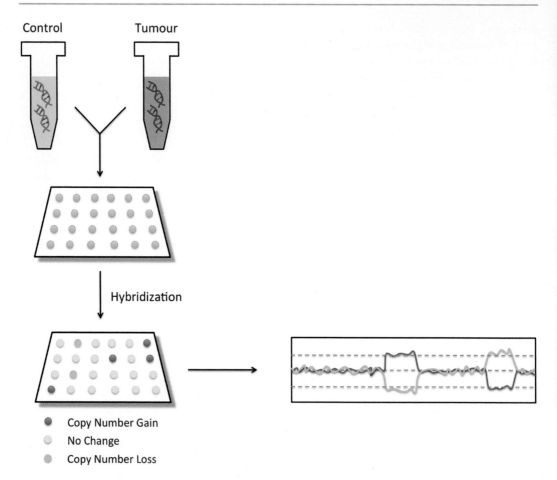

Fig. 7.3 Overview of aCGH. Genomic DNA from two samples (e.g., tumor and normal) are labeled with different fluorophores, which are then hybridized onto a cDNA microarray. Copy number status is indicated through the ratio of the Cy5/ Cy3 fluorescence: *red* represents a gain of copy number in the tumor samples, *green* represents a loss of copy number in the tumor samples, and *yellow* represents no copy number differences between normal and tumor samples

of interest is released and profiled using a microarray (ChIP-Chip) [6]. Various methods for analyzing ChIP-Chip data exist [59, 104–108]. Model-based analysis of tiling arrays (MAT) normalizes probes by considering probe sequence for GC contents as well as the copy number of probes across the array [106]. Some methods use a hidden Markov model (HMM) approach, whereas others use a sliding window-based approach for identifying areas enriched for ChIP [104–108]. Taking intensity values from each probe directly as a potential DNA–protein interaction point would result in a high number of false-positives; hence, a sliding window approach is often suggested for analysis of ChIP-Chip data where a fixed window moves along the genome and summarizes all probes within that window. Any peaks identified from this summarized window approach will be regarded as binding sites.

Similarly, microarrays can be used to study epigenetic changes and specifically DNA methylation. Methylated DNA fragments can be enriched through various methods (Table 7.3). DNA fragments enriched for methylation are hybridized to a microarray for global detection. Following data acquisition, probe intensities need to be normalized. Various methods exist for normalizing methylation data including RMA (described above), which is often used for

Table 7.3 The different approaches to enrich for methylated DNA fragments

Enrichment approaches	Description
Bisulfite treatment	Treatment of genomic DNA with sodium bisulfite will convert unmethylated cytosine to uracil but leave methylated cytosine the same. These can be identified as SNPs through either array- or NGS-based approaches
Methylation-sensitive restriction enzyme enrichment (MSRE)	Restriction enzymes can target either methylated or unmethylated DNA, hence enriching for either the unmethylated or methylated fractions, respectively, upon PCR amplification
Methylated DNA immunoprecipitation (MeDIP)	5-methylcytosine-specific antibody targets and immunoprecipitates methylated DNA

Table 7.4 Sliding window selection methods

Authors	Method description
Cawley et al. (2004)	Rank probe signals within 1,000-base-pair sliding window using Mann–Whitney U test [104]
Li et al. (2005)	Use two-hidden-state HMM to estimate enrichment probability at each probe location [108]
Keles et al. (2004)	Use a sliding window of mean Welch's t statistics to identify enrichment regions [107]
Ji and Wong (2005)	Weigh observed probe variance and pooled variances using empirical Bayes shrinkage [105]
Johnson et al. (2006)	Calculate trimmed mean (removes top and bottom 10 %) of all t values within 600-base-pair window [106]

analyzing mRNA expression data [45, 90], and MAT and Potter, which incorporate signal intensity, sequence, and copy number of all probes into the normalization model [106, 109]. Similar to ChIP-Chip analysis, a sliding window approach is used to summarize probe-level values by genomic regions (Table 7.4). Selection of sliding window method depends on informatic resources, biological questions, and the types of data being interrogated.

Advantages and Limitations of Microarrays

RNA Applications

The emergence of RNA microarrays has dictated much of the research done over the past decade, offering an efficient and high-throughput genome-wide view of transcriptome as opposed to predecessor techniques such as reverse-transcription PCR (RT-PCR), expressed sequence tag (EST) analysis, and serial analysis of gene expression (SAGE) [110–113]. However, a fundamental limitation of RNA microarrays is that they can only measure the abundance of probes that are present on the array. Therefore, isoform-specific expression, discovery of novel transcripts, profiling of noncoding elements, and identification of RNA sequence variants were not possible. Of these, isoform-specific expression and profiling of noncoding elements can be achieved by using a combination of less popular splicing/junction arrays and tiling arrays; however, their accuracy due to cross-hybridization potential remains unclear [114–116]. With the advent of next-generation sequencing technologies, RNA-sequencing (RNA-seq) has overcome these issues by simultaneously sequencing all the transcribed contents of DNA. The sequenced RNA molecules are termed as "sequence reads" (30–400 bp long depending upon the sequencing technology). The sequence reads are either post-processed to create de novo transcriptome assembly [117–119] or aligned against a reference genome to estimate abundance of known transcribed element [120–124]. This fine-scale coverage of genome-wide transcription landscape offers nucleotide-level view and therefore helps determine the structure and function of all RNA elements beyond the well-annotated genes. Compared to microarrays, RNA-seq certainly offers a much wider view and complexity of transcriptome. However, it requires processing and interpretation of large volumes of read data using bioinformatics tools that are very much in development. Furthermore, to determine the splicing of rare transcripts and RNA variants requires greater coverage, resulting in higher cost and analysis burden. In a nutshell, the ultimate parameter to determine the method of choice lies in the biological question, where microarrays are a preferred and cost-effective solution with well-established bioinformatics pipelines or when profiling of only known genes is required. Furthermore, when studying samples representing heterogeneous population, more clinically relevant information may be achieved by running microarrays on large number of samples than RNA-seq on fewer samples, in the same budget.

DNA Applications

Microarrays have been widely applied to multiple aspects of high-throughput genome research such as copy number analyses and genotyping of mutations and polymorphisms. As for RNA analysis, DNA microarray analysis is fundamentally limited because one can only measure what is on the array and in many applications the design requires a priori knowledge of the genome. If, for example, screening for novel DNA variants, one is limited to a specific gene or genomic region or multiple microarrays have to be used which can make it a costly process. This has changed with the introduction of next-generation sequencing (NGS) technology; the 1000 Genomes Project reported twice as many potentially functional DNA variants as were previously identified in their pilot study [125]. Further with microarrays, not all types of aberrations can be discovered. It is not even possible to screen for certain structural variants (SVs), like translocations and indels, using microarrays. By contrast, with NGS technology, these can be readily detected [126]. Also unlike microarrays, NGS offers single nucleotide resolution making it possible to find base-pair-level breakpoints [127]. Another application of DNA NGS is the identification of novel sequence insertions (e.g., viral integration) [128],

which is not possible with microarrays. In conclusion, with the introduction of NGS technology, it is thus not only possible to explore known variance at a large scale, but it also provides a platform for the discovery of novel variation at the entire genome level.

Epigenetic Applications

In addition to RNA and DNA profiling, studies of the epigenome are also gaining popularity as high-throughput detection technology advances. Microarrays have been traditionally used for the interrogation of epigenetic changes and are rather attractive to the field because of its affordability and the established and mature bioinformatics pipeline [129]. Various methylation detection methods have been developed including bisulfite conversion, methylation-sensitive restriction enzyme digestion, and affinity-based method [130]. Bisulfite conversion works by treating genomic DNA with sodium bisulfite where unmethylated cytosine is converted to uracil but methylated cytosine remains as a cytosine. PCR amplification will then replace uracils with thymines. From there, amplified DNA can either be profiled using pyrosequencing [131], Sanger sequencing [132], or Illumina bead arrays [133, 134]. To study methylation polymorphisms, genomic DNA often undergoes bisulfite treatment followed by hybridization to an Illumina bead array. Bisulfite-treated DNA is targeted by two primers (labeled with different fluorescent tags) using the Illumina bead array where one targets the unmethylated fragments and the other targets the methylated fragments [130]. This method is best for studying methylation polymorphisms on a known set of methylated loci on a larger sample size. It provides more quantitative measure of cytosine methylation [130]. However, it has lower coverage in comparison to other array-based technologies and requires sophistication and knowledge in the evaluation and design of the differentially labeled primers. As a result, to gain knowledge from a whole-genome perspective, next-generation sequencing (NGS) is used to study organisms with both small and large genomes. One advantage of NGS is that DNA can be sequenced directly, hence bypassing the labor-intensive and bias-prone PCR amplification and DNA labeling [130]. The read counts provide quantitative measures of the abundances of methylated sequences. Unlike array-based technologies, no a priori information is needed for NGS technologies and hybridization-induced biases are unlikely to be present for NGS data [130]. Another technique for studying DNA methylation patterns is methylation-sensitive restriction enzyme enrichment (MSRE) [135–140]. Samples are digested with a set of restriction enzymes that cut either methylated or unmethylated fragments; hence, upon PCR amplification, it enriches for DNA fractions that have not been cut by restriction enzymes. The enriched fragments can be profiled using both array and NGS methods. Methylated DNA sequences can also be enriched using affinity-based method. One such method is called methylated DNA immunoprecipitation (MeDIP), which targets and immunoprecipitates methylated DNA using 5-methylcytosine-specific antibody [141–146]. Similarly with MSRE, MeDIP-enriched DNA can also be analyzed using both microarray and NGS methods. Affymetrix provides short oligonucleotide tiling arrays that contain 25-bp long probes [130, 138]. These arrays are one-channel arrays and DNA from one sample is hybridized to one array. This type of array gives high specificity but suffers from lower sensitivity and higher noise [130, 141]. Each sample is hybridized to one array and comparison can be made across different arrays following normalization. Conversely, NimbleGen and Agilent offer long oligonucleotide arrays with probes that are 60-mers. NimbleGen arrays use an adaptive photolithographic method and can hold up to two million features, and Agilent arrays use inkjet technology and could hold up to ~240,000 features [130, 147]. Both Agilent and NimbleGen arrays are two-channel arrays where two samples can be labeled with different fluorescent dyes and hybridized on the same array. These arrays with longer probes yield higher sensitivity in comparison to the short oligonucleotide arrays but suffer from low specificity and

low probe density [148]. These are things that researchers need to consider before choosing the array platform they wish to employ.

A Case Study: Breast Cancer

Cell-Line Profiling

Cell-line models have been fundamental to understanding behavior of cancer, its types/subtypes, and response to treatment. While some researchers argue that cell-line models are not always true representative of primary tissues and may accumulate mutations specific to their growth cultures [149–151], cell lines continue to provide accurate insights into cancer biology at an affordable price [152–154]. Microarray profiling of genomic and transcriptomic features across a large compendium of breast cancer cell lines has enabled scientists to understand the similarities and differences between the cell-line models and primary tumors [153, 154]. Using DNA microarrays, profiling of 51 breast cell lines revealed a large number of genomic aberrations as present in the primary breast tumors as well. Likewise, RNA microarray profiling of the same 51 cell lines demonstrated distinctive expression clusters. These clusters were largely similar to the previously known human breast cancer molecular subtypes [155] with an exception of HER2-positive subtype. The authors further analyzed HER2-amplified cell lines following treatment with trastuzumab and observed variable levels of sensitivity, which is consistent with the variable response to trastuzumab in HER2-positive patients [156]. Such microarray analyses at genomic and transcriptomic levels highlight the promising potential of cell lines for the discovery of biologically and clinically relevant molecular features. For instance, disease subtype-specific cell lines can be used to test both the efficacy of new treatments and prognostic and predictive assessment of novel targets. Further, the convenience and affordability of cell lines combined with microarray profiling makes it an ideal choice for studying biological phenomena and generation of new hypotheses.

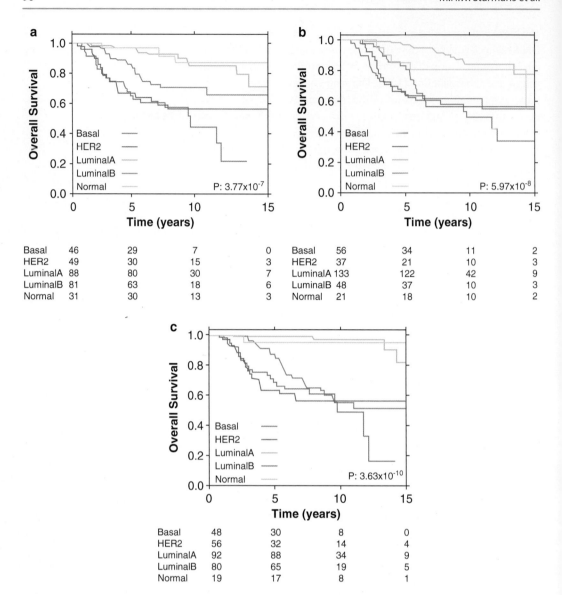

Basal	46	29	7	0
HER2	49	30	15	3
LuminalA	88	80	30	7
LuminalB	81	63	18	6
Normal	31	30	13	3

Basal	56	34	11	2
HER2	37	21	10	3
LuminalA	133	122	42	9
LuminalB	48	37	10	3
Normal	21	18	10	2

Basal	48	30	8	0
HER2	56	32	14	4
LuminalA	92	88	34	9
LuminalB	80	65	19	5
Normal	19	17	8	1

Fig. 7.4 Kaplan–Meier analysis of patients belonging to different subtypes of breast cancer using NKI cohort ($n=295$). (**a**, **b**, **c**) Subtype prediction was conducted using the gene sig- natures of Sorlie et al., Hu et al., and Parker et al., respectively. Groups were compared using log-rank test. Implementation of these classifiers was reused from Weigelt et al.

Primary Tumor Profiling

Microarray-based expression profiling has resulted in five well-established molecular sub- types of breast cancer: basal, HER2, luminal A, luminal B, and normal-like breast cancers [155]. These subtypes are associated with differential prognosis and response to treatment (Fig. 7.4). As shown in Fig. 7.4, patients presenting basal and

HER2 breast cancers have significantly shorter 5-year survival compared to luminal A, luminal B, and normal-like breast cancers. Since their dis- covery, a number of studies have focused on iden- tifying gene signatures that can distinctly classify patients into these subtypes [157–159]. These sig- natures are composed of 50–500 genes, along with centroids for every gene in each of the five subtypes. The centroids serve as a representative profile of each subtype and are used to estimate correlation with a new patient's expression profile, thereby determining patient's molecular subgroup. Detailed inspection of cross-classifier predictions has revealed that, apart from basal-type cancers, the concordance between these classifiers remains clinically unacceptable [160]. For instance, patients who demonstrate HER2 protein overexpression (by immunohistochemistry) are likely to benefit from targeted therapy with trastuzumab. However, if a microarray classifier misclassifies these patients, they would not benefit from the most appropriate treatment regime. Although genes underlying these subtypes manifest differential activity and relate with key cancer pathways, their ability to successfully guide therapeutic decisions has been largely unsuccessful.

To date, there are two clinically approved gene expression-based biomarkers for breast cancer prognosis: Oncotype DX [161] and MammaPrint [162]. Oncotype DX assay is RT-PCR based, while MammaPrint is the only microarray-based gene expression signature available for breast cancer clinical use. MammaPrint is a 70-gene signature that assesses the risk of recurrence in early stage breast cancer patients. These genes were identified on a series of 117 primary breast cancer patients with lymph node-negative status (discovery cohort) and validated on 295 patients (NKI cohort). Of these, 151 patients were lymph node negative (including 61 patients from the discovery cohort) and 144 were lymph node positive [162, 163]. The 70-gene signature was able to accurately identify patients at a higher risk of recurrence (Fig. 7.5a, b; poor prognosis group). The Kaplan–Meier analysis indicates the patients, which are likely to benefit from aggressive therapy (poor prognosis group). On the other hand, the good prognosis group comprises patients that could avoid overtreatment. Further prospective validation of MammaPrint is being conducted through a number of clinical trials such as ISPY-I/II and MINDACT [164, 165]. On molecular level, the two outcome groups exhibit distinct patterns of gene expression (Fig. 7.5c). As shown in the heatmap, patients with high risk of recurrence cluster together and are char-

acterized by a combination of over- and under-expressed genes, and vice versa. In terms of functional interpretation, recent studies have shown that these 70 genes are regulated by key tumorigenesis-associated genes including CDKN2A, JUN, MYC, RB1, and TP53 [166]. This is where high-throughput nature of microarrays serves as a very useful tool as it enables researchers to characterize the signature genes by integrating activity of known gene–gene interactions as well as cancer-associated genes. In general, microarray-based gene expression activity landscape for any given prognostic signature serves two important functions beyond biomarker discovery: (1) it can shed light on the underlying tumor biology of patients with differential outcome and/or response to treatment, and (2) the signature genes along with their interaction partners serve as potential targets towards the discovery of cancer drugs.

From a clinical perspective, MammaPrint test can be applied to breast cancer patients (invasive carcinoma) satisfying the eligibility criteria as outlined in Table 7.5. If a patient satisfies these criteria, MammaPrint test kit can be ordered through its marketing company Agendia. The protocol involves extraction of tumor biopsy specimens (fresh or paraffin embedded) and submission to Agendia for subsequent microarray profiling of 70 genes. The test in turn correlates the expression profile of the 70 genes for that patient with a preestablished good prognosis profile. Depending upon the strength of similarity between the patient's profile and the representative good prognosis profile, patient's risk group is determined. This dichotomous classification system means that if a patient is labeled as low-risk, there is a 10 % chance of tumor recurrence within 10 years without hormonal therapy or chemotherapy. However, if a patient is labeled as high-risk, there is a 29 % chance of recurrence within 10 years without hormonal therapy or chemotherapy. The risk classification, in combination with other risk factors, can guide oncologists on the most optimal treatment choices. For instance, patients classed as high-risk groups are prime candidates for aggressive chemotherapy to reduce the risk of metastasis.

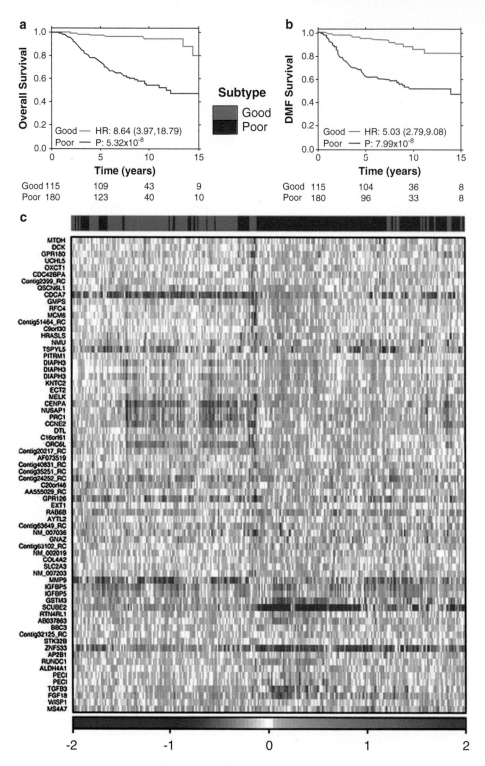

Fig. 7.5 (**a**, **b**) Kaplan–Meier analysis of patients belonging to low- and high-risk prognosis groups using NKI cohort ($n = 295$). (**a**) and (**b**) represent overall and distant metastasis-free (DMF) survival, respectively. Groups were compared using log-rank test. (**c**) Heatmap of expression profiles of 70 genes in NKI cohort. *Rows* represent genes (HGNC gene symbol, and probe name where

gene symbol was not available). *Columns* represent patients' gene expression levels for 70 genes. Ward's hierarchical clustering was performed using Pearson correlation as distance metric across rows and columns. The covariate *bar* across the *top* represents good (*blue*) and poor (*red*) prognosis groups. Re-annotated NKI dataset was used from Weigelt, B et al.

Table 7.5 Eligibility criteria for the MammaPrint testing in invasive breast cancer

Region	Tumor stage	Tumor size (cm)	Lymph node	Estrogen receptor
US	1, 2	<5	Negative	Negative, positive
Internationally	1, 2	<5	Negative, positive ($\leq$3 nodes)	Negative, positive

The Future of Microarrays

While sequencing-based methods continue to gain traction in the research community, it is likely that microarray technologies will be in use for many years. Their combination of low prices, high reproducibility, and well-characterized bioinformatics pipelines makes them ideal for quality control pipelines and for clinical diagnostics. Indeed, it remains standard for next-generation sequencing studies to include DNA arrays alongside whole-genome sequencing studies as both a quality assurance [167–169] and to help in the detection of cellular heterogeneity [170, 171].

References

1. Fodor SP, et al. Light-directed, spatially addressable parallel chemical synthesis. Science. 1991;251:767–73.
2. Schena M, Shalon D, Davis RW, Brown PO. Quantitative monitoring of gene expression patterns with a complementary DNA microarray. Science. 1995;270:467–70.
3. Shalon D, Smith SJ, Brown PO. A DNA microarray system for analyzing complex DNA samples using two-color fluorescent probe hybridization. Genome Res. 1996;6:639–45.
4. Lockhart DJ, et al. Expression monitoring by hybridization to high-density oligonucleotide arrays. Nat Biotechnol. 1996;14:1675–80.
5. MacBeath G. Protein microarrays and proteomics. Nat Genet. 2002;32(Suppl):526–32.
6. Pollack JR, et al. Genome-wide analysis of DNA copy-number changes using cDNA microarrays. Nat Genet. 1999;23:41–6.
7. Heinrichs S, Look AT. Identification of structural aberrations in cancer by SNP array analysis. Genome Biol. 2007;8:219.
8. Laird PW. Principles and challenges of genome-wide DNA methylation analysis. Nat Rev Genet. 2010;11:191–203.
9. Shoemaker DD, et al. Experimental annotation of the human genome using microarray technology. Nature. 2001;409:922–7.
10. Hughes TR, et al. Expression profiling using microarrays fabricated by an ink-jet oligonucleotide synthesizer. Nat Biotechnol. 2001;19:342–7.
11. Searles RP. Arrays for the masses-setting up a microarray facility. In: Blalock E, editor. A beginner's guide to microarrays. Boston: Kluwer; 2003. p. 123–49.
12. Dalma-Weiszhausz DD, Warrington J, Tanimoto EY, Miyada CG. The Affymetrix GeneChip platform: an overview. Methods Enzymol. 2006;410:3–28.
13. Tomiuk S, Hofmann K. Microarray probe selection strategies. Brief Bioinform. 2001;2:329–40.
14. Chou CC, Chen CH, Lee TT, Peck K. Optimization of probe length and the number of probes per gene for optimal microarray analysis of gene expression. Nucleic Acids Res. 2004;32:e99.
15. Mah N, et al. A comparison of oligonucleotide and cDNA-based microarray systems. Physiol Genomics. 2004;16:361–70.
16. Miller MB, Tang YW. Basic concepts of microarrays and potential applications in clinical microbiology. Clin Microbiol Rev. 2009;22:611–33.
17. Hekstra D, Taussig AR, Magnasco M, Naef F. Absolute mRNA concentrations from sequence-specific calibration of oligonucleotide arrays. Nucleic Acids Res. 2003;31:1962–8.
18. Held GA, Grinstein G, Tu Y. Modeling of DNA microarray data by using physical properties of hybridization. Proc Natl Acad Sci U S A. 2003;100:7575–80.
19. Yang YH, Speed T. Design issues for cDNA microarray experiments. Nat Rev Genet. 2002;3:579–88.
20. Nygaard V, Hovig E. Options available for profiling small samples: a review of sample amplification technology when combined with microarray profiling. Nucleic Acids Res. 2006;34:996–1014.
21. Kurimoto K, Saitou M. Single-cell cDNA microarray profiling of complex biological processes of differentiation. Curr Opin Genet Dev. 2010;20:470–7.
22. The International Human Genome Sequencing Consortium. Help in accessing human genome information. Science. 2000;289:1471b.
23. Lander ES, et al. Initial sequencing and analysis of the human genome. Nature. 2001;409:860–921.
24. Halgren RG, Fielden MR, Fong CJ, Zacharewski TR. Assessment of clone identity and sequence fidelity for 1189 IMAGE cDNA clones. Nucleic Acids Res. 2001;29:582–8.
25. Knight J. When the chips are down. Nature. 2001;410:860–1.
26. Dai M, et al. Evolving gene/transcript definitions significantly alter the interpretation of GeneChip data. Nucleic Acids Res. 2005;33:e175.
27. Tsai J, et al. RESOURCERER: a database for annotating and linking microarray resources within and across species. Genome Biol. 2001;2: SOFTWARE0002.

28. Elo LL, et al. Integrating probe-level expression changes across generations of Affymetrix arrays. Nucleic Acids Res. 2005;33:e193.

29. Carter SL, Eklund AC, Mecham BH, Kohane IS, Szallasi Z. Redefinition of Affymetrix probe sets by sequence overlap with cDNA microarray probes reduces cross-platform inconsistencies in cancer-associated gene expression measurements. BMC Bioinformatics. 2005;6:107.

30. Consortium M, et al. The MicroArray Quality Control (MAQC) project shows inter- and intraplatform reproducibility of gene expression measurements. Nat Biotechnol. 2006;24:1151–61.

31. Shi L, et al. The MicroArray Quality Control (MAQC)-II study of common practices for the development and validation of microarray-based predictive models. Nat Biotechnol. 2010;28: 827–38.

32. Tan PK, et al. Evaluation of gene expression measurements from commercial microarray platforms. Nucleic Acids Res. 2003;31:5676–84.

33. Tumor Analysis Best Practices Working Group. Expression profiling—best practices for data generation and interpretation in clinical trials. Nat Rev Genet. 2004;5:229–37.

34. Starmans MH, et al. Exploiting the noise: improving biomarkers with ensembles of data analysis methodologies. Genome Med. 2012;4:84.

35. Dupuy A, Simon RM. Critical review of published microarray studies for cancer outcome and guidelines on statistical analysis and reporting. J Natl Cancer Inst. 2007;99:147–57.

36. Coombes KR, Wang J, Baggerly KA. Microarrays: retracing steps. Nat Med. 2007;13:1276–7. author reply 1277–1278.

37. Edgar R, Domrachev M, Lash AE. Gene Expression Omnibus: NCBI gene expression and hybridization array data repository. Nucleic Acids Res. 2002;30: 207–10.

38. Brazma A, et al. ArrayExpress—a public repository for microarray gene expression data at the EBI. Nucleic Acids Res. 2003;31:68–71.

39. Brazma A, et al. Minimum information about a microarray experiment (MIAME)-toward standards for microarray data. Nat Genet. 2001;29:365–71.

40. Piwowar HA, Day RS, Fridsma DB. Sharing detailed research data is associated with increased citation rate. PLoS One. 2007;2:e308.

41. Ioannidis JP, et al. Repeatability of published microarray gene expression analyses. Nat Genet. 2009;41: 149–55.

42. Goodman L. Unlimited access—limitless success. Genome Res. 2001;11:637–8.

43. Gentleman RC, et al. Bioconductor: open software development for computational biology and bioinformatics. Genome Biol. 2004;5:R80.

44. Gupta V, et al. Directly labeled mRNA produces highly precise and unbiased differential gene expression data. Nucleic Acids Res. 2003;31:e13.

45. Irizarry RA, et al. Summaries of Affymetrix GeneChip probe level data. Nucleic Acids Res. 2003;31:e15.

46. Babak T, Zhang W, Morris Q, Blencowe BJ, Hughes TR. Probing microRNAs with microarrays: tissue specificity and functional inference. RNA. 2004;10: 1813–9.

47. Liu C-G, et al. An oligonucleotide microchip for genome wide microRNA profiling in human and mouse tissues. Proc Natl Acad Sci U S A. 2004;101:9740–4.

48. Schmittgen TD, Jiang J, Liu Q, Yang L. A high-throughput method to monitor the expression of microRNA precursors. Nucleic Acids Res. 2004;32:e43.

49. Irizarry RA, et al. Exploration, normalization, and summaries of high density oligonucleotide array probe level data. Biostatistics. 2003;4:249–64.

50. Durbin BP, Rocke DM. Variance-stabilizing transformations for two-color microarrays. Bioinformatics. 2004;20:660–7.

51. Edwards D. Non-linear normalization and background correction in one-channel cDNA microarray studies. Bioinformatics. 2003;19:825–33.

52. Gilad Y, Oshlack A, Smyth GK, Speed TP, White KP. Expression profiling in primates reveals a rapid evolution of human transcription factors. Nature. 2006;440:242–5.

53. Huber W, von Heydebreck A, Sultmann H, Poustka A, Vingron M. Variance stabilization applied to microarray data calibration and to the quantification of differential expression. Bioinformatics. 2002;18: S96–104.

54. Kooperberg C, Fazzio TG, Delrow JJ, Tsukiyama T. Improved background correction for spotted DNA microarrays. J Comput Biol. 2002;9:55–66.

55. Peart MJ, et al. Identification and functional significance of genes regulated by structurally different histone deacetylase inhibitors. Proc Natl Acad Sci U S A. 2005;102:3697–702.

56. Smyth GK. Limma: linear models for microarray data. In: Gentleman R, Carey V, Dudoit S, Irizarry R, Huber W, editors. Bioinformatics and computational biology solutions using R and Bioconductor. New York: Springer; 2005. p. 397–420.

57. Sarkar D, et al. Quality assessment and data analysis for microRNA expression arrays. Nucleic Acids Res. 2009;37:e17.

58. Meyer SU, Pfaffl MW, Ulbrich SE. Normalization strategies for microRNA profiling experiments: a 'normal' way to a hidden layer of complexity? Biotechnol Lett. 2010;32:1777–88.

59. Ketela T, et al. A comprehensive platform for highly multiplexed mammalian functional genetic screens. BMC Genomics. 2011;12:213.

60. Oeffinger M, et al. Comprehensive analysis of diverse ribonucleoprotein complexes. Nat Methods. 2007;4:951–6.

61. Niranjanakumari S, Lasda E, Brazas R, Garcia-Blanco MA. Reversible cross-linking combined with

immunoprecipitation to study RNA-protein interactions in vivo. Methods. 2002;26:182–90.

62. Khalil AM, et al. Many human large intergenic noncoding RNAs associate with chromatin-modifying complexes and affect gene expression. Proc Natl Acad Sci U S A. 2009;106:11667–72.

63. Rinn JL, et al. Functional demarcation of active and silent chromatin domains in human HOX loci by noncoding RNAs. Cell. 2007;129:1311–23.

64. Tenenbaum SA, Carson CC, Lager PJ, Keene JD. Identifying mRNA subsets in messenger ribonucleoprotein complexes by using cDNA arrays. Proc Natl Acad Sci U S A. 2000;97:14085–90.

65. Gerber AP, Luschnig S, Krasnow MA, Brown PO, Herschlag D. Genome-wide identification of mRNAs associated with the translational regulator PUMILIO in Drosophila melanogaster. Proc Natl Acad Sci U S A. 2006;103:4487–92.

66. Guttman M, et al. Chromatin signature reveals over a thousand highly conserved large non-coding RNAs in mammals. Nature. 2009;458:223–7.

67. López de Silanes I, Zhan M, Lal A, Yang X, Gorospe M. Identification of a target RNA motif for RNA-binding protein HuR. Proc Natl Acad Sci U S A. 2004;101:2987–92.

68. Dong S, et al. Flexible use of high-density oligonucleotide arrays for single-nucleotide polymorphism discovery and validation. Genome Res. 2001;11:1418–24.

69. Lisitsyn N, Wigler M. Cloning the differences between two complex genomes. Science. 1993;259:946–51.

70. Huang LE, Gu J, Schau M, Bunn HF. Regulation of hypoxia-inducible factor 1 is mediated by an O2-dependent degradation domain via the ubiquitin-proteasome pathway. Proc Natl Acad Sci. 1998;95:7987–92.

71. Gu J, Parthasarathi S, Varela-Echavarría A, Ron Y, Dougherty JP. Mutations of conserved cysteine residues in the CWLC motif of the oncoretrovirus SU protein affect maturation and translocation. Virology. 1995;206:885–93.

72. Wang Y, et al. Precision and functional specificity in mRNA decay. Proc Natl Acad Sci U S A. 2002;99:5860–5.

73. Chu E, Allegra CJ. The role of thymidylate synthase as an RNA binding protein. Bioessays. 1996;18:191–8.

74. Chu E, et al. Identification of in vivo target RNA sequences bound by thymidylate synthase. Nucleic Acids Res. 1996;24:3222–8.

75. Derrigo M, Cestelli A, Savettieri G, Di Liegro I. RNA-protein interactions in the control of stability and localization of messenger RNA (review). Int J Mol Med. 2000;5:111–23.

76. Mikulits W, et al. Isolation of translationally controlled mRNAs by differential screening. FASEB J. 2000;14:1641–52.

77. Sheikh MS, Fornace AJ. Regulation of translation initiation following stress. Oncogene. 1999;18:6121–8.

78. Arava Y, et al. Genome-wide analysis of mRNA translation profiles in Saccharomyces cerevisiae. Proc Natl Acad Sci U S A. 2003;100:3889–94.

79. Ju J, et al. Simultaneous gene expression analysis of steady-state and actively translated mRNA populations from osteosarcoma MG-63 cells in response to IL-1alpha via an open expression analysis platform. Nucleic Acids Res. 2003;31:5157–66.

80. Kudo K, et al. Translational control analysis by translationally active RNA capture/microarray analysis (TrIP-Chip). Nucleic Acids Res. 2010;38:e104.

81. Morris DR. Growth control of translation in mammalian cells. Prog Nucleic Acid Res Mol Biol. 1995;51:339–63.

82. Zong Q, Schummer M, Hood L, Morris DR. Messenger RNA translation state: the second dimension of high-throughput expression screening. Proc Natl Acad Sci U S A. 1999;96:10632–6.

83. Altshuler D, et al. An SNP map of the human genome generated by reduced representation shotgun sequencing. Nature. 2000;407:513–6.

84. Lucito R, et al. Genetic analysis using genomic representations. Proc Natl Acad Sci U S A. 1998;95:4487–92.

85. Vos P, et al. AFLP: a new technique for DNA fingerprinting. Nucleic Acids Res. 1995;23:4407–14.

86. Kennedy GC, et al. Large-scale genotyping of complex DNA. Nat Biotechnol. 2003;21:1233–7.

87. Carvalho B, Bengtsson H, Speed TP, Irizarry RA. Exploration, normalization, and genotype calls of high-density oligonucleotide SNP array data. Biostatistics. 2007;8:485–99.

88. Affymetrix. BRLMM: an Improved Genotype Calling Method for the GeneChip® Human Mapping 500K Array Set. 2006.

89. Affymetrix. BRLMM-P: a Genotype Calling Method for the SNP 5.0 Array. 2007.

90. Carvalho BS, Louis TA, Irizarry RA. Quantifying uncertainty in genotype calls. Bioinformatics. 2010; 26:242–9.

91. Korn JM, et al. Integrated genotype calling and association analysis of SNPs, common copy number polymorphisms and rare CNVs. Nat Genet. 2008;40:1253–60.

92. Dugad R, Desai UB. A tutorial on hidden Markov models. Research memorandum, Department of Electrical Engineering, Indian Institute of Technology, Bombay Technical Report No. SPANN-96.1; 1996.

93. Colella S, et al. QuantiSNP: an objective Bayes hidden-Markov model to detect and accurately map copy number variation using SNP genotyping data. Nucleic Acids Res. 2007;35:2013–25.

94. Nannya Y, et al. A robust algorithm for copy number detection using high-density oligonucleotide single nucleotide polymorphism genotyping arrays. Cancer Res. 2005;65:6071–9.

95. Wang K, et al. PennCNV: an integrated hidden Markov model designed for high-resolution copy number variation detection in whole-genome SNP genotyping data. Genome Res. 2007;17:1665–74.

96. Zhao X, et al. An integrated view of copy number and allelic alterations in the cancer genome using single nucleotide polymorphism arrays. Cancer Res. 2004;64:3060–71.

97. Bengtsson H, Irizarry R, Carvalho B, Speed TP. Estimation and assessment of raw copy numbers at the single locus level. Bioinformatics. 2008;24: 759–67.

98. Bengtsson H, Wirapati P, Speed TP. A single-array preprocessing method for estimating full-resolution raw copy numbers from all Affymetrix genotyping arrays including GenomeWideSNP 5 & 6. Bioinformatics. 2009;25:2149–56.

99. Hupé P, Stransky N, Thiery J-P, Radvanyi F, Barillot E. Analysis of array CGH data: from signal ratio to gain and loss of DNA regions. Bioinformatics. 2004;20:3413–22.

100. LaFramboise T, Winckler W, Thomas RK. A flexible rank-based framework for detecting copy number aberrations from array data. Bioinformatics. 2009;25: 722–8.

101. Yavaş G, Koyutürk M, Ozsoyoğlu M, Gould MP, Laframboise T. COKGEN: a software for the identification of rare copy number variation from SNP microarrays. Pac Symp Biocomput. 2010;371–82. ISBN: 978-981-4299-47-3.

102. Fridlyand J, Snijders AM, Pinkel D, Albertson DG, Jain AN. Hidden Markov models approach to the analysis of array CGH data. J Multivariate Anal. 2004;90:132–53.

103. Olshen AB, Venkatraman ES, Lucito R, Wigler M. Circular binary segmentation for the analysis of array-based DNA copy number data. Biostatistics. 2004;5:557–72.

104. Cawley S, et al. Unbiased mapping of transcription factor binding sites along human chromosomes 21 and 22 points to widespread regulation of noncoding RNAs. Cell. 2004;116:499–509.

105. Ji H, Wong WH. TileMap: create chromosomal map of tiling array hybridizations. Bioinformatics. 2005;21:3629–36.

106. Johnson WE, et al. Model-based analysis of tiling-arrays for ChIP-chip. Proc Natl Acad Sci U S A. 2006;103:12457–62.

107. Keleş S, van der Laan MJ, Dudoit S, Cawley SE. Multiple testing methods for ChIP-chip high density oligonucleotide array data. J Comput Biol. 2006;13: 579–613.

108. Li W, Meyer CA, Liu XS. A hidden Markov model for analyzing ChIP-chip experiments on genome tiling arrays and its application to p53 binding sequences. Bioinformatics. 2005;21 Suppl 1:i274–82.

109. Potter DP, Yan P, Huang THM, Lin S. Probe signal correction for differential methylation hybridization experiments. BMC Bioinformatics. 2008;9:453.

110. VanGuilder HD, Vrana KE, Freeman WM. Twenty-five years of quantitative PCR for gene expression analysis. Biotechniques. 2008;44:619–26.

111. Adams MD, et al. Complementary DNA sequencing: expressed sequence tags and human genome project. Science. 1991;252:1651–6.

112. Velculescu VE, Zhang L, Vogelstein B, Kinzler KW. Serial analysis of gene expression. Science. 1995;270:484–7.

113. Schulze A, Downward J. Navigating gene expression using microarrays—a technology review. Nat Cell Biol. 2001;3:E190 5.

114. Draghici S, Khatri P, Eklund AC, Szallasi Z. Reliability and reproducibility issues in DNA microarray measurements. Trends Genet. 2006;22: 101–9.

115. Vartanian K, et al. Gene expression profiling of whole blood: comparison of target preparation methods for accurate and reproducible microarray analysis. BMC Genomics. 2009;10:2.

116. Wren JD, Kulkarni A, Joslin J, Butow RA, Garner HR. Cross-hybridization on PCR-spotted microarrays. IEEE Eng Med Biol Mag. 2002;21:71–5.

117. Grabherr MG, et al. Full-length transcriptome assembly from RNA-Seq data without a reference genome. Nat Biotechnol. 2011;29:644–52.

118. Zerbino DR, Birney E. Velvet: algorithms for de novo short read assembly using de Bruijn graphs. Genome Res. 2008;18:821–9.

119. Trapnell C, et al. Transcript assembly and quantification by RNA-Seq reveals unannotated transcripts and isoform switching during cell differentiation. Nat Biotechnol. 2010;28:511–5.

120. Langmead B, Trapnell C, Pop M, Salzberg SL. Ultrafast and memory-efficient alignment of short DNA sequences to the human genome. Genome Biol. 2009;10:R25.

121. Clement NL, et al. The GNUMAP algorithm: unbiased probabilistic mapping of oligonucleotides from next-generation sequencing. Bioinformatics. 2010;26: 38–45.

122. Li H, Ruan J, Durbin R. Mapping short DNA sequencing reads and calling variants using mapping quality scores. Genome Res. 2008;18:1851–8.

123. David M, Dzamba M, Lister D, Ilie L, Brudno M. SHRiMP2: sensitive yet practical SHort Read Mapping. Bioinformatics. 2011;27:1011–2.

124. Ozols RF, et al. Phase III trial of carboplatin and paclitaxel compared with cisplatin and paclitaxel in patients with optimally resected stage III ovarian cancer: a gynecologic oncology group study. J Clin Oncol. 2003;21:3194–200.

125. Abecasis GR, et al. A map of human genome variation from population-scale sequencing. Nature. 2010;467:1061–73.

126. Xi R, Kim TM, Park PJ. Detecting structural variations in the human genome using next generation sequencing. Brief Funct Genomics. 2010;9:405–15.

127. Sobreira NL, et al. Characterization of complex chromosomal rearrangements by targeted capture and next-generation sequencing. Genome Res. 2011;21:1720–7.

128. Naeem R, Rashid M, Pain A. READSCAN: a fast and scalable pathogen discovery program with accurate genome relative abundance estimation. Bioinformatics. 2013;29:391–2.

129. Hurd PJ, Nelson CJ. Advantages of next-generation sequencing versus the microarray in epigenetic research. Brief Funct Genomic Proteomic. 2009;8:174–83.

130. Zilberman D, Henikoff S. Genome-wide analysis of DNA methylation patterns. Development. 2007;134: 3959–65.

131. Tost J, Gut IG. Analysis of gene-specific DNA methylation patterns by pyrosequencing technology. Methods Mol Biol. 2007;373:89–102.

132. Eckhardt F, et al. DNA methylation profiling of human chromosomes 6, 20 and 22. Nat Genet. 2006; 38:1378–85.

133. Bibikova M, et al. High-throughput DNA methylation profiling using universal bead arrays. Genome Res. 2006;16:383–93.

134. Fan J-B, et al. Illumina universal bead arrays. Methods Enzymol. 2006;410:57–73.

135. Khulan B, et al. Comparative isoschizomer profiling of cytosine methylation: the HELP assay. Genome Res. 2006;16:1046–55.

136. Lippman Z, Gendrel A-V, Colot V, Martienssen R. Profiling DNA methylation patterns using genomic tiling microarrays. Nat Methods. 2005;2:219–24.

137. Rollins RA, et al. Large-scale structure of genomic methylation patterns. Genome Res. 2006;16: 157–63.

138. Schumacher A, et al. Microarray-based DNA methylation profiling: technology and applications. Nucleic Acids Res. 2006;34:528–42.

139. Tompa R, et al. Genome-wide profiling of DNA methylation reveals transposon targets of CHROMOMETHYLASE3. Curr Biol. 2002;12: 65–8.

140. Yuan E, et al. A single nucleotide polymorphism chip-based method for combined genetic and epigenetic profiling: validation in decitabine therapy and tumor/normal comparisons. Cancer Res. 2006;66: 3443–51.

141. Keshet I, et al. Evidence for an instructive mechanism of de novo methylation in cancer cells. Nat Genet. 2006;38:149–53.

142. Reynaud C, et al. Monitoring of urinary excretion of modified nucleosides in cancer patients using a set of six monoclonal antibodies. Cancer Lett. 1992;61: 255–62.

143. Weber M, et al. Chromosome-wide and promoter-specific analyses identify sites of differential DNA methylation in normal and transformed human cells. Nat Genet. 2005;37:853–62.

144. Weber M, et al. Distribution, silencing potential and evolutionary impact of promoter DNA methylation in the human genome. Nat Genet. 2007;39:457–66.

145. Zhang X, et al. Genome-wide high-resolution mapping and functional analysis of DNA methylation in arabidopsis. Cell. 2006;126:1189–201.

146. Zilberman D, Gehring M, Tran RK, Ballinger T, Henikoff S. Genome-wide analysis of Arabidopsis thaliana DNA methylation uncovers an interdependence between methylation and transcription. Nat Genet. 2007;39:61–9.

147. Wolber PK, Collins PJ, Lucas AB, De Witte A, Shannon KW. The Agilent in situ-synthesized microarray platform. Methods Enzymol. 2006;410:28–57.

148. Kreil DP, Russell RR, Russell S. Microarray oligonucleotide probes. Methods Enzymol. 2006;410: 73–98.

149. Mehta JP, O'Driscoll L, Barron N, Clynes M, Doolan P. A microarray approach to translational medicine in breast cancer: how representative are cell line models of clinical conditions? Anticancer Res. 2007;27:1295–300.

150. Gillet JP, Varma S, Gottesman MM. The clinical relevance of cancer cell lines. J Natl Cancer Inst. 2013;105:452–8.

151. Gillet JP, et al. Redefining the relevance of established cancer cell lines to the study of mechanisms of clinical anti-cancer drug resistance. Proc Natl Acad Sci U S A. 2011;108:18708–13.

152. Bignell GR, et al. Signatures of mutation and selection in the cancer genome. Nature. 2010;463:893–8.

153. Chin K, et al. Genomic and transcriptional aberrations linked to breast cancer pathophysiologies. Cancer Cell. 2006;10:529–41.

154. Neve RM, et al. A collection of breast cancer cell lines for the study of functionally distinct cancer subtypes. Cancer Cell. 2006;10:515–27.

155. Sorlie T, et al. Gene expression patterns of breast carcinomas distinguish tumor subclasses with clinical implications. Proc Natl Acad Sci U S A. 2001;98:10869–74.

156. Montemurro F, et al. Outcome of patients with HER2-positive advanced breast cancer progressing during trastuzumab-based therapy. Oncologist. 2006;11:318–24.

157. Hu Z, et al. The molecular portraits of breast tumors are conserved across microarray platforms. BMC Genomics. 2006;7:96.

158. Parker JS, et al. Supervised risk predictor of breast cancer based on intrinsic subtypes. J Clin Oncol. 2009;27:1160–7.

159. Sorlie T, et al. Repeated observation of breast tumor subtypes in independent gene expression data sets. Proc Natl Acad Sci U S A. 2003;100:8418–23.

160. Weigelt B, et al. Breast cancer molecular profiling with single sample predictors: a retrospective analysis. Lancet Oncol. 2010;11:339–49.

161. Paik S, et al. A multigene assay to predict recurrence of tamoxifen-treated, node-negative breast cancer. N Engl J Med. 2004;351:2817–26.

162. van de Vijver MJ, et al. A gene-expression signature as a predictor of survival in breast cancer. N Engl J Med. 2002;347:1999–2009.

163. van 't Veer LJ, et al. Gene expression profiling predicts clinical outcome of breast cancer. Nature. 2002;415:530–6.

164. Cardoso F, et al. Clinical application of the 70-gene profile: the MINDACT trial. J Clin Oncol. 2008;26: 729–35.
165. Cardoso F, Piccart-Gebhart M, Van't Veer L, Rutgers E, Consortium T. The MINDACT trial: the first prospective clinical validation of a genomic tool. Mol Oncol. 2007;1:246–51.
166. Tian S, et al. Biological functions of the genes in the mammaprint breast cancer profile reflect the hallmarks of cancer. Biomark Insights. 2010;5:129–38.
167. The Cancer Genome Atlas Research Network. Comprehensive molecular characterization of human colon and rectal cancer. Nature. 2012;487:330–7.
168. Baca SC, et al. Punctuated evolution of prostate cancer genomes. Cell. 2013;153:666–77.
169. Network TCGA. Comprehensive molecular portraits of human breast tumours. Nature. 2012;490: 61–70.
170. Carter SL, et al. Absolute quantification of somatic DNA alterations in human cancer. Nat Biotechnol. 2012;30:413–21.
171. Quon G, et al. Computational purification of individual tumor gene expression profiles leads to significant improvements in prognostic prediction. Genome Med. 2013;5:29.

Proteomics in Cancer Diagnostics

8

Kevin P. Conlon, Delphine Rolland,
and Kojo S.J. Elenitoba-Johnson

Overview

Proteomics is the term used to describe the large-scale interrogation of proteins in cells, in tissues, or in an organism. Proteomics provides unparalleled opportunities to annotate protein expression, localization, interaction, modification, and function. Accordingly, proteomics techniques have been instrumental in the discovery of the function of proteins and their dysregulation in diseased states. Proteomics permit a refined view of disease biomarkers, protein-protein interactions involved in signaling, and the characterization of drug targets. Recently, mass spectrometry (MS)-driven proteomics approaches have been incorporated into routine clinical diagnostics.

Protein Microarrays

Principle of Protein Microarrays

Technologies that are well-established for DNA/RNA applications have been adapted for protein-based research resulting in the creation of protein microarrays. Protein microarrays permit interactions between proteins and capture reagents such as antibodies on a solid matrix. These may be configured as forward-phase arrays or reverse-phase arrays, depending on whether the sample is captured from a solution phase or bound to solid-phase matrixes such as membranes or glass (Fig. 8.1).

Forward-phase microarrays permit the simultaneous analysis of several parameters per sample. In forward-phase microarrays, specific proteins are selectively isolated from biological samples such as serum, plasma, cell lysates, or cell culture supernatants by using well-characterized capture agents such as antibodies, full-length proteins, or active protein domains that are immobilized onto a solid surface. Each spot of the array contains one type of immobilized antibody or bait molecule. Each array may be incubated with one sample and the bound analytes are visualized either by direct labeling of the analytes or by using labeled secondary antibodies. Strategies for signal detection include fluorescence, chemiluminescence, and colorimetry. Current microarray configurations permit the interrogation and screening of several analytes in one experiment. The concept of planar microarray-based systems has been successfully miniaturized and operationalized into a bead-based microarray system where each bead is coupled to a specific bait molecule. This bead-based microarray system provides an advantageous alternative since it is more flexible, robust, highly scalable, and amenable to automation.

For reverse-phase microarrays, multiple samples (tissues or cell lysates) are immobilized as

K.P. Conlon, B.Sc. • D. Rolland, Ph.D.
K.S.J. Elenitoba-Johnson, M.D. (✉)
Department of Pathology, University of Michigan
Medical School, 2037 BSRB, 109 Zina Pitcher Place,
Ann Arbor, MI 48109, USA
e-mail: kojoelen@umich.edu

G.M. Yousef and S. Jothy (eds.), *Molecular Testing in Cancer*,
DOI 10.1007/978-1-4899-8050-2_8, © Springer Science+Business Media New York 2014

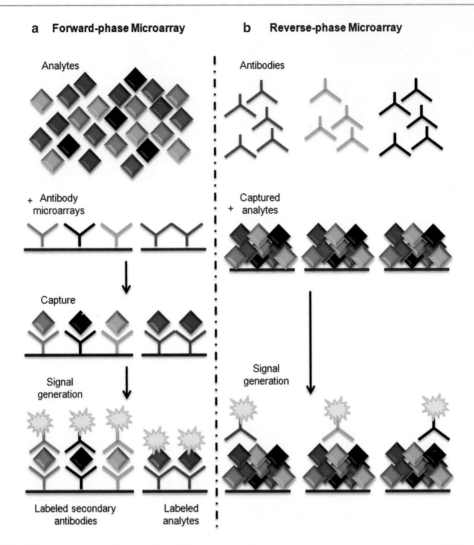

Fig. 8.1 Difference between forward-phase and reverse-phase protein microarrays. (**a**) Forward-phase microarray: capture antibodies are first immobilized on the slide surface. These immobilized antibodies are used to capture the antigens they recognize in a test sample. (**b**) Reverse-phase microarray: complex samples are immobilized on the surface and targeted by antibodies

distinct regularly distributed spots in rows and columns on a solid support such that the array contains numerous spots representing the proteome of different samples. Each microarray is incubated with one highly specific detection molecule or antibody, measuring a single analyte with direct comparison of the analyte across multiple samples. This approach allows the detection of sets of proteins present in large collections of tissue or cell samples.

Clinical Applications of Protein Microarrays

The applications of forward-phase microarrays are mainly in use for the detection of different protein classes such as cytokines and chemokines, signaling molecules, and/or cancer biomarkers. Many clinical applications of protein microarrays are for the diagnosis of infectious diseases or conditions associated with immune dysfunction. For example, the AtheNA Multi-Lyte® Test System (Zeus Scientific) has been used for the diagnosis of *Borrelia burgdorferi* infection by a multiplex sandwich immunoassay which quantitatively detects distinct IgG antibody to Vlse-1 and distinct IgM antibody to pepC10. Another example is the BioPlex™ 2200 ANA Screen (Bio-Rad Laboratories) which detects autoantibodies in serum or plasma and has found application as an aid in the diagnosis of systemic diseases such as systemic lupus erythematosus, mixed connective tissue disease, undifferentiated connective tissue disease, Sjogren's syndrome, scleroderma, dermatomyositis, polymyositis, rheumatoid arthritis, CREST syndrome, and Raynaud's disease.

Mass Spectrometry-Based Proteomic Analysis

Introduction to Mass Spectrometry

Instrumentation

A mass spectrometer can be broken down into four components: an ionization source, ion optics, the mass analyzer, and the detector. The ionization source allows ions from the sample to enter the mass spectrometer either by direct ionization of the sample or by permitting ions already formed in the sample to be released. The ion optics guide the charged analytes from the source to the mass analyzer without contacting internal components of the mass spectrometer which would neutralize the ion resulting in its loss. The mass analyzer selects and controls ions based on their mass-to-charge ratio (m/z). The detector indicates the relative signal intensity of the ions selected in the mass analyzer.

Ionization Source
MALDI
J.J. Thomson (1897) is credited with conducting the first mass spectrometry (MS) experiment in the early 1900s. Initially these MS-based efforts were limited to applications in analytical chemistry, but advances have broadened its applicability to a number of diverse fields including clinical

testing. Two different soft ionization techniques pioneered in the late 1980s facilitated the use of MS-based approaches in the examination of proteins and peptides. The first was matrix-assisted laser desorption/ionization (MALDI) [11, 23] (Fig. 8.2a). MALDI-based proteomic involves the co-crystallization of a protein/peptide sample on a suitable solid matrix. The vaporization and ionization of the protein/peptide sample is achieved by pulse irradiation of the surface with a laser. This technique generates ions that are ejected from the solid support into the gas phase and directed into the mass analyzer for analysis, filtering, and detection.

Electrospray Ionization
Electrospray ionization (ESI) [5] was another technique developed during this time which releases ions from solution into the gaseous phase at atmospheric pressure through ion desolvation (Fig. 8.2b). As the sample solution elutes under pressure from the ESI needle, a high voltage is applied to the tip forcing the spray into a Taylor cone and driving the ions in solution into smaller droplets which are desolvated using heat or dry gas as they pass into the mass spectrometer through the heated capillary tube. The process is generally thought to occur as a result of Coulombic explosion whereby ions of the same polarity are forced together as the solvent evaporates until the concentration of the ions exceeds the surface tension of the droplet and explodes leaving only charged ions to enter the mass analyzer.

Ion Optics
Ions are drawn into the mass spectrometer and guided to the mass analyzer by a series of ion optics using a combination of RF and DC voltages or magnetic fields under a vacuum gradient. Voltages are adjusted such that ions of opposite charge to the target analytes and neutrals are lost along the way and ions of interest are focused into a narrow beam.

Mass Analyzers
The mass analyzer measures and manipulates ions based upon their mass-to-charge ratios (m/z) ultimately directing the selected ions to an electron

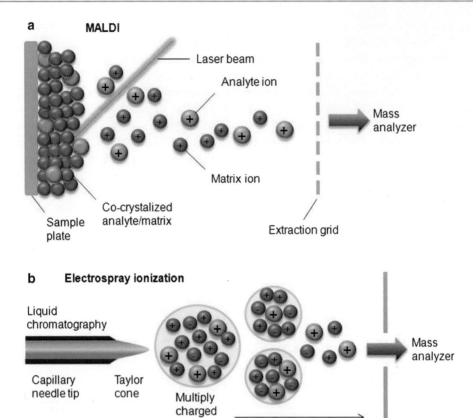

Fig. 8.2 Principles of operation of matrix-assisted laser desorption/ionization (MALDI) and electrospray ionization (ESI). (**a**) MALDI: The protein/peptide sample is co-crystallized with a matrix, then the vaporization and ionization of the protein/peptide sample is achieved by pulse irradiation of the surface with a laser. The matrix material heavily absorbs UV laser light, leading to the ablation of the upper layer of the matrix. This process generates ions that usually are accelerated into a mass analyzer for analysis. (**b**) ESI: The liquid containing the analyte is dispersed by electrospray into a fine aerosol. Via evaporation and the Coulomb explosion, large charged droplets are sequentially blown apart to form smaller droplets until reaching a certain droplet size limit, leaving only the discrete peptide sample ions to enter the mass analyzer

multiplier for detection. There are many types of mass analyzers; but three commonly used for proteomic analysis are time-of-flight (TOF), ion trap, and quadrupoles.

Time-of-Flight

In a TOF mass spectrometer, ions are accelerated down a flight tube by an electric field of known strength to impart the same kinetic energy to all ions in the field. The velocity of each ion then depends on its mass-to-charge ratio causing differences in transit time with lighter ions having a higher velocity than heavier ions. The time it takes each ion to reach the detector is measured, and from this time and the known experimental parameters, the mass-to-charge ratio of the ion can be determined.

Ion Traps

Ion traps come in various configurations but generally use alternating voltages to trap ions in the presence of helium gas in a stable oscillating trajectory based upon their m/z. Changes in voltage can induce resonance excitation causing the precursor ions to be ejected sequentially towards the detector in a controlled manner. Voltages can then be changed to impart sufficient kinetic energy to create collisions between the precursor ion and helium gas to generate smaller fragment or product ions (MS/MS), which are then directed to the detector. Newer variants such as Orbitrap offer much greater mass accuracy and confidence in the structural data obtained.

Quadrupoles

Quadrupoles are made up of a series of four parallel rods through which RF currents are applied to transmit ions over a range. A combination of RF and DC voltages can be applied to provide selection based upon the *m/z*. Only ions of a certain *m/z* will be transmitted for a given ratio of voltages; ions not selected will have unstable trajectories and collide with the rods. A triple quadrupole mass spectrometer is a series of three quadrupoles where the first (Q1) and third (Q3) act as mass filters. The middle quadrupole acts as a collision cell using a gas such as Ar for collision-induced dissociation (CID) of selected precursor ion(s) transmitted from Q1 producing fragment or product ions which are passed on to Q3 to be scanned or filtered.

These mass analyzers differ considerably in their ability to detect low abundance ions (sensitivity) and discriminate between ions with different *m/z* values (resolution), the extent to which the exact mass can be determined (mass accuracy), and the minimum and maximum *m/z* limit of the mass analyzer (mass range). They also differ in their capacity to perform tandem mass analysis (MS/MS) whereby a precursor ion is isolated and then fragmented into product ions which are further analyzed. Peptide fragmentation occurs in a predictable manner yielding structural information such as the amino acid sequence of the peptide or characterization of posttranslational protein modifications. Hybrid instruments containing different types of mass analyzers such as a quadrupole TOF can combine their strengths to enhance their individual characteristics. Selection of an ion source and mass analyzer depends on the specific application.

Identification Strategies

Mass spectrometry-driven proteomics is generally approached in either a top-down or bottom-up fashion. Top-down proteomics analyzes intact proteins or polypeptides eliminating the need to use a proteolytic enzyme and preserving the intact structural information of the molecule. Bottom-up proteomics is more commonly employed and uses a proteolytic enzyme such as trypsin, which cleaves C-terminal to arginine and lysine residues [16], to digest complex protein mixtures into peptides. These peptides are then separated by liquid chromatography (LC) and analyzed by tandem mass spectrometry (MS/MS). Precursor and product masses obtained can then be matched against translated genomic databases modified "in silico" to the specific cleavage of the proteolytic enzyme used producing theoretical precursor and product masses for each peptide (Fig. 8.3). The experimentally determined values are matched to the theoretical values of the peptides in the database. Numerous algorithms are employed to identify and provide a confidence score for the proteins and peptides matched. Some of the parameters considered for assigning a confidence score to each protein and peptide identified include the correctness of the match, uniqueness of the peptide sequence to a particular protein, overlapping or longer peptide sequences, and the number of times a peptide sequence is identified in a given sample.

Quantitative Mass Spectrometry-Based Proteomics

The ability to identify and quantitatively measure protein levels both globally and in a targeted fashion is an important component of mass spectrometry-based proteomics. Global quantitation of protein levels can be achieved via stable isotope labeling of proteins/peptides, using heavy peptides as standards and through label-free quantitation. Isotope labels can be introduced metabolically (i.e., in vivo), chemically, or enzymatically (i.e., in vitro).

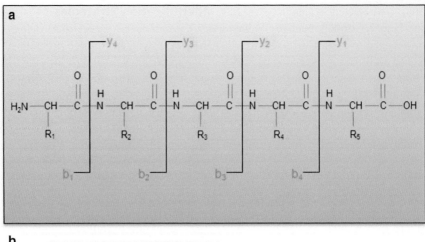

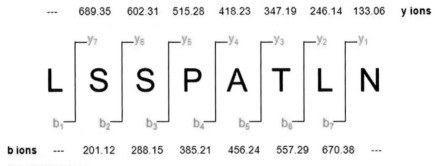

Fig. 8.3 Predicted precursor and product ions. (**a**) Tandem mass spectrometry (MS/MS) performed with low collision energies, as with ion traps and triple quadrupole mass spectrometers, fragment peptides in a predictable manner. The example peptide shows the predicted break points along the backbone under these conditions and provides the nomenclature for the C-terminal *b* ions and N-terminal *y* ions generated from this fragmentation. (**b**) The predicted precursor and product ions (*b* and *y*) for the trypsin autolysis peptide LSSPATLN are shown

In Vivo Quantification

The in vivo technique stable isotope labeling with amino acids in cell culture (SILAC) involves metabolic labeling of two distinct cellular populations in culture media deficient in a natural amino acid. Cells are maintained in culture for 6–7 passages in the presence of stable isotopes of the deficient amino acids (heavy Arg, Lys, Leu, or Ile). The two populations metabolically incorporate separate "light" and "heavy" isotopes into their cellular proteins after which they are combined in a 1:1 ratio and subjected to proteolytic digestion and analysis by mass spectrometry. Corresponding peptides from each sample co-elute during liquid chromatography and relative quantification is done by measuring the ratio of the "light" and "heavy" isotope from matching peptide/proteins. The requirement for viable cells to be maintained for 6–7 passages makes the usefulness of this technique in clinically relevant scenarios unlikely.

In Vitro Quantification

The in vitro methods for labeling include isotope-coded affinity tagging (ICAT) and isobaric tags for relative and absolute quantitation (iTRAQ) as well as tandem mass tag (TMT). These methods can be adapted to clinical scenarios since cell viability is not required for labeling. In the ICAT labeling method, cysteine residues are derivatized with a reagent containing either a "light" or "heavy"

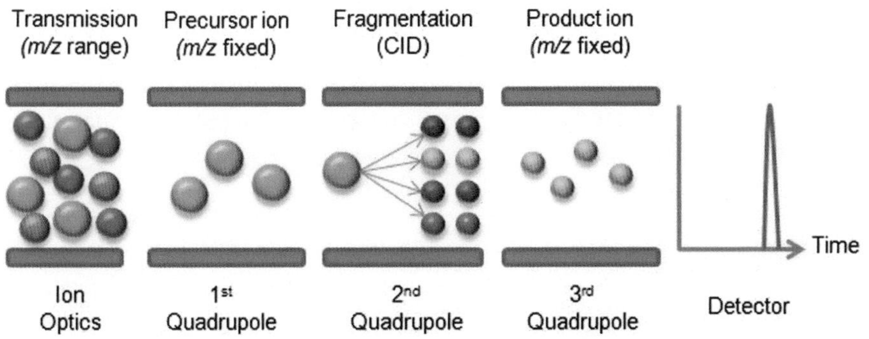

Transmission
(*m/z* range)

Precursor ion
(*m/z* fixed)

Fragmentation
(CID)

Product ion
(*m/z* fixed)

Time

Ion
Optics

1st
Quadrupole

2nd
Quadrupole

3rd
Quadrupole

Detector

Fig. 8.4 Multiple reaction monitoring (MRM) using a triple quadrupole mass spectrometer. Multiple co-eluting charged analytes enter the mass spectrometer from the chromatographic system and are transmitted to the first quadrupole (Q1) using the ion optics. Ionized peptide precursors with specific predefined mass-to-charge ratios (*m/z*) are selected in the first quadrupole (Q1) and transmitted to the second quadrupole (Q2) where collision-induced dissociation (CID) causes peptide fragmentation. Detection and quantification of the target analyte are achieved following selective transmission in the third quadrupole (Q3) of a predefined product ion to the detector

isotope in separate samples as well as a biotin group after which the samples are combined in a 1:1 ratio and digested with trypsin. The biotin group is used for affinity purification of the cysteine-derivatized peptides followed by mass spectrometry analysis. Sample complexity is greatly reduced with this approach; however, no quantitative information is available for peptides that do not contain a cysteine and is limited to binary comparisons between samples. The iTRAQ method is another in vitro labeling approach which tags the N-terminus amino acid of all peptides with varying masses in up to eight different biological samples providing simultaneous identification and relative quantification. Similarly, the TMT method labels primary amines with tags of varying mass allowing identification and measurement of protein expression in up to ten conditions simultaneously.

Label-Free Quantification

Label-free quantitation methods which do not require additional sample preparation and can be employed in either in vivo or in vitro scenarios are gaining popularity and are increasingly being employed as an alternative to label-based approaches. These techniques do not require isotopic labeling, but instead directly compare signal intensities across different mass spectrometry runs using either the signal intensity of peptide precursors or the number of fragment spectra identifying peptides of a given protein.

Targeted Quantification

Absolute quantification (AQUA) is a targeted approach using isotope-labeled synthetic peptides as standards spiked at known concentrations into a sample preparation. Quantitation is achieved by comparing the mass spectrometric signal intensity, area, or area ratio of the synthetic peptide(s) to its endogenous counterpart in the sample. Alternatively, all peptides in a sample can be compared to the synthetic peptide to obtain qualitative information on relative protein abundance.

Multiple Reaction Monitoring

Multiple reaction monitoring (MRM) and selected reaction monitoring (SRM) are terms often used interchangeably to refer to a targeted proteomic mass spectrometry technique where specific peptide ions from complex sample matrixes undergo selection—fragmentation—selection based upon their *m/z* using quadrupole mass analyzers (Fig. 8.4) [13]. Samples are typically digested with trypsin and separated by nano-LC eluting into the source of a triple quadrupole mass spectrometer where precursor peptide ions with predetermined m/z values are allowed to pass through the first quadrupole (Q1). Ions selected in Q1 are transmitted to the second quadrupole (Q2) where CID of the precursor ions occurs. Specific collision energies are applied to each precursor ion entering Q2 to generate sufficient velocity for peptide bonds to break as they collide with neutral gas molecules such as helium or argon that are pumped into the chamber. These product ions derived from the fragments of the precursor are transmitted to the third quadrupole (Q3) where specific predetermined product ions are passed to the electron multiplier for detection and positive identification of the target analyte. The power of MRM experiments is in allowing numerous proteins of interest to be selectively identified and quantitated in complex biological backgrounds.

Protein Posttranslational Modification Analysis by Mass Spectrometry

Phosphoproteomics

Phosphoproteomics involves the large-scale study of the phosphorylation state and specific modification sites of proteins within a protein sample obtained from tissues, cells, organelles, complex protein mixtures, or singular proteins. Reversible protein phosphorylations at serine, threonine, and tyrosine residues represent fundamental and highly evolutionarily conserved types of posttranslational protein modifications which control essential cellular processes including metabolism, growth, cell cycle, motility, and differentiation [10, 20]. The Human Genome Project identified more than 520 protein kinases and 130 protein phosphatases with tight and reversible control of protein phosphorylation. Deregulation of protein phosphorylation underlies the pathogenesis of many human diseases including diabetes, cardiovascular diseases [27], immune disorders [15], and cancer [2]. Recently, there has been an exponential increase of interest in tyrosine kinases (TKs) due to the remarkably successful introduction of specific tyrosine kinase inhibitors (TKIs) for the treatment of cancer. Indeed, many TKIs have been approved by the US Food and Drug Administration (FDA) as routine therapeutic options for certain human cancers [4].

Due to the low stoichiometry of phosphorylation as a posttranslational modification, strategies for enrichment of the phosphoproteome are required prior to analysis to improve opportunities to detect phosphorylation by mass spectrometry. Several methods are well-described for phosphopeptide or phosphoprotein enrichment such as strong cation exchange chromatography (SCX), immobilized metal affinity chromatography (IMAC), metal oxide affinity chromatography (MOAC) [14], and immunoaffinity purification (IAP) with high affinity anti-phosphotyrosine antibodies [19]. The first three methods are used for global phosphorylation enrichment and enrich for proteins that are phosphorylated at tyrosine, serine, or threonine residues. With the identification and quantification of phosphorylated peptides extracted from samples, intracellular signaling networks can be generated to highlight pathophysiological mechanisms. Global phosphoproteomics provides insights into pathways involved in physiologic or pathologic cellular responses that occur during the initiation or maintenance of disease phenotypes. Such knowledge has proven valuable in the development of targeted therapeutics for management of several conditions.

Glycoproteomics

Glycosylation represents the most common of all known posttranslational modifications, and like the majority of cell surface proteins, receptor TKs also are glycoproteins with asparagine-(N)-linked oligosaccharides (N-glycans). Since glycopeptides often constitute a minor proportion of complex peptide mixtures, several strategies have been developed to reduce the sample complexity and enrich glycoprotein content. One glycoprotein enrichment method is lectin affinity chromatography. In 2003, Zhang et al. suggested a new method for the selective isolation of N-glycosyl peptides [28]. This method for glycoprotein capture involves glycoprotein oxidation which converts the *cis*-diol groups of carbohydrates to aldehydes. These aldehydes are then derivatized with hydrazide groups immobilized on a solid support to form covalent hydrazone bonds. After protease digestion with trypsin, N-glycopeptides are released using peptide N-glycosidases (PNGase F). The identification and quantification of N-glycopeptides lead to characterization of proteins that are mainly expressed at the plasma membrane and, therefore, could be useful as potential diagnostic biomarkers.

Clinical Applications of Qualitative Mass Spectrometry Proteomic Analysis

Amyloid Typing by Mass Spectrometry

Amyloidosis is an accumulation of amorphous insoluble protein deposits in extracellular space. Apple-green birefringence on Congo red staining has traditionally been used as the method of detection. The advent of mass spectrometry has permitted MS-based proteomics to be utilized in combination with tissue microdissection for the diagnosis and typing of amyloidosis [6, 25]. With this approach, specific clinical variants of amyloidosis have been correlated with the predominant protein components within the amyloid deposits in the tissue specimens. Using MS-based proteomics, various forms of amyloidosis have been defined, including AL amyloidosis (lambda/kappa light chain), heavy chain amyloidosis, AA amyloidosis, fibrinogen-a-amyloidosis, LECT2 amyloidosis, and other types. The accuracy and sensitivity of this approach may rationalize its replacement of Congo red staining as the method of choice for the diagnosis of amyloid.

Imaging Mass Spectrometry

Imaging mass spectrometry entails the use of MALDI-TOF MS for profiling and imaging proteins directly from tissue sections [22]. This application provides specific in situ information on the composition, relative abundance, and spatial distribution of peptides and proteins in the analyzed tissue section. An area of a tissue section to be analyzed is coated uniformly with a matrix solution by air spraying which becomes physically bound and co-crystallized with the tissue. The co-crystallized area is subjected to MALDI using a discrete Cartesian pattern of laser shot spots. The distance between the spots is fixed and depends on the chosen resolution which typically ranges from 10 to 100 μm. From the intensity of a given m/z value monitored in each spectrum, a two-dimensional ion density image is reconstructed using specialized software. When full images are not required, but rather data from discrete targeted areas within the tissue are needed, a histology-directed profiling approach can be employed. Several studies have shown the potential of imaging mass spectrometry for molecular profiling and biomarker identification of prostate cancer [7, 21], prediction of the response to neoadjuvant chemotherapy and radiation or HER2 status in breast cancer [1, 18], classification and survival prediction in lung cancer [9], and determination of molecular tumor margins [17]. The principal drawbacks of imaging mass spectrometry are the fact that almost 90 % of the observed signals are below m/z of 30,000 with poor resolution of signal above m/z of 50,000.

Clinical Applications of Multiple Reaction Monitoring Mass Spectrometry

As reviewed above, MRM or SRM is a method of analysis performed on a triple quadrupole mass spectrometer that permits selective analysis of specific analytes. Prostate-specific antigen (PSA) is a biomarker used in the diagnosis and surveillance of prostate cancer. In 2009, Fortin et al. published a sensitive SRM assay to detect PSA in the sera of patients with either benign prostate hyperplasia or prostate cancer [8]. They demonstrated a limit of detection of the PSA peptide LSEPAELTDAVK of 1.5 ng/mL by SRM mass spectrometry. The PSA levels measured by SRM mass spectrometry were validated using the VIDAS TPSA ELISA (bio-Mérieux) with a reliable correlation between these two technologies ($r^2 = 0.99$). Several other studies established SRM mass spectrometry assays as a useful method to detect and quantify different biomarkers such as C-reactive protein (CRP) [12] and inter-α-trypsin inhibitor heavy chain 4 (ITIH4) [24]. A proof-of-principle study demonstrated the potential of SRM mass spectrometry to profile and quantify a high-frequency KRAS missense mutation in colorectal and pancreatic tumors [26]. Given the frequent role of chimeric oncogenic fusions in the pathogenesis and diagnosis of cancers, MRM could potentially play a prominent role in the sensitive and specific identification of cancers. In this regard, Conlon et al. have demonstrated the ability of MRM to accurately identify chimeric fusion proteins found in several different forms of human cancer. In particular, a tryptic fusion peptide characteristic of NPM-ALK-positive anaplastic large cell lymphoma (ALCL) was used to interrogate tissue biopsy material from patients with ALCL (Fig. 8.5). These studies offer promise that chimeric

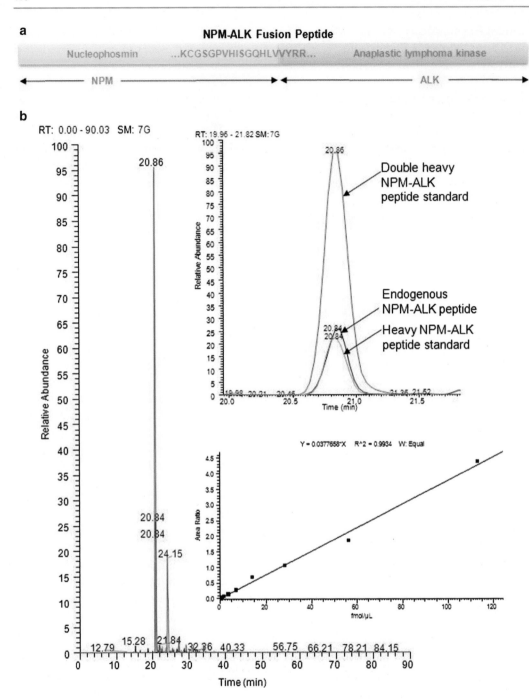

Fig. 8.5 An extracted ion chromatogram showing a targeted quantitative approach of the NPM-ALK fusion peptide using MRM mass spectrometry and stable isotopic standards. (**a**) An illustration of the tryptic NPM-ALK fusion peptide showing the amino acids contributed by each protein. (**b**) A single chromatographic run of a sample spiked with stable isotopic NPM-ALK fusion peptide standards is shown with retention times indicated at the top of the peaks. The inset to the upper right shows an expanded view of the NPM-ALK fusion peptide signal. The inset to the lower right shows a standard curve derived from the sample of interest after dividing it into separate aliquots and spiking each with an isotopic "double heavy" NPM-ALK fusion peptide at a constant concentration and an isotopic "heavy" NPM-ALK fusion peptide at varying concentrations. The co-eluting endogenous peptide signal from each injection is then compared to the curve generated to determine the concentration

fusion peptides can be used as cancer-specific biomarkers that might be applicable in clinical contexts using MRM mass spectrometry [3].

Conclusion

Proteomic approaches are poised to play a prominent role in routine cancer diagnostics. The rapid development of sophisticated and user-friendly technologies with high sensitivity and specificity will promote the deployment of proteomic approaches in the clinical laboratory.

References

1. Bauer JA, Chakravarthy AB, et al. Identification of markers of taxane sensitivity using proteomic and genomic analyses of breast tumors from patients receiving neoadjuvant paclitaxel and radiation. Clin Cancer Res. 2010;16(2):681–90.
2. Blume-Jensen P, Hunter T. Oncogenic kinase signalling. Nature. 2001;411(6835):355–65.
3. Conlon KP, Basrur V, et al. Fusion peptides from oncogenic chimeric proteins as putative specific biomarkers of cancer. Mol Cell Proteomics. 2013.
4. Druker BJ, Guilhot F, et al. Five-year follow-up of patients receiving imatinib for chronic myeloid leukemia. N Engl J Med. 2006;355(23):2408–17.
5. Fenn JB, Mann M, et al. Electrospray ionization for mass spectrometry of large biomolecules. Science. 1989;246(4926):64–71.
6. Figueroa JJ, Peter Bosch E, et al. Amyloid-like IgM deposition neuropathy: a distinct clinico-pathologic and proteomic profiled disorder. J Peripher Nerv Syst. 2012;17(2):182–90.
7. Flatley B, Malone P, et al. MALDI mass spectrometry in prostate cancer biomarker discovery. Biochim Biophys Acta. 2013. pii: S1570-9639(13)00252-5.
8. Fortin T, Salvador A, et al. Clinical quantitation of prostate-specific antigen biomarker in the low nanogram/milliliter range by conventional bore liquid chromatography-tandem mass spectrometry (multiple reaction monitoring) coupling and correlation with ELISA tests. Mol Cell Proteomics. 2009;8(5):1006–15.
9. Groseclose MR, Massion PP, et al. High-throughput proteomic analysis of formalin-fixed paraffin-embedded tissue microarrays using MALDI imaging mass spectrometry. Proteomics. 2008;8(18):3715–24.
10. Hunter T. Signaling—2000 and beyond. Cell. 2000;100(1):113–27.
11. Karas M, Bachamann D, et al. Matrix-assisted ultraviolet laser desorption of non-volatile compounds. Int J Mass Spectrom Ion Proc. 1989;78:53–68.
12. Kuhn E, Wu J, et al. Quantification of C-reactive protein in the serum of patients with rheumatoid arthritis using multiple reaction monitoring mass spectrometry and 13C-labeled peptide standards. Proteomics. 2004;4(4):1175–86.
13. Lange V, Picotti P, et al. Selected reaction monitoring for quantitative proteomics: a tutorial. Mol Syst Biol. 2008;4:222.
14. Larsen MR, Thingholm TE, et al. Highly selective enrichment of phosphorylated peptides from peptide mixtures using titanium dioxide microcolumns. Mol Cell Proteomics. 2005;4(7):873–86.
15. Matsuo K, Arito M, et al. Arthritogenicity of annexin VII revealed by phosphoproteomics of rheumatoid synoviocytes. Ann Rheum Dis. 2011;70(8):1489–95.
16. Olsen JV, Ong SE, et al. Trypsin cleaves exclusively C-terminal to arginine and lysine residues. Mol Cell Proteomics. 2004;3(6):608–14.
17. Oppenheimer SR, Mi D, et al. Molecular analysis of tumor margins by MALDI mass spectrometry in renal carcinoma. J Proteome Res. 2010;9(5):2182–90.
18. Rauser S, Marquardt C, et al. Classification of HER2 receptor status in breast cancer tissues by MALDI imaging mass spectrometry. J Proteome Res. 2010;9(4):1854–63.
19. Rush J, Moritz A, et al. Immunoaffinity profiling of tyrosine phosphorylation in cancer cells. Nat Biotechnol. 2005;23(1):94–101.
20. Schlessinger J. Cell signaling by receptor tyrosine kinases. Cell. 2000;103(2):211–25.
21. Schwamborn K, Krieg RC, et al. Identifying prostate carcinoma by MALDI-Imaging. Int J Mol Med. 2007;20(2):155–9.
22. Stoeckli M, Chaurand P, et al. Imaging mass spectrometry: a new technology for the analysis of protein expression in mammalian tissues. Nat Med. 2001;7(4):493–6.
23. Tanaka K, Waki H, et al. Protein and polymer analysis up to m/z 100 000 by ionization time-flight mass spectrometry. Rapid Commun Mass Spectrom. 1988;2(151–2).
24. van den Broek I, Sparidans RW, et al. Quantitative assay for six potential breast cancer biomarker peptides in human serum by liquid chromatography coupled to tandem mass spectrometry. J Chromatogr B Analyt Technol Biomed Life Sci. 2010;878(5–6):590–602.
25. Vrana JA, Gamez JD, et al. Classification of amyloidosis by laser microdissection and mass spectrometry-based proteomic analysis in clinical biopsy specimens. Blood. 2009;114(24):4957–9.
26. Wang Q, Chaerkady R, et al. Mutant proteins as cancer-specific biomarkers. Proc Natl Acad Sci U S A. 2011;A108(6):2444–9.
27. Zahedi RP, Lewandrowski U, et al. Phosphoproteome of resting human platelets. J Proteome Res. 2008;7(2):526–34.
28. Zhang H, Li XJ, et al. Identification and quantification of N-linked glycoproteins using hydrazide chemistry, stable isotope labeling and mass spectrometry. Nat Biotechnol. 2003;21(6):660–6.

Circulating Tumor Cells: A Noninvasive Liquid Biopsy in Cancer

Evi S. Lianidou

Introduction

Circulating tumor cells (CTC) were first described by Thomas Ashworth, an Australian physician, in 1869 [1], while in 1889 Steve Paget in the very first historical issue of Lancet described "The Seed and Soil Hypothesis," a hypothesis revisited many years later by Fidler [2]. During the last decade, the critical role that CTC play in the metastatic spread of cancer has been widely recognized [3–5]. The clinical importance of CTC detection and enumeration has been established in several clinical studies, and a correlation with decreased progression-free survival (PFS) and overall survival (OS) has been shown in many types of solid cancers.

CTC analysis provides a unique source of cancer cells that can be used as a noninvasive liquid biopsy for the continuous follow-up of cancer patients, when the primary tumor is already surgically removed. CTC are outstanding tools for understanding tumor biology and tumor cell dissemination and their molecular characterization offers an exciting approach to better understand the biology of metastasis and resistance to established therapies [6, 7]. However, since CTC are circulating in peripheral blood at low concentra-

tions in most cases, the amount of available sample for analysis is very limited and this, together with their heterogeneity, presents a formidable analytical and technical challenge for their isolation, detection, and molecular characterization. The emerging interest in the analysis of CTC is reflected in the growing number of publications in this field (Fig. 9.1).

Clinical Significance of CTC

Breast Cancer

Very recently, the first comprehensive meta-analysis of published literature on the prognostic relevance of CTC in patients with early-stage and metastatic breast cancer (MBC) clearly indicated that the detection of CTC is a reliable prognostic factor [8].

Metastatic Breast Cancer

In patients with MBC, Cristofanilli and colleagues have clearly shown many years ago by using the CellSearch system (Veridex, USA) that CTC represent an independent prognostic factor for PFS and overall survival (OS) and that a cut-off of 5 CTC/7.5 ml of blood in MBC patients was highly predictive of clinical outcome [9]. This seminal paper led to the FDA clearance of the CellSearch assay that revolutionized the clinical applications of CTC in many types of cancer, since it is standardized, semiautomated, and not subjected to pre-analytical errors.

E.S. Lianidou, Ph.D. (✉)
Laboratory of Analytical Chemistry,
Department of Chemistry, University
of Athens, Athens 15771, Greece
e-mail: lianidou@chem.uoa.gr

G.M. Yousef and S. Jothy (eds.), *Molecular Testing in Cancer*,
DOI 10.1007/978-1-4899-8050-2_9, © Springer Science+Business Media New York 2014

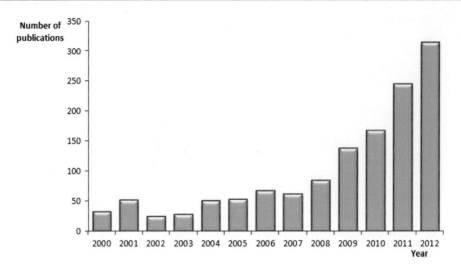

Fig. 9.1 CTC detection and analysis is a fast emerging field that has the potential to contribute to cancer patient diagnosis, prognosis, and response to therapy, as well as for accelerating oncologic drug development

Since then, a plethora of clinical studies have verified the importance of CTC enumeration in MBC [10–14].

Could CTC clearance be used as a "surrogate" marker for potentially improved survival of breast cancer patients? In the official website of the National Institutes of Health, a search (Nov 2012) on clinical studies, based on the key word "Circulating Tumor Cells," revealed 479 ongoing clinical studies, while the combination "Circulating Tumor Cells and breast cancer" revealed 116 ongoing clinical studies. These trials have different designs in various patient populations but are expected to be the pivotal trials for CTC implementation in the routine management of breast cancer patients [15].

For all these reasons, the American Society of Clinical Oncology (ASCO) cited CTC and disseminated tumor cells (DTC) for the first time in its 2007 recommendations on tumor markers, but in the category of insufficient evidence to support routine use in clinical practice [16]. Very recently, the American Joint Committee on Cancer has proposed a new category, M0(i+), for TNM staging in BC defined as *"no clinical or radiographic evidence of distant metastases, but deposits of molecularly or microscopically detected tumor cells (no larger than 0.2 mm) in blood, bone marrow, or other non-regional nodal*

tissue in a patient without symptoms or signs of metastases."

Early Breast Cancer

In bone marrow the detection of DTC in breast cancer patients at the time of primary diagnosis has been confirmed to be of prognostic significance by a large pooled analysis by Braun and colleagues already in 2005 [17]. The heterogeneity of DTC has already been shown many years ago [18, 19]. Since then, the prognostic impact of DTC in breast cancer patients has been shown in numerous studies [20, 21]. According to the results recently reported by the Norwegian group in Oslo, the presence of DTC after neoadjuvant chemotherapy indicated a high risk for disease relapse and death, irrespective of the DTC status before treatment. These findings support the potential use of DTC analysis as a monitoring tool during follow-up, for the selection of patients who are candidates for secondary treatment intervention within clinical trials [22]. Janni and colleagues recently reported that the persistence of DTC after adjuvant therapy in breast cancer patients significantly predicted an increased risk for subsequent relapse and death and can serve as a clinically useful monitoring tool [23]. However, bone marrow sampling is very invasive and patients do not easily accept repeated follow-up examinations. The analysis of CTC in peripheral blood represents a noninvasive alternative to bone marrow analysis of DTC.

In peripheral blood the prognostic value of *CK-19* mRNA-positive CTC in axillary lymph node-negative breast cancer patients, based on a nested RT-PCR, was already shown in 2002 [24]. Later on, by using a real-time RT-qPCR assay for *CK-19* RNA [25, 26], CTC detection was shown to be an independent prognostic factor for reduced disease-free and overall survival before [27], during [28], and after [29] chemotherapy in early breast cancer. Detection of *CK-19* mRNA-positive CTC before adjuvant chemotherapy predicted poor clinical outcome mainly in patients with ER-negative, triple-negative, and HER-2-positive early-stage breast cancer [30]. When the prognostic significance of *CK-19* mRNA-positive CTC in peripheral blood of women with early-stage breast cancer after the completion of adjuvant chemotherapy was evaluated, it was found that the detection of *CK-19* mRNA-positive CTC in the blood after adjuvant chemotherapy was an independent risk factor indicating the presence of chemotherapy-resistant residual disease [29]. However, when the prognostic value of DTC and CTC was compared in early breast cancer by using another method, it was reported that only the presence of DTC was highly predictive for OS [31]. When CTC were prospectively detected before and after neoadjuvant chemotherapy in a phase II trial it was found that detection of one or more CTC in 7.5 ml of blood before neoadjuvant chemotherapy can accurately predict OS [32]. A more recent study investigating the value of CTC detection during the first 5 years of follow-up in predicting late disease relapse has shown that persistent detection of *CK-19* mRNA-positive CTC during the first 5 years of follow-up was associated with an increased risk of late disease relapse and death in patients with operable breast cancer and indicated the presence of chemo- and hormonotherapy-resistant residual disease. This may be useful when deciding on subsequent adjuvant systemic therapy [33]. Lucci et al. prospectively collected data on CTC at the time of definitive surgery from chemonaïve patients with stage 1–3 breast cancer. They enumerated CTC

and assessed outcomes at a median follow-up of 35 months. According to their findings, the presence of one or more CTC predicted early recurrence and decreased overall survival in chemonaïve patients with non-metastatic breast cancer [34].

Ductal Carcinoma In Situ (DCIS)

Despite the general belief that only invasive cancers are assumed to shed isolated tumor cells into the bloodstream and infiltrate lymph nodes, latest studies indicated that tumor cell dissemination may occur before stromal invasion, i.e., in DCIS. This can be explained by that these cells have started already to disseminate from preinvasive mammary lesions or represent the earliest step of microinvasion in a preinvasive lesion [35, 36]. The clinical relevance of these cells has to be further evaluated.

Colorectal Cancer

A very recent systematic review and meta-analysis that investigated the prognostic value of CTC and DTC in patients with resectable colorectal liver metastases or widespread metastatic colorectal cancer (mCRC), and was based on data reported in 12 studies representing 1,329 patients, showed that the detection of CTC in peripheral blood of patients with resectable colorectal liver metastases or widespread mCRC is associated with disease progression and poor survival [37].

Metastatic Colorectal Cancer

Cohen and colleagues were the first to show in 2008 that the number of CTC before and during treatment was an independent predictor of PFS and OS in patients with mCRC. In this prospective multicenter study, CTC were enumerated in the peripheral blood of 430 patients with mCRC at baseline and after starting first-, second-, or third-line therapy by using the CellSearch system. This study led to the FDA clearance of the CellSearch assay for mCRC [38].

CTC enumeration before and during treatment independently predicts PFS and OS in advanced colorectal cancer (CRC) patients treated with chemotherapy plus targeted agents and provides additional information to CT imaging [39]. Recent data support the clinical utility of CTC enumeration in improving the clinician's ability to accurately assess oxaliplatin-based chemotherapy treatment benefit and in expediting the identification of effective treatment regimens for individual patients [40]. By using immunomagnetic enrichment for CTC followed by real-time RT-qPCR analysis of the tumor-associated genes *KRT19*, *MUC1*, *EPCAM*, *CEACAM5*, and *BIRC5*, de Albuquerque and colleagues have shown that CTC detection during treatment was significantly correlated with radiographic findings at the 6-month staging and patients with CTC positivity at baseline had a significant shorter median PFS compared with patients with no CTC. This study showed a strong correlation between CTC detection and radiographic disease progression in patients receiving chemotherapy for CRC [41].

Jiao and colleagues found that surgical resection of metastases, but not radiofrequency ablation, immediately decreases CTC levels. In patients with colorectal liver metastases, CTC appear localized to the hepatic (and pulmonary) macrocirculations. This may explain why metastases in sites other than the liver and lungs are infrequently observed in cancer [42]. The qualitative and quantitative detection of CTC in the central and mesenteric venous blood compartments was investigated to elucidate the patterns of hematogenous tumor cell dissemination in patients with CRC. This study has shown that qualitative and quantitative detection of CTC is higher in the mesenteric venous blood compartments of patients with CRC [43].

Non-metastatic Colorectal Cancer

Currently one of the challenges facing medical oncologists is the identification of patients at higher risk of recurrence after primary CRC resection. CTC may represent a surrogate marker of an early disease spread in patients without overt metastases. However, the prognostic significance of CTC in non-metastatic CRC is less clear than in mCRC. A recent review examined the possible clinical significance of CTC in non-metastatic CRC (TNM stage I–III) with the primary focus on detection methods and prognosis. According to the findings reported in this review, the presence of CTC in peripheral blood is a potential marker of poor disease-free survival in patients with non-metastatic CRC. The low abundance of CTC in non-metastatic CRC requires very sensitive and specific detection methods. An international consensus on choice of detection method and markers is needed before incorporating CTC into risk stratification in the clinical setting [44].

Gazzaniga and colleagues have recently come to the conclusion that CTC detection might help in the selection of high-risk stage II CRC patient candidates for adjuvant chemotherapy, after enumerating CTC with the FDA-cleared CellSearch system. They detected CTC in 22 % of patients with a significant correlation with regional lymph nodes involvement and stage of disease [45].

Prostate Cancer

Although the metastatic cascade in prostate cancer is yet to be fully understood, monitoring CTC and quantifying the load of tumor cell dissemination can be used for estimating prognosis and monitoring treatment success [46]. Unmet needs in prostate cancer drug development and patient management are the ability to monitor treatment effects and to identify therapeutic targets at the time treatment is being considered. CTC enumeration at baseline and posttreatment is of prognostic value, with no threshold effect, and the shedding of cells into the circulation represents an intrinsic property of the tumor, distinct from extent of disease. The clinical utility of monitoring CTC changes with treatment, as an efficacy-response surrogate biomarker of survival, is currently being tested in large phase III trials, with the novel antiandrogen therapies abiraterone acetate (AA) and MDV3100. Molecular determinants can be identified and characterized in CTC as potential predictive biomarkers of tumor sensitivity to a therapeutic modality [47].

Metastatic Prostate Cancer

In 2001, Moreno and colleagues investigated the diurnal variations in CTC in metastatic carcinoma of the prostate and concluded that CTC levels can be quantified in the circulation of patients with metastatic prostate cancer and that the change in the number of CTC correlates with disease progression with no diurnal variations [48]. In 2007, Danila and colleagues evaluated the association of baseline CTC number with clinical characteristics and survival in patients with castrate metastatic disease considered for different hormonal and cytotoxic therapies. Baseline CTC was predictive of survival, with no threshold effect. The shedding of cells into the circulation represents an intrinsic property of the tumor, distinct from extent of disease, and provides unique information relative to prognosis [49].

In 2008, de Bono and colleagues showed that CTC enumeration by using the CellSearch platform has prognostic and predictive value in patients with metastatic castration-resistant prostate cancer (CRPC) and is an independent predictor of overall survival. Their data led to the FDA clearance of this assay for the evaluation of CRPC [50]. CTC numbers, analyzed as a continuous variable, predict OS and provide independent prognostic information to time to disease progression; CTC dynamics following therapy need to be evaluated as an intermediate end point of outcome in randomized phase III trials and can be used to monitor disease status [51, 52].

Real-time PCR assays of Kallikrein gene mRNAs are highly concordant with CellSearch CTC results in patients with CRPC. *KLK2/3* (KLK3 is also known as PSA)-expressing CTC are common in men with CRPC and bone metastases but are rare in patients with metastases diagnosed only in soft tissues and patients with localized cancer [53].

Resel and colleagues analyzed the correlation between CTC and PSA level, Gleason score, and TNM stage in patients with metastatic hormone-sensitive prostate cancer and reported that CTC count in peripheral blood could provide a method for correctly staging prostate cancer and for assessing the prognosis of metastatic hormone-sensitive cancer [54]. Combination of CTC and PSA velocity or doubling-time assessments may offer insights into the prognosis and management of advanced prostate cancer [55].

Early-Stage Prostate Cancer

Within 10 years of radical prostatectomy up to 30 % of prostate cancer patients will have a rise in PSA, requiring radiation therapy. However, with current technology, distinction between local and distant recurrent prostate cancer is not possible. This lack of an accurate test constrains the decision whether to offer systemic or local treatment. CTC and DTC have been detected in prostate cancer and may be new surrogate candidates. The current prognostic significance of CTC/DTC in prostate cancer patients has been recently extensively reviewed [56]. Lowes and colleagues hypothesized that tests for detecting CTC in the blood may assist with clinical decision-making and investigated in a pilot study whether CTC could be detected in early-stage prostate cancer patients receiving salvage radiotherapy using the CellSearch system. Their results demonstrated that CTC can be detected in early-stage cancer and suggest the possibility that posttreatment reduction in CTC levels may be indicative of radiation therapy response [57].

Molecular Characterization of CTC and Individualized Treatment

Molecular characterization of CTC is very important to increase the diagnostic specificity of CTC assays and to investigate therapeutic targets and their downstream pathways in CTC [58]. Molecular characterization of CTC is now a hot research topic and a lot of interesting information is exponentially accumulating in a number of cancers. As an example, to improve patient selection, assessing mutation status in CTC, which possibly better represent metastases than the primary tumor, could be advantageous [59]. We strongly believe that this information will have a great impact on the clinical management of patients, hopefully sooner than anticipated.

Breast Cancer

HER-2 and ER/PR Status in CTC

According to accumulating data CTC may have a different hormone receptor and HER-2 status than the primary tumor. There is a growing body of evidence that the HER-2 status can change during disease recurrence or progression in breast cancer patients. Based on this, it is clear that reevaluation of HER-2 status by assessment of HER-2 expression on CTC is a strategy with potential clinical application. Monitoring of HER-2 expression on CTC might be useful in trials with anti-HER-2 therapies. An optimal individualized treatment could then be selected by characterizing ERα and HER-2 status in CTC and comparing it to the primary tumor [60].

It was shown in 2004 that HER-2 gene amplification by FISH is present in CTC and that administration of trastuzumab could eliminate CTC since a high proportion of these cells expressed the HER-2 receptor [61, 62]. Recently, Georgoulias and colleagues have shown in a pilot randomized study that the administration of trastuzumab can eliminate chemotherapy-resistant *CK19* mRNA-positive CTC, reduce the risk of disease recurrence, and prolong the DFS [63].

The existence of tumor-initiating cells in breast cancer has profound implications for cancer therapy. Magnifico and colleagues investigated the sensitivity of tumor-initiating cells isolated from HER-2 overexpressing carcinoma cell lines to trastuzumab and they provided evidence for the therapeutic efficacy of trastuzumab in debulking and targeting tumor-initiating cells of HER-2 overexpressing tumors [64]. HER-2-positive CTC were detected in DCIS/LCIS or M0 breast cancer irrespective of the primary tumor HER-2 status. Nevertheless,

their presence was more common in women with HER-2-positive disease [65].

In a prospective study, Fehm and colleagues reported that HER-2-positive CTC could be detected in a relevant number of patients with HER-2-negative primary tumors [66]. The same investigators reported that most of the CTC were "triple-negative." Since the expression profile between CTC and the primary tumor differs, the consequence for the selection of adjuvant treatment has to be evaluated [67].

According to findings reported by Rack and colleagues, trastuzumab is effective in clearing HER-2-positive cells from bone marrow during recurrence-free follow-up of breast cancer patients. Given the heterogeneity of minimal residual disease, these patients might benefit from a combination of targeted treatment approaches [60].

Estrogen receptor (ER)-positive breast cancer often recurs many years after the initial diagnosis, and understanding the patterns of timing of relapse could identify patients who need more aggressive treatment. Reliable prediction of early treatment failure may identify patients who require adjuvant therapy to prevent the early onset of distant metastases. When *CK-19* mRNA-positive cells were prospectively and longitudinally detected in 119 patients with estrogen and/or progesterone receptor-positive tumors during the period of tamoxifen administration, multivariate analysis revealed that the detection of *CK-19* mRNA-positive cells during the administration of tamoxifen was associated with an increased risk of relapse [28]. Exploiting the molecular differences between early versus late recurrences may also guide the development of effective novel drug combinations in this group of patients. Towards this goal, a recent study by Liu and colleagues provided clear evidence that robust molecular differences exist between ER-positive breast cancers that recur early on versus much later, despite adjuvant tamoxifen; this group analyzed gene-expression data from breast tumor biopsies, and then correlated them with the development of distant metastases. What emerged was a 91-gene classifier that reliably separates early recurrences (distant relapse ≤3 years from diagnosis) from late recurrences (≥10 years) [68].

Epithelial–Mesenchymal Transition and Stem Cell Markers

The persistence of CTC in breast cancer patients might be associated with stem cell-like tumor cells which have been proposed to be the active source of metastatic spread in primary tumors [69]. Current models suggest that the invasive phenotype appears to be associated with an epithelial–mesenchymal transition (EMT), which enables detachment of tumor cells from a primary site and migration. The reverse process of mesenchymal–epithelial transition (MET) might play a crucial role in the further steps of metastasis when CTC settle down in distant organs and establish metastasis. Nevertheless, the exact mechanisms and interplay of EMT and MET are only partially understood and their relevance in cancer patients is unclear. A subset of CTC shows EMT and stem cell characteristics. Research groups have just started to apply EMT-related markers in their studies of CTC in cancer patients. In a recent review, the current state of investigations on CTC in the context of research on EMT/MET is discussed in detail [70].

Aktas and colleagues reported that a major proportion of CTC of MBC patients show EMT and tumor stem cell characteristics [71]. Moreover CTC co-expressing TWIST and vimentin, suggestive of EMT, were identified in patients with metastatic and early breast cancer patients. The high incidence of these cells in patients with metastatic compared to early-stage breast cancer strongly supports the hypothesis that EMT is involved in the metastatic potential of CTC [72]. A recent study showed that a subset of primary breast cancer patients shows EMT and stem cell characteristics but the currently used detection methods for CTC are not efficient to identify the subgroup of CTC which underwent EMT [73].

Activated Kinases and Angiogenic Molecules

It was also shown by immunofluorescence that CTC express receptors and activated signaling kinases of the EGFR/HER-2/PI3K/Akt pathway, which could be used as targets for their effective elimination [74] as well as pFAK, HIF-1 alpha, VEGF, and VEGF2 [75]. These data could explain the metastatic potential of these cells and may provide a therapeutic target for their elimination.

Colorectal Cancer

Molecular characterization of CTC could provide important information for improving the management of CRC patients. In mCRC, the presence of *KRAS* and *BRAF* mutations is currently assessed in the primary tumor, since it has been shown to reflect anti-EGFR therapy efficacy. The mutation status of *KRAS* and *BRAF* in CRC patients matching primary tumors, liver metastasis, and CTC was very recently investigated, and it was interesting to find discordance between primary tumors, CTC, and metastatic tumors [76].

Gasch and colleagues isolated CTC from patients with metastatic and non-metastatic CRC and further assessed EGFR expression, *EGFR* gene amplification, and *KRAS*, *BRAF*, and *PIK3CA* mutations in single CTC. They demonstrated a considerable intra- and interpatient heterogeneity of EGFR expression and genetic alterations in *EGFR*, *KRAS*, and *PIK3CA* in CTC, possibly explaining the variable response rates to EGFR inhibition in patients with CRC [77]. Barbazán and colleagues isolated CTC by EpCAM-based immunobeads and performed whole transcriptome amplification and hybridization onto cDNA microarrays. They found 410 genes that characterized the CTC population, that were related to cell movement and adhesion, cell death and proliferation, and cell signaling and interaction. When the expression of genes related to the main cellular functions characterizing the CTC population was evaluated by RT-qPCR in an independent series of mCRC patients, controls showed a correlation of CTC-gene expression with clinical parameters and prognosis significance [78].

A very recent and interesting study by the group of M. Mori has shown that Plastin3 is a novel marker for CTC undergoing EMT and is associated with CRC prognosis. They found that PLS3 was expressed in mCRC cells but not in normal circulation and by using fluorescent immune-cytochemistry, they clearly showed that PLS3 was expressed in EMT-induced CTC in peripheral blood from patients with CRC with distant metastasis. PLS3-expressing cells were detected in the peripheral blood of approximately one-third of an independent set of 711 Japanese patients with CRC. Multivariate analysis showed that PLS3-positive CTC was independently associated with prognosis and that the association between PLS3-positive CTC and prognosis was particularly strong in patients with Duke B and Duke C [79].

Prostate Cancer

To improve future drug development and patient management for patients with CRPC, surrogate biomarkers that are linked to relevant outcomes are urgently needed. This area is rapidly evolving, with recent trials incorporating the detection of CTC, imaging, and patient-reported outcome biomarkers [80].

In CRPC persistence of ligand-mediated androgen receptor signaling has been documented. Abiraterone acetate (AA) is an androgen biosynthesis inhibitor shown to prolong life in patients with CRPC already treated with chemotherapy. AA treatment resulted in dramatic declines in PSA only in a subset of patients and no declines in others, suggesting the presence of molecular determinants of sensitivity in tumors. Androgen deprivation therapy is initially effective in treating metastatic prostate cancer, and secondary hormonal therapies are being tested to suppress androgen receptor (AR) reactivation in CRPC.

Danila and colleagues studied the role of transmembrane protease, serine 2 (TMPRSS2)-v-ets erythroblastosis virus E26 oncogene homolog (ERG) fusion, an androgen-dependent growth factor, in CTC as a biomarker of sensitivity to AA. Molecular profiles of CTC with an analytically valid assay identified the presence of the prostate cancer-specific TMPRSS2-ERG fusion but did not predict for response to AA treatment. This finding demonstrates the role of CTC as

surrogate tissue that can be obtained in a routine practice setting [81].

Miyamoto and colleagues presented data that prostate-specific antigen/prostate-specific membrane antigen (PSA/PSMA)-based measurements of AR signaling in CTC enable real-time quantitative monitoring of intra-tumoral AR signaling. This finding indicates that measuring AR signaling within CTC may help to guide therapy in metastatic prostate cancer and highlights the use of CTC as liquid biopsy [82].

FISH analysis of CTC has been shown to be a valuable, noninvasive surrogate for routine tumor profiling. Leversha and colleagues assessed the feasibility of characterizing gene copy number alteration by FISH in CTC in patients with progressive metastatic CRPC. They have shown that FISH analysis of CTC can be a valuable, noninvasive surrogate for routine tumor profiling. The finding that as many as 50 % of these patients have substantial amplification of the AR locus indicates that androgen signaling continues to play an important role in late-stage prostate cancer [83]. Recent results by Darshan and colleagues suggest that monitoring AR subcellular localization in the CTC of CRPC patients might predict clinical responses to taxane chemotherapy [84].

Coding mutations in the AR gene have been identified in tissue samples from patients with advanced prostate cancer and represent a possible mechanism underlying the development of CRPC. AR mutations have been identified in CTC-enriched peripheral blood samples from CRPC patients. This approach has the potential to open new perspectives in understanding CTC and the mechanisms for tumor progression and metastasis in CRPC [85]. It was also recently shown that the majority (>80 %) of CTC in patients with metastatic CRPC co-express epithelial proteins such as EpCAM, cytokeratins, and E-cadherin, with mesenchymal proteins including vimentin, N-cadherin, and O-cadherin, and the stem cell marker CD133 [86].

BRCA1 allelic imbalances were detected among CTC in multifocal prostate cancer. By using FISH analysis of primary tumors and lymph node sections, and CTC from peripheral blood Bednarz and colleagues found that 14 % of 133 tested patients carried monoallelic BRCA1 loss in at least one tumor focus. BRCA1 losses appeared in a minute fraction of cytokeratin- and vimentin-positive CTC. Small subpopulations of prostate cancer cells bearing BRCA1 losses might be one confounding factor initiating tumor dissemination and might provide an early indicator of shortened DFS [87].

Hormone-driven expression of the ERG oncogene after fusion with TMPRSS2 occurs in 30–70 % of therapy-naive prostate cancers. Attard et al. have used multicolor FISH to show that CRPC CTC, metastases, and prostate tissue invariably had the same ERG gene status as therapy-naive tumors and reported a significant association between ERG rearrangements in therapy-naive tumors, CRPC, and CTC and magnitude of PSA decline ($P=0.007$) in CRPC patients treated with abiraterone acetate [88].

Little information exists regarding the utility of CTC enumeration in hormone-sensitive prostate cancer. Goodman and colleagues enumerated CTC in 33 consecutive patients undergoing androgen deprivation therapy and their data revealed that initial CTC values predict the duration and magnitude of response to hormonal therapy. CTC enumeration may identify patients at risk of progression to CRPC before initiation of androgen deprivation therapy [89].

Stott and colleagues developed a quantitative automated imaging system for analysis of prostate CTC, taking advantage of PSA. The specificity of PSA staining enabled optimization of criteria for baseline image intensity, morphometric measurements, and integration of multiple signals in a three-dimensional microfluidic device. The prostate cancer-specific TMPRSS2-ERG fusion was detectable in RNA extracted from CTC from patients with metastatic disease, and dual staining of captured CTC for PSA and the cell division marker Ki67 indicated a broad range for the proportion of proliferating cells among CTC. This method for analysis of CTC will facilitate the application of noninvasive tumor sampling to direct targeted therapies in advanced prostate cancer and warrants the initiation of long-term clini-cal studies to test the importance of CTC in invasive local disease [90].

Circulating endothelial cells, CTC, and tissue factor levels alone and combined can predict OS in CRPC patients treated with docetaxel-based therapy [91]. Coumans and colleagues evaluated the association between circulating objects positive for epithelial cell adhesion molecules and cytokeratin (EpCAM+CK+) that are not counted as CTC and survival in patients with prostate cancer and came to the conclusion that each EpCAM+CK+CD45− circulating object showed a strong association with overall survival ($P<0.001$). This class included small tumor microparticles (S-TMP), which did not require a nucleus and thus are unable to metastasize [92].

Quality Control in CTC Analysis

Since the detection of CTC has been shown to be of considerable utility in the clinical management of patients with solid cancers, a plethora of analytical systems for their isolation and detection have been developed and are still under development and their number is increasing at an exponential rate [93–96]. Since CTC are very rare (1 CTC in 10^6–10^7 leukocytes) [97], in most cases they are specifically detected by using a combination of two steps: (a) isolation-enrichment and (b) detection. The detailed presentation of these systems is beyond the scope of this review.

All these advanced technologies recently developed for CTC isolation and detection are very promising for providing useful assays for oncological drug development, monitoring the course of disease in cancer patients, and in understanding the biology of cancer progression. However, comparison of different methods for CTC enumeration and characterization by using the same samples and quality control is an important issue for the clinical use of CTC analysis as a liquid biopsy. Following the path to regulatory and general clinical acceptance for technologies currently under development and standardization of CTC detection and characterization methodologies are important for the incorporation of CTC into prospective clinical trials.

Critical issues concerning the standardized detection of CTC include (a) the standardization of the pre-analytical phase such as sampling itself (e.g., sample volume, avoidance of epidermal epithelial cells co-sampling in case that epithelial markers such as *CK-19* will be later used for CTC detection), sample shipping (stability of CTC under different conditions), and storage conditions (use of preservatives, or anticoagulants); (b) standardization of CTC isolation through use of spiking controls in peripheral blood; (c) standardization of detection systems; and (d) interlaboratory and intra-laboratory comparison studies for the same samples. The development of international standards for CTC enumeration and characterization is also very important especially in imaging detection systems that are observer-dependent [94, 95].

However, the phenotypic heterogeneity of CTC and their low numbers in the blood stream of patients, together with differences in pre-analytical sample processing, has led to the collection and accumulation of inconsistent data among independent studies [95]. There is still a lot to be done for the automation, standardization, quality control, and accreditation of analytical methodologies used for CTC isolation, detection, and molecular characterization.

Conclusions: Future Directions

The main implication of CTC analysis is based on their unique potential to offer a minimally invasive "liquid biopsy" sample, easily obtainable at multiple time points during the course of the disease which can provide valuable information on the very early assessment of treatment efficacy and can help towards establishing individualized treatment approaches that will improve efficacy with less cost and side effects for cancer patients.

Further research on the molecular characterization of CTC will provide important information for the identification of therapeutic targets and understanding resistance to therapies. The molecular characterization of CTC and DTC at the single cell level is very promising and highly challenging especially in combination with next generation sequencing technologies [98–101]. Even if this is still far from being considered to be applied in a routine clinical setting, it holds a great promise for the future management of cancer patients.

The detection rates of CTC using different analytical systems vary considerably and there is a clear need for an external quality control system for CTC enumeration and validation of findings for the same samples by participating laboratories. Microscopic detection systems used in CTC cytological methods are highly observer-dependent, so the development of international standards for CTC enumeration and characterization is of utmost importance in this case. Cross validation of findings between different labs, using the same or different detection and enumeration platforms, is urgently needed. Especially the application of modern powerful technologies such as next generation sequencing in CTC analysis will enable the elucidation of molecular pathways in CTC and lead to the design of novel molecular therapies targeting specifically CTC.

One of the main clinical issues that are currently being addressed in CTC is to evaluate whether CTC detection can lead to a change in the management of cancer patients and can result in improved clinical outcome. This has not yet been fully proved. Therefore, the challenge of using CTC as novel tumor biomarkers is currently evaluated in clinical trials. In conclusion, the clinical use of CTC as a "liquid biopsy" for selection of patients and real-time monitoring of therapies will have a major impact in personalized medicine.

References

1. Ashworth TR. A case of cancer in which cells similar to those in the tumours were seen in the blood after death. Med J Aust. 1869;14:146–7.
2. Fidler IJ. The pathogenesis of cancer metastasis: the 'seed and soil' hypothesis revisited. Nat Rev Cancer. 2003;3:453–8.
3. Alix-Panabieres C, Pantel K. Circulating tumor cells: liquid biopsy of cancer. Clin Chem. 2013;59:110–8.

4. Lianidou ES, Markou A. Circulating tumor cells as emerging tumor biomarkers in breast cancer. Clin Chem Lab Med. 2011;49:1579–90.

5. Pantel K, Alix-Panabieres C, Riethdorf S. Cancer micrometastases. Nat Rev Clin Oncol. 2009;6:339–51.

6. Aguirre-Ghiso JA, Bragado P, Sosa MS. Metastasis awakening: targeting dormant cancer. Nat Med. 2013;19:276–7.

7. Polzer B, Klein CA. Metastasis awakening: the challenges of targeting minimal residual cancer. Nat Med. 2013;19:274–5.

8. Zhang L, Riethdorf S, Wu G, Wang T, Yang K, Peng G, et al. Meta-analysis of the prognostic value of circulating tumor cells in breast cancer. Clin Cancer Res. 2012;18:5701–10.

9. Cristofanilli M, Budd GT, Ellis MJ, Stopeck A, Matera J, Miller MC, et al. Circulating tumor cells, disease progression, and survival in metastatic breast cancer. N Engl J Med. 2004;351:781–91.

10. Pierga JY, Hajage D, Bachelot T, Delaloge S, Brain E, Campone M, et al. High independent prognostic and predictive value of circulating tumor cells compared with serum tumor markers in a large prospective trial in first-line chemotherapy for metastatic breast cancer patients. Ann Oncol. 2012;23:618–24.

11. Giordano A, Egleston BL, Hajage D, Bland J, Hortobagyi GN, Reuben JM, et al. Establishment and validation of circulating tumor cell-based prognostic nomograms in first-line metastatic breast cancer patients. Clin Cancer Res. 2013;19:1596–602.

12. Giordano A, Cristofanilli M. CTCs in metastatic breast cancer. Recent Results Cancer Res. 2012;195:193–201.

13. Muller V, Riethdorf S, Rack B, Janni W, Fasching PA, Solomayer E, et al. Prognostic impact of circulating tumor cells assessed with the Cell Search System and AdnaTest Breast in metastatic breast cancer patients: the DETECT study. Breast Cancer Res. 2012;14:R118.

14. Wallwiener M, Hartkopf AD, Baccelli I, Riethdorf S, Schott S, Pantel K, et al. The prognostic impact of circulating tumor cells in subtypes of metastatic breast cancer. Breast Cancer Res Treat. 2013;137: 503–10.

15. Bidard FC, Fehm T, Ignatiadis M, Smerage JB, Alix-Panabieres C, Janni W, et al. Clinical application of circulating tumor cells in breast cancer: overview of the current interventional trials. Cancer Metastasis Rev. 2013;32(1–2):179–88.

16. Harris L, Fritsche H, Mennel R, Norton L, Ravdin P, Taube S, et al. American Society of Clinical Oncology 2007 update of recommendations for the use of tumor markers in breast cancer. J Clin Oncol. 2007;25:5287–312.

17. Braun S, Vogl FD, Naume B, Janni W, Osborne MP, Coombes RC, et al. A pooled analysis of bone marrow micrometastasis in breast cancer. N Engl J Med. 2005;353:793–802.

18. Braun S, Hepp F, Sommer HL, Pantel K. Tumor-antigen heterogeneity of disseminated breast cancer cells: implications for immunotherapy of minimal residual disease. Int J Cancer. 1999;84:1–5.

19. Klein CA, Schmidt-Kittler O, Schardt JA, Pantel K, Speicher MR, Riethmuller G. Comparative genomic hybridization, loss of heterozygosity, and DNA sequence analysis of single cells. Proc Natl Acad Sci U S A. 1999;96:4494–9.

20. Synnestvedt M, Borgen E, Wist E, Wiedswang G, Weyde K, Risberg T, et al. Disseminated tumor cells as selection marker and monitoring tool for secondary adjuvant treatment in early breast cancer. Descriptive results from an intervention study. BMC Cancer. 2012;12:616.

21. Synnestvedt M, Borgen E, Schlichting E, Schirmer CB, Renolen A, Giercksky KE, et al. Disseminated tumour cells in the bone marrow in early breast cancer: morphological categories of immunocytochemically positive cells have different impact on clinical outcome. Breast Cancer Res Treat. 2013;138:485–97.

22. Mathiesen RR, Borgen E, Renolen A, Lokkevik E, Nesland JM, Anker G, et al. Persistence of disseminated tumor cells after neoadjuvant treatment for locally advanced breast cancer predicts poor survival. Breast Cancer Res. 2012;14:R117.

23. Janni W, Vogl FD, Wiedswang G, Synnestvedt M, Fehm T, Juckstock J, et al. Persistence of disseminated tumor cells in the bone marrow of breast cancer patients predicts increased risk for relapse—a European pooled analysis. Clin Cancer Res. 2011;17: 2967–76.

24. Stathopoulou A, Vlachonikolis I, Mavroudis D, Perraki M, Kouroussis C, Apostolaki S, et al. Molecular detection of cytokeratin-19-positive cells in the peripheral blood of patients with operable breast cancer: evaluation of their prognostic significance. J Clin Oncol. 2002;20:3404–12.

25. Stathopoulou A, Gizi A, Perraki M, Apostolaki S, Malamos N, Mavroudis D, et al. Real-time quantification of CK-19 mRNA-positive cells in peripheral blood of breast cancer patients using the lightcycler system. Clin Cancer Res. 2003;9:5145–51.

26. Stathopoulou A, Ntoulia M, Perraki M, Apostolaki S, Mavroudis D, Malamos N, et al. A highly specific real-time RT-PCR method for the quantitative determination of CK-19 mRNA positive cells in peripheral blood of patients with operable breast cancer. Int J Cancer. 2006;119:1654–9.

27. Xenidis N, Perraki M, Kafousi M, Apostolaki S, Bolonaki I, Stathopoulou A, et al. Predictive and prognostic value of peripheral blood cytokeratin-19 mRNA-positive cells detected by real-time polymerase chain reaction in node-negative breast cancer patients. J Clin Oncol. 2006;24:3756–62.

28. Xenidis N, Markos V, Apostolaki S, Perraki M, Pallis A, Sfakiotaki G, et al. Clinical relevance of circulating CK-19 mRNA-positive cells detected during the adjuvant tamoxifen treatment in patients with early breast cancer. Ann Oncol. 2007;18: 1623–31.

29. Xenidis N, Ignatiadis M, Apostolaki S, Perraki M, Kalbakis K, Agelaki S, et al. Cytokeratin-19 mRNA-positive circulating tumor cells after adjuvant chemotherapy in patients with early breast cancer. J Clin Oncol. 2009;27:2177–84.

30. Ignatiadis M, Xenidis N, Perraki M, Apostolaki S, Politaki E, Kafousi M, et al. Different prognostic value of cytokeratin-19 mRNA positive circulating tumor cells according to estrogen receptor and HER2 status in early-stage breast cancer. J Clin Oncol. 2007;25:5194–202.

31. Benoy IH, Elst H, Philips M, Wuyts H, Van DP, Scharpe S, et al. Real-time RT-PCR detection of disseminated tumour cells in bone marrow has superior prognostic significance in comparison with circulating tumour cells in patients with breast cancer. Br J Cancer. 2006;94:672–80.

32. Pierga JY, Bidard FC, Mathiot C, Brain E, Delaloge S, Giachetti S, et al. Circulating tumor cell detection predicts early metastatic relapse after neoadjuvant chemotherapy in large operable and locally advanced breast cancer in a phase II randomized trial. Clin Cancer Res. 2008;14:7004–10.

33. Saloustros E, Perraki M, Apostolaki S, Kallergi G, Xyrafas A, Kalbakis K, et al. Cytokeratin-19 mRNA-positive circulating tumor cells during follow-up of patients with operable breast cancer: prognostic relevance for late relapse. Breast Cancer Res. 2011;13:R60.

34. Lucci A, Hall CS, Lodhi AK, Bhattacharyya A, Anderson AE, Xiao L, et al. Circulating tumour cells in non-metastatic breast cancer: a prospective study. Lancet Oncol. 2012;13:688–95.

35. Banys M, Gruber I, Krawczyk N, Becker S, Kurth R, Wallwiener D, et al. Hematogenous and lymphatic tumor cell dissemination may be detected in patients diagnosed with ductal carcinoma in situ of the breast. Breast Cancer Res Treat. 2012;131:801–8.

36. Sanger N, Effenberger KE, Riethdorf S, Van Haasteren V, Gauwerky J, Wiegratz I, et al. Disseminated tumor cells in the bone marrow of patients with ductal carcinoma in situ. Int J Cancer. 2011;129:2522–6.

37. Groot KB, Rahbari NN, Buchler MW, Koch M, Weitz J. Circulating tumor cells and prognosis of patients with resectable colorectal liver metastases or widespread metastatic colorectal cancer: a meta-analysis. Ann Surg Oncol. 2013;20(7):2156–65.

38. Cohen SJ, Punt CJ, Iannotti N, Saidman BH, Sabbath KD, Gabrail NY, et al. Relationship of circulating tumor cells to tumor response, progression-free survival, and overall survival in patients with metastatic colorectal cancer. J Clin Oncol. 2008;26:3213–21.

39. Tol J, Koopman M, Miller MC, Tibbe A, Cats A, Creemers GJ, et al. Circulating tumour cells early predict progression-free and overall survival in advanced colorectal cancer patients treated with chemotherapy and targeted agents. Ann Oncol. 2010;21:1006–12.

40. Matsusaka S, Suenaga M, Mishima Y, Kuniyoshi R, Takagi K, Terui Y, et al. Circulating tumor cells as a surrogate marker for determining response to chemotherapy in Japanese patients with metastatic colorectal cancer. Cancer Sci. 2011;102:1188–92.

41. de Albuquerque A, Kubisch I, Stolzel U, Ernst D, Boese-Landgraf J, Breier G, et al. Prognostic and predictive value of circulating tumor cell analysis in colorectal cancer patients. J Transl Med. 2012;10:222.

42. Jiao LR, Apostolopoulos C, Jacob J, Szydlo R, Johnson N, Tsim N, et al. Unique localization of circulating tumor cells in patients with hepatic metastases. J Clin Oncol. 2009;27:6160–5.

43. Rahbari NN, Bork U, Kircher A, Nimitz T, Scholch S, Kahlert C, et al. Compartmental differences of circulating tumor cells in colorectal cancer. Ann Surg Oncol. 2012;19:2195–202.

44. Thorsteinsson M, Jess P. The clinical significance of circulating tumor cells in non-metastatic colorectal cancer—a review. Eur J Surg Oncol. 2011;37: 459–65.

45. Gazzaniga P, Gianni W, Raimondi C, Gradilone A, Lo Russo G, Longo F, et al. Circulating tumor cells in high-risk nonmetastatic colorectal cancer. Tumour Biol. 2013;34(5):2507–9.

46. Schilling D, Todenhofer T, Hennenlotter J, Schwentner C, Fehm T, Stenzl A. Isolated, disseminated and circulating tumour cells in prostate cancer. Nature Reviews Urology 9, 448–463 (August 2012).

47. Danila DC, Fleisher M, Scher HI. Circulating tumor cells as biomarkers in prostate cancer. Clin Cancer Res. 2011;17:3903–12.

48. Moreno JG, O'Hara SM, Gross S, Doyle G, Fritsche H, Gomella LG, et al. Changes in circulating carcinoma cells in patients with metastatic prostate cancer correlate with disease status. Urology. 2001;58: 386–92.

49. Danila DC, Heller G, Gignac GA, Gonzalez-Espinoza R, Anand A, Tanaka E, et al. Circulating tumor cell number and prognosis in progressive castration-resistant prostate cancer. Clin Cancer Res. 2007;13:7053–8.

50. de Bono JS, Scher HI, Montgomery RB, Parker C, Miller MC, Tissing H, et al. Circulating tumor cells predict survival benefit from treatment in metastatic castration-resistant prostate cancer. Clin Cancer Res. 2008;14:6302–9.

51. Scher HI, Jia X, de Bono JS, Fleisher M, Pienta KJ, Raghavan D, et al. Circulating tumour cells as prognostic markers in progressive, castration-resistant prostate cancer: a reanalysis of IMMC38 trial data. Lancet Oncol. 2009;10:233–9.

52. Olmos D, Arkenau HT, Ang JE, Ledaki I, Attard G, Carden CP, et al. Circulating tumour cell (CTC) counts as intermediate end points in castration-resistant prostate cancer (CRPC): a single-centre experience. Ann Oncol. 2009;20:27–33.

53. Helo P, Cronin AM, Danila DC, Wenske S, Gonzalez-Espinoza R, Anand A, et al. Circulating prostate tumor cells detected by reverse transcription-PCR in men with localized or castration-refractory prostate cancer: concordance with Cell Search assay and association with bone metastases and with survival. Clin Chem. 2009;55:765–73.

54. Resel FL, San Jose ML, Galante RI, Moreno SJ, Olivier GC. Prognostic significance of circulating tumor cell count in patients with metastatic hormone-sensitive prostate cancer. Urology. 2012;80:1328–32.

55. Saad F, Pantel K. The current role of circulating tumor cells in the diagnosis and management of bone metastases in advanced prostate cancer. Future Oncol. 2012;8:321–31.

56. Doyen J, Alix-Panabieres C, Hofman P, Parks SK, Chamorey E, Naman H, et al. Circulating tumor cells in prostate cancer: a potential surrogate marker of survival. Crit Rev Oncol Hematol. 2012;81:241–56.

57. Lowes LE, Lock M, Rodrigues G, D'Souza D, Bauman G, Ahmad B, et al. Circulating tumour cells in prostate cancer patients receiving salvage radiotherapy. Clin Transl Oncol. 2012;14:150–6.

58. Lianidou ES, Markou A, Strati A. Molecular characterization of circulating tumor cells in breast cancer: challenges and promises for individualized cancer treatment. Cancer Metastasis Rev. 2012;31:663–71.

59. Maheswaran S, Sequist LV, Nagrath S, Ulkus L, Brannigan B, Collura CV, et al. Detection of mutations in EGFR in circulating lung-cancer cells. N Engl J Med. 2008;359:366–77.

60. Rack B, Juckstock J, Gunthner-Biller M, Andergassen U, Neugebauer J, Hepp P, et al. Trastuzumab clears HER2/neu-positive isolated tumor cells from bone marrow in primary breast cancer patients. Arch Gynecol Obstet. 2012;285:485–92.

61. Bozionellou V, Mavroudis D, Perraki M, Papadopoulos S, Apostolaki S, Stathopoulos E, et al. Trastuzumab administration can effectively target chemotherapy-resistant cytokeratin-19 messenger RNA-positive tumor cells in the peripheral blood and bone marrow of patients with breast cancer. Clin Cancer Res. 2004;10:8185–94.

62. Meng S, Tripathy D, Shete S, Ashfaq R, Haley B, Perkins S, et al. HER-2 gene amplification can be acquired as breast cancer progresses. Proc Natl Acad Sci U S A. 2004;101:9393–8.

63. Georgoulias V, Bozionelou V, Agelaki S, Perraki M, Apostolaki S, Kallergi G, et al. Trastuzumab decreases the incidence of clinical relapses in patients with early breast cancer presenting chemotherapy-resistant CK-19mRNA-positive circulating tumor cells: results of a randomized phase II study. Ann Oncol. 2012;23:1744–50.

64. Magnifico A, Albano L, Campaner S, Delia D, Castiglioni F, Gasparini P, et al. Tumor-initiating cells of HER2-positive carcinoma cell lines express the highest oncoprotein levels and are sensitive to trastuzumab. Clin Cancer Res. 2009;15:2010–21.

65. Ignatiadis M, Rothe F, Chaboteaux C, Durbecq V, Rouas G, Criscitiello C, et al. HER2-positive circulating tumor cells in breast cancer. PLoS One. 2011;6:e15624.

66. Fehm T, Muller V, Aktas B, Janni W, Schneeweiss A, Stickeler E, et al. HER2 status of circulating tumor cells in patients with metastatic breast cancer: a prospective, multicenter trial. Breast Cancer Res Treat. 2010;124:403–12.

67. Fehm T, Hoffmann O, Aktas B, Becker S, Solomayer EF, Wallwiener D, et al. Detection and characterization of circulating tumor cells in blood of primary breast cancer patients by RT-PCR and comparison to status of bone marrow disseminated cells. Breast Cancer Res. 2009;11:R59.

68. Liu M, Dixon J, Xuan J. Molecular signaling distinguishes early ER-positive breast cancer recurrences despite adjuvant tamoxifen. San Antonio Breast Cancer Symposium; 2011:Abstract S1–8.

69. Wicha MS, Hayes DF. Circulating tumor cells: not all detected cells are bad and not all bad cells are detected. J Clin Oncol. 2011;29:1508–11.

70. Thiery JP, Lim CT. Tumor dissemination: an EMT affair. Cancer Cell. 2013;23:272–3.

71. Aktas B, Tewes M, Fehm T, Hauch S, Kimmig R, Kasimir-Bauer S. Stem cell and epithelial-mesenchymal transition markers are frequently overexpressed in circulating tumor cells of metastatic breast cancer patients. Breast Cancer Res. 2009;11:R46.

72. Kallergi G, Papadaki MA, Politaki E, Mavroudis D, Georgoulias V, Agelaki S. Epithelial to mesenchymal transition markers expressed in circulating tumour cells of early and metastatic breast cancer patients. Breast Cancer Res. 2011;13:R59.

73. Kasimir-Bauer S, Hoffmann O, Wallwiener D, Kimmig R, Fehm T. Expression of stem cell and epithelial-mesenchymal transition markers in primary breast cancer patients with circulating tumor cells. Breast Cancer Res. 2012;14:R15.

74. Kallergi G, Agelaki S, Kalykaki A, Stournaras C, Mavroudis D, Georgoulias V. Phosphorylated EGFR and PI3K/Akt signaling kinases are expressed in circulating tumor cells of breast cancer patients. Breast Cancer Res. 2008;10:R80.

75. Kallergi G, Markomanolaki H, Giannoukaraki V, Papadaki MA, Strati A, Lianidou ES, et al. Hypoxia-inducible factor-1alpha and vascular endothelial growth factor expression in circulating tumor cells of breast cancer patients. Breast Cancer Res. 2009; 11:R84.

76. Mostert B, Jiang Y, Sieuwerts AM, Wang H, Bolt-de VJ, Biermann K, et al. KRAS and BRAF mutation status in circulating colorectal tumor cells and their correlation with primary and metastatic tumor tissue. Int J Cancer. 2013;133:130–41.

77. Gasch C, Bauernhofer T, Pichler M, Langer-Freitag S, Reeh M, Seifert AM, et al. Heterogeneity of epidermal growth factor receptor status and mutations of KRAS/PIK3CA in circulating tumor cells of patients with colorectal cancer. Clin Chem. 2013;59:252–60.

78. Barbazan J, Alonso-Alconada L, Muinelo-Romay L, Vieito M, Abalo A, Alonso-Nocelo M, et al. Molecular characterization of circulating tumor cells in human metastatic colorectal cancer. PLoS One. 2012;7:e40476.

79. Yokobori T, Iinuma H, Shimamura T, Imoto S, Sugimachi K, Ishii H, et al. Plastin3 is a novel marker for circulating tumor cells undergoing the epithelial-mesenchymal transition and is associated with colorectal cancer prognosis. Cancer Res. 2013;73: 2059–69.

80. Scher HI, Morris MJ, Larson S, Heller G. Validation and clinical utility of prostate cancer biomarkers. Nat Rev Clin Oncol. 2013;10:225–34.

81. Danila DC, Anand A, Sung CC, Heller G, Leversha MA, Cao L, et al. TMPRSS2-ERG status in circulating tumor cells as a predictive biomarker of sensitivity in castration-resistant prostate cancer patients treated with abiraterone acetate. Eur Urol. 2011;60:897–904.

82. Miyamoto DT, Lee RJ, Stott SL, Ting DT, Wittner BS, Ulman M, et al. Androgen receptor signaling in circulating tumor cells as a marker of hormonally responsive prostate cancer. Cancer Discov. 2012;2: 995–1003.

83. Leversha MA, Han J, Asgari Z, Danila DC, Lin O, Gonzalez-Espinoza R, et al. Fluorescence in situ hybridization analysis of circulating tumor cells in metastatic prostate cancer. Clin Cancer Res. 2009;15: 2091–7.

84. Darshan MS, Loftus MS, Thadani-Mulero M, Levy BP, Escuin D, Zhou XK, et al. Taxane-induced blockade to nuclear accumulation of the androgen receptor predicts clinical responses in metastatic prostate cancer. Cancer Res. 2011;71:6019–29.

85. Jiang Y, Palma JF, Agus DB, Wang Y, Gross ME. Detection of androgen receptor mutations in circulating tumor cells in castration-resistant prostate cancer. Clin Chem. 2010;56:1492–5.

86. Armstrong AJ, Marengo MS, Oltean S, Kemeny G, Bitting RL, Turnbull JD, et al. Circulating tumor cells from patients with advanced prostate and breast cancer display both epithelial and mesenchymal markers. Mol Cancer Res. 2011;9:997–1007.

87. Bednarz N, Eltze E, Semjonow A, Rink M, Andreas A, Mulder L, et al. BRCA1 loss preexisting in small subpopulations of prostate cancer is associated with advanced disease and metastatic spread to lymph nodes and peripheral blood. Clin Cancer Res. 2010;16: 3340–8.

88. Attard G, Swennenhuis JF, Olmos D, Reid AH, Vickers E, A'Hern R, et al. Characterization of ERG, AR and PTEN gene status in circulating tumor cells from patients with castration-resistant prostate cancer. Cancer Res. 2009;69:2912–8.

89. Goodman Jr OB, Symanowski JT, Loudyi A, Fink LM, Ward DC, Vogelzang NJ. Circulating tumor cells as a predictive biomarker in patients with hormone-sensitive prostate cancer. Clin Genitourin Cancer. 2011;9:31–8.

90. Stott SL, Lee RJ, Nagrath S, Yu M, Miyamoto DT, Ulkus L, et al. Isolation and characterization of circulating tumor cells from patients with localized and metastatic prostate cancer. Sci Transl Med. 2010,2: 25ra23.

91. Strijbos MH, Gratama JW, Schmitz PI, Rao C, Onstenk W, Doyle GV, et al. Circulating endothelial cells, circulating tumour cells, tissue factor, endothelin-1 and overall survival in prostate cancer patients treated with docetaxel. Eur J Cancer. 2010;46: 2027–35.

92. Coumans FA, Doggen CJ, Attard G, de Bono JS, Terstappen LW. All circulating EpCAM + CK + CD45- objects predict overall survival in castration-resistant prostate cancer. Ann Oncol. 2010;21:1851–7.

93. Pantel K, Alix-Panabieres C. Detection methods of circulating tumor cells. J Thorac Dis. 2012;4:446–7.

94. Lianidou ES, Markou A. Circulating tumor cells in breast cancer: detection systems, molecular characterization, and future challenges. Clin Chem. 2011;57: 1242–55.

95. Parkinson DR, Dracopoli N, Petty BG, Compton C, Cristofanilli M, Deisseroth A, et al. Considerations in the development of circulating tumor cell technology for clinical use. J Transl Med. 2012;10:138.

96. Yu M, Stott S, Toner M, Maheswaran S, Haber DA. Circulating tumor cells: approaches to isolation and characterization. J Cell Biol. 2011;192:373–82.

97. Tibbe AG, Miller MC, Terstappen LW. Statistical considerations for enumeration of circulating tumor cells. Cytometry A. 2007;71:154–62.

98. Klein CA, Seidl S, Petat-Dutter K, Offner S, Geigl JB, Schmidt-Kittler O, et al. Combined transcriptome and genome analysis of single micrometastatic cells. Nat Biotechnol. 2002;20:387–92.

99. Stoecklein NH, Klein CA. Genetic disparity between primary tumours, disseminated tumour cells, and manifest metastasis. Int J Cancer. 2010;126:589–98.

100. Fuhrmann C, Schmidt-Kittler O, Stoecklein NH, Petat-Dutter K, Vay C, Bockler K, et al. High-resolution array comparative genomic hybridization of single micrometastatic tumor cells. Nucleic Acids Res. 2008;36:e39.

101. Heitzer E, Auer M, Gasch C, Pichler M, Ulz P, Hoffmann EM, et al. Complex tumor genomes inferred from single circulating tumor cells by array-CGH and next-generation sequencing. Cancer Res. 2013;73(10):2965–75.

Part II

Molecular Applications in Various Malignancies

Molecular Testing in Hematologic Malignancies

10

Amir Behdad, Bryan L. Betz, Megan S. Lim, and Nathanael G. Bailey

Abbreviations

ALK+ALCL	Anaplastic large cell lymphoma ALK positive
ALL/LBL	Lymphoblastic leukemia/lymphoma
AML	Acute myeloid leukemia
APL	Acute promyelocytic leukemia
ATRA	All-trans retinoic acid
BL	Burkitt lymphoma
bZIP	Basic leucine zipper
CLL	Chronic lymphocytic leukemia
CM	Cutaneous mastocytosis
CML	Chronic myelogenous leukemia
D	Ig/TCR diversity region gene
DHL	Double-hit lymphoma
DLBCL	Diffuse large B-cell lymphoma
DSB	Double-strand break
ET	Essential thrombocythemia
FISH	Fluorescence in situ hybridization
FL	Follicular lymphoma
HCL	Hairy cell leukemia
Ig	Immunoglobulin
IS	International scale
ITD	Internal tandem duplication
J	Ig/TCR joining region gene
LPL	Lymphoplasmacytic lymphoma
MALT	Mucosa-associated lymphoid tissue
M-bcr	Major breakpoint region in *BCR*
m-bcr	minor breakpoint region in *BCR*
μ-bcr	micro breakpoint region in *BCR*
MCL	Mantle cell lymphoma
MDS	Myelodysplastic syndrome
MMR	Major molecular response
MPN	Myeloproliferative neoplasm
MRD	Minimal residual disease
NPM1c+	Cytoplasmic localization of NPM1 protein
PCM	Plasma cell myeloma
PCR	Polymerase chain reaction
Ph+	Philadelphia chromosome positive
PMF	Primary myelofibrosis
PV	Polycythemia vera
RT-PCR	Reverse transcription polymerase chain reaction
SM	Systemic mastocytosis
SNP-A	Single nucleotide polymorphism array
TCR	T-cell receptor
TKD	Tyrosine kinase domain
TKI	Tyrosine kinase inhibitor
V	Ig/TCR variable region gene
WHO	World Health Organization

A. Behdad, M.D. • B.L. Betz, Ph.D.
M.S. Lim, M.D., Ph.D. • N.G. Bailey, M.D. (✉)
Department of Pathology, University of Michigan
Medical School, M5242 Medical Science I,
1301 Catherine St, Ann Arbor, MI 48109, USA
e-mail: abehdad@med.umich.edu;
bbetz@med.umich.edu; meganlim@med.umich.edu;
ngbailey@med.umich.edu

G.M. Yousef and S. Jothy (eds.), *Molecular Testing in Cancer*,
DOI 10.1007/978-1-4899-8050-2_10, © Springer Science+Business Media New York 2014

Myeloid Neoplasms

Myeloid neoplasms are a heterogeneous group of disorders involving precursors of granulocytes, monocytes, erythrocytes, and platelets. Myeloid neoplasms may manifest with abnormally high numbers of circulating mature cells, may exhibit ineffective hematopoiesis and cytopenias, or may be characterized by a proliferation of immature cells. Genetic testing of myeloid neoplasms is critically important, as many entities are defined by the genetic aberrations that they harbor, and therapy may change dramatically depending upon genetic findings. Table 10.1 gives an overview of genetic tests that are commonly performed to evaluate myeloid neoplasms. These tests are discussed in detail in the subsequent sections.

Myeloproliferative Neoplasms

Chronic Myelogenous Leukemia

Chronic myelogenous leukemia (CML) is defined and caused by the *BCR-ABL1* gene fusion, which is formed by the translocation of chromosomes 9 and 22. The fusion of *BCR* and *ABL1* leads to constitutive activation of the ABL1 tyrosine kinase [1], resulting in panmyelosis with marked proliferation of granulocytes and their precursors. While all CML cases harbor the *BCR-ABL1* fusion, it is important to note that this fusion is not unique to CML, as it is present in a large percentage (20–30 %) of adult de novo B lymphoblastic leukemia/lymphoma (B-ALL/LBL) [2].

CML is paradigmatic of a neoplasm with a defined, targeted therapy. The development of

Table 10.1 Established molecular tests for the assessment of the myeloid neoplasms

Molecular marker	Neoplasm	Specimen type	Molecular assay	Clinical utility
BCR-ABL1	CML, B-ALL	Blood or BM	RT-PCR[a]; FISH	Diagnosis, MRD, therapy
BCR-ABL1 kinase mutation	CML, B-ALL	Blood or BM	Sequencing	Therapy
JAK2 V617F	PV, PMF, ET	Blood or BM	PCR	Diagnosis
JAK2 exon 12	PV	Blood or BM	PCR/sequencing	Diagnosis
MPL	PMF, ET	Blood or BM	PCR/sequencing	Diagnosis
KIT D816V	Mastocytosis	BM	PCR	Diagnosis
PDGFRA, *PDGFRB*	M/L NE	Blood or BM	FISH	Diagnosis, therapy
FGFR1	M/L NE	Blood or BM	FISH	Diagnosis
PML-RARA	AML	Blood or BM	RT-PCR[a], FISH	Diagnosis, MRD, therapy
MLL rearrangement	AML	Blood or BM	FISH	Diagnosis
RUNX1-RUNX1T1, *CBFB-MYH11*	AML	Blood or BM	FISH, RT-PCR	Diagnosis
FLT3-ITD	AML	Blood or BM	PCR	Diagnosis
NPM1	AML	Blood or BM	PCR	Diagnosis, +/− MRD
CEBPA	AML	Blood or BM	Sequencing	Diagnosis

CML chronic myelogenous leukemia, *ALL* acute lymphoblastic leukemia, *BM* bone marrow, *PCR* polymerase chain reaction, *RT-PCR* reverse transcription polymerase chain reaction, *FISH* fluorescence in situ hybridization, *MRD* minimal residual disease, *PV* polycythemia vera, *PMF* primary myelofibrosis, *ET* essential thrombocythemia, *M/L NE* myeloid/lymphoid neoplasms with eosinophilia
[a]These assays are commonly performed quantitatively; the other listed PCR assays are typically qualitative

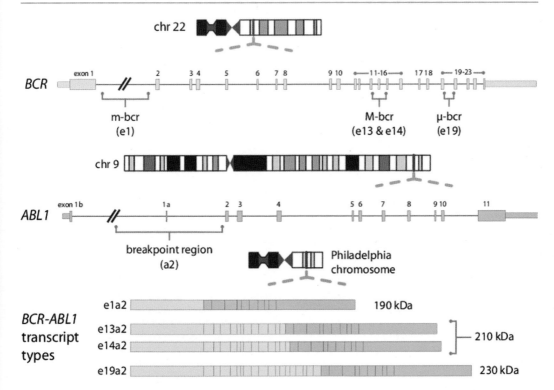

Fig. 10.1 The t(9;22)(q34;q11) translocation and associated BCR-ABL1 fusion products. The translocation of chromosomes 9 and 22 leads to the juxtaposition of the *BCR* and *ABL1* genes and is cytogenetically recognizable by the presence of the Philadelphia (Ph) chromosome. A large breakpoint region upstream of *ABL1* exon 2 is joined with one of several *BCR* breakpoint regions. In CML the M-bcr (major) breakpoint region is most common (~98 % cases) and leads to juxtaposition of either *BCR* exon 13 or 14 to *ABL1* exon 2, producing e13a2 or e14a2 transcripts and a 210 kDa BCR-ABL1 fusion protein (p210). This transcript is also found in B-ALL/LBL. Fusion of the *BCR* minor breakpoint region (m-bcr) with *ABL1* exon 2 leads to e1a2 transcripts and a 190 kDa protein (p190). This transcript is associated with B-ALL/LBL and only rarely occurs in CML. The micro breakpoint region (μ-bcr) is rare and juxtaposes *BCR* exon 19 with *ABL1* exon 2, resulting in e19a2 transcript and a 230 kDa (p230) protein

imatinib (STI571) and other tyrosine kinase inhibitors (TKI) with activity against *BCR-ABL1* has revolutionized the treatment of CML [3, 4]. The efficacy of treatment can be monitored by assessing the levels of *BCR-ABL1* transcripts in affected patients [5]. Over time, resistance to TKI therapy develops, frequently due to *ABL1* kinase mutations. Some mutations impart resistance to certain TKIs and susceptibility to others, and so the identification of the specific mutation present in a patient's tumor allows personalized selection of a targeted TKI [6]. In CML, molecular testing is crucial at all stages of therapy, from establish-

ing the diagnosis through monitoring and prediction of response to therapy.

There are several variants of the *BCR-ABL1* fusion transcript [7, 8] (Fig. 10.1). The breakpoint in *ABL1* almost always occurs upstream of the second exon, leading to juxtaposition of exon 2 (a2) with one of several possible *BCR* exons. Several breakpoint regions are common in *BCR*. The most common region in CML is called the major breakpoint region (M-bcr) and leads to juxtaposition of either exon 13 (e13 or b2) or exon 14 (e14 or b3) with a2, generating e13a2 or e14a2 transcripts that produce a protein with a

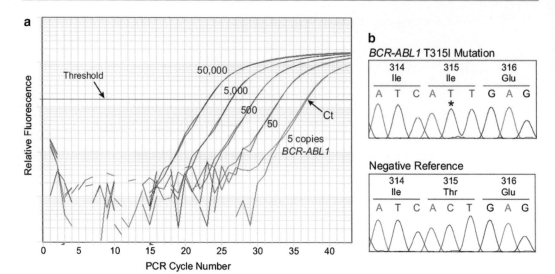

Fig. 10.2 Molecular tests for BCR-ABL1. (**a**) Quantitative *BCR-ABL1* testing. Real-time reverse transcription PCR (RT-PCR) is a sensitive means to detect and quantify *BCR-ABL1* transcripts across a 4–6 log range of *BCR-ABL1* levels. Amplification products can be detected during each PCR cycle using a fluorescent probe specific to the PCR product. The accumulated fluorescence in log(10) value is plotted against the number of PCR cycles. For a given specimen, the PCR cycle number is measured when the increase in fluorescence is exponential and exceeds a threshold. This point is called the quantification or threshold cycle (Ct), which is inversely proportional to the amount of PCR target in the specimen (i.e., lower Ct values indicate greater amount of target). Calibration standards of known quantity are used in standard curves to calculate the amount of target in a tested specimen. Shown are real-time RT-PCR plots of calibration standards for *BCR-ABL1* quantitation. Note that PCR increases the amount of amplification product by a factor of 2 with each PCR cycle. Therefore specimens that produce a Ct value that is 1 cycle lower are expected to have a twofold higher concentration of target. Specimens that differ in target concentration by a factor of 10 (as shown) are expected to be 3.3 cycles apart ($2^{3.3} = 10$). Note the calibration samples with 500 and 50 copies of *BCR-ABL1* produced Ct values of 29.7 and 33.0, respectively. (**b**) *ABL1* kinase mutation testing. A variety of substitution mutations within the ABL1 kinase domain of BCR-ABL1 can lead to differential resistance to TKI therapies. Sanger sequencing of this region within the *BCR-ABL1* transcript is a preferred method to detect the variety of mutations. Shown is a sequencing trace of a C to T nucleotide transition leading to a threonine (Thr) to isoleucine (Ile) substitution at amino acid 315 (T315I). A wild-type trace is included for reference

molecular weight of 210 kDa (p210). B-ALL/LBL cases frequently have a structurally different *BCR-ABL1* fusion involving the minor breakpoint region (m-bcr), with juxtaposition of *BCR* exon 1 (e1) with a2 (e1a2). This e1a2 product produces the p190 fusion protein and is uncommon in CML. A third far more rare fusion event involves the micro breakpoint region (μ-bcr) in *BCR*, leading to exon 19 fusion with a2 and a protein product designated p230. The p230 product is associated with a "chronic neutrophilic leukemia" phenotype [9], but is considered a CML variant in the World Health Organization (WHO) classification [10]. Other extremely rare variants have been identified, but these are uncommonly encountered in clinical practice [11].

Although *BCR-ABL1* fusions typically occur through formation of the Philadelphia chromosome, which is readily detectable by metaphase cytogenetics, approximately 5 % of *BCR-ABL1* fusions are cytogenetically cryptic [10]; therefore, more sensitive techniques are mandatory to fully exclude CML in suspicious cases (Fig. 10.2). Fluorescence in situ hybridization (FISH) identifies essentially all *BCR-ABL1* fusion variants, and dual-color, dual-fusion assay designs have excellent sensitivity and specificity at diagnosis [12]. The utility of FISH in the follow-up setting is limited, and reverse transcription polymerase chain reaction (RT-PCR) testing is the mainstay for disease monitoring. RT-PCR assays generally detect both the M-bcr and m-bcr rearrangements, which together account for nearly all *BCR-ABL1* fusion events [11]. Once the diagnosis of CML has been established, TKI therapy is initiated and *BCR-ABL1* transcripts are monitored by quantitative RT-PCR every 3 months [13]. The goal of TKI therapy is to induce a complete cytogenetic response and, ideally, a major molecular response (MMR), which is assessed by quantifying *BCR-ABL1* transcript levels. An MMR is defined by a greater than 3 log reduction of *BCR-ABL1* mRNA from a standardized baseline level in the international scale (IS). The IS is itself derived from patient values in the International Randomized Study of Interferon and STI571 (IRIS) trial [5]; by definition, an MMR exists at IS values of <0.1 %. Laboratories establish a conversion factor for their individual quantitative *BCR-ABL1* assay in order to translate their result to an IS value, which then allows patients to be monitored across laboratories and institutions.

If an appropriate initial response to TKI therapy is not obtained at 3 months, if there are increasing (log-fold change) *BCR-ABL1* transcripts later in therapy, or if there is other evidence of disease progression, then *ABL1* kinase domain mutation testing is considered [14]. TKI resistance is multifactorial; approximately half to three fourths of patients have *ABL1* kinase mutations that contribute to resistance [15]. Numerous secondary *ABL1* kinase domain mutations have been described [6]; therefore, Sanger sequencing is used to allow unbiased detection of all the possible variants [6]. Individual *ABL1* mutations may lead to resistance against some TKIs but preserved susceptibility to others. One of the most notorious mutations involves a substitution of isoleucine for the threonine at position 315 (T315I), which imparts resistance to imatinib, dasatinib, and nilotinib [13]. Recently, novel TKIs have been developed that have shown promise in targeting the T315I mutation [16]. Identification of *ABL1* mutations allows appropriate, patient-specific selection of TKIs with activity against the particular resistance mutation that a patient's tumor harbors and helps select patients for whom hematopoietic stem cell transplantation is appropriate.

BCR-ABL1-Negative Myeloproliferative and Myelodysplastic/Myeloproliferative Neoplasms

By definition, all non-CML myeloproliferative neoplasms (MPNs) lack *BCR-ABL1* fusion. The most common *BCR-ABL1*-negative MPNs are polycythemia vera (PV), primary myelofibrosis (PMF), and essential thrombocythemia (ET), all of which are characterized by uncontrolled proliferation of one or more hematopoietic lineages. PV leads to marked proliferation of red blood cells and is essentially defined by the presence of a mutation in Janus kinase 2 (*JAK2*), a tyrosine kinase important in cytokine signal transduction. *JAK2* V617F is the most common mutation in PV, present in approximately 95 % of cases [17–19]. The remaining 5 % of cases typically have other mutations in *JAK2*, most often in exon 12 [20]. Both PMF and ET may also have *JAK2* V617F mutations, although at a much lower frequency than in PV (approximately 40–50 %) [17–19, 21]. *JAK2* exon 12 mutations are not present in these disorders; however, myeloproliferative leukemia virus oncogene (*MPL*), which encodes the thrombopoietin receptor, is occasionally mutated in PMF and ET (approximately 5 % of patients) [22].

Although JAK inhibitors are now available, the primary clinical utility of *JAK2* and *MPL* testing is diagnostic. There are many reactive causes of thrombocytosis and erythrocytosis, and the identification of a *JAK2* or *MPL* mutation is helpful to establish the presence of an MPN [10]. JAK inhibition is not analogous to *BCR-ABL1*-targeted therapy. Both patients with and without *JAK2* mutations may derive some benefit from JAK inhibition, and the currently available JAK inhibitors have little effect on the size of the mutant clone and do not induce "molecular remissions" in *JAK2*-mutated patients [23]. Therefore, quantitative serial assessment of *JAK2*V617F is not currently indicated for therapeutic monitoring [24].

Myelodysplastic/myeloproliferative neoplasms (MDS/MPN) are clonal myeloid disorders that exhibit a combination of both proliferative and dysplastic hematopoiesis. By definition, these disorders lack *BCR-ABL1* fusion, and tests for this translocation are a necessary part of the workup of MDS/MPNs. The two historically best understood disorders in this category are typified by a monocytic expansion: chronic myelomonocytic leukemia (CMML) and juvenile myelomonocytic leukemia (JMML). Aside from exclusion of *BCR-ABL1*, molecular testing has not been a prominent part of the routine evaluation of CMML. CMML is genetically heterogeneous, with common mutations involving *TET2, KRAS, NRAS, CBL, SRSF2*, and *ASXL1* [25–28]. Studies have suggested that identification of *ASXL1* mutations may inform prognostic stratification [29]. In JMML, mutations in genes involved in the RAS signaling pathway are present in most cases. Commonly mutated genes in JMML include *NF1, PTPN11, NRAS, KRAS*, and *CBL* [30]. The current WHO diagnostic criteria are not fully specific for JMML, as some viral illnesses may exhibit similar features. Therefore, revised diagnostic criteria for JMML have been proposed that incorporate molecular testing of these genes [31]. Atypical chronic myeloid leukemia (*BCR-ABL1* negative) (aCML) is an MDS/MPN that harbors *SETBP1* mutations in approximately 25 % of cases [32]. Recently, the entities of aCML and chronic neutrophilic leukemia (CNL), a rare MPN, have been somewhat unified by the identification of activating mutations in *CSF3R* in a combined 59 % of patients with these uncommon neoplasms [33]. *CSF3R* mutations appear particularly prevalent in CNL, present in 8 of 9 cases [33]. As CNL is extremely challenging to distinguish from reactive neutrophilia, identification of a somatic mutation is diagnostically helpful and suggests the utility of targeted therapies directed at this dysregulated signaling pathway [33].

Mastocytosis

Mastocytosis is an MPN characterized by a neoplastic proliferation of mast cells. Many clinical subtypes of mastocytosis exist, broadly categorized into cutaneous mastocytosis (CM) and systemic mastocytosis (SM) [10]. Activating point mutations of *KIT*, a receptor tyrosine kinase, are frequently present in the neoplastic cells. In adults with systemic mastocytosis, approximately 95 % of cases have a single aspartate to valine substitution at position 816 (D816V) [10, 34], and detection of the *KIT* D816V mutation is a minor criterion for establishing a diagnosis of SM [10]. Identification of the *KIT* D816V mutation requires use of an assay with a very low limit of detection, such as allele-specific polymerase chain reaction (PCR), due to the low numbers of neoplastic mast cells typically found in bone marrow aspirates of patients with SM. Other less common *KIT* mutations exist in SM, and they are more frequent than D816V in pediatric patients with CM [35, 36]. However, assays for non-D816V *KIT* mutations are not frequently performed when evaluating for mastocytosis given their rarity in SM and the typically indolent course of CM.

Myeloid/Lymphoid Neoplasms with Eosinophilia and Rearranged PDGFRA, PDGFRB, and FGFR1

A subset of myeloid and, less commonly, lymphoid neoplasms associated with eosinophilia have rearrangements involving *PDGFRA*, *PDGFRB*, or *FGFR1* [10]. Identification of neoplasms with *PDGFRA* or *PDGFRB* rearrangements is particularly important, as they respond exquisitely to imatinib [37, 38], and the clinical consequences of unchecked eosinophilia can be severe. These gene fusions can (and in the case of *PDGFRA* must) be identified by FISH or other molecular techniques. A cytogenetically cryptic interstitial deletion on chromosome 4 leads to the fusion of *PDGFRA* with a nearby gene, *FIP1L1*. This leads to loss of the intervening material, including the gene *CHIC2*. Common FISH designs for translocations (dual-color fusion, break-apart) are not optimal to detect this rearrangement given the close proximity of the fused genes. Therefore, the typical FISH strategy for *FIP1L1-PDGFRA* identification detects the loss of the *CHIC2* gene [39]. *PDGFRB* has multiple translocation partners, and so a break-apart FISH strategy can be employed to detect rearrangements.

FGFR1 rearrangements are often associated with an immature lymphoid neoplasm with an aggressive clinical course [40]. *FGFR1* rearrangements are not targeted by imatinib but may respond to novel TKI therapies [41].

Myelodysplastic Syndromes

Myelodysplastic syndromes (MDS) are clonal myeloid neoplasms characterized by ineffective hematopoiesis and peripheral cytopenias, often with subsequent bone marrow failure or acute leukemic transformation. Cytogenetic abnormalities are detectable in approximately 45 % of patients by metaphase cytogenetics [42] and typically consist of gains or losses of large regions of chromosomes. These karyotypically recognizable abnormalities allow risk stratification of patients with MDS and are incorporated into widely used clinical algorithms to determine appropriate therapy [43–45]. FISH assays are often used to identify many of the more common genetic alterations (del (5q)/-5, del(7q)/-7, del(20q), +8), and the identification of a clonal abnormality can be very helpful in morphologically challenging cases. However, in the setting of an adequate cytogenetic analysis with normal results, the additional use of FISH does not detect a significant number of cryptic abnormalities [46]. Routine use of MDS FISH is therefore not indicated: FISH analysis should be reserved for specimens with inadequate growth for cytogenetic analysis or perhaps for cases with morphologic features suggestive of an MDS with isolated del(5q) (anemia with or without thrombocytosis, <5 % blasts, no Auer rods, increased monolobate megakaryocytes) and a normal karyotype [10].

In contrast with FISH, unbiased genome-wide analytic techniques such as single nucleotide polymorphism arrays (SNP-A) may significantly improve detection of clonality in MDS [47–49]. SNP-A analysis has a much higher resolution than metaphase cytogenetics and can identify karyotypically silent aberrations such as copy-neutral loss of heterozygosity (acquired uniparental disomy), which may be functionally equivalent to a deletion [48]. Appropriate incor-

poration of these technologies into clinical practice remains a challenge, although clinically relevant prognostic information can be obtained [47]. In addition to the well-established copy number alterations present in MDS, the prognostic and therapeutic significance of single gene mutations is currently being explored. One large study has suggested that mutations of *TP53*, *EZH2*, *ETV6*, *RUNX1*, or *ASXL1* are associated with poor outcome, independent of cytogenetic risk category [50]. The discovery of mutations in multiple spliceosome genes in MDS [27] further adds to our understanding of the disease and provides more genes that may be relevant for risk stratification in the future [51, 52].

Acute Myeloid Leukemia

Acute myeloid leukemia (AML) is the most common group of acute leukemia affecting the adult population. Better understanding of the molecular pathogenesis of this heterogeneous group of diseases has led to the utilization of cytogenetic abnormalities and single gene mutations, in conjunction with morphology, for subclassification of AML [10].

Recurrent Cytogenetic Abnormalities in AML

Pretreatment chromosomal abnormalities are the most important predictor of outcome and are detected in over half of adult AML [10, 53–59]. The 2008 WHO classification recognizes distinct AML entities based on these recurrent cytogenetic abnormalities. Table 10.2 summarizes these subgroups and their predicted prognosis. A pretreatment cytogenetic analysis is a mandatory part of the diagnostic workup of any suspected case of AML. FISH on metaphase cells can help confirm cytogenetic abnormalities identified in a karyotype. Much like in MDS, routine FISH analysis for recurrent genetic abnormalities is not necessary in the setting of a successful conventional cytogenetic analysis [60, 61]. However, in cases where the cytogenetic analysis fails or is of poor quality, or in cases with morphologic

Table 10.2 Cytogenetic abnormalities defining the WHO category of "acute myeloid leukemia with recurrent genetic abnormalities" [10]

Abnormality	Prognosis
t(8;21)(q22;q22); *RUNX1-RUNX1T1*	Favorable
inv(16)(p13.1q22) or t(16;16)(p13.1;q22); *CBFB-MYH11*	Favorable
t(15;17)(q22;q12); *PML-RARA*	Favorable
t(9;11)(p22;q23); *MLLT3-MLL*	Intermediate
t(6;9)(p23;q34); *DEK-NUP214*	Unfavorable
inv(3)(q21q26.2) or t(3;3)(q21;q26.2); *RPN1-MECOM(EVI1)*	Unfavorable
t(1;22)(p13;q13); *RBM15-MKL1*	Not different

suspicion for a specific undetected cytogenetic aberration, interphase FISH can be useful to detect abnormalities such as *RUNX1-RUNX1T1*, *CBFB-MYH11*, and *MLL* rearrangements [61]. RT-PCR assays to detect recurrent fusion genes have also been developed [62]; however, with the notable exception of *PML-RARA*, these are not routinely used for diagnosis or monitoring.

Acute Promyelocytic Leukemia

One of the most common recurrent cytogenetic abnormalities in AML is t(15; 17), *PML-RARA*, accounting for approximately 10–12 % of AMLs. This rearrangement approximates the myeloid transcription factor *RARA* (retinoic acid receptor, alpha) to *PML* (promyelocytic leukemia), typically giving rise to two new fusion transcripts, *PML-RARA* and *RARA-PML*. The PML-RARA chimeric protein leads to a myeloid differentiation block that is the hallmark of acute promyelocytic leukemia (APL) and is critical for its pathogenesis and is the basis for its treatment [63, 64]. All-trans retinoic acid (ATRA), a vitamin A-derived substance, unblocks and promotes terminal cell differentiation of the myeloid lineage by promoting degradation of the PML-RARA fusion protein [65, 66].

Given the availability of targeted therapy with a very high cure rate and the high incidence of catastrophic hemorrhagic events early in the disease course, the accurate and rapid diagnosis of APL is extremely important. Empiric ATRA

therapy should be initiated if the morphologic or clinical features suggest APL [67]. However, confirmation of the diagnosis requires proof of the presence of *PML-RARA*. Conventional cytogenetic methods detect 70–90 % of cases, while sensitive FISH and RT-PCR techniques are thought to detect close to 100 % of translocations [68, 69]. In addition to higher sensitivity, FISH and RT-PCR can be performed expeditiously, which is particularly important in APL. Rare cases harbor cryptic *PML-RARA*, where FISH is negative and RT-PCR methods detect the rearrangement [70]; therefore, testing by multiple modalities should be pursued in suspicious cases.

A therapeutic objective in APL is molecular remission, currently defined as negative qualitative PCR status at the end of consolidation therapy [71]. Earlier testing for *PML-RARA* transcripts after the induction phase of therapy is not indicated. Patients with detectable *PML-RARA* transcripts in two consecutive assays following consolidation will relapse, and so therapeutic intervention is necessary in this setting [67]. Quantitative transcript values, utilizing real-time RT-PCR methods, are currently reported by some laboratories and have been used in clinical trials for the detection of minimal residual disease (MRD) [72].

A small subset of APLs lack the classical t(15;17) and may be caused by an alternative fusion between *RARA* and other nuclear protein genes, including *ZBTB16* (*PLZF*, located at 11q23), *NUMA1* (located at 11q13), *NPM1* (located at 5q35), and *STAT5B* (located at 17q11.2) [73, 74]. The *NUMA1* and *NPM1* subtypes are responsive to therapy with ATRA, whereas *ZBTB16-RARA* and *STAT5B-RARA* are associated with a poor prognosis and lack of response to retinoids [75]. Conventional karyotyping plays an important role in detection of these translocations and also in detecting complex rearrangements involving more than two chromosomes.

Core Binding Factor AML

Two other AML groups with recurrent cytogenetic abnormalities, t(8;21) and inv(16)/t(16;16), collectively constitute the category of core binding factor (CBF) AML and together account for approximately 10–15 % of AMLs. CBF, an important transcription factor in hematopoiesis, is a heterodimer composed of a DNA-binding protein encoded by *RUNX1* (*CBFA2, AML1*) and a non-DNA-binding protein encoded by *CBFB*. t(8;21) (q22;q22) and inv(16) (p13.1q22)/t(16;16) (p13.1;q22) create *RUNX1-RUNX1T1*(*AML1-ETO*) and *CBFB-MYH11* fusion genes, respectively, disrupting the function of CBF and leading to impaired differentiation [76]. These two rearrangements predict favorable outcomes and can be detected using conventional cytogenetic or FISH techniques. Inv(16), in particular, may be cytogenetically cryptic, and so alternative (FISH) detection strategies should be considered in cases with suspicious morphologic features (i.e., myelomonocytic differentiation and abnormal eosinophils) and normal cytogenetic results [61].

MLL gene (11q23) rearrangements can be seen in AML, often in cases with monoblastic differentiation. In AML, the most frequent *MLL* translocation partner is *MLLT3* (*AF9*), although numerous *MLL* fusion partners exist. In general, *MLL* rearrangements are associated with a poor prognosis; however, the t(9;11), *MLLT3-MLL* fusion has a slightly better prognosis than the others [10]. Conventional cytogenetics does not detect all *MLL* translocations, and FISH may be necessary to identify them in selected cases [77].

In addition to the detection of recurrent cytogenetic abnormalities, karyotyping may identify MDS-like cytogenetic abnormalities. These cytogenetic abnormalities are summarized in Table 10.3 and are sufficient for the diagnosis of AML with MDS-related features, even in the absence of morphologic evidence of dysplasia [10]. These cytogenetic changes are predictive for adverse outcomes and are usually associated with resistance to standard treatment [78–80]. Identification of cytogenetic abnormalities is not required for diagnosis of AML with MDS-related features; however, studies have suggested that the presence of cytogenetic abnormalities is more prognostically significant than morphologic dysplasia alone [81].

Table 10.3 Cytogenetic abnormalities sufficient to diagnose WHO category of "acute myeloid leukemia with myelodysplasia-related changes" [10]

Complex karyotype (defined as 3 or more unrelated abnormalities, none of which can be a rearrangement of "AML with recurrent genetic abnormalities")
Unbalanced abnormalities
−7 or del(7q)
−5 or del(5q)
i(17q) or t(17p)
−13 or del(13q)
del(11q)
del(12p) or t(12p)
del(9q)
idic(X)(q13)
Balanced abnormalities
t(11;16)(q23;p13.3)a
t(3;21)(q26.2;q22.1)a
t(1;3)(p36.3;q21.1)
t(2;11)(p21;q23)a
t(5;12)(q33;p12)
t(5;7)(q33;q11.2)
t(5;17)(q33;p13)
t(5;10)(q33;q21)
t(3;5)(q25;q34)

Gene Mutations in AML

In addition to structural chromosomal abnormalities, single gene mutations play an important role in the pathogenesis of AML, and their detection is prognostically and therapeutically important in the large fraction of AML patients without recurrent cytogenetic abnormalities. Among these, mutations of fms-related tyrosine kinase 3 (*FLT3*), nucleophosmin (*NPM1*), and CCAAT/enhancer-binding protein alpha (*CEBPA*) are the most clinically established, and assays to detect them are routinely performed in molecular laboratories (Fig. 10.3).

The *FLT3* gene, located at the long arm of chromosome 13, encodes a receptor tyrosine kinase that is constitutively activated through mutation in approximately one third of AML patients. Patients with *FLT3* mutation may be candidates for experimental treatment with TKI [82]; however, *FLT3* is currently most important as a prognostic marker. Two types of functionally important *FLT3* mutations have been identified:

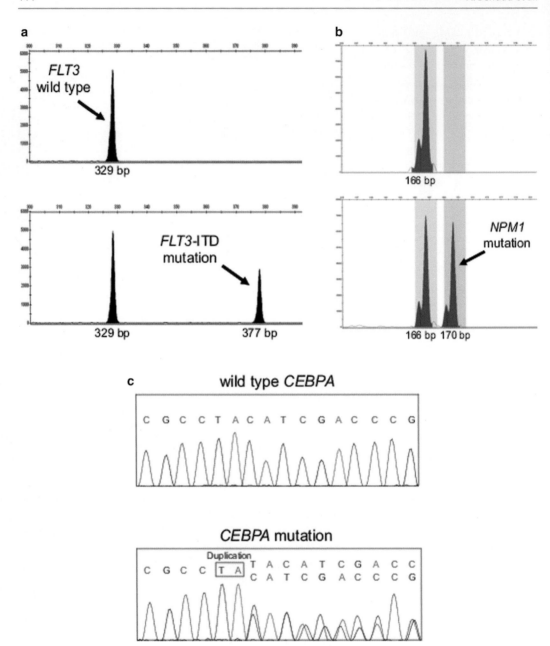

Fig. 10.3 Molecular tests for AML prognosis. Examples of mutation positive (*bottom*) and negative (*top*) cases are shown. (**a**) *FLT3* internal tandem duplication (*FLT3-ITD*) mutations can be detected by PCR amplicon sizing using capillary electrophoresis. The wild-type *FLT3* PCR fragment in this assay is 329 base pairs (bp) in length. Note the second PCR fragment of larger size in the bottom case, which is consistent with the presence of an ITD insertion mutation of 48 bp. (**b**) *NPM1* mutations can also be detected by PCR amplicon sizing. These mutations result in a net 4 bp insertion and are indicated by a PCR fragment that is 4 bp larger than the wild-type fragment. (**c**) *CEBPA* mutation testing requires a technology like Sanger sequencing that can detect the diverse variety of mutations that span the entire gene. Overlapping peaks in the DNA sequence chromatogram indicate the presence of a mutation. In this case it is a duplication of 2 nucleotides (TA) leading to a frameshift in the N-terminus region of the *CEBPA* protein. A second mutation was also observed in the C-terminus region (not shown), which is consistent with double (biallelic) *CEBPA* mutations in this case

(1) an internal tandem duplication (ITD), of the juxtamembrane domain-coding sequence occurring between exons 14 and 15 [83], and (2) a missense point mutation that alters an aspartic acid residue at position 835 (D835) in the tyrosine kinase domain (TKD) located at exon 20 [84]. The *FLT3*-ITD and D835 mutations occur in approximately 30 % and 7 % of patients with AML, respectively. The presence of *FLT3*-ITD is clearly associated with a worse prognosis [84–86], particularly at high mutant allele burdens [87, 88], and it may be the most clinically significant single gene mutation in AML. The importance of *FLT3* TKD mutations, on the other hand, is not entirely clear, with mixed reports of their impact on prognosis [89–92].

The *FLT3*-ITD can be identified utilizing a PCR-based assay with fragment size analysis to detect a product size expansion of anywhere from 6 to several hundred bases. The D835 wild-type sequence contains an EcoRV restriction site, which is eliminated in the setting of mutation. These two assays can be combined into a multiplexed PCR with subsequent restriction endonuclease digestion of the PCR product and analysis by capillary electrophoresis [93]. Figure 10.3 depicts an example of *FLT3*-ITD-positive AML.

AML with *NPM1* or *CEBPA* mutation represent separate provisional entities in the 2008 WHO classification [10]. Both of these mutations are thought to be associated with favorable outcomes; however, their favorable association is eliminated when they co-occur with *FLT3*. NPM1 is a chaperone protein that regulates assembly and shuttling of proteins between the nucleus and cytoplasm and is predominantly expressed in the nucleolus [94, 95]. *NPM1* mutation was first discovered after the observation that a subset of AML with normal karyotype showed abnormal localization of NPM1 protein within the cytoplasm of blasts (NPM1c+) [96]. Molecular analysis of these cases revealed a mutation of the *NPM1* gene in nearly all cases. The most common type of *NPM1* mutation (type A), encountered in 70–80 % of the cases with NPM1c+, is a tetranucleotide sequence insertion at positions 956–959 in exon 12. This insert causes a frameshift sequence alteration in the C-terminus of the protein, which eliminates the nucleolar localization signal and generates a novel nuclear export signal, with consequent cytoplasmic localization of the protein [97]. Alternative mutations include different tetranucleotide sequence insertions in the same location as the type A mutation and rare mutations in exon 9 or 11. The mechanism of leukemogenesis by mutated *NPM1* is thought to be due to mislocalization of the ARF tumor suppressor protein, a key regulator of p53-dependent cell cycle arrest [98]. In the clinical laboratory, the majority of *NPM1* mutations can be detected using a PCR-based assay, amplifying exon 12 from genomic DNA with subsequent fragment size analysis (see Fig. 10.3). The mutations are always heterozygous and are, in general, mutually exclusive with other recurrent cytogenetic abnormalities [99].

CEBPA is a single exon gene located at chromosome 19q13.1 that encodes a basic leucine zipper (bZIP) transcription factor with an important role in the differentiation of myeloid cells. *CEBPA* contains different start codons located in the same open reading frame, generating two isoforms: p42, which promotes myeloid differentiation, and p30, which promotes proliferation [100]. *CEBPA* mutations typically occur in either the N-terminus or C-terminus regions. N-terminal mutations are frequently frameshift mutations that eliminate the possibility of p42 production, only allowing formation of the pro-proliferative p30 isoform. The C-terminal mutations are often in-frame insertions and deletions that impair the DNA-binding bZIP domain [101, 102]. These two types of mutation frequently co-occur on different alleles, eliminating normal p42 CEBPA function [100]. In other cases, only a single *CEBPA* mutation is present; however, the favorable outcome associated with *CEBPA* mutations is thought to be limited to the cases with biallelic mutation [103]. Multiplex PCR techniques or direct sequencing of PCR product has been used for the detection of the mutations. While the multiplex PCR assay may have higher analytical sensitivity, it may miss a subset of mutations such as multiple base pair substitution or point mutations [104]. Since the analytical sensitivity is generally not an issue at time of diagnosis in AML, a direct sequencing assay to detect *CEBPA* mutations is commonly utilized (Fig. 10.3). *CEBPA* and *NPM1* mutations are thought to be mutually exclusive [99], while *FLT3*-ITD and *CEBPA* biallelic mutations can rarely occur in the same tumor population. The prognosis in such cases is similar to that of cases with *FLT3*-ITD [103].

Mutations in *KIT* are frequently present in CBF AML [105–109]. Most of these mutations cluster in exons 8 and 17, and the D816 residue in exon 17, characteristically mutated in SM, is also one of the most frequently mutated sites in CBF AML [106, 107, 109]. The presence of a *KIT* mutation is clearly associated with a worse prognosis in the normally favorable-risk subset of CBF AML patients with t(8;21), and some studies have suggested a negative impact in inv(16) AML, although this finding has not been uniform [105–109].

Through integration of cytogenetic and molecular analysis, well-defined prognostic risk groups have been established in AML (see Table 10.4) [54, 56, 59, 105, 110, 111]. These risk groups guide therapeutic decision-making, as patients with favorable genetic risk factors are typically not transplanted in the first complete remission,

Table 10.4 Cytogenetic and molecular risk groups in acute myeloid leukemia [54, 56, 59, 105, 110, 111]

Risk category	Cytogenetic and molecular features
Favorable	t(8;21) without *KIT* mutation
	t(15;17)
	inv(16)/t(16;16)
	Intermediate-risk cytogenetics without *FLT3*-ITD and with either *NPM1* or biallelic *CEBPA* mutation
Intermediate	t(8;21) with *KIT* mutation
	t(9;11)
	Other cytogenetics, including normal karyotype
Poor	inv(3)/t(3;3)
	t(6;9)
	11q23 abnormalities other than t(9;11)
	t(9;22)
	-5, del(5q)
	-7, del(7q)
	-17, 17p abnormalities
	Complex cytogenetics (>3 abnormalities)

while early hematopoietic stem cell transplantation is frequently used for patients with poor-risk features [60]. Although *FLT3*, *NPM1*, and *CEBPA* are the most commonly assayed genes in AML, they are by no means the only genes important in AML pathogenesis. Many other genes are recurrently mutated in AML and reported to have prognostic relevance. With the recent development of high-throughput sequencing technology, it is becoming feasible to perform targeted resequencing of a panel of genes associated with AML outcomes. Translating this newfound ability to generate information about multiple genes into meaningful information for patients remains a major challenge. However, in the near future it is anticipated that panels of genes will be routinely analyzed at diagnosis, allowing more accurate risk stratification and personalized treatment selection [105].

Lymphoid Malignancies

Lymphoblastic Leukemia/Lymphoma

Lymphoblastic leukemia/lymphoma (ALL/LBL) is a heterogeneous group of precursor B-cell and T-cell malignancies which result from various genetic alterations that cause a block in lymphoid differentiation, exaggerated proliferation, and enhanced cell survival. ALL/LBL is more common in children than in adults, constituting 25 % of childhood malignancies with a cure rate approaching 80 % [112]. Previously, these neoplasms were categorized solely based upon their morphologic and immunophenotypic characteristics. However, in the last 2 decades, our understanding of the underlying genetic basis of these neoplasms has improved and has led to the discovery of prognostically and therapeutically important subgroups. The 2008 WHO classification recognizes distinct categories of B-ALL/LBL with recurrent genetic abnormalities [10]. Table 10.5 summarizes the cytogenetic abnormalities recognized by 2008 WHO as distinct entities with their common age group and prognosis. Conventional metaphase cytogenetics and FISH are routinely used to identify these

Table 10.5 Cytogenetic abnormalities defining the WHO category of "B-ALL/LBL with recurrent genetic abnormalities" [10]

Abnormality	Age group	Prognosis[a]
t(9;22); *BCR-ABL1*	Adult > children	Unfavorable
t(v;11q23); *MLL* rearranged	Infants > adults	Unfavorable
t(12;21); *ETV6-RUNX1* (*TEL-AML1*)	Children	Favorable
Hyperdiploidy[b]	Children	Favorable
Hypodiploidy[c]	Adult, children[d]	Unfavorable
t(5;14); *IL3-IGH*	Adult, children	Not different
t(1;19); *TCF3-PBX1*	Children > adults	? Not different[e]

ALL lymphoblastic leukemia, *LBL* lymphoblastic lymphoma
[a] Prognosis is compared to B-ALL/LBL, not otherwise specified
[b] Blasts contain >50 and <66 chromosomes without other structural alterations
[c] Blasts contain <46 chromosomes without other structural alterations
[d] Near haploid is limited to children and has worst prognosis
[e] Earlier studies indicated poor prognosis, but not with new intensive therapies

numerical and structural chromosomal abnormalities. Of note, the t(12;21) leading to *ETV6-RUNX1* fusion, which is associated with a good prognosis in childhood B-ALL/LBL, is cytogenetically cryptic and requires FISH or RT-PCR for detection [113].

The most common and therapeutically important genetic subgroup of B-ALL/LBL in adults is defined by the presence of *BCR-ABL1*. *BCR-ABL1* occurs in 20–30 % of adult ALL/LBL overall [114], but it is far less common in the pediatric population (2–4 %) [115]. The presence of *BCR-ABL1*, or the Philadelphia chromosome (Ph+), in ALL of any age group is associated with adverse outcomes and shortened survival [115–118]. In addition to its prognostic impact, the presence of *BCR-ABL1* rearrangement has therapeutic importance. First- and second-generation TKIs were developed to target the BCR-ABL1 fusion protein and are often utilized in the treatment of Ph+ ALL [119]. Similar to CML, development of resistance is observed.

Among the three described breakpoint cluster regions in the *BCR* gene, two are seen in B-ALL: M-bcr and m-bcr. As described previously, these two breakpoints within *BCR* produce two fusion proteins differing in size. The p190 isoform is encountered in most pediatric patients and about half of adult Ph+ B-ALLs, [120, 121], whereas p210, common in CML, is seen in about half of adult Ph+ B-ALL.

Molecular techniques for detection of *BCR-ABL1* rearrangements, MRD, and TKI resistance are discussed in the CML section.

In addition to chromosomal abnormalities, genome-wide analysis has led to discovery of copy number abnormalities (CNA) of genes involved in development, cell cycle regulation, and differentiation of B-cells [122, 123]. *IKZF1* encodes the Ikaros transcription factor, which plays a role in B-cell development. *IKZF1* deletion is seen in over 80 % of Ph+ B-ALL and is associated with poor outcomes [124–126]. *PAX5* mutations are the most common somatic mutation in pediatric B-ALL, encountered in about a third of patients [122], but are not thought to be an independent predictor of outcome [127]. Other gene alterations implicated in B-ALL pathogenesis include *IKZF3* (Aiolos), *LEF1*, *EBF1*, *RB1*, *TCF3*, *CDKN2A/CDKN2B*, *PTEN*, and *BTG1* [122, 128]. It remains to be seen whether testing for alterations of any of these genes will be a routine part of clinical practice.

T-ALL/LBL accounts for 15 % of pediatric and 25 % of adult lymphoblastic leukemia [129]. Eighty to ninety percent of lymphoblastic lymphomas, on the other hand, are of T-cell lineage. More than 50 % of T-ALL/LBLs have cytogenetic abnormalities that range from recurrent translocations detected by conventional cytogenetics to cryptic deletions, disclosed only by FISH [130]. The translocations in T-ALL/LBL often involve breakpoints involving T-cell receptor (TCR) loci on 14q11 (*TRA* and *TRD*) and 7q34 (*TRB*), bringing transcription factors such as *TAL1*, *TLX1*(*HOX11*), *TLX3*, *LMO2*, and *LYL1* under the control of the TCR enhancer regions [130–135]. The most common of the cryptic deletions are deletions of 9p21 and 1p32 which may occur with other genetic abnormalities [130].

NOTCH1 activation has been implicated in the pathogenesis of T-ALL/LBL [136]. NOTCH proteins are transmembrane receptors that play an important role in cell regulation and T-cell development. *NOTCH1* can be a fusion partner with *TRB* in the rare t(7; 9), but the majority of *NOTCH1* alterations are activating mutations, encountered in over half of T-ALL/LBL [137]. Given the high prevalence of these mutations, it has been hypothesized that they are one of the early events in T-ALL/LBL development and may be important as future therapeutic targets, as NOTCH signaling could be decreased through gamma secretase inhibitors and other strategies [138].

Identification of Immunoglobulin and T-Cell Receptor Rearrangements

B-cells and T-cells are unique in that they contain genes (immunoglobulin (Ig) genes in B-cells, TCR genes in T-cells) that undergo somatic recombination under normal physiologic conditions. Each Ig gene and each TCR gene contains multiple variable (V) and joining (J) gene segments. The Ig heavy chain locus (*IGH*), TCR beta locus (*TRB*), and TCR delta locus (*TRD*) additionally contain diversity (D) gene segments that sit between the V and J genes. Through a process mediated by recombination activating gene proteins (RAG1 and RAG2) [139], early in B- and T-cell development, Ig or TCR genes undergo V-(D)J rearrangement, which juxtaposes random V, D, and J gene segments together by excising intervening V, D, or J gene segments and noncoding DNA (Fig. 10.4). At the coding junctions where the V, D, and J genes are brought together, additional diversity is generated by loss of nucleotides and incorporation of random, nontemplated nucleotides by terminal deoxynucleo-

tidyl transferase (TdT). Through this process, Ig and TCR diversity is formed that is needed to generate the broad repertoire of antigen recognition necessary for effective immunity. When B-cells recognize antigen in a T-cell-dependent process, they go through the germinal center reaction. In the germinal center, affinity maturation proceeds through the generation of an additional level of Ig diversity by activation-induced cytidine deaminase (AID)-dependent somatic hypermutation [140]. As a result of these processes, a population of reactive, polyclonal B-cells or T-cells contains myriad unique V-(D)J rearrangements which differ from one another in length and base composition.

This property of reactive lymphoid populations can be easily harnessed to identify a clonal lymphoproliferation. As lymphomas are derived from a single cell, a lymphomatous neoplastic clonal expansion would be expected to share a common V-(D)J rearrangement. Therefore, detection of a dominant V-(D)J rearrangement is a surrogate for identification of a clonal population of lymphocytes. Historically, V-(D)J rearrangements have been detected by Southern blot hybridization [141, 142]. This method was limited by its laborious nature, long analysis time, and requirement of a large (~5 μg) amount of high-quality DNA, precluding testing of formalin-fixed, paraffin-embedded tissues. Southern blot analysis has largely been supplanted in clinical pathology laboratories by PCR-based analysis of Ig and TCR loci.

Numerous multiplexed PCR primer sets have been reported that allow for detection of the majority of Ig and TCR rearrangements [143–151]. Due to its relative structural simplicity, the TCR gamma locus (*TRG*) is most frequently analyzed in suspected T-cell lymphoproliferations. Both TCR αβ- and TCR γδ-expressing T-cells are expected to have rearranged *TRG*, as *TRD* and *TRG* rearrangements occur before those at *TRB* and TCR alpha (*TRA*) in T-cell ontogeny [152]. Many *TRG* rearrangements are nonproductive, and so biallelic rearrangements are frequently identified [153]. *TRB* has become feasible to assess by PCR, and its more complex genomic architecture is advantageous in decreasing the

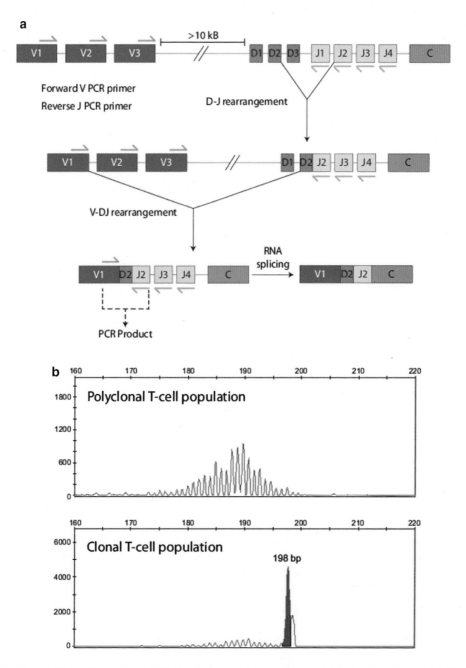

Fig. 10.4 Lymphoid clonality testing. (**a**) Idealized schematic representation of an immunoglobulin/T-cell receptor (Ig/TCR) locus. Forward and reverse primers bind to variable (V) gene segments and joining (J) gene segments, respectively. In the germline (i.e., nonlymphoid) configuration, no PCR product is generated due to the large distance between PCR primers. A J gene segment and diversity (D) gene segment are first joined together. The intervening, unused D and J gene segments Fig. 10.4 (continued) are excised. A similar process then occurs between the V gene segments and the D-J rearranged sequence. This final rearrangement brings the V and J forward and reverse primers near one another and allows generation of a PCR product. Because different V, D, and J gene segments are recombined in each lymphocyte, Ig/TCR diversity is generated by this process. Additional junctional diversity of the Ig/TCR is generated by the addition and deletion of random nucleotides at the D-J and V-DJ junctions (not depicted in the schematic). Because of the combinatorial and junctional diversity generated during physiologic B-cell and T-cell development, a polyclonal, reactive population of lymphocytes will generate multiple PCR products of varying sizes. (**b**) Examples of polyclonal and monoclonal T-cell populations by PCR analysis. When analyzed by capillary electrophoresis, as depicted in the first panel, a polyclonal population generates a pseudo-Gaussian distribution of peaks. No single peak is significantly larger than any of the others, and this is the expected result in a reactive population with numerous small T-cell clones. The second panel depicts a clonal T-cell population, which generates a dominant peak in the PCR assay. Note that some polyclonal T-cells are also present in this specimen (small peaks present to the left of the clonal peak)

likelihood of "pseudoclonal" results. However, rare γδ T-cell lymphomas may lack *TRB* rearrangements, and so sensitivity may not be as great as with a *TRG* assay. *TRD* is located within the *TRA* locus and both copies are deleted in most αβ T-cell lymphomas, severely limiting its utility in diagnosis [153]. *TRA* is highly complex, precluding the design of multiplexed PCR assays for this region.

IGH is the most commonly assayed immunoglobulin gene, as all mature B-cells express a functional IGH protein. In contrast with TCR assays, Ig assays may be affected by somatic hypermutation. If the primer binding sites have undergone mutation, it is possible that no product will be generated and the assay will appear falsely negative. This problem is particularly prevalent in germinal center-derived lymphomas, such as follicular lymphoma (FL) and some diffuse large B-cell lymphomas (DLBCL), where somatic hypermutation is ongoing [154]. This can be ameliorated to some degree by using multiple primer sets for *IGH* that avoid the area near the complementarity determining region 3 (CDR3), a major site of hypermutation in *IGH* (i.e., examining frameworks 1 and 2 in addition to framework 3). Alternatively, examining a light chain locus for clonality could yield greater sensitivity for rearrangements. *IGK* and *IGL* are amenable to PCR clonality testing [144]. Essentially every mature B-cell rearranges *IGK*; therefore, examining it for rearrangements can be useful and may detect rearrangements missed by examining *IGH* alone [154]. Given that all lambda light chain expressing lymphomas also contain rearrangements of *IGH* and *IGK* (and that the more common kappa light chain expressing lymphomas generally lack *IGL* rearrangement), examining *IGL* for rearrangement is not especially useful [154].

Clonality testing is generally performed by sizing PCR products detected by capillary electrophoresis (Fig. 10.4). This method distinguishes products based only on size: distinct clones with varying sequence but the same number of nucleotides are not discriminated from one another. A polyclonal population of lymphocytes will demonstrate a pseudo-Gaussian distribution, with the most abundant peaks surrounding the "germline" rearrangement size (i.e., without significant loss or non-templated gain of nucleotides). Clonal peaks are seen either in isolation or as predominant over the background polyclonal distribution. Criteria for interpretation as a "positive" result for clonality have been published [145, 155–157], but no consensus exists. The significance of a peak can vary dramatically based upon clinical context: a "clonal" peak in a TCR assay from a skin biopsy containing very few T-cells may be entirely insignificant, while a similar peak from a piece of tissue containing an overt lymphoma likely represents a true clonal result. It is extremely important to recognize that in clinical specimens with few lymphocytes, a "jackpot" phenomenon may occur with stochastic over-amplification of a single Ig or TCR rearrangement early during the PCR that leads to a spurious "pseudoclonal" appearance. Performance of clonality assays in duplicate is a necessary step to help reduce misinterpretation of these artifacts as monoclonal populations [158]. Even in the absence of an artifactual explanation for a clonal result, it is vital to remember that clonality is not synonymous with malignancy and that all Ig and TCR clonality results should ultimately be interpreted in light of the patient's other clinical and histologic features. Also importantly, the identification of Ig or TCR rearrangement cannot be confidently used to assign lineage to a neoplasm: T-cell lymphoblastic leukemias may harbor Ig rearrangements [159], B-ALLs frequently have TCR rearrangements [160], and either may be seen in AMLs [161].

Translocations in Lymphoma

Given that the production of physiologic Ig and TCR rearrangements requires DNA double-strand breaks (DSBs) and subsequent repair, it is perhaps not surprising that errors in this process occur. In experimental models, the induction of DSBs at *IGH* leads to aberrant gene fusions at hundreds of thousands of sites [162, 163]. If one of these abnormal gene fusions exerts a selection advantage, a lymphoma may eventually form following the acquisition of additional mutational events. Several B-cell lymphomas are strongly associated with the presence of an abnormal Ig gene fusion, including *BCL2* in FL [164], *CCND1* in mantle cell lymphoma (MCL) [165, 166], and *MYC* in Burkitt lymphoma (BL) [167, 168]. In general, Ig fusions differ from most gene fusions seen in acute leukemias in which a qualitatively abnormal novel protein is produced. In Ig fusions, on the other hand, a qualitatively normal gene is translocated so that it is under the influence of the Ig enhancer regions, which leads to marked upregulation of the normal protein product. This characteristic frequently limits the utility of PCR-based detection of Ig-associated rearrangements, as the breakpoints may be quite variable.

BCL2 Translocations

BCL2 encodes an anti-apoptotic protein that is aberrantly upregulated as a result of its juxtaposition to the *IGH* enhancer on chromosome 14. As a consequence of this deregulation, cell survival is enhanced [169]. *IGH-BCL2* fusion is present in approximately 90 % of FL [170, 171] and in approximately 20 % of DLBCL, predominantly in those with a germinal center immunophenotype [171–173]. From a practical standpoint, the diagnosis of FL is straightforward in lymph node biopsies, and documentation of *BCL2* rearrangement is not needed in most cases. However, in non-nodal sites or in cases with atypical morphologic or immunophenotypic features, documentation of *IGH-BCL2* can be a useful diagnostic adjunctive assay. Although the breakpoint in the *IGH* locus is generally near the *IGHJ* gene segments, multiple breakpoint regions are present in *BCL2*, occurring in three primary areas: the major breakpoint region (MBR), minor cluster region (mcr), and 3′ of the MBR [174–177]. Interphase FISH analysis using dual-color, dual-fusion probes for *IGH-BCL2* rearrangement identifies the vast majority of *IGH-BCL2* fusions [178]. Multiplexed PCR assays have been designed to capture the majority of *IGH-BCL2* rearrangements [144]; however, given the heterogeneity at the molecular level, even assays that evaluate all three breakpoint regions lack sensi-

tivity when compared with interphase FISH, detecting only 60–80 % of rearrangements in FISH-positive cases [179, 180]. PCR has an advantage over FISH in that it has a much lower limit of detection. For patients with PCR-detectable *IGH-BCL2* rearrangements, PCR positivity can be used as a marker for MRD following chemotherapy; however, the conclusion of studies has been mixed regarding the prognostic significance of MRD detection in FL [181, 182], and assessment of MRD is not recommended outside of a clinical trial setting [183].

The absence of *BCL2* translocation in lymphomas morphologically consistent with FL can be informative in certain clinical settings. In a younger patient with morphologic features of FL and limited stage disease, the absence of a detectable *BCL2* translocation would support a diagnosis of "pediatric-type" FL, which appears to have an indolent clinical course [184, 185]. Similarly, low-stage extranodal FL such as those located primarily in the testis [186, 187], ovary [188], and salivary gland [189] are typically negative for *BCL2* rearrangements with favorable outcomes. Primary cutaneous follicle center lymphomas (PCFCL) frequently lack *BCL2* rearrangements, although the frequency of the rearrangement is variably reported in the literature, ranging from being present in 0–40 % of cases [190–192]. Secondary cutaneous involvement by systemic FL must be excluded if an *IGH-BCL2* fusion is identified in a cutaneous B-cell lymphoma of germinal center derivation.

CCND1 Translocations

The vast majority of MCLs (>95 %) [193–196] contain *IGH-CCND1* fusions, leading to increased expression of cyclin D1 and subsequent cell cycle progression [197]. Many *CCND1* breaks occur at the major translocation cluster (MTC) [198], but this region contains only 40 % of all breakpoints. The remaining breakpoints are widely dispersed, which severely limits the sensitivity of PCR-based strategies for detection of *IGH-CCND1* [154]. In contrast, FISH is highly sensitive for *CCND1* translocations [193, 196] and is the technique of choice for documentation of *CCND1* translocation (in addition to cyclin D1 protein overexpression). FISH for *CCND1* is commonly performed as part of a "chronic lymphocytic leukemia (CLL) FISH panel" to exclude MCL, as MCL and CLL are immunophenotypically similar. If a tumor has typical morphologic and immunophenotypic features of MCL, the absence of cyclin D1 overexpression or detectable *IGH-CCND1* fusion does not exclude the diagnosis: "cyclin D1-negative" MCL have been described [194], and many of these tumors have rearrangements involving *CCND2* [199]. Identification of these cases is challenging in routine clinical practice.

MYC Translocations

BL is characterized by *MYC* translocations to *IG* genes [10] and is an aggressive tumor that frequently occurs in children and young adults. *MYC* is most commonly translocated to the *IGH* locus, but rearrangements with *IGK* and *IGL* also occur [167, 168]. All of the translocations have the common effect of abnormally upregulating MYC, leading to increased proliferation and dysregulation of many other cellular processes [200]. Both the *MYC* and *IG* breakpoints are heterogeneous [201–203] and vary among clinical subtypes of BL (i.e., endemic vs. sporadic vs. immunodeficiency associated) [204]. Therefore, *MYC* rearrangement detection by PCR is not feasible in the clinical setting. A break-apart FISH strategy would be expected to identify the vast majority of MYC translocations and is widely used clinically [205, 206]; however, rare variant breakpoints may still generate normal results with this approach [205]. Break-apart FISH does not identify the translocation partner, which may be important in BL. It has become clear that *MYC* in BL characteristically has an *IG* gene translocation partner, while *MYC* translocations in DLBCL cases often occur with non-*IG* genes [207]. Fusion FISH probe sets could be used to specifically identify the translocation partner in the absence of metaphase cytogenetics. As implied above, although characteristic in BL, identification of a *MYC* translocation is not at all specific, as they are present in 5–10 % of DLBCL [207–209]. Conversely, given the limitations of FISH and the recognition of alternative mechanisms of MYC deregulation [210], absence of an identifiable *MYC* translocation does not preclude a diagnosis of bona fide BL in an appropriate setting [10].

Double-Hit Aggressive B-Cell Lymphomas

A subset of large B-cell lymphomas harbor both a *MYC* translocation and another recurrent translocation, most often *IGH-BCL2*, but sometimes *BCL6*. These lymphomas are often called double-hit lymphomas (DHL) and have an aggressive clinical course with poor response to typical DLBCL chemotherapeutic regimens (R-CHOP) [211–213] (Fig. 10.5). DHL lymphomas with *IGH-BCL2* and *MYC* translocations are the best characterized variant; DHL with *BCL6* and *MYC* translocations appear to have similarly poor outcomes [214], and "triple-hit" lymphomas with rearrangements of all three genes are occasionally encountered [211]. Appropriate selection of patients with morphologic DLBCL for further FISH testing is critical given the important prognostic and therapeutic implication of identifying a DHL. Proliferation as assessed by Ki-67 lacks sufficient sensitivity and specificity to be useful in this determination [212, 215, 216]. MYC and BCL2 protein overexpression may better select appropriate patients for subsequent FISH testing and could possibly even supplant FISH testing for DHL, although further studies are needed [215, 217–219].

MALT1 Translocation

Extranodal marginal zone lymphomas of mucosa-associated lymphoid tissue (MALT lymphomas) that occur in the stomach and lung are frequently associated with t(11;18), *BIRC3(API2)-MALT1* fusion [220, 221]. The chimeric BIRC3-MALT1 protein activates NF-κB signaling and leads to increased cell survival [222]. In the stomach,

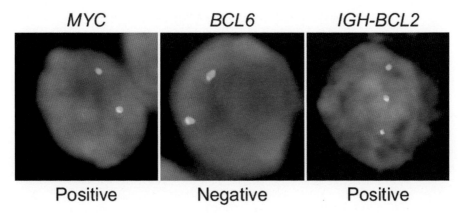

Positive   Negative   Positive

Fig. 10.5 Identification of a double-hit lymphoma by fluorescence in situ hybridization (FISH). *MYC* rearrangements may involve a variety of translocation partners, including *IGH, IGK, IGL*, and other non-*IG* genes. Therefore a break-apart FISH probe strategy is used that will detect any *MYC* rearrangement, regardless of the partner gene. Fluorescently labeled red and green probes are designed on opposite sides of the *MYC* gene breakpoint region. With this design, a normal *MYC* gene is observed as overlapping or adjacent red and green fluorescent signals, while a rearranged *MYC* gene is indicated by split red and green signals. *BCL6* rearrangements also involve a variety of partner genes and are identified using a similar break-apart strategy. The *IGH-BCL2* translocation is conserved in B-cell lymphoma and is usually detected with a dual-fusion probe strategy. This design utilizes a green probe specific to the *IGH* locus and a red probe specific to the *BCL2* gene, each spanning the respective breakpoint regions. Individual green and red probe signals indicate a lack of translocation. Colocalization of green and red probes is observed when an *IGH-BCL2* translocation is present. This case harbored both a *MYC* rearrangement and an *IGH-BCL2* translocation. *BCL6* rearrangement was not observed

MALT lymphomas are highly associated with infection by *Helicobacter pylori*, and *H. pylori* eradication is typically the initial therapeutic option in gastric MALT lymphoma, as a significant number of cases regress with antibiotic treatment [223]. However, the presence of *BIRC3-MALT1* fusion predicts for lack of response to *H. pylori* eradication [224–226], and therefore, testing for *BIRC3-MALT1* fusion by FISH or molecular techniques is recommended at diagnosis of gastric MALT lymphoma so that alternative therapies can be considered [223].

ALK + ALCL, most commonly with *NPM1* [228], which occurs in approximately 80 % of patients [229]. In the remaining cases, numerous other translocation partners are implicated, all of which lead to constitutive *ALK* activation [230]. The diagnosis of ALK + ALCL is often straightforward through the use of immunohistochemistry for ALK protein expression, which is essentially never seen in postnatal tissue [231]. However, in selected cases *ALK* may be assessed for rearrangements through breakapart FISH probes.

ALK Translocation

ALK-positive anaplastic large cell lymphoma (ALK + ALCL) is a mature T-cell lymphoma characterized by CD30 expression and *ALK* translocation with increased ALK protein expression [10]. Its incidence is highest in childhood and adolescence [227]. *ALK* encodes a receptor tyrosine kinase that is deregulated and activated through translocation in

TCL1 Translocation

T-cell prolymphocytic leukemia (T-PLL) is an aggressive mature T-cell neoplasm characterized by marked lymphocytosis and organomegaly [10]. The histopathologic and immunophenotypic features may show some overlap with other mature T-cell neoplasms with leukemic presentation, such as adult T-cell leukemia/lymphoma and Sézary syndrome.

Table 10.6 Genetic abnormalities associated with lymphoid neoplasms

Abnormality	Lymphoma	Detection method
IGH-BCL2	FL, subset DLBCL	FISH, PCR
IGH-CCND1	MCL, subset PCM	FISH
MYC rearrangement	BL, subset DLBCL	FISH
BIRC3(API2)-MALT1	Gastric/pulmonary MALT	FISH
ALK rearrangement	ALCL	IHC, FISH
TRA-TCL1	T-PLL	FISH
BRAF V600E	HCL	PCR
MYD88 L265P	LPL, subset DLBCL	PCR

FISH fluorescence in situ hybridization, PCR polymerase chain reaction, IHC immunohistochemistry, FL follicular lymphoma, DLBCL diffuse large B-cell lymphoma, MCL mantle cell lymphoma, PCM plasma cell myeloma, BL Burkitt lymphoma, MALT extranodal marginal zone lymphoma of mucosa-associated lymphoid tissue, ALCL anaplastic large cell lymphoma, T-PLL T-cell prolymphocytic leukemia, HCL hairy cell leukemia, LPL lymphoplasmacytic lymphoma

T-PLL frequently has rearrangements of TRA with the TCL1A/TCL1B locus [232, 233] through inv(14) or t(14; 14). Other cases involve TRA translocation with a gene homologous to TCL1A, MTCP1, which is located at Xq28 [234]. These rearrangements are readily identified by FISH analysis, often through a break-apart probe strategy targeting TCL1 or TRA, which allows for diagnostic confirmation of T-PLL.

Single Gene Mutations

Hairy cell leukemia (HCL) and lymphoplasmacytic lymphoma (LPL), two low-grade mature B-cell neoplasms, harbor highly recurrent point mutations, BRAF V600E and MYD88 L265P, respectively [235, 236]. The fact that both occur at a single codon makes them highly amenable to testing in a molecular diagnostics laboratory. HCL can usually be easily diagnosed through morphologic and immunophenotypic analysis [10]; however, the presence of BRAF V600E (which occurs in >95 % of HCL cases) essentially excludes other lymphomas that may mimic HCL, such as HCL-variant [237], and documentation of its presence may be helpful in patients with disease refractory to standard treatments, as BRAF inhibitors are approved for non-hematologic malignancies and anecdotal reports of response in HCL exist

[238]. LPL exhibits extensive morphologic overlap with other low-grade B-cell lymphomas with plasmacytic differentiation, and it has often been considered a "diagnosis of exclusion" [10]. MYD88 L265P is present in 70–90 % of LPL [235, 239, 240], and while not entirely specific, its presence is highly suggestive of LPL in the appropriate setting. Diagnostically important genetic abnormalities in lymphoma are summarized in Table 10.6.

While not as high prevalence as these examples, many other genes have recently been found to be recurrently mutated at a substantial frequency in lymphomas. Splenic marginal zone lymphoma (SMZL) has recurrent mutations in NOTCH2 in approximately 25 % of cases [241, 242], leading to increased NOTCH signaling. This finding suggests NOTCH inhibition as a possible therapeutic approach in SMZL. Genes involved in epigenetic regulation such as EZH2, MLL2, CREBBP, and EP300 are often mutated in germinal center-derived neoplasms such as FL and some DLBCLs [243–246]. DLBCLs that are not derived from germinal centers frequently have aberrations of genes that lead to NF-κB activation, such as CARD11, CD79A, CD79B, MYD88, and TNFAIP3 [247–251]. Comprehensive testing for many of these aberrations will be feasible in the near future and may lead to more rational, targeted therapies for patients with these lymphomas.

CLL Prognostication

CLL is a mature lymphoma that typically has a leukemic (blood and bone marrow involvement) presentation. The clinical course is heterogeneous: some patients have stable disease for years, while others have a more progressive course. FISH analysis reveals the presence of cytogenetic abnormalities in the majority of CLL cases, and patients can be risk stratified by their cytogenetic abnormalities [252]. 13q14 deletions are the most commonly identified abnormality and, in isolation, indicate a good prognosis. CLL with abnormalities of trisomy 12 have a more intermediate prognosis, while deletions of 11q23 and 17p (targeting *ATM* and *TP53*) [253] indicate more aggressive behavior [252]. Because identification of patients with 11q23 and 17p may be important therapeutically, FISH profiling of CLL is recommended prior to the initiation of therapy [254–256]. In the future, risk stratification may be further informed by the addition of mutational analysis for genes recurrently mutated in CLL (e.g., *NOTCH1*, *SF3B1*, *MYD88*, *BIRC3*, *TP53*) [257]; however, this analysis is outside of the scope of that offered by most laboratories today.

In addition to the utility of FISH testing, analysis of the *IGHV* region is prognostic in CLL. Patients with unmutated (defined as ≥98 % germline sequence homology) [258, 259] *IGHV* have a poorer outcome than those with evidence of hypermutation. Similar findings have been reported in MCL. Although classically thought of as a neoplasm of naïve B-cells, some MCL have hypermutated immunoglobulin genes. These uncommon hypermutated MCLs frequently have leukemic and splenic involvement, without significant lymphadenopathy, and may have a more indolent clinical course than those with unmutated *IGHV* [260].

Plasma Cell Myeloma

Many genetic aberrations have been identified in plasma cell myeloma (PCM), and testing by both metaphase cytogenetics and FISH is routinely performed at diagnosis. Two major genetic categories

have been described: tumors with a hyperdiploid genome characterized by numerous trisomies of odd-numbered chromosomes and a relatively favorable prognosis and non-hyperdiploid tumors with frequent *IGH* translocations and generally poorer outcomes [261]. A cytogenetically cryptic t(4;14) (p16;q32) translocation deregulates both *FGFR3* and *WHSC1* (*MMSET*) in PCM through their juxtaposition with the *IGH* enhancer [262]. This translocation is often associated with chromosome 13 monosomy/13q deletion [261] and typically has an aggressive clinical course [263]. In addition to their presence in MCL, *IGH-CCND1* translocations with slightly different breakpoints are frequent in PCM and are associated with good to intermediate survival, lymphoplasmacytoid morphology, and aberrant CD20 expression [261]. A t(14;16) leading to *IGH-MAF* fusion is somewhat less common than rearrangements involving either *CCND1* or *FGFR3/WHSC1* [10]. *IGH-MAF* has been reported to be associated with a poor prognosis [263], although this is controversial [264]. Secondary genetic events with prognostic importance include both 17p (*TP53*) deletion and alterations of chromosome 1 (leading to 1p loss and 1q gain) [261]. *TP53* deletions are associated with a poor prognosis [263, 265]. The impact of chromosome 1 abnormalities in PCM is unclear: some studies have suggested that they are poor prognostic indicators [266–268], while others have failed to confirm a worse prognosis when 1q gain is detected by FISH [265, 269].

Conclusions

Rapid technologic advances and scientific insights into the genetic basis of hematologic malignancies have led to significant opportunities for the molecular diagnostics laboratory. The expansion of multiple molecular testing modalities including FISH, PCR, targeted sequencing, whole exome sequencing, and microarrays has greatly impacted the clinical significance of molecular testing. Similarly, with the availability of multiple testing modalities and their respective sample requirements and turnaround times, adequate communication regarding appropriateness for testing and reflex testing algorithms is becoming increasingly important. Furthermore, the incorporation of high-content data generated by whole exome sequencing, SNP microarrays, or other "omics" platforms necessitates implementation of appropriate resources to develop a bioinformatics component to the integrated molecular diagnostics laboratory. Emerging technologies and genetic alterations involving microRNAs, long noncoding RNAs, and epigenetics will continue to provide opportunities for the molecular diagnostics laboratory to continually adapt to the rapidly evolving technologic environment. Ultimately, molecular testing will continue to play a critical role in the identification of the genetic basis of hematologic malignancy and will allow selection of therapeutic agents for personalized/precision medicine for patients.

References

1. Ren R. Mechanisms of BCR-ABL in the pathogenesis of chronic myelogenous leukaemia. Nat Rev Cancer. 2005;5:172–83.
2. Faderl S, Kantarjian HM, Talpaz M, Estrov Z. Clinical significance of cytogenetic abnormalities in adult acute lymphoblastic leukemia. Blood. 1998;91:3995–4019.
3. Druker BJ, Tamura S, Buchdunger E, Ohno S, Segal GM, Fanning S, et al. Effects of a selective inhibitor of the Abl tyrosine kinase on the growth of Bcr-Abl positive cells. Nat Med. 1996;2:561–6.
4. Deininger M, Buchdunger E, Druker BJ. The development of imatinib as a therapeutic agent for chronic myeloid leukemia. Blood. 2005;105:2640–53.
5. Hughes TP, Kaeda J, Branford S, Rudzki Z, Hochhaus A, Hensley ML, et al. Frequency of major molecular responses to imatinib or interferon alfa plus cytarabine in newly diagnosed chronic myeloid leukemia. N Engl J Med. 2003;349:1423–32.
6. Soverini S, Hochhaus A, Nicolini FE, Gruber F, Lange T, Saglio G, et al. BCR-ABL kinase domain mutation analysis in chronic myeloid leukemia patients treated with tyrosine kinase inhibitors: recommendations from an expert panel on behalf of European LeukemiaNet. Blood. 2011;118:1208–15.
7. Deininger MWN, Goldman JM, Melo JV. The molecular biology of chronic myeloid leukemia. Blood. 2000;96:3343–56.
8. Kurzrock R, Gutterman JU, Talpaz M. The molecular genetics of Philadelphia chromosome–positive leukemias. N Engl J Med. 1988;319:990–8.
9. Pane F, Frigeri F, Sindona M, Luciano L, Ferrara F, Cimino R, et al. Neutrophilic-chronic myeloid leukemia: a distinct disease with a specific molecular marker (BCR/ABL with C3/A2 junction). Blood. 1996;88:2410–4.
10. Swerdlow SH, International Agency for Research on Cancer, World Health Organization. WHO classification of tumours of haematopoietic and lymphoid tissues. 4th ed. Lyon, France: International Agency for Research on Cancer; 2008.
11. Barnes DJ, Melo JV. Cytogenetic and molecular genetic aspects of chronic myeloid leukaemia. Acta Haematol. 2002;108:180–202.
12. Primo D, Tabernero MD, Rasillo A, Sayagues JM, Espinosa AB, Chillon MC, et al. Patterns of BCR//ABL gene rearrangements by interphase fluorescence in situ hybridization (FISH) in BCR//ABL+ leukemias: incidence and underlying genetic abnormalities. Leukemia. 2003;17:1124–9.
13. Baccarani M, Pileri S, Steegmann J-L, Muller M, Soverini S, Dreyling M, et al. Chronic myeloid leukemia: ESMO Clinical Practice Guidelines for diagnosis, treatment and follow-up. Ann Oncol. 2012;23:vii72–7.
14. Saglio G, Fava C. Practical monitoring of chronic myelogenous leukemia: when to change treatment. J Natl Compr Cancer Netw. 2012;10:121–9.
15. Milojkovic D, Apperley J. Mechanisms of resistance to imatinib and second-generation tyrosine inhibitors in chronic myeloid leukemia. Clin Cancer Res. 2009;15:7519–27.
16. Cortes JE, Kantarjian H, Shah NP, Bixby D, Mauro MJ, Flinn I, et al. Ponatinib in refractory Philadelphia chromosome–positive leukemias. N Engl J Med. 2012;367:2075–88.
17. Baxter EJ, Scott LM, Campbell PJ, East C, Fourouclas N, Swanton S, et al. Acquired mutation of the tyrosine kinase JAK2 in human myeloproliferative disorders. Lancet. 2005;365:1054–61.
18. Levine RL, Wadleigh M, Cools J, Ebert BL, Wernig G, Huntly BJP, et al. Activating mutation in the tyrosine kinase JAK2 in polycythemia vera, essential thrombocythemia, and myeloid metaplasia with myelofibrosis. Cancer Cell. 2005;7:387–97.
19. Kralovics R, Passamonti F, Buser AS, Teo S-S, Tiedt R, Passweg JR, et al. A gain-of-function mutation of JAK2 in myeloproliferative disorders. N Engl J Med. 2005;352:1779–90.
20. Scott LM, Tong W, Levine RL, Scott MA, Beer PA, Stratton MR, et al. JAK2 Exon 12 mutations in polycythemia vera and idiopathic erythrocytosis. N Engl J Med. 2007;356:459–68.
21. Jones AV, Kreil S, Zoi K, Waghorn K, Curtis C, Zhang L, et al. Widespread occurrence of the JAK2 V617F mutation in chronic myeloproliferative disorders. Blood. 2005;106:2162–8.
22. Pardanani AD, Levine RL, Lasho T, Pikman Y, Mesa RA, Wadleigh M, et al. MPL515 mutations in myeloproliferative and other myeloid disorders: a study of 1182 patients. Blood. 2006;108:3472–6.

23. Tefferi A. JAK inhibitors for myeloproliferative neoplasms: clarifying facts from myths. Blood. 2012;119:2721–30.

24. Barosi G, Mesa R, Finazzi G, Harrison C, Kiladjian J-J, Lengfelder E, et al. Revised response criteria for polycythemia vera and essential thrombocythemia: a ELN and IWG-MRT consensus project. Blood. 2013;121:4778–81.

25. Abdel-Wahab O, Mullally A, Hedvat C, Garcia-Manero G, Patel J, Wadleigh M, et al. Genetic characterization of TET1, TET2, and TET3 alterations in myeloid malignancies. Blood. 2009;114:144–7.

26. Kohlmann A, Grossmann V, Klein H-U, Schindela S, Weiss T, Kazak B, et al. Next-generation sequencing technology reveals a characteristic pattern of molecular mutations in 72.8% of chronic myelomonocytic leukemia by detecting frequent alterations in TET2, CBL, RAS, and RUNX1. J Clin Oncol. 2010;28:3858–65.

27. Yoshida K, Sanada M, Shiraishi Y, Nowak D, Nagata Y, Yamamoto R, et al. Frequent pathway mutations of splicing machinery in myelodysplasia. Nature. 2011;478:64–9.

28. Gelsi-Boyer V, Trouplin V, Adélaïde J, Bonansea J, Cervera N, Carbuccia N, et al. Mutations of polycomb-associated gene ASXL1 in myelodysplastic syndromes and chronic myelomonocytic leukaemia. Br J Haematol. 2009;145:788–800.

29. Itzykson R, Kosmider O, Renneville A, Gelsi-Boyer V, Meggendorfer M, Morabito M, et al. Prognostic score including gene mutations in chronic myelomonocytic leukemia. J Clin Oncol. 2013;31:2428–36.

30. Loh ML, Sakai DS, Flotho C, Kang M, Fliegauf M, Archambeault S, et al. Mutations in CBL occur frequently in juvenile myelomonocytic leukemia. Blood. 2009;114:1859–63.

31. Chan RJ, Cooper T, Kratz CP, Weiss B, Loh ML. Juvenile myelomonocytic leukemia: a report from the 2nd international JMML symposium. Leuk Res. 2009;33:355–62.

32. Piazza R, Valletta S, Winkelmann N, Redaelli S, Spinelli R, Pirola A, et al. Recurrent SETBP1 mutations in atypical chronic myeloid leukemia. Nat Genet. 2013;45:18–24.

33. Maxson JE, Gotlib J, Pollyea DA, Fleischman AG, Agarwal A, Eide CA, et al. Oncogenic CSF3R mutations in chronic neutrophilic leukemia and atypical CML. N Engl J Med. 2013;368:1781–90.

34. Longley BJ, Tyrrell L, Lu SZ, Ma YS, Langley K, Ding TG, et al. Somatic c-KIT activating mutation in urticaria pigmentosa and aggressive mastocytosis: establishment of clonality in a human mast cell neoplasm. Nat Genet. 1996;12:312–4.

35. Bodemer C, Hermine O, Palmerini F, Yang Y, Grandpeix-Guyodo C, Leventhal PS, et al. Pediatric mastocytosis is a clonal disease associated with D816V and other activating c-KIT mutations. J Invest Dermatol. 2010;130:804–15.

36. Longley Jr BJ, Metcalfe DD, Tharp M, Wang X, Tyrrell L, Lu SZ, et al. Activating and dominant inactivating c-KIT catalytic domain mutations in distinct clinical forms of human mastocytosis. Proc Natl Acad Sci U S A. 1999;96:1609–14.

37. Baccarani M, Cilloni D, Rondoni M, Ottaviani E, Messa F, Merante S, et al. The efficacy of imatinib mesylate in patients with FIP1L1-PDGFRalpha-positive hypereosinophilic syndrome. Results of a multicenter prospective study. Haematologica. 2007;92:1173–9.

38. Apperley JF, Gardembas M, Melo JV, Russell-Jones R, Bain BJ, Baxter EJ, et al. Response to imatinib mesylate in patients with chronic myeloproliferative diseases with rearrangements of the platelet-derived growth factor receptor beta. N Engl J Med. 2002;347:481–7.

39. Fink SR, Belongie KJ, Paternoster SF, Smoley SA, Pardanani AD, Tefferi A, et al. Validation of a new three-color fluorescence in situ hybridization (FISH) method to detect CHIC2 deletion, FIP1L1/PDGFRA fusion and PDGFRA translocations. Leuk Res. 2009;33:843–6.

40. Macdonald D, Reiter A, Cross NC. The 8p11 myeloproliferative syndrome: a distinct clinical entity caused by constitutive activation of FGFR1. Acta Haematol. 2002;107:101–7.

41. Chen J, DeAngelo DJ, Kutok JL, Williams IR, Lee BH, Wadleigh M, et al. PKC412 inhibits the zinc finger 198-fibroblast growth factor receptor 1 fusion tyrosine kinase and is active in treatment of stem cell myeloproliferative disorder. Proc Natl Acad Sci U S A. 2004;101:14479–84.

42. Schanz J, Tüchler H, Solé F, Mallo M, Luño E, Cervera J, et al. New comprehensive cytogenetic scoring system for primary myelodysplastic syndromes (MDS) and oligoblastic acute myeloid leukemia after mds derived from an international database merge. J Clin Oncol. 2012;30:820–9.

43. Greenberg P, Cox C, LeBeau MM, Fenaux P, Morel P, Sanz G, et al. International scoring system for evaluating prognosis in myelodysplastic syndromes. Blood. 1997;89:2079–88.

44. Malcovati L, Germing U, Kuendgen A, Della Porta MG, Pascutto C, Invernizzi R, et al. Time-dependent prognostic scoring system for predicting survival and leukemic evolution in myelodysplastic syndromes. J Clin Oncol. 2007;25:3503–10.

45. Greenberg PL, Tuechler H, Schanz J, Sanz G, Garcia-Manero G, Solé F, et al. Revised international prognostic scoring system for myelodysplastic syndromes. Blood. 2012;120:2454–65.

46. Coleman JF, Theil KS, Tubbs RR, Cook JR. Diagnostic yield of bone marrow and peripheral blood FISH panel testing in clinically suspected myelodysplastic syndromes and/or acute myeloid leukemia: a prospective analysis of 433 cases. Am J Clin Pathol. 2011;135:915–20.

47. Tiu RV, Gondek LP, O'Keefe CL, Elson P, Huh J, Mohamedali A, et al. Prognostic impact of SNP array karyotyping in myelodysplastic syndromes and related myeloid malignancies. Blood. 2011;117: 4552–60.

48. Gondek LP, Tiu R, O'Keefe CL, Sekeres MA, Theil KS, Maciejewski JP. Chromosomal lesions and uniparental disomy detected by SNP arrays in MDS, MDS/MPD, and MDS-derived AML. Blood. 2008;111:1534–42.

49. Mohamedali A, Gäken J, Twine NA, Ingram W, Westwood N, Lea NC, et al. Prevalence and prognostic significance of allelic imbalance by single-nucleotide polymorphism analysis in low-risk myelodysplastic syndromes. Blood. 2007;110:3365–73.

50. Bejar R, Stevenson K, Abdel-Wahab O, Galili N, Nilsson B, Garcia-Manero G, et al. Clinical effect of point mutations in myelodysplastic syndromes. N Engl J Med. 2011;364:2496–506.

51. Papaemmanuil E, Cazzola M, Boultwood J, Malcovati L, Vyas P, Bowen D, et al. Somatic SF3B1 mutation in myelodysplasia with ring sideroblasts. N Engl J Med. 2011;365:1384–95.

52. Thol F, Kade S, Schlarmann C, Löffeld P, Morgan M, Krauter J, et al. Frequency and prognostic impact of mutations in SRSF2, U2AF1, and ZRSR2 in patients with myelodysplastic syndromes. Blood. 2012;119:3578–84.

53. Byrd JC, Mrozek K, Dodge RK, Carroll AJ, Edwards CG, Arthur DC, et al. Pretreatment cytogenetic abnormalities are predictive of induction success, cumulative incidence of relapse, and overall survival in adult patients with de novo acute myeloid leukemia: results from Cancer and Leukemia Group B (CALGB 8461). Blood. 2002;100:4325–36.

54. Grimwade D, Walker H, Oliver F, Wheatley K, Harrison C, Harrison G, et al. The importance of diagnostic cytogenetics on outcome in AML: analysis of 1,612 patients entered into the MRC AML 10 trial. The Medical Research Council Adult and Children's Leukæmia Working Parties. Blood. 1998;92:2322–33.

55. Keating MJ, Smith TL, Kantarjian H, Cork A, Walters R, Trujillo JM, et al. Cytogenetic pattern in acute myelogenous leukemia: a major reproducible determinant of outcome. Leukemia. 1988;2:403–12.

56. Slovak ML, Kopecky KJ, Cassileth PA, Harrington DH, Theil KS, Mohamed A, et al. Karyotypic analysis predicts outcome of preremission and postremission therapy in adult acute myeloid leukemia: a Southwest Oncology Group/Eastern Cooperative Oncology Group Study. Blood. 2000;96:4075–83.

57. Yunis JJ, Brunning RD, Howe RB, Lobell M. High-resolution chromosomes as an independent prognostic indicator in adult acute nonlymphocytic leukemia. N Engl J Med. 1984;311:812–8.

58. Mrozek K, Heerema NA, Bloomfield CD. Cytogenetics in acute leukemia. Blood Rev. 2004;18: 115–36.

59. Grimwade D, Hills RK, Moorman AV, Walker H, Chatters S, Goldstone AH, et al. Refinement of cytogenetic classification in acute myeloid leukemia: determination of prognostic significance of rare recurring chromosomal abnormalities among 5876 younger adult patients treated in the United Kingdom Medical Research Council trials. Blood. 2010;116: 354–65.

60. Döhner H, Estey EH, Amadori S, Appelbaum FR, Büchner T, Burnett AK, et al. Diagnosis and management of acute myeloid leukemia in adults: recommendations from an international expert panel, on behalf of the European LeukemiaNet. Blood. 2010;115:453–74.

61. Fröhling S, Skelin S, Liebisch C, Scholl C, Schlenk RF, Döhner H, et al. Comparison of cytogenetic and molecular cytogenetic detection of chromosome abnormalities in 240 consecutive adult patients with acute myeloid leukemia. J Clin Oncol. 2002;20: 2480–5.

62. van Dongen JJ, Macintyre EA, Gabert JA, Delabesse E, Rossi V, Saglio G, et al. Standardized RT-PCR analysis of fusion gene transcripts from chromosome aberrations in acute leukemia for detection of minimal residual disease. Report of the BIOMED-1 Concerted Action: investigation of minimal residual disease in acute leukemia. Leukemia. 1999;13:1901–28.

63. Grignani F, Ferrucci PF, Testa U, Talamo G, Fagioli M, Alcalay M, et al. The acute promyelocytic leukemia-specific PML-RAR alpha fusion protein inhibits differentiation and promotes survival of myeloid precursor cells. Cell. 1993;74:423–31.

64. Lengfelder E, Saussele S, Weisser A, Buchner T, Hehlmann R. Treatment concepts of acute promyelocytic leukemia. Crit Rev Oncol Hematol. 2005;56: 261–74.

65. Warrell Jr RP, Frankel SR, Miller Jr WH, Scheinberg DA, Itri LM, Hittelman WN, et al. Differentiation therapy of acute promyelocytic leukemia with tretinoin (all-trans-retinoic acid). N Engl J Med. 1991; 324:1385–93.

66. de Thé H, Chen Z. Acute promyelocytic leukaemia: novel insights into the mechanisms of cure. Nat Rev Cancer. 2010;10:775–83.

67. Sanz MA, Grimwade D, Tallman MS, Lowenberg B, Fenaux P, Estey EH, et al. Management of acute promyelocytic leukemia: recommendations from an expert panel on behalf of the European LeukemiaNet. Blood. 2009;113:1875–91.

68. Berger R, Le Coniat M, Derre J, Vecchione D, Jonveaux P. Cytogenetic studies in acute promyelocytic leukemia: a survey of secondary chromosomal abnormalities. Genes Chromosom Cancer. 1991;3: 332–7.

69. Brockman SR, Paternoster SF, Ketterling RP, Dewald GW. New highly sensitive fluorescence in situ hybridization method to detect PML/RARA fusion in acute promyelocytic leukemia. Cancer Genet Cytogenet. 2003;145:144–51.

70. Kim MJ, Cho SY, Kim MH, Lee JJ, Kang SY, Cho EH, et al. FISH-negative cryptic PML-RARA rearrangement detected by long-distance polymerase chain reaction and sequencing analyses: a case study and review of the literature. Cancer Genet Cytogenet. 2010;203:278–83.

71. Lo-Coco F, Ammatuna E. Front line clinical trials and minimal residual disease monitoring in acute promyelocytic leukemia. Curr Top Microbiol Immunol. 2007;313:145–56.

72. Grimwade D, Jovanovic JV, Hills RK, Nugent EA, Patel Y, Flora R, et al. Prospective minimal residual disease monitoring to predict relapse of acute promyelocytic leukemia and to direct pre-emptive arsenic trioxide therapy. J Clin Oncol. 2009;27:3650–8.

73. Grimwade D, Biondi A, Mozziconacci MJ, Hagemeijer A, Berger R, Neat M, et al. Characterization of acute promyelocytic leukemia cases lacking the classic t(15;17): results of the European Working Party. Groupe Francais de Cytogenetique Hematologique, Groupe de Francais d'Hematologie Cellulaire, UK Cancer Cytogenetics Group and BIOMED 1 European Community-Concerted Action "Molecular Cytogenetic Diagnosis in Haematological Malignancies". Blood. 2000;96:1297–308.

74. Zelent A, Guidez F, Melnick A, Waxman S, Licht JD. Translocations of the RARalpha gene in acute promyelocytic leukemia. Oncogene. 2001;20:7186–203.

75. Grimwade D, Mrozek K. Diagnostic and prognostic value of cytogenetics in acute myeloid leukemia. Hematol Oncol Clin North Am. 2011;25:1135 –61, vii.

76. Speck NA, Gilliland DG. Core-binding factors in haematopoiesis and leukaemia. Nat Rev Cancer. 2002;2:502–13.

77. Shih LY, Liang DC, Fu JF, Wu JH, Wang PN, Lin TL, et al. Characterization of fusion partner genes in 114 patients with de novo acute myeloid leukemia and MLL rearrangement. Leukemia. 2006;20: 218–23.

78. Arber DA, Stein AS, Carter NH, Ikle D, Forman SJ, Slovak ML. Prognostic impact of acute myeloid leukemia classification. Importance of detection of recurring cytogenetic abnormalities and multilineage dysplasia on survival. Am J Clin Pathol. 2003;119: 672–80.

79. Gahn B, Haase D, Unterhalt M, Drescher M, Schoch C, Fonatsch C, et al. De novo AML with dysplastic hematopoiesis: cytogenetic and prognostic significance. Leukemia. 1996;10:946–51.

80. Miyazaki Y, Kuriyama K, Miyawaki S, Ohtake S, Sakamaki H, Matsuo T, et al. Cytogenetic heterogeneity of acute myeloid leukaemia (AML) with trilineage dysplasia: Japan Adult Leukaemia Study Group-AML 92 study. Br J Haematol. 2003;120: 56–62.

81. Miesner M, Haferlach C, Bacher U, Weiss T, Macijewski K, Kohlmann A, et al. Multilineage dysplasia (MLD) in acute myeloid leukemia (AML) correlates with MDS-related cytogenetic abnormalities and a prior history of MDS or MDS/MPN but has no independent prognostic relevance: a comparison of 408 cases classified as "AML not otherwise specified" (AML-NOS) or "AML with myelodysplasia-related changes" (AML-MRC). Blood. 2010;116: 2742–51.

82. Zauli G, Voltan R, Tisato V, Secchiero P. State of the art of the therapeutic perspective of sorafenib against hematological malignancies. Curr Med Chem. 2012;19:4875–84.

83. Nakao M, Yokota S, Iwai T, Kaneko H, Horiike S, Kashima K, et al. Internal tandem duplication of the flt3 gene found in acute myeloid leukemia. Leukemia. 1996;10:1911–8.

84. Yamamoto Y, Kiyoi H, Nakano Y, Suzuki R, Kodera Y, Miyawaki S, et al. Activating mutation of D835 within the activation loop of FLT3 in human hematologic malignancies. Blood. 2001;97:2434–9.

85. Kottaridis PD, Gale RE, Frew ME, Harrison G, Langabeer SE, Belton AA, et al. The presence of a FLT3 internal tandem duplication in patients with acute myeloid leukemia (AML) adds important prognostic information to cytogenetic risk group and response to the first cycle of chemotherapy: analysis of 854 patients from the United Kingdom Medical Research Council AML 10 and 12 trials. Blood. 2001;98:1752–9.

86. Thiede C, Steudel C, Mohr B, Schaich M, Schakel U, Platzbecker U, et al. Analysis of FLT3-activating mutations in 979 patients with acute myelogenous leukemia: association with FAB subtypes and identification of subgroups with poor prognosis. Blood. 2002;99:4326–35.

87. Whitman SP, Archer KJ, Feng L, Baldus C, Becknell B, Carlson BD, et al. Absence of the wild-type allele predicts poor prognosis in adult de novo acute myeloid leukemia with normal cytogenetics and the internal tandem duplication of FLT3: a cancer and leukemia group B study. Cancer Res. 2001;61: 7233–9.

88. Gale RE, Green C, Allen C, Mead AJ, Burnett AK, Hills RK, et al. The impact of FLT3 internal tandem duplication mutant level, number, size, and interaction with NPM1 mutations in a large cohort of young adult patients with acute myeloid leukemia. Blood. 2008;111:2776–84.

89. Bacher U, Haferlach C, Kern W, Haferlach T, Schnittger S. Prognostic relevance of FLT3-TKD mutations in AML: the combination matters—an analysis of 3082 patients. Blood. 2008;111: 2527–37.

90. Yanada M, Matsuo K, Suzuki T, Kiyoi H, Naoe T. Prognostic significance of FLT3 internal tandem duplictation and tyrosine kinase domain mutations

for acute myeloid leukemia: a meta-analysis. Leukemia. 2005;19:1345–9.

91. Mead AJ, Linch DC, Hills RK, Wheatley K, Burnett AK, Gale RE. FLT3 tyrosine kinase domain mutations are biologically distinct from and have a significantly more favorable prognosis than FLT3 internal tandem duplications in patients with acute myeloid leukemia. Blood. 2007;110:1262–70.

92. Whitman SP, Ruppert AS, Radmacher MD, Mrózek K, Paschka P, Langer C, et al. FLT3 D835/I836 mutations are associated with poor disease-free survival and a distinct gene-expression signature among younger adults with de novo cytogenetically normal acute myeloid leukemia lacking FLT3 internal tandem duplications. Blood. 2008;111:1552–9.

93. Murphy KM, Levis M, Hafez MJ, Geiger T, Cooper LC, Smith BD, et al. Detection of FLT3 internal tandem duplication and D835 mutations by a multiplex polymerase chain reaction and capillary electrophoresis assay. J Mol Diagn. 2003;5:96–102.

94. Cordell JL, Pulford KA, Bigerna B, Roncador G, Banham A, Colombo E, et al. Detection of normal and chimeric nucleophosmin in human cells. Blood. 1999;93:632–42.

95. Borer RA, Lehner CF, Eppenberger HM, Nigg EA. Major nucleolar proteins shuttle between nucleus and cytoplasm. Cell. 1989;56:379–90.

96. Falini B, Mecucci C, Tiacci E, Alcalay M, Rosati R, Pasqualucci L, et al. Cytoplasmic nucleophosmin in acute myelogenous leukemia with a normal karyotype. N Engl J Med. 2005;352:254–66.

97. Falini B, Nicoletti I, Martelli MF, Mecucci C. Acute myeloid leukemia carrying cytoplasmic/mutated nucleophosmin (NPMc+ AML): biologic and clinical features. Blood. 2007;109:874–85.

98. Colombo E, Martinelli P, Zamponi R, Shing DC, Bonetti P, Luzi L, et al. Delocalization and destabilization of the Arf tumor suppressor by the leukemia-associated NPM mutant. Cancer Res. 2006;66: 3044–50.

99. Falini B, Martelli MP, Bolli N, Sportoletti P, Liso A, Tiacci E, et al. Acute myeloid leukemia with mutated nucleophosmin (NPM1): is it a distinct entity? Blood. 2011;117:1109–20.

100. Nerlov C. C/EBP alpha mutations in acute myeloid leukaemias. Nat Rev Cancer. 2004;4:394–400.

101. Pabst T, Mueller BU, Zhang P, Radomska HS, Narravula S, Schnittger S, et al. Dominant-negative mutations of CEBPA, encoding CCAAT/enhancer binding protein-alpha (C/EBP alpha), in acute myeloid leukemia. Nat Genet. 2001;27:263–70.

102. Gombart AF, Hofmann WK, Kawano S, Takeuchi S, Krug U, Kwok SH, et al. Mutations in the gene encoding the transcription factor CCAAT/enhancer binding protein alpha in myelodysplastic syndromes and acute myeloid leukemias. Blood. 2002;99: 1332–40.

103. Dufour A, Schneider F, Metzeler KH, Hoster E, Schneider S, Zellmeier E, et al. Acute myeloid leukemia with biallelic CEBPA gene mutations and normal karyotype represents a distinct genetic entity associated with a favorable clinical outcome. J Clin Oncol. 2010;28:570–7.

104. Ahn JY, Seo K, Weinberg O, Boyd SD, Arber DA. A comparison of two methods for screening CEBPA mutations in patients with acute myeloid leukemia. J Mol Diagn. 2009;11:319–23.

105. Patel JP, Gönen M, Figueroa ME, Fernandez H, Sun Z, Racevskis J, et al. Prognostic relevance of integrated genetic profiling in acute myeloid leukemia. N Engl J Med. 2012;366:1079–89.

106. Paschka P, Marcucci G, Ruppert AS, Mrózek K, Chen H, Kittles RA, et al. Adverse prognostic significance of KIT mutations in adult acute myeloid leukemia with inv(16) and t(8;21): a cancer and leukemia group B study. J Clin Oncol. 2006;24: 3904–11.

107. Cairoli R, Beghini A, Grillo G, Nadali G, Elice F, Ripamonti CB, et al. Prognostic impact of c-KIT mutations in core binding factor leukemias: an Italian retrospective study. Blood. 2006;107:3463–8.

108. Schnittger S, Kohl TM, Haferlach T, Kern W, Hiddemann W, Spiekermann K, et al. KIT-D816 mutations in AML1-ETO-positive AML are associated with impaired event-free and overall survival. Blood. 2006;107:1791–9.

109. Care RS, Valk PJM, Goodeve AC, Abu-Duhier FM, Geertsma-Kleinekoort WMC, Wilson GA, et al. Incidence and prognosis of c-KIT and FLT3 mutations in core binding factor (CBF) acute myeloid leukaemias. Br J Haematol. 2003;121:775–7.

110. Mrózek K, Marcucci G, Nicolet D, Maharry KS, Becker H, Whitman SP, et al. Prognostic significance of the European LeukemiaNet standardized system for reporting cytogenetic and molecular alterations in adults with acute myeloid leukemia. J Clin Oncol. 2012;30:4515–23.

111. Schlenk RF, Döhner K, Krauter J, Fröhling S, Corbacioglu A, Bullinger L, et al. Mutations and treatment outcome in cytogenetically normal acute myeloid leukemia. N Engl J Med. 2008;358: 1909–18.

112. Pui CH, Sandlund JT, Pei D, Campana D, Rivera GK, Ribeiro RC, et al. Improved outcome for children with acute lymphoblastic leukemia: results of Total Therapy Study XIIIB at St Jude Children's Research Hospital. Blood. 2004;104:2690–6.

113. Romana SP, Coniat ML, Berger R. t(12;21): a new recurrent translocation in acute lymphoblastic leukemia. Genes Chromosom Cancer. 1994;9:186–91.

114. Moorman AV, Harrison CJ, Buck GA, Richards SM, Secker-Walker LM, Martineau M, et al. Karyotype is an independent prognostic factor in adult acute lymphoblastic leukemia (ALL): analysis of cytogenetic data from patients treated on the Medical Research Council (MRC) UKALLXII/Eastern Cooperative Oncology Group (ECOG) 2993 trial. Blood. 2007;109:3189–97.

115. Pui CH, Crist WM, Look AT. Biology and clinical significance of cytogenetic abnormalities in childhood acute lymphoblastic leukemia. Blood. 1990;76: 1449–63.

116. Secker-Walker LM, Craig JM, Hawkins JM, Hoffbrand AV. Philadelphia positive acute lymphoblastic leukemia in adults: age distribution, BCR breakpoint and prognostic significance. Leukemia. 1991;5:196–9.

117. Secker-Walker LM, Prentice HG, Durrant J, Richards S, Hall E, Harrison G. Cytogenetics adds independent prognostic information in adults with acute lymphoblastic leukaemia on MRC trial UKALL XA. MRC Adult Leukaemia Working Party. Br J Haematol. 1997;96:601–10.

118. Faderl S, Kantarjian HM, Thomas DA, Cortes J, Giles F, Pierce S, et al. Outcome of Philadelphia chromosome-positive adult acute lymphoblastic leukemia. Leuk Lymphoma. 2000;36:263–73.

119. Hunger SP. Tyrosine kinase inhibitor use in pediatric Philadelphia chromosome-positive acute lymphoblastic anemia. Hematol Am Soc Hematol Educ Program. 2011;2011:361–5.

120. Gleissner B, Gokbuget N, Bartram CR, Janssen B, Rieder H, Janssen JW, et al. Leading prognostic relevance of the BCR-ABL translocation in adult acute B-lineage lymphoblastic leukemia: a prospective study of the German Multicenter Trial Group and confirmed polymerase chain reaction analysis. Blood. 2002;99:1536–43.

121. Cazzaniga G, Lanciotti M, Rossi V, Di Martino D, Arico M, Valsecchi MG, et al. Prospective molecular monitoring of BCR/ABL transcript in children with Ph+ acute lymphoblastic leukaemia unravels differences in treatment response. Br J Haematol. 2002; 119:445–53.

122. Mullighan CG, Goorha S, Radtke I, Miller CB, Coustan-Smith E, Dalton JD, et al. Genome-wide analysis of genetic alterations in acute lymphoblastic leukaemia. Nature. 2007;446:758–64.

123. Strefford JC, Worley H, Barber K, Wright S, Stewart AR, Robinson HM, et al. Genome complexity in acute lymphoblastic leukaemia is revealed by array-based comparative genomic hybridization. Oncogene. 2007;26:4306–18.

124. Mullighan CG, Miller CB, Radtke I, Phillips LA, Dalton J, Ma J, et al. BCR-ABL1 lymphoblastic leukaemia is characterized by the deletion of Ikaros. Nature. 2008;453:110–4.

125. Mullighan CG, Su X, Zhang J, Radtke I, Phillips LA, Miller CB, et al. Deletion of IKZF1 and prognosis in acute lymphoblastic leukemia. N Engl J Med. 2009;360:470–80.

126. Yang YL, Hung CC, Chen JS, Lin KH, Jou ST, Hsiao CC, et al. IKZF1 deletions predict a poor prognosis in children with B-cell progenitor acute lymphoblastic leukemia: a multicenter analysis in Taiwan. Cancer Sci. 2011;102:1874–81.

127. Iacobucci I, Lonetti A, Paoloni F, Papayannidis C, Ferrari A, Storlazzi CT, et al. The PAX5 gene is frequently rearranged in BCR-ABL1-positive acute lymphoblastic leukemia but is not associated with outcome. A report on behalf of the GIMEMA Acute Leukemia Working Party. Haematologica. 2010;95: 1683–90.

128. Iacobucci I, Papayannidis C, Lonetti A, Ferrari A, Baccarani M, Martinelli G. Cytogenetic and molecular predictors of outcome in acute lymphocytic leukemia: recent developments. Curr Hematol Malig Rep. 2012;7:133–43.

129. Pui CH, Relling MV, Downing JR. Acute lymphoblastic leukemia. N Engl J Med. 2004;350: 1535–48.

130. Graux C, Cools J, Michaux L, Vandenberghe P, Hagemeijer A. Cytogenetics and molecular genetics of T-cell acute lymphoblastic leukemia: from thymocyte to lymphoblast. Leukemia. 2006;20:1496–510.

131. Bernard OA, Busson-LeConiat M, Ballerini P, Mauchauffe M, Della Valle V, Monni R, et al. A new recurrent and specific cryptic translocation, t(5;14) (q35;q32), is associated with expression of the Hox11L2 gene in T acute lymphoblastic leukemia. Leukemia. 2001;15:1495–504.

132. Finger LR, Kagan J, Christopher G, Kurtzberg J, Hershfield MS, Nowell PC, et al. Involvement of the TCL5 gene on human chromosome 1 in T-cell leukemia and melanoma. Proc Natl Acad Sci U S A. 1989;86:5039–43.

133. Hatano M, Roberts CW, Minden M, Crist WM, Korsmeyer SJ. Deregulation of a homeobox gene, HOX11, by the t(10;14) in T cell leukemia. Science. 1991;253:79–82.

134. Mellentin JD, Smith SD, Cleary ML. lyl-1, a novel gene altered by chromosomal translocation in T cell leukemia, codes for a protein with a helix-loop-helix DNA binding motif. Cell. 1989;58:77–83.

135. Royer-Pokora B, Loos U, Ludwig WD. TTG-2, a new gene encoding a cysteine-rich protein with the LIM motif, is overexpressed in acute T-cell leukaemia with the t(11;14)(p13;q11). Oncogene. 1991;6: 1887–93.

136. Aster JC, Pear WS, Blacklow SC. Notch signaling in leukemia. Annu Rev Pathol. 2008;3:587–613.

137. Weng AP, Ferrando AA, Lee W, Morris JPT, Silverman LB, Sanchez-Irizarry C, et al. Activating mutations of NOTCH1 in human T cell acute lymphoblastic leukemia. Science. 2004;306:269–71.

138. Real PJ, Tosello V, Palomero T, Castillo M, Hernando E, de Stanchina E, et al. Gamma-secretase inhibitors reverse glucocorticoid resistance in T cell acute lymphoblastic leukemia. Nat Med. 2009;15: 50–8.

139. Oettinger MA, Schatz DG, Gorka C, Baltimore D. RAG-1 and RAG-2, adjacent genes that synergistically activate V(D)J recombination. Science. 1990;248: 1517–23.

140. Muramatsu M, Kinoshita K, Fagarasan S, Yamada S, Shinkai Y, Honjo T. Class switch recombination and hypermutation require activation-induced cytidine deaminase (AID), a potential RNA editing enzyme. Cell. 2000;102:553–63.

141. Arnold A, Cossman J, Bakhshi A, Jaffe ES, Waldmann TA, Korsmeyer SJ. Immunoglobulin-gene rearrangements as unique clonal markers in human lymphoid neoplasms. N Engl J Med. 1983; 309:1593–9.

142. Cleary ML, Chao J, Warnke R, Sklar J. Immunoglobulin gene rearrangement as a diagnostic criterion of B-cell lymphoma. Proc Natl Acad Sci U S A. 1984;81:593–7.

143. Davis MM, Chien YH, Gascoigne NR, Hedrick SM. A murine T cell receptor gene complex: isolation, structure and rearrangement. Immunol Rev. 1984;81: 235–58.

144. van Dongen JJ, Langerak AW, Bruggemann M, Evans PA, Hummel M, Lavender FL, et al. Design and standardization of PCR primers and protocols for detection of clonal immunoglobulin and T-cell receptor gene recombinations in suspect lymphoproliferations: report of the BIOMED-2 Concerted Action BMH4-CT98-3936. Leukemia. 2003;17: 2257–317.

145. Greiner TC, Rubocki RJ. Effectiveness of capillary electrophoresis using fluorescent-labeled primers in detecting T-cell receptor gamma gene rearrangements. J Mol Diagn. 2002;4:137–43.

146. Vega F, Medeiros LJ, Jones D, Abruzzo LV, Lai R, Manning J, et al. A novel four-color PCR assay to assess T-cell receptor gamma gene rearrangements in lymphoproliferative lesions. Am J Clin Pathol. 2001;116:17–24.

147. Luo V, Lessin SR, Wilson RB, Rennert H, Tozer C, Benoit B, et al. Detection of clonal T-cell receptor gamma gene rearrangements using fluorescent-based PCR and automated high-resolution capillary electrophoresis. Mol Diagn. 2001;6:169–79.

148. Cushman-Vokoun AM, Connealy S, Greiner TC. Assay design affects the interpretation of T-cell receptor gamma gene rearrangements: comparison of the performance of a one-tube assay with the BIOMED-2-based TCRG gene clonality assay. J Mol Diagn. 2010;12:787–96.

149. Bottaro M, Berti E, Biondi A, Migone N, Crosti L. Heteroduplex analysis of T-cell receptor gamma gene rearrangements for diagnosis and monitoring of cutaneous T-cell lymphomas. Blood. 1994;83: 3271–8.

150. Brisco MJ, Tan LW, Orsborn AM, Morley AA. Development of a highly sensitive assay, based on the polymerase chain reaction, for rare B-lymphocyte clones in a polyclonal population. Br J Haematol. 1990;75:163–7.

151. Aubin J, Davi F, Nguyen-Salomon F, Leboeuf D, Debert C, Taher M, et al. Description of a novel FR1 IgH PCR strategy and its comparison with three other strategies for the detection of clonality in B cell malignancies. Leukemia. 1995;9:471–9.

152. Blom B, Verschuren MC, Heemskerk MH, Bakker AQ, van Gastel-Mol EJ, Wolvers-Tettero IL, et al. TCR gene rearrangements and expression of the pre-T cell receptor complex during human T-cell differentiation. Blood. 1999;93:3033–43.

153. Bruggemann M, White H, Gaulard P, Garcia-Sanz R, Gameiro P, Oeschger S, et al. Powerful strategy for polymerase chain reaction-based clonality assessment in T-cell malignancies Report of the BIOMED-2 Concerted Action BHM4 CT98-3936. Leukemia. 2007;21:215–21.

154. Evans PA, Pott C, Groenen PJ, Salles G, Davi F, Berger F, et al. Significantly improved PCR-based clonality testing in B-cell malignancies by use of multiple immunoglobulin gene targets. Report of the BIOMED-2 Concerted Action BHM4-CT98-3936. Leukemia. 2007;21:207–14.

155. Kuo FC, Hall D, Longtine JA. A novel method for interpretation of T-cell receptor γ gene rearrangement assay by capillary Gel electrophoresis based on normal distribution. J Mol Diag. 2007;9:12–9.

156. Lee S-C, Berg KD, Racke FK, Griffin CA, Eshleman JR. Pseudo-spikes are common in histologically benign lymphoid tissues. J Mol Diag. 2000;2: 145–52.

157. Langerak AW, Groenen PJTA, Bruggemann M, Beldjord K, Bellan C, Bonello L, et al. EuroClonality/BIOMED-2 guidelines for interpretation and reporting of Ig/TCR clonality testing in suspected lymphoproliferations. Leukemia. 2012;26:2159–71.

158. Elenitoba-Johnson KSJ, Bohling SD, Mitchell RS, Brown MS, Robetorye RS. PCR analysis of the immunoglobulin heavy chain gene in polyclonal processes can yield pseudoclonal bands as an artifact of low B cell number. J Mol Diag. 2000;2:92–6.

159. Szczepański T, Pongers-Willemse MJ, Langerak AW, Harts WA, Wijkhuijs AJM, van Wering ER, et al. Ig heavy chain gene rearrangements in T-cell acute lymphoblastic leukemia exhibit predominant Dh6-19 and Dh7-27 gene usage, can result in complete V-D-J rearrangements, and are rare in T-cell receptor β lineage. Blood. 1999;93:4079–85.

160. Szczepański T, Beishuizen A, Pongers-Willemse MJ, Hählen K, Van Wering ER, Wijkhuijs AJ, et al. Cross-lineage T cell receptor gene rearrangements occur in more than ninety percent of childhood precursor-B acute lymphoblastic leukemias: alternative PCR targets for detection of minimal residual disease. Leukemia. 1999;13:196–205.

161. Boeckx N, Willemse MJ, Szczepański T, van der Velden VH, Langerak AW, Vandekerckhove P, et al. Fusion gene transcripts and Ig/TCR gene rearrangements are complementary but infrequent targets for PCR-based detection of minimal residual disease in acute myeloid leukemia. Leukemia. 2002;16:368–75.

162. Chiarle R, Zhang Y, Frock RL, Lewis SM, Molinie B, Ho YJ, et al. Genome-wide translocation sequencing

reveals mechanisms of chromosome breaks and rearrangements in B cells. Cell. 2011;147:107–19.

163. Klein IA, Resch W, Jankovic M, Oliveira T, Yamane A, Nakahashi H, et al. Translocation-capture sequencing reveals the extent and nature of chromosomal rearrangements in B lymphocytes. Cell. 2011;147:95–106.

164. Tsujimoto Y, Cossman J, Jaffe E, Croce CM. Involvement of the bcl-2 gene in human follicular lymphoma. Science. 1985;228:1440–3.

165. Motokura T, Bloom T, Kim HG, Juppner H, Ruderman JV, Kronenberg HM, et al. A novel cyclin encoded by a bcl1-linked candidate oncogene. Nature. 1991;350:512–5.

166. Tsujimoto Y, Yunis J, Onorato-Showe L, Erikson J, Nowell PC, Croce CM. Molecular cloning of the chromosomal breakpoint of B-cell lymphomas and leukemias with the t(11;14) chromosome translocation. Science. 1984;224:1403–6.

167. Dalla-Favera R, Bregni M, Erikson J, Patterson D, Gallo RC, Croce CM. Human c-myc onc gene is located on the region of chromosome 8 that is translocated in Burkitt lymphoma cells. Proc Natl Acad Sci U S A. 1982;79:7824–7.

168. Taub R, Kirsch I, Morton C, Lenoir G, Swan D, Tronick S, et al. Translocation of the c-myc gene into the immunoglobulin heavy chain locus in human Burkitt lymphoma and murine plasmacytoma cells. Proc Natl Acad Sci U S A. 1982;79:7837–41.

169. Nuñez G, London L, Hockenbery D, Alexander M, McKearn JP, Korsmeyer SJ. Deregulated Bcl-2 gene expression selectively prolongs survival of growth factor-deprived hematopoietic cell lines. J Immunol. 1990;144:3602–10.

170. Horsman DE, Gascoyne RD, Coupland RW, Coldman AJ, Adomat SA. Comparison of cytogenetic analysis, southern analysis, and polymerase chain reaction for the detection of t(14; 18) in follicular lymphoma. Am J Clin Pathol. 1995;103:472–8.

171. Weiss LM, Warnke RA, Sklar J, Cleary ML. Molecular analysis of the t(14;18) chromosomal translocation in malignant lymphomas. N Engl J Med. 1987;317:1185–9.

172. Huang JZ, Sanger WG, Greiner TC, Staudt LM, Weisenburger DD, Pickering DL, et al. The t(14;18) defines a unique subset of diffuse large B-cell lymphoma with a germinal center B-cell gene expression profile. Blood. 2002;99:2285–90.

173. Iqbal J, Sanger WG, Horsman DE, Rosenwald A, Pickering DL, Dave B, et al. BCL2 translocation defines a unique tumor subset within the germinal center B-cell-like diffuse large B-cell lymphoma. Am J Pathol. 2004;165:159–66.

174. Bakhshi A, Jensen JP, Goldman P, Wright JJ, McBride OW, Epstein AL, et al. Cloning the chromosomal breakpoint of t(14;18) human lymphomas: clustering around JH on chromosome 14 and near a transcriptional unit on 18. Cell. 1985;41:899–906.

175. Buchonnet G, Lenain P, Ruminy P, Lepretre S, Stamatoullas A, Parmentier F, et al. Characterisation of BCL2-JH rearrangements in follicular lymphoma: PCR detection of 3′ BCL2 breakpoints and evidence of a new cluster. Leukemia. 2000;14:1563–9.

176. Cleary ML, Galili N, Sklar J. Detection of a second t(14;18) breakpoint cluster region in human follicular lymphomas. J Exp Med. 1986;164:315–20.

177. Cleary ML, Smith SD, Sklar J. Cloning and structural analysis of cDNAs for bcl-2 and a hybrid bcl-2/immunoglobulin transcript resulting from the t(14;18) translocation. Cell. 1986;47:19–28.

178. Frater JL, Tsiftsakis EK, Hsi ED, Pettay J, Tubbs RR. Use of novel t(11;14) and t(14;18) dual-fusion fluorescence in situ hybridization probes in the differential diagnosis of lymphomas of small lymphocytes. Diagn Mol Pathol. 2001;10:214–22.

179. Belaud-Rotureau MA, Parrens M, Carrere N, Turmo M, Ferrer J, de Mascarel A, et al. Interphase fluorescence in situ hybridization is more sensitive than BIOMED-2 polymerase chain reaction protocol in detecting IGH-BCL2 rearrangement in both fixed and frozen lymph node with follicular lymphoma. Hum Pathol. 2007;38:365–72.

180. Espinet B, Bellosillo B, Melero C, Vela MC, Pedro C, Salido M, et al. FISH is better than BIOMED-2 PCR to detect IgH/BCL2 translocation in follicular lymphoma at diagnosis using paraffin-embedded tissue sections. Leuk Res. 2008;32:737–42.

181. Rambaldi A, Carlotti E, Oldani E, Della Starza I, Baccarani M, Cortelazzo S, et al. Quantitative PCR of bone marrow BCL2/IgH+ cells at diagnosis predicts treatment response and long-term outcome in follicular non-Hodgkin lymphoma. Blood. 2005;105:3428–33.

182. van Oers MH, Tonnissen E, Van Glabbeke M, Giurgea L, Jansen JH, Klasa R, et al. BCL-2/IgH polymerase chain reaction status at the end of induction treatment is not predictive for progression-free survival in relapsed/resistant follicular lymphoma: results of a prospective randomized EORTC 20981 phase III intergroup study. J Clin Oncol. 2010;28:2246–52.

183. Dreyling M, Ghielmini M, Marcus R, Salles G, Vitolo U. Newly diagnosed and relapsed follicular lymphoma: ESMO Clinical Practice Guidelines for diagnosis, treatment and follow-up. Ann Oncol. 2011;22 Suppl 6:vi59–63.

184. Liu Q, Salaverria I, Pittaluga S, Jegalian AG, Xi L, Siebert R, et al. Follicular lymphomas in children and young adults: a comparison of the pediatric variant with usual follicular lymphoma. Am J Surg Pathol. 2013;37:333–43.

185. Louissaint Jr A, Ackerman AM, Dias-Santagata D, Ferry JA, Hochberg EP, Huang MS, et al. Pediatric-type nodal follicular lymphoma: an indolent clonal proliferation in children and adults with high proliferation index and no BCL2 rearrangement. Blood. 2012;120:2395–404.

186. Bacon CM, Ye H, Diss TC, McNamara C, Kueck B, Hasserjian RP, et al. Primary follicular lymphoma of the testis and epididymis in adults. Am J Surg Pathol. 2007;31:1050–8.

187. Finn LS, Viswanatha DS, Belasco JB, Snyder H, Huebner D, Sorbara L, et al. Primary follicular lymphoma of the testis in childhood. Cancer. 1999;85:1626–35.

188. Ozsan N, Bedke BJ, Law ME, Inwards DJ, Ketterling RP, Knudson RA, et al. Clinicopathologic and genetic characterization of follicular lymphomas presenting in the ovary reveals 2 distinct subgroups. Am J Surg Pathol. 2011;35:1691–9.

189. Kojima M, Nakamura S, Ichimura K, Shimizu K, Itoh H, Masawa N. Follicular lymphoma of the salivary gland: a clinicopathological and molecular study of six cases. Int J Surg Pathol. 2001;9:287–93.

190. Kim BK, Surti U, Pandya A, Cohen J, Rabkin MS, Swerdlow SH. Clinicopathologic, immunophenotypic, and molecular cytogenetic fluorescence in situ hybridization analysis of primary and secondary cutaneous follicular lymphomas. Am J Surg Pathol. 2005;29:69–82.

191. Streubel B, Scheucher B, Valencak J, Huber D, Petzelbauer P, Trautinger F, et al. Molecular cytogenetic evidence of t(14;18)(IGH;BCL2) in a substantial proportion of primary cutaneous follicle center lymphomas. Am J Surg Pathol. 2006;30:529–36.

192. Vergier B, Belaud-Rotureau MA, Benassy MN, Beylot-Barry M, Dubus P, Delaunay M, et al. Neoplastic cells do not carry bcl2-JH rearrangements detected in a subset of primary cutaneous follicle center B-cell lymphomas. Am J Surg Pathol. 2004;28:748–55.

193. Li J-Y, Gaillard F, Moreau A, Harousseau J-L, Laboisse C, Milpied N, et al. Detection of translocation t(11;14)(q13;q32) in mantle cell lymphoma by fluorescence in situ hybridization. Am J Pathol. 1999;154:1449–52.

194. Rosenwald A, Wright G, Wiestner A, Chan WC, Connors JM, Campo E, et al. The proliferation gene expression signature is a quantitative integrator of oncogenic events that predicts survival in mantle cell lymphoma. Cancer Cell. 2003;3:185–97.

195. Royo C, Salaverria I, Hartmann EM, Rosenwald A, Campo E, Beà S. The complex landscape of genetic alterations in mantle cell lymphoma. Semin Cancer Biol. 2011;21:322–34.

196. Vaandrager JW, Schuuring E, Zwikstra E, de Boer CJ, Kleiverda KK, van Krieken JH, et al. Direct visualization of dispersed 11q13 chromosomal translocations in mantle cell lymphoma by multicolor DNA fiber fluorescence in situ hybridization. Blood. 1996;88:1177–82.

197. Musgrove EA, Caldon CE, Barraclough J, Stone A, Sutherland RL. Cyclin D as a therapeutic target in cancer. Nat Rev Cancer. 2011;11:558–72.

198. de Boer CJ, Loyson S, Kluin PM, Kluin-Nelemans HC, Schuuring E, van Krieken JH. Multiple break-

points within the BCL-1 locus in B-cell lymphoma: rearrangements of the cyclin D1 gene. Cancer Res. 1993;53:4148–52.

199. Salaverria I, Royo C, Carvajal-Cuenca A, Clot G, Navarro A, Valera A, et al. CCND2 rearrangements are the most frequent genetic events in cyclin D1-mantle cell lymphoma. Blood. 2013;121:1394–402.

200. Meyer N, Penn LZ. Reflecting on 25 years with MYC. Nat Rev Cancer. 2008;8:976–90.

201. Joos S, Falk MH, Lichter P, Haluska FG, Henglein B, Lenoir GM, et al. Variable breakpoints in Burkitt lymphoma cells with chromosomal t(8;14) translocation separate c-myc and the IgH locus up to several hundred kb. Hum Mol Genet. 1992;1:625–32.

202. Joos S, Haluska FG, Falk MH, Henglein B, Hameister H, Croce CM, et al. Mapping chromosomal breakpoints of Burkitt's t(8;14) translocations far upstream of c-myc. Cancer Res. 1992;52:6547–52.

203. Zeidler R, Joos S, Delecluse HJ, Klobeck G, Vuillaume M, Lenoir GM, et al. Breakpoints of Burkitt's lymphoma t(8;22) translocations map within a distance of 300 kb downstream of MYC. Genes Chromosom Cancer. 1994;9:282–7.

204. Neri A, Barriga F, Knowles DM, Magrath IT, Dalla-Favera R. Different regions of the immunoglobulin heavy-chain locus are involved in chromosomal translocations in distinct pathogenetic forms of Burkitt lymphoma. Proc Natl Acad Sci U S A. 1988;85:2748–52.

205. Haralambieva E, Schuuring E, Rosati S, van Noesel C, Jansen P, Appel I, et al. Interphase fluorescence in situ hybridization for detection of 8q24/MYC breakpoints on routine histologic sections: validation in Burkitt lymphomas from three geographic regions. Genes Chromosom Cancer. 2004;40:10–8.

206. Ventura RA, Martin-Subero JI, Jones M, McParland J, Gesk S, Mason DY, et al. FISH analysis for the detection of lymphoma-associated chromosomal abnormalities in routine paraffin-embedded tissue. J Mol Diagn. 2006;8:141–51.

207. Hummel M, Bentink S, Berger H, Klapper W, Wessendorf S, Barth TF, et al. A biologic definition of Burkitt's lymphoma from transcriptional and genomic profiling. N Engl J Med. 2006;354:2419–30.

208. Dave SS, Fu K, Wright GW, Lam LT, Kluin P, Boerma EJ, et al. Molecular diagnosis of Burkitt's lymphoma. N Engl J Med. 2006;354:2431–42.

209. Kramer MH, Hermans J, Wijburg E, Philippo K, Geelen E, van Krieken JH, et al. Clinical relevance of BCL2, BCL6, and MYC rearrangements in diffuse large B-cell lymphoma. Blood. 1998;92:3152–62.

210. Leucci E, Cocco M, Onnis A, De Falco G, van Cleef P, Bellan C, et al. MYC translocation-negative classical Burkitt lymphoma cases: an alternative pathogenetic mechanism involving miRNA deregulation. J Pathol. 2008;216:440–50.

211. Aukema SM, Siebert R, Schuuring E, van Imhoff GW, Kluin-Nelemans HC, Boerma EJ, et al. Double-hit B-cell lymphomas. Blood. 2011;117:2319–31.
212. Snuderl M, Kolman OK, Chen YB, Hsu JJ, Ackerman AM, Dal Cin P, et al. B-cell lymphomas with concurrent IGH-BCL2 and MYC rearrangements are aggressive neoplasms with clinical and pathologic features distinct from Burkitt lymphoma and diffuse large B-cell lymphoma. Am J Surg Pathol. 2010;34:327–40.
213. Tomita N, Tokunaka M, Nakamura N, Takeuchi K, Koike J, Motomura S, et al. Clinicopathological features of lymphoma/leukemia patients carrying both BCL2 and MYC translocations. Haematologica. 2009;94:935–43.
214. Pillai RK, Sathanoori M, Van Oss SB, Swerdlow SH. Double-hit B-cell lymphomas with BCL6 and MYC translocations are aggressive, frequently extranodal lymphomas distinct from BCL2 double-hit B-cell lymphomas. Am J Surg Pathol. 2013;37: 323–32.
215. Johnson NA, Slack GW, Savage KJ, Connors JM, Ben-Neriah S, Rogic S, et al. Concurrent expression of MYC and BCL2 in diffuse large B-cell lymphoma treated with rituximab plus cyclophosphamide, doxorubicin, vincristine, and prednisone. J Clin Oncol. 2012;30:3452–9.
216. Kluk MJ, Chapuy B, Sinha P, Roy A, Dal Cin P, Neuberg DS, et al. Immunohistochemical detection of MYC-driven diffuse large B-cell lymphomas. PLoS One. 2012;7:e33813.
217. Green TM, Young KH, Visco C, Xu-Monette ZY, Orazi A, Go RS, et al. Immunohistochemical double-hit score is a strong predictor of outcome in patients with diffuse large B-cell lymphoma treated with rituximab plus cyclophosphamide, doxorubicin, vincristine, and prednisone. J Clin Oncol. 2012;30: 3460–7.
218. Horn H, Ziepert M, Becher C, Barth TF, Bernd HW, Feller AC, et al. MYC status in concert with BCL2 and BCL6 expression predicts outcome in diffuse large B-cell lymphoma. Blood. 2013;121:2253–63.
219. Hu S, Xu-Monette ZY, Tzankov A, Green T, Wu L, Balasubramanyam A, et al. MYC/BCL2 protein co-expression contributes to the inferior survival of activated B-cell subtype of diffuse large B-cell lymphoma and demonstrates high-risk gene expression signatures: a report from The International DLBCL Rituximab-CHOP Consortium Program Study. Blood. 2013;121:4021–31.
220. Ye H, Liu H, Attygalle A, Wotherspoon AC, Nicholson AG, Charlotte F, et al. Variable frequencies of t(11;18)(q21;q21) in MALT lymphomas of different sites: significant association with CagA strains of H pylori in gastric MALT lymphoma. Blood. 2003;102:1012–8.
221. Streubel B, Simonitsch-Klupp I, Mullauer L, Lamprecht A, Huber D, Siebert R, et al. Variable frequencies of MALT lymphoma-associated genetic aberrations in MALT lymphomas of different sites. Leukemia. 2004;18:1722–6.
222. Rosebeck S, Madden L, Jin X, Gu S, Apel IJ, Appert A, et al. Cleavage of NIK by the API2-MALT1 fusion oncoprotein leads to noncanonical NF-κB activation. Science. 2011;331:468–72.
223. Ruskone-Fourmestraux A, Fischbach W, Aleman BM, Boot H, Du MQ, Megraud F, et al. EGILS consensus report. Gastric extranodal marginal zone B-cell lymphoma of MALT. Gut. 2011;60:747–58.
224. Nakamura S, Sugiyama T, Matsumoto T, Iijima K, Ono S, Tajika M, et al. Long-term clinical outcome of gastric MALT lymphoma after eradication of Helicobacter pylori: a multicentre cohort follow-up study of 420 patients in Japan. Gut. 2012;61: 507–13.
225. Liu H, Ye H, Ruskone-Fourmestraux A, De Jong D, Pileri S, Thiede C, et al. T(11;18) is a marker for all stage gastric MALT lymphomas that will not respond to H. pylori eradication. Gastroenterology. 2002;122:1286–94.
226. Wündisch T, Thiede C, Morgner A, Dempfle A, Gunther A, Liu H, et al. Long-term follow-up of gastric MALT lymphoma after Helicobacter pylori eradication. J Clin Oncol. 2005;23:8018–24.
227. Stein H, Foss HD, Durkop H, Marafioti T, Delsol G, Pulford K, et al. CD30(+) anaplastic large cell lymphoma: a review of its histopathologic, genetic, and clinical features. Blood. 2000;96:3681–95.
228. Morris SW, Kirstein MN, Valentine MB, Dittmer KG, Shapiro DN, Saltman DL, et al. Fusion of a kinase gene, ALK, to a nucleolar protein gene, NPM, in non-Hodgkin's lymphoma. Science. 1994; 263:1281–4.
229. Falini B, Bigcrna B, Fizzotti M, Pulford K, Pileri SA, Delsol G, et al. ALK expression defines a distinct group of T/null lymphomas ("ALK lymphomas") with a wide morphological spectrum. Am J Pathol. 1998;153:875–86.
230. Amin HM, Lai R. Pathobiology of ALK+ anaplastic large-cell lymphoma. Blood. 2007;110:2259–67.
231. Pulford K, Lamant L, Morris SW, Butler LH, Wood KM, Stroud D, et al. Detection of anaplastic lymphoma kinase (ALK) and nucleolar protein nucleophosmin (NPM)-ALK proteins in normal and neoplastic cells with the monoclonal antibody ALK1. Blood. 1997;89:1394–404.
232. Russo G, Isobe M, Gatti R, Finan J, Batuman O, Huebner K, et al. Molecular analysis of a t(14;14) translocation in leukemic T-cells of an ataxia telangiectasia patient. Proc Natl Acad Sci U S A. 1989;86: 602–6.
233. Pekarsky Y, Hallas C, Isobe M, Russo G, Croce CM. Abnormalities at 14q32.1 in T cell malignancies involve two oncogenes. Proc Natl Acad Sci U S A. 1999;96:2949–51.
234. Stern MH, Soulier J, Rosenzwajg M, Nakahara K, Canki-Klain N, Aurias A, et al. MTCP-1: a novel gene on the human chromosome Xq28 translocated

to the T cell receptor alpha/delta locus in mature T cell proliferations. Oncogene. 1993;8:2475–83.

235. Treon SP, Xu L, Yang G, Zhou Y, Liu X, Cao Y, et al. MYD88 L265P somatic mutation in Waldenstrom's macroglobulinemia. N Engl J Med. 2012;367: 826–33.

236. Tiacci E, Trifonov V, Schiavoni G, Holmes A, Kern W, Martelli MP, et al. BRAF mutations in hairy-cell leukemia. N Engl J Med. 2011;364:2305–15.

237. Xi L, Arons E, Navarro W, Calvo KR, Stetler-Stevenson M, Raffeld M, et al. Both variant and IGHV4-34-expressing hairy cell leukemia lack the BRAF V600E mutation. Blood. 2012;119:3330–2.

238. Dietrich S, Glimm H, Andrulis M, von Kalle C, Ho AD, Zenz T. BRAF inhibition in refractory hairy-cell leukemia. N Engl J Med. 2012;366:2038–40.

239. Jimenez C, Sebastian E, del Carmen Chillon M, Giraldo P, Mariano Hernandez J, Escalante F, et al. MYD88 L265P is a marker highly characteristic of, but not restricted to, Waldenstrom's macroglobulinemia. Leukemia. 2013;27:1722–8.

240. Xu L, Hunter ZR, Yang G, Zhou Y, Cao Y, Liu X, et al. MYD88 L265P in Waldenstrom macroglobulinemia, immunoglobulin M monoclonal gammopathy, and other B-cell lymphoproliferative disorders using conventional and quantitative allele-specific polymerase chain reaction. Blood. 2013;121: 2051–8.

241. Kiel MJ, Velusamy T, Betz BL, Zhao L, Weigelin HG, Chiang MY, et al. Whole-genome sequencing identifies recurrent somatic NOTCH2 mutations in splenic marginal zone lymphoma. J Exp Med. 2012;209:1553–65.

242. Rossi D, Trifonov V, Fangazio M, Bruscaggin A, Rasi S, Spina V, et al. The coding genome of splenic marginal zone lymphoma: activation of NOTCH2 and other pathways regulating marginal zone development. J Exp Med. 2012;209:1537–51.

243. Morin RD, Johnson NA, Severson TM, Mungall AJ, An J, Goya R, et al. Somatic mutations altering EZH2 (Tyr641) in follicular and diffuse large B-cell lymphomas of germinal-center origin. Nat Genet. 2010;42:181–5.

244. Morin RD, Mendez-Lago M, Mungall AJ, Goya R, Mungall KL, Corbett RD, et al. Frequent mutation of histone-modifying genes in non-Hodgkin lymphoma. Nature. 2011;476:298–303.

245. Pasqualucci L, Trifonov V, Fabbri G, Ma J, Rossi D, Chiarenza A, et al. Analysis of the coding genome of diffuse large B-cell lymphoma. Nat Genet. 2011;43:830–7.

246. Pasqualucci L, Dominguez-Sola D, Chiarenza A, Fabbri G, Grunn A, Trifonov V, et al. Inactivating mutations of acetyltransferase genes in B-cell lymphoma. Nature. 2011;471:189–95.

247. Davis RE, Ngo VN, Lenz G, Tolar P, Young RM, Romesser PB, et al. Chronic active B-cell-receptor signalling in diffuse large B-cell lymphoma. Nature. 2010;463:88–92.

248. Lenz G, Davis RE, Ngo VN, Lam L, George TC, Wright GW, et al. Oncogenic CARD11 mutations in human diffuse large B cell lymphoma. Science. 2008;319:1676–9.

249. Compagno M, Lim WK, Grunn A, Nandula SV, Brahmachary M, Shen Q, et al. Mutations of multiple genes cause deregulation of NF-kappaB in diffuse large B-cell lymphoma. Nature. 2009;459: 717–21.

250. Kato M, Sanada M, Kato I, Sato Y, Takita J, Takeuchi K, et al. Frequent inactivation of A20 in B-cell lymphomas. Nature. 2009;459:712–6.

251. Ngo VN, Young RM, Schmitz R, Jhavar S, Xiao W, Lim KH, et al. Oncogenically active MYD88 mutations in human lymphoma. Nature. 2011;470: 115–9.

252. Döhner H, Stilgenbauer S, Benner A, Leupolt E, Kröber A, Bullinger L, et al. Genomic aberrations and survival in chronic lymphocytic leukemia. N Engl J Med. 2000;343:1910–6.

253. Edelmann J, Holzmann K, Miller F, Winkler D, Bühler A, Zenz T, et al. High-resolution genomic profiling of chronic lymphocytic leukemia reveals new recurrent genomic alterations. Blood. 2012;120: 4783–94.

254. Eichhorst B, Dreyling M, Robak T, Montserrat E, Hallek M, Group ObotEGW. Chronic lymphocytic leukemia: ESMO Clinical Practice Guidelines for diagnosis, treatment and follow-up. Ann Oncol. 2011;22:vi50–4.

255. Ghielmini M, Vitolo U, Kimby E, Montoto S, Walewski J, Pfreundschuh M, et al. ESMO Guidelines consensus conference on malignant lymphoma 2011 part 1: diffuse large B-cell lymphoma (DLBCL), follicular lymphoma (FL) and chronic lymphocytic leukemia (CLL). Ann Oncol. 2013;24:561–76.

256. Hallek M, Cheson BD, Catovsky D, Caligaris-Cappio F, Dighiero G, Döhner H, et al. Guidelines for the diagnosis and treatment of chronic lymphocytic leukemia: a report from the International Workshop on Chronic Lymphocytic Leukemia updating the National Cancer Institute–Working Group 1996 guidelines. Blood. 2008;111:5446–56.

257. Rossi D, Rasi S, Spina V, Bruscaggin A, Monti S, Ciardullo C, et al. Integrated mutational and cytogenetic analysis identifies new prognostic subgroups in chronic lymphocytic leukemia. Blood. 2013;121: 1403–12.

258. Damle RN, Wasil T, Fais F, Ghiotto F, Valetto A, Allen SL, et al. Ig V gene mutation status and CD38 expression as novel prognostic indicators in chronic lymphocytic leukemia: presented in part at the 40th annual meeting of the American society of hematology, held in Miami beach, FL, December 4-8, 1998. Blood. 1999;94:1840–7.

259. Hamblin TJ, Davis Z, Gardiner A, Oscier DG, Stevenson FK. Unmutated Ig VH genes are associated with a more aggressive form of chronic lymphocytic leukemia. Blood. 1999;94:1848–54.

260. Navarro A, Clot G, Royo C, Jares P, Hadzidimitriou A, Agathangelidis A, et al. Molecular subsets of mantle cell lymphoma defined by the IGHV mutational status and SOX11 expression have distinct biologic and clinical features. Cancer Res. 2012;72:5307–16.

261. Fonseca R, Bergsagel PL, Drach J, Shaughnessy J, Gutierrez N, Stewart AK, et al. International Myeloma Working Group molecular classification of multiple myeloma: spotlight review. Leukemia. 2009;23:2210–21.

262. Chesi M, Nardini E, Lim RS, Smith KD, Kuehl WM, Bergsagel PL. The t(4;14) translocation in myeloma dysregulates both FGFR3 and a novel gene, MMSET, resulting in IgH/MMSET hybrid transcripts. Blood. 1998;92:3025–34.

263. Fonseca R, Blood E, Rue M, Harrington D, Oken MM, Kyle RA, et al. Clinical and biologic implications of recurrent genomic aberrations in myeloma. Blood. 2003;101:4569–75.

264. Avet-Loiseau H, Malard F, Campion L, Magrangeas F, Sebban C, Lioure B, et al. Translocation t(14;16) and multiple myeloma: is it really an independent prognostic factor? Blood. 2011;117:2009–11.

265. Avet-Loiseau H, Attal M, Moreau P, Charbonnel C, Garban F, Hulin C, et al. Genetic abnormalities and survival in multiple myeloma: the experience of the Intergroupe Francophone du Myelome. Blood. 2007;109:3489–95.

266. Hanamura I, Stewart JP, Huang Y, Zhan F, Santra M, Sawyer JR, et al. Frequent gain of chromosome band 1q21 in plasma-cell dyscrasias detected by fluorescence in situ hybridization: incidence increases from MGUS to relapsed myeloma and is related to prognosis and disease progression following tandem stem-cell transplantation. Blood. 2006;108: 1724–32.

267. Shaughnessy Jr JD, Zhan F, Burington BE, Huang Y, Colla S, Hanamura I, et al. A validated gene expression model of high-risk multiple myeloma is defined by deregulated expression of genes mapping to chromosome 1. Blood. 2007;109:2276–84.

268. Rosinol L, Carrio A, Blade J, Queralt R, Aymerich M, Cibeira MT, et al. Comparative genomic hybridisation identifies two variants of smoldering multiple myeloma. Br J Haematol. 2005;130:729–32.

269. Fonseca R, Wier SAV, Chng WJ, Ketterling R, Lacy MQ, Dispenzieri A, et al. Prognostic value of chromosome 1q21 gain by fluorescent in situ hybridization and increase CKS1B expression in myeloma. Leukemia. 2006;20:2034–40.

Molecular Testing in Breast Cancer

11

Dimitrios Zardavas, Debora Fumagalli,
and Christos Sotiriou

Introduction

The advent of microarray technologies has enabled us to interrogate the expression levels of thousands of genes in a single experiment, thus opening the door towards refined molecular characterization and classification of breast cancer [1]. The initial studies using microarray identified four main intrinsic subtypes [2–5]: luminal A tumors, being estrogen receptor (ER) and/or progesterone receptor (PgR) positive, slowly proliferating, and low grade; luminal B tumors, being ER and/or PgR positive, highly proliferating, and high grade; HER2-enriched tumors, showing an amplification of the HER2 oncogene as well as other genes in the same amplicon; and basal-like tumors, overlapping to a major extent with ER/PgR/HER2-negative tumors (the triple-negative phenotype) and showing characteristics of basal-origin, such as positivity for basal cytokeratins. Subsequent studies identified additional subtypes, mostly within the heterogeneous group of the basal-like tumors. Examples include (1) the claudin low tumors, characterized by a gene expression profile similar to that of mammary stem cells (immune response genes, mesenchymal features, and enrichment for epithelial-to-mesenchymal transition markers) [6], and (2) the molecular apocrine tumors, characterized by androgen receptor (AR) positivity and subsequent activation of the AR-signaling pathway [7].

Identifying distinct molecular subtypes of the disease represents a major breakthrough in the field of breast cancer, since different molecular characteristics have been found to underlie these phenotypes (Table 11.1). Indeed, studies coupling genome copy number analyses with gene expression profiling have revealed that recurrent DNA copy number aberrations (CNA) differ between the different breast cancer subtypes [8, 9]. These findings improve our understanding of the pathophysiology of the disease, and they indicate that the molecular subtypes of breast cancer develop along distinct genetic pathways. Moreover, clinically relevant information can be derived, since some of these CNAs have been shown either to hold prognostic relevance or to include genes that could be therapeutically targeted [8, 9]. Recent large-scale studies of next-generation sequencing (NGS) of breast cancer genomes have highlighted the vast molecular heterogeneity governing this disease; they have also associated the molecular subtypes with distinct mutational profiles, which in turn can potentially provide additional therapeutic targets [10–15].

The aforementioned intrinsic molecular subtypes were identified by using DNA microarray platforms, this being an impediment to their clinical implementation. To overcome this hurdle, immunohistochemical (IHC) surrogates have been proposed (Table 11.2). However, these show

D. Zardavas, M.D. • D. Fumagalli, M.D.
C. Sotiriou, M.D., Ph.D. (✉)
Institut Jules Bordet, Université Libre de Bruxelles,
Brussels, Belgium
e-mail: christos.sotiriou@bordet.be

Table 11.1 Patterns of molecular alterations across different molecular subtypes of breast cancer

Molecular subtype	Copy number aberrations	Mutations (%)
Luminal A	*Increased copy number*: 1q and 16p *Decreased copy number*: 16q *High-level amplifications*: 8p11-12, 11q13-14, 12q13-14, 17q11-12, 17q21-24, and 20q13	PIK3CA(45 %), GATA3(14 %), MAP3K1 (13 %), TP53(12 %), CDH1(9 %), MLL3 (8 %), MAP2K4(7 %), NCOR1(5 %), RUNX1(4 %), PTEN(4 %), CTCF(4 %), TBX3(3 %), SF3B1(3 %), CBFB(2 %), FOXA1(2 %), NF1(2 %), PTPRD(2 %), CDKN1B(1 %), AFF2(1 %), PIK3R1 (0.4 %), RB1(0.4 %), PTPN22(0.4 %)
Luminal B	*Increased copy number*: 1q, 8q, 17q, and 20q *Decreased copy number*: 1p, 8p, 13q, 16q, 17p, and 22q *High-level amplifications*: 8p11-12, 8q, and 11q13-14	TP53(29 %), PIK3CA(29 %), GATA3(15 %), MLL3(6 %), MAP3K1(5 %), CDH1(5 %), PTEN(4 %), TBX3(4 %), NF1(4 %), PTPRD (4 %), RB1(3 %), MAP2K4(2 %), PIK3R1 (2 %), AKT1(2 %), RUNX1(2 %), CBFB(2 %), NCOR1(2 %), CTCF(2 %), FOXA1(2 %), AFF2(2 %), PTPN22(2 %), CDKN1B(1 %)
HER2-enriched	*Increased copy number*: 1q, 7p, 8q, 16p, and 20q *Decreased copy number*: 1p, 8p, 13q, and 18q *High-level amplifications*: 17q	TP53(72 %), PIK3CA(39 %), MLL3(7 %), AFF2(5 %), PTPN22(5 %), CDH1(5 %), MAP3K1(4 %), PIK3R1(4 %), RUNX1(4 %), SF3B1(4 %), PTPRD(4 %), MAP2K4 (2 %), GATA3(2 %), PTEN(2 %), AKT1 (2 %), CBFB(2 %), CTCF(2 %), FOXA1 (2 %), CDKN1B(2 %)
Basal-like	*Increased copy number*: 3q, 8q, and 10p *Decreased copy number*: 3p, 4p, 4q, 5q, 12q, 13q, 14q, and 15q *High-level amplifications*: rare	TP53(80 %), PIK3CA(9 %), MLL3(5 %), RB1(4 %), AFF2 (4 %), GATA3(2 %), NCOR1(2 %), NF1(2 %), PTEN(1 %), TBX3(1 %), CTCF(1 %), SF3B1(1 %), PTPRD(1 %)

AFF2 AF4/FMR2 family member 2, *AKT1* V-Akt murine thymoma viral oncogene homolog 1, *CBFB* core-binding factor subunit beta, *CDH1* cadherin 1, type 1, E-cadherin (epithelial), *CDKN1B* cyclin-dependent kinase inhibitor 1B (p27Kip1), *CTCF* CCCTC-binding factor (zinc finger protein), *FOXA1* forkhead box A1, *GATA3* GATA-binding protein 3, *MAP3K1* mitogen-activated protein kinase kinase kinase 1, E3 ubiquitin protein ligase, *MAP2K4* mitogen-activated protein kinase kinase 4, *MLL3* myeloid/lymphoid or mixed-lineage leukemia 3, *NCOR1* nuclear receptor corepressor 1, *NF1* neurofibromin 1, *PIK3CA* phosphatidylinositol-4,5-bisphosphate 3-kinase, catalytic subunit alpha, *PIK3R1* phosphoinositide-3-kinase, regulatory subunit 1 (alpha), *PTEN* phosphatase and tensin homolog, *PTPN22* protein tyrosine phosphatase, non-receptor type 22 (lymphoid), *PTPRD* protein tyrosine phosphatase, receptor type D, *RB1* retinoblastoma 1, *RUNX1* runt-related transcription factor 1, *SF3B1* splicing factor 3b, subunit 1, 155 kDa, *TBX3* T-box 3, *TP53* tumor protein p53

Table 11.2 Molecular subtypes of breast cancer and their immunohistochemical (IHC) surrogates

Molecular subtype	IHC surrogate
Luminal A	ER(+) and/or PgR(+), HER2(−), Ki67 < 14 % (St Gallen) or ER(+), PR ≤ 20 %, HER2(−), Ki67 < 14 % (Prat A et al.) or ER(+) and/or PgR(+), HER2(−) (Blows FM et al.)
Luminal B	ER(+) and/or PgR(+), HER2(−), Ki67 ≥ 14 % (St Gallen) or ER(+), PgR > 20 %, HER2(−), Ki67 ≥ 14 % (Prat A et al.) or ER(+) and/or PgR(+), HER2(+) (Blows FM et al.)
HER2	ER(+/−), PgR(+/−), HER2(+) (St Gallen) or ER(−), PgR(−), HER2(+) (Blows FM et al.)
Basal-like	ER(−), PgR(−), HER2(−) (St Gallen) or ER(−), PgR(−), HER2(−), CK5/6(+) and/or EGFR (+) (Blows FM et al.)

CK cytokeratin, *EGFR* epidermal growth factor receptor, *ER* estrogen receptor, *HER2* human epidermal receptor 2, *Ki67* antigen KI-67, *PgR* progesterone receptor

Table 11.3 Molecular tests implemented in clinical practice for breast cancer and the information they provide

Molecular test	Classification	Prognostic value		Predictive value	
		Early stage	Metastatic stage	Early stage	Metastatic stage
Steroid receptors status (ER/PgR IHC)	Yes	Yes	Yes	Yes (endocrine therapy)	Yes (endocrine therapy)
HER2 status (IHC and/or FISH, CISH)	Yes	Yes	Yes	Yes (HER2 blockade)	Yes (HER2 blockade)
Ki67 (IHC)	Yes	Yes	NA	Generic chemosensitivity	NA
Oncotype DX	No	Yes	NA	Generic chemosensitivity	NA
MammaPrint	No	Yes	NA	Generic chemosensitivity	NA
Genomic grade index (GGI)	Yes	Yes	NA	Generic chemosensitivity	NA
EndoPredict	No	Yes	NA	NA	NA
PAM50/ROR	Yes	Yes	NA	Generic chemosensitivity	NA
CellSearch	No	Yes	Yes	Under investigation	Under investigation
BRCA1/2 mutation analysis	Yes	Under investigation	NA	Under investigation (platinum compounds)	Potentially yes (PARP inhibitors/ platinum compounds)

BRCA1/2 breast cancer 1/2, early onset, *CISH* chromogenic in situ hybridization, *ER* estrogen receptor, *FISH* fluorescence in situ hybridization, *HER2* human epidermal receptor 2, *IHC* immunohistochemistry, *NA* not available, *PgR* progesterone receptor

suboptimal concordance with microarray results, the most important areas of uncertainty being as follows: (1) the discrimination between luminal A and B subtypes. Because proliferation-related genes are the driving factor to define them, they constitute a continuum rather than a binary set of characteristics Ki67, and, more recently, PgR expression levels have been proposed as IHC markers to discriminate between these two subtypes [16, 17]; (2) the lack of concordance between HER2-positive cases as defined by IHC and microarray platforms, with only 70 % of HER2-enriched cases by microarray showing IHC HER2 overexpression; and (3) the lack of concordance between basal-like tumors and cases of the triple-negative phenotype [18].

In recent years, accumulating molecular biology data have been generated in the field of breast cancer, promising to improve all aspects of what has been called "personalized cancer medicine," namely, better characterization, improved prognostication, accurate prediction of response to therapeutics, and sensitive monitoring of the disease [19]. In the following sections, we provide a thorough overview of the different molecular

tests already implemented in clinical practice for breast cancer patients (Table 11.3), as well as information about promising emerging methods of molecular testing.

Molecular Tests in Clinical Practice for Breast Cancer

Estrogen and Progesterone Receptors

It has been known for more than 40 years now that most human breast cancers (up to 80 %) depend on estrogen and/or progesterone for growth and that this effect is mediated through their corresponding receptors, ER and PgR [20]. So far, two isoforms of ER have been identified: ER-α and ER-ß [21]. Both of them are transcription factors binding estradiol and mediating the actions of estrogen, but they differ in their transcriptional properties [22, 23]. Not much is known about the function of ER-ß, and the majority of available clinical data and guidelines presented here pertain to ER-α. PgR also exists as

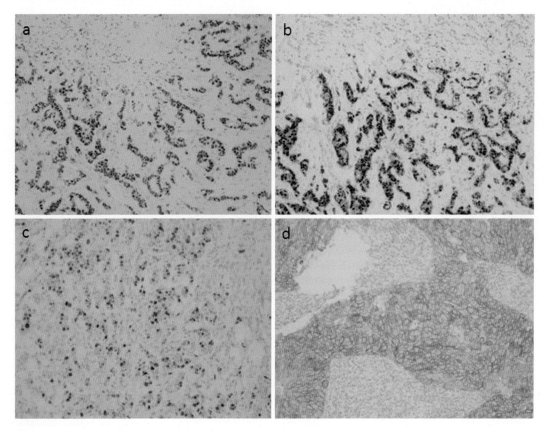

Fig. 11.1 Photomicrograph of IHC assessment of ER (**a**), PgR (**b**), Ki67 (**c**), and HER2 (**d**) in representative cases of invasive ductal carcinoma of the breast (magnification ×20)

two isoforms, A and B; however, little is known about their relative biological and clinical significance [24].

Originally, ER and PgR were quantified by using ligand-binding assays (LBAs), i.e., assays based on the competitive binding of a radiolabeled steroid ligand to the receptors [25]. Since the early 1990s, LBAs have been replaced by immunohistochemistry (IHC) (Fig. 11.1). IHC provides information about both the percentage of positive cells and the intensity of staining within individual cells and has several advantages over LBAs, such as its simplicity and wider applicability. However, several reports have shown that ER and PgR assays can vary from one laboratory to another, and this in relation to several factors, such as specimen handling, tissue fixation, antigen retrieval, and antibody type [26–28].

To improve the accuracy of ER and PgR assays, a panel of the American Society of Clinical Oncology (ASCO) and College of American Pathologist (CAP) has issued recommendations on ER and PgR testing and reporting in breast cancer [29]. According to these guidelines, breast cancers that have >1 % of cells staining positive for ER and/or PgR should be considered as ER and/or PgR positive. The quantification of ER and/or PgR mRNA by reverse transcriptase-polymerase chain reaction (RT-PCR), per se or as part of a multigene assay (see below), constitutes another measurement option, but it is currently not recommended to replace IHC [30].

The prognostic significance of hormone receptor expression is ambiguous. Much evidence has shown that patients with stage I, ER-positive breast cancer who receive no systemic therapy after surgery have a 5–10 % lower likelihood of recurrence at 5 years than patients with ER-negative disease [31–33]. However, the advantage of ER positivity in terms of risk of relapse and death diminishes over time, probably as an effect of the benefits of adjuvant chemotherapy in hormone receptor-negative cancers [34–36]. The independent prognostic contribution of PgR expression has also been evaluated; clinical evidence suggests that patients with ER/PgR-positive breast cancers have a better prognosis than patients with ER-positive and PgR-negative cancers, who in turn have a better prognosis than ER/PgR-negative ones [37, 38].

ER is the most important predictive biomarker in breast cancer as a predictor of response to endocrine therapy. Tamoxifen, a selective ER modulator, represents an established adjuvant endocrine therapy. In women with ER-positive breast cancer, adjuvant tamoxifen has been shown to decrease the annual odds of recurrence by 39 % and the annual odds of death by 31 %, and this irrespective of age, lymph node involvement, menopausal status, and the use of chemotherapy [39]. In postmenopausal women, several studies have shown that, compared to long-term tamoxifen therapy, the use of a third-generation aromatase inhibitor (AI) lowers the risk of ipsilateral, contralateral, and distant relapse when used as initial adjuvant therapy, sequential therapy, or extended therapy [40–51]. In premenopausal women, tamoxifen remains the standard of care, and the role of ovarian suppression is under investigation [52–54].

Besides the presence of ER, evidence suggests that ER quantitative expression levels could predict the magnitude of benefit from endocrine therapy [55, 56]. In the rare ER-negative, PgR-positive breast cancers, limited benefit from tamoxifen has been reported, but hormone treatment is widely recommended anyway [57].

Great efforts have been invested to identify which patients with ER-positive early breast cancer could benefit from additional adjuvant chemotherapy. This has given rise to a series of multigene signatures, which can be of help in treatment decision-making, as discussed below [58]. Clinical evidence has been generated to support the hypothesis that ER status predicts the response to neoadjuvant chemotherapy; specifically, ER-negative breast cancers seem more likely to achieve a pathologic complete response (pCR) after chemotherapy than ER-positive ones [59, 60].

Breast cancer patients with metastatic disease expressing hormone receptors are candidates for initial endocrine treatment. In recent years, AIs have become standard first-line treatment in postmenopausal women based on the results of several randomized trials showing their enhanced efficacy over tamoxifen [61–65]. Of interest, data show that in the metastatic setting, response to antiestrogens is better among patients expressing both ER and PgR than in patients with ER-positive cancers lacking PgR expression [66].

Because of the data discussed above, current guidelines recommend performing ER and PgR testing for all newly diagnosed breast cancers, as well as for any local or distant recurrence. Moreover, patients with hormone receptor-positive disease should receive hormonal therapy unless otherwise contraindicated [67].

Human Epidermal Growth Factor Receptor 2

The human epidermal growth factor receptor 2 (HER2) is a transmembrane glycoprotein belonging to the epidermal growth factor receptor (ErbB) family that plays a role in cell growth, differentiation, adhesion, and motility [68, 69]. HER2 is expressed at low levels in a variety of normal epithelia, including breast duct epithelium, but amplification of the gene and concomitant protein overexpression are present in up to 30 % of primary breast cancers [70].

HER2 testing has become an integral part of the diagnostic workup of all patients with primary breast cancers and those with newly recurrent metastasis. Usually, HER2 status is first assessed by IHC (Fig. 11.1); in cases of equivocal protein expression levels, *HER2* gene copy number is defined using fluorescent in situ hybridization (FISH) or chromatin in situ hybridization (CISH). Defining HER2 status based on mRNA assays is currently not recommended.

Performing IHC for HER2 poses several challenges, because both accurate and semiquantitative assessments are critical. Despite the tight association existing between *HER2* gene amplification and protein overexpression [71], several reports have shown that IHC can have variable ability to identify *HER2*-amplified tumors and that discordance rates may represent up to 20 % if HER2 testing is performed in low volume, local laboratories [72–75]. In order to overcome these problems, ASCO and CAP have released guidelines for HER2 testing in breast cancer; of note, the guidelines require laboratories be validated for HER2 testing before they start performing the assays [76].

The value of HER2 as a prognostic marker is controversial. Available evidence shows that HER2 overexpression in patients with breast cancer who did not receive adjuvant systemic therapy is associated with poor prognosis in both node-negative and node-positive disease [70, 77–80]. However, most of these studies were conducted before trastuzumab was approved for use in the adjuvant treatment of high-risk patients with HER2-positive breast cancer (see below). For this reason, an ASCO expert panel recommended against the use of HER2 amplification and/or overexpression solely to determine prognosis in patients with early breast cancer [81].

The major utility of HER2 amplification and/or overexpression is as a predictive marker for chemotherapy, targeted therapy, and endocrine therapy. Retrospective analyses have demonstrated that HER2-positive breast cancers are more sensitive to anthracycline-based adjuvant regimens than to non-anthracycline-based ones [82–85] and that the dose of doxorubicin may be important in defining the efficacy of the treatment [82, 86]. The role of topoisomerase IIa and polysomy of chromosome 17 in conferring this sensitivity has been investigated [87, 88]. HER2-positive breast cancers seem to benefit from the administration of paclitaxel [89], while they seem relatively resistant to cyclophosphamide-based regimens [90–92].

HER2 status serves as a predictive factor for response to trastuzumab, the humanized monoclonal antibody directed against the extracellular domain of the HER2 receptor. Trastuzumab was first shown to improve response rates, time to progression, and overall survival in patients with HER2-positive metastatic breast cancers, either alone or in combination with chemotherapy [93–95]. The results of pivotal randomized clinical trials have also shown that in the adjuvant setting, trastuzumab significantly reduces the risk of recurrence and mortality of patients with HER2-positive early-stage breast cancer, independently of ER status, tumor size, or nodal status [96–101]. Consequently, trastuzumab has become one of the most successful targeted drugs.

Adding trastuzumab to neoadjuvant chemotherapy regimens has shown to improve the rate of pCR [102, 103]. Moreover, in two recent independent, multicentric, neoadjuvant clinical trials, a significantly higher pCR rate was observed with dual anti-HER2 blockade (i.e., trastuzumab and either the tyrosine-kinase inhibitor lapatinib or the monoclonal antibody pertuzumab), confirming the relevance of neoadjuvant HER2-targeted treatment for HER2-positive breast cancers [104, 105].

Several HER2-blocking agents with diverse mechanisms of actions are under clinical development for HER2-overexpressing breast cancers and promise to improve the management of this breast cancer subtype [106, 107]. Of interest, some of these agents seem active in patients expressing truncated cytoplasmic HER2 receptors (p95HER2), which seems to confer resistance to trastuzumab [108].

There is also evidence suggesting that HER2 positivity may predict for resistance to some endocrine therapies; however, the data are controversial, and HER2 expression is currently not considered an exclusion criterion for the use of endocrine treatment in patients with hormone receptor-positive breast cancers [67].

It is worth mentioning that uncertainty about the threshold currently used to define HER2 positivity has recently arisen because of data showing a significant benefit from trastuzumab for patients defined as HER2 negative on central testing [109–111]. Several studies have addressed whether circulating HER2 protein extracellular domain levels could better predict response to HER2-directed treatment; the results are controversial [112] and, until more information is available, a change in standard practice is not warranted.

Ki67

Ki67 antigen, initially identified 30 years ago [113], represents a biological marker commonly assessed in breast cancer, influencing treatment decisions for endocrine therapy and chemotherapy of the primary tumor. Evidence supports the involvement of this protein in polymerase I-dependent rRNA synthesis, without a fully clear picture to the present day about its functional importance [114, 115]. Ki67 is assessed with immunohistochemistry (IHC) using several antibodies (MM-1, Ki-S5, SP-6), among which MIB-1 has predominated daily practice (Fig. 11.1). Overall, the measurement is based on the percentage of breast cancer cells stained in their nuclei by the antibody, a strenuous and poorly reproducible task. To overcome these hurdles, automated readers have been developed, which can be applied to both tumor biopsies and fine needle aspirates [116, 117].

Evidence supporting the clinical usefulness of Ki67 assessment has been generated and sustains this biological marker as valuable tool for IHC approximation of molecular subtyping of breast cancer and as a prognostic and predictive biomarker. The Ki67 labeling index has been shown to enable the distinction between luminal A and B subtypes, with the best Ki67 index cutoff point for this purpose being 14 % [16]. Multiple studies have reported the prognostic impact of Ki67 in the setting of early-stage breast cancer. Meta-analyses have been also conducted and indicate that Ki67 positivity is a negative prognosticator in terms of both disease-free survival (DFS) and overall survival (OS) [118, 119].

Data supporting a predictive role for Ki67 in the adjuvant, neoadjuvant, and metastatic settings have been generated, though not always consistently. In the adjuvant setting, the findings of the randomized trials assessing the predictive role of

Ki67 can be summarized as follows: (1) Ki67 positivity might predict a benefit for adjuvant letrozole compared with adjuvant tamoxifen, as shown by the Breast International Group's BIG 1–98 trial, which randomized 4,922 patients to receive tamoxifen or letrozole in four different arms [116]. Using 11 % as a Ki67 cutoff point, the magnitude of treatment benefit achieved by letrozole compared to tamoxifen was higher in the subgroup of patients with high Ki67 expression levels (HR [Let:Tam] = 0.53; 95 % CI, 0.39–0.72) than what was estimated for patients with low Ki67 expression levels (HR [Let:Tam] = 0.81; 95 % CI, 0.57–1.15), with the p value for Ki67 and treatment interaction being 0.09; (2) Ki67 positivity might predict a benefit from adjuvant taxanes, as indicated by the Breast Cancer International Research Group (BCIRG) 001 and the PACS01 trials [120, 121]. BCIRG 001 randomized patients to receive doxorubicin and cyclophosphamide with either fluorouracil (FAC) or docetaxel (TAC) and stratified them into the four intrinsic subtypes. For the subgroup of luminal B breast cancer patients (defined as hormone receptor positive, HER2 positive, and/or Ki67 > 11 %), the taxane-containing regimen showed improvement over the taxane-free one, with a 3-year DFS of 85.2 % for TAC and 79.0 % for FAC chemotherapy (HR = 0.66; 95 % CI, 0.46–0.95, p = 0.025) [120]. PACS01 randomized patients to receive six cycles of fluorouracil, epirubicin, and cyclophosphamide (FEC) or three cycles of FEC followed by three cycles of docetaxel. Using a Ki67 cut point of 20 % or more to indicate Ki67 positivity, the docetaxel-containing chemotherapy was associated with reduced HR for relapse in the ER-positive/Ki67-positive group of patients (HR = 0.51; 95 % CI, 0.26–1.01) compared with ER-positive/Ki67-negative patients (HR = 1.03; 95 % CI, 0.69–1.55) [121]. (3) High Ki67 does not predict benefit of chemotherapy over hormonal treatment alone, as indicated by the International Breast Cancer Study Group (IBCSG) trials VIII and IX [122].

In the neoadjuvant setting, several studies have associated Ki67 with response to chemotherapy, defined as either clinical or pathologic response.

However, these results are inconsistent, with two neoadjuvant chemotherapy studies failing to show a correlation between Ki67 levels and sensitivity to treatment [123, 124]. Importantly, there is no data to support using Ki67 expression levels to predict for response to specific chemotherapy regimens. In terms of Ki67 as a predictive biomarker for response to neoadjuvant endocrine therapy, two studies with monotherapy, assessing tamoxifen ($n=54$) and letrozole ($n=63$), respectively, were negative ($p=0.08$ and not reported, respectively) [125, 126].

The potential predictive role of Ki67 in the metastatic setting has been less extensively studied. Two studies associated Ki67 expression status with either response rate to endocrine therapy ($p=0.024$) [127] or time to endocrine therapy failure ($p=0.047$) in univariate analysis [128], with lack of evidence for a predictive role of Ki67 in multivariate analysis performed in the second study ($p=0.16$). Another study assessing trastuzumab with or without chemotherapy in HER2-positive metastatic breast cancer patients ($n=74$) failed to show an association of Ki67 with time to treatment failure in both univariate and multivariate analysis [129].

Gene Prognostic Signatures

Gene expression profiling studies have been conducted in an attempt to improve the prognostication conferred by standard clinicopathologic parameters assessed in patients with early-stage breast cancer. These studies have led to the generation of gene signatures currently commercially available, which will be described in this section. Interestingly, some of these gene signatures have been retrospectively evaluated as potential predictive biomarkers, and they have been shown to assess generic chemosensitivity. This chemosensitivity assessment mostly derives from their ability to quantify the proliferation status of breast cancer cells [1].

Oncotype DX®

This is a 21-gene, quantitative reverse transcriptase-polymerase chain reaction (qRT-PCR)-based assay, initially developed to assess the risk of recurrence in women with lymph node-negative, ER-positive, tamoxifen-treated breast cancers [130]. This gene signature was developed by selecting genes from among a list of 250 candidates identified on the basis of existing biologic knowledge, the so-called "candidate-gene" approach. The Oncotype DX® assay provides a "recurrence score" (RS), which is a continuous variable that assigns patients to three different risk groups according to the probability of recurrence at 10 years: low risk, intermediate risk, and high risk, with 10-year distant recurrence rates of 7 %, 14 %, and 30 %, respectively, according to the initial discovery study assessing a cohort of patients enrolled in the National Surgical Adjuvant Breast and Bowel Project trial B-14 [130]. A subsequent study assessed Oncotype DX® in patients enrolled in the Arimidex, Tamoxifen, Alone or in Combination (ATAC) trial and showed statistically significant prognostication for both lymph node-negative ($p<0.001$) and lymph node-positive disease ($p=0.002$) [131].

Additional confirmation for RS being prognostic for lymph node-positive breast cancer patients treated with tamoxifen has been generated [132]. Retrospective analyses have associated RS with clinical outcome, showing that it provides prognostication independently of standard clinicopathologic parameters [133]. Importantly, one randomized phase III clinical trial, TAILORx (Trial Assigning Individualized Options for Treatment) (NCT00310180), is prospectively assessing the clinical utility of Oncotype DX®. Patients with node-negative, hormone receptor-positive breast cancer showing an intermediate RS have been randomized to receive endocrine therapy alone or endocrine therapy plus chemotherapy. The primary research question is whether patients with intermediate RS can be safely spared adjuvant chemotherapy.

MammaPrint®

This is a 70-gene microarray platform/qRT-PCR-based assay, initially identified by scientists from the Netherlands Cancer Institute, who retrospectively investigated a cohort of 78 untreated patients with lymph node-negative breast cancer with tumor size <5 cm [134]. MammaPrint® was derived using the "top-down" approach, since it was developed by directly comparing global gene expression data between patient groups with different clinical outcomes without making a priori biological assumptions. The prognostic ability of this multigene prognosticator was subsequently validated by two independent retrospective studies [135, 136].

A randomized phase III clinical trial, MINDACT (Microarray in Node Negative and 0–3 Positive Lymph Node Disease May Avoid Chemotherapy Trial) (NCT00433589), is also prospectively assessing the clinical value of MammaPrint®. Breast cancer patients with node negative or with up to three infiltrated lymph nodes, any hormone receptor status, and discordant risk stratification as assessed by MammaPrint® and Adjuvant Online have been randomized to receive treatment on the basis of genomic or clinical risk, respectively. The primary research question is whether patients with low genomic but high clinical risk can safely avoid adjuvant chemotherapy.

MapQuant Dx™

Sotiriou et al. used the "bottom-up" discovery strategy to capture histological grade through a characteristic gene expression profile [137]. A 97-gene signature was generated, called the genomic grade index (GGI), consisting of proliferation and cell-cycle genes. Among 570 early-stage breast cancer patients, GGI consistently discriminated low-grade from high-grade breast cancer tumors. Importantly, GGI was able to classify grade II tumors into two separate groups of low and high genomic grade, exhibiting statistically significant different clinical outcomes ($p < 0.001$). These findings are clinically relevant: they indicate GGI's ability to provide accurate prognostication for grade II tumors, which constitute an area of uncertainty for clinical decision-making because of high interobserver discrepancy rates. Of note, the prognostic value of GGI was recently demonstrated in a cohort of 166 patients with invasive lobular breast cancer: in multivariate analysis, GGI was associated with invasive DFS ($p < 0.001$) and OS ($p = 0.01$), outperforming histological grade and providing additional prognostication in comparison to standard clinicopathologic variables, including nodal status [138].

EndoPredict®

This is an 11-gene qRT-PCR-based assay, assessing 8 cancer-related and 3 normalization genes in paraffin-embedded tumor tissue, providing a final EndoPredict (EP) score ranging from 0 to 15. The EP score was combined with nodal status and tumor size into a comprehensive clinico-genomic score, EPclin, the prognostication ability of which has been assessed in patients from the Austrian Breast and Colorectal Cancer Study Group (ABCSG)-6 and ABCSG-8 trials [139]. EPclin discriminated two prognostic groups with different clinical outcomes in terms of 10-year distant recurrence rates ($p < 0.001$ in both trials). Importantly, a retrospective analysis of 1,702 postmenopausal patients with ER-positive/HER2-negative breast cancer treated only with endocrine treatment showed that EPclin outperformed National Comprehensive Cancer Center Network, German S3, and St Gallen guidelines in terms of prognostic ability [140]. Lastly, a comparison between EndoPredict® and Oncotype DX® was performed among 34 hormone receptor-positive breast cancer patients: significant but moderate concordance (76 %) and moderate correlation (Pearson coefficient 0.65, $p < 0.01$) were reported [141].

PAM50/ROR

This is a 50-gene intrinsic subtype predictor that was developed using microarray analysis and qRT-PCR data in a training set of 189 lymph node-negative and lymph node-positive breast cancer samples [142]. A risk of relapse score (ROR) was provided, taking into account the PAM50-assigned intrinsic subtype, tumor size, and histologic grade. With respect to accurate prognostication, this combined clinico-genomic assay outperformed both clinico-pathologic and subtype-based prognostic classification in a lymph node-negative, untreated cohort of patients. The ROR score showed potential to accurately prognosticate patients with ER-positive, tamoxifen-treated early-stage breast cancer [143]. In another study, PAM50 prognostication was compared to that of IHC in a cohort of patients enrolled in the NCIC CTG MA.12 study, evaluating tamoxifen versus placebo in premenopausal breast cancer patients [144]. PAM50-based intrinsic subtype classification was found to be prognostic for both DFS ($p = 0.0003$) and overall survival (OS; $p = 0.0002$), whereas IHC-based classification was not.

IHC4

IHC4 (AQUA® Technology) is a recurrence risk signature using the protein expression of four well-established prognostic markers, i.e., ER, PgR, HER2, and Ki67, as assessed by central IHC testing. The prognostication ability of IHC4 was compared to Oncotype DX® in a cohort of 1,125 patients with ER-positive breast cancer from the ATAC trial, with the two tests providing similar prognostic information [145]. In the same study, further validation of IHC4 was derived from a second cohort of 786 ER-positive breast cancer patients, where it was found to be significantly prognostic.

Gene Signatures of Specific Pathway Activation Status

Diverse oncogenic molecular alterations have been observed in human cancer, with some of them aggregating in the same signaling pathway. This is best exemplified by alterations affecting different molecular components of the PI3K signaling pathway, such as PTEN loss, *PIK3CA*, and/or *Akt1* mutations [146]. Such alterations influence the functional output of the corresponding signaling pathway, which can be captured by either gene transcription analysis or specific phospho-antibodies assessing downstream molecules that serve as readouts of the pathway activation status. This raises the prospect of assessing oncogenic pathway activation status as a potential predictive biomarker of response to targeted therapeutics. A recent example has been the development of a PI3K/mTOR-pathway gene signature (PIK3CA-GS), indicating low functional output of the pathway [147]. Clinical data have recently been generated suggesting that the PIK3CA-GS can serve as a predictive biomarker for response to everolimus, an mTOR inhibitor, in ER-positive breast cancer [148].

Detection and Enumeration of Circulating Tumor Cells

Enumeration of circulating tumor cells (CTCs) is another molecular test applied in clinical practice in the metastatic setting of breast cancer. Among several CTC detection methods, to date CellSearch® (Veridex, Warren, NJ, USA) is the only one to have received US Food and Drug Administration (FDA) approval for the monitoring of patients with metastatic breast cancer [149]. This is an automated enrichment and immune staining system used to isolate and enumerate CTCs, using antibody-coated magnetic beads to separate epithelial cell adhesion molecule

(EpCAM)-expressing epithelial cells from whole blood. After this first enrichment step, triple fluorescence staining follows: nucleic acid dye (4',6-diamidino-2-phenylindole dihydrochloride, or DAPI) stains cellular nuclei, antibodies specific for cytokeratins 8, 18, and 19 (pan-CK) define epithelial cells, and CD45 identifies leucocytes. According to this protocol, a CTC is defined as a cell positively stained for DAPI and pan-CK, but not for CD45 [150].

The number of CTCs detected in patients with metastatic breast cancer has been shown to be an independent prognostic factor of clinical outcome according to several studies. A prospective, multicenter study assessed the potential of prognostic relevance of CTCs in 177 patients with measurable metastatic disease burden [149]. Using a cutoff of ≥ 5 CTCs/7.5 mL of blood, CTCs were found to be an independent prognosticator for both progression-free survival (PFS) and OS. Following from the same study, evidence indicating the potential superiority of CTCs enumeration over traditional radiologic assessment for prognostication in the metastatic setting has been generated in a subgroup of 138 of the original 177 patients [151]. A retrospective analysis of 115 metastatic breast cancer patients with CTC counting and [(18) F]-fluorodeoxyglucose (FDG) positron emission tomography (PET)/computed tomography (CT) performed at baseline and at 9–12 weeks during therapy showed that in univariate analysis, mid-therapy CTC count levels ($p < 0.001$) and FDG-PET/CT response ($p = 0.001$) predicted OS, with the former being the only significant prognostic factor in a multivariate analysis ($p = 0.004$) [152]. Lastly, a prospective study of CTC detection by CellSearch® in 267 patients with metastatic breast cancer on first-line treatment confirmed the prognostic relevance of CTC isolation and enumeration. CTCs ≥ 5/7.5 mL of blood was a statistically significant prognostic factor for PFS and OS on multivariate analysis ($p = 0.03$). Of note, the seventh edition of the American Joint Committee on Cancer Staging Manual (2010) defined a new M0(i+) stage of disease, acknowledging the clinical relevance of micrometastatic disease, which is defined as molecularly or microscopically detected cancer cells, with CTCs being part of it [153].

BRCA1/2 Mutational Testing

BRCA1/2 (breast cancer 1/2, early onset) represent the two most extensively studied breast cancer susceptibility genes, with genetic assessment of their mutational status currently implemented in clinical practice. *BRCA1* germline mutations confer a 50–70 % lifetime risk for development of invasive breast cancer, with the corresponding risk for *BRCA2* mutations reaching 40–60 %. In terms of selection of patients to be offered *BRCA1/2* mutational analysis, several guidelines have been developed, encompassing aspects of both family history and certain clinicopathologic characteristics of breast cancer disease. Regarding the method of assessment of the *BRCA1/2* mutational status, full gene sequencing is one option. However, the predominance of specific founder mutations within populations of certain ethnic origin (e.g., the 185delAG and 5382insC *BRCA1* mutations and the 6174delT *BRCA2* mutation within the Ashkenazi Jewish population) offers a simpler and less expensive form of targeted gene sequencing [154].

There is accumulating evidence that *BRCA1/2* mutational status can impact the clinical management of breast cancer patients. The prognostic impact of *BRCA1/2* germline mutations is still unclear, with most but not all of the studies reporting deleterious effects. A meta-analysis of 11 studies reported the negative prognostic impact of *BRCA1* germline mutations for newly diagnosed breast cancer patients in terms of both short-term and long-term OS rates, as compared to *BRCA* wild-type patients (HR = 1.92 [95 % CI = 1.45–2.53]; 1.33 [1.12–1.58], respectively) [155]. In the same study, *BRCA2* was shown to provide no prognostic information. The issue of the prognostic impact of *BRCA1/2* mutational status will be addressed by the POSH (Prospective study of Outcomes in Sporadic versus Hereditary breast cancer) study, which is prospectively identifying and following a cohort of 3,000 newly diagnosed early-onset (i.e., <40 years old) breast cancer patients [156].

BRCA1/2 mutational status can influence locoregional treatment decision-making. Indeed, *BRCA*-related breast cancer has been associated with increased rates of both ipsilateral and, more consistently, contralateral breast cancer recurrence. Prophylactic contralateral mastectomy has been shown to significantly decrease the risk of contralateral breast cancer and increase the DFS, with data about its effects on overall survival still missing. In terms of locoregional radiotherapy, no evidence exists to support a tailored approach for patients with germline *BRCA* mutations.

BRCA1/2 mutational status holds the potential to influence the choice of systemic treatment in breast cancer. Preclinical evidence supports a sensitivity of such tumors to DNA damaging agents, such as platinum compounds [157], with preliminary clinical data confirming this in the neoadjuvant setting [158]. Preliminary clinical data suggest a potential innate resistance of *BRCA*-related breast cancer to taxanes in the metastatic and neoadjuvant settings [159, 160]. Currently, there is an ongoing phase II clinical trial (NCT00321633) randomizing *BRCA1* and/or *BRCA2-mutation* carriers with metastatic breast cancer to receive either carboplatin or docetaxel chemotherapy (with the addition of trastuzumab for the HER2-overexpressing cases).

Lastly, knowing a patient's *BRCA1/2* mutational status can open new therapeutic avenues, exploiting the concept of synthetic lethality, according to which two different gene defects lead to cellular death, whereas each one of them separately does not. Poly (ADP-ribose) polymerase (PARP) represents an important mediator of single-stranded DNA repair pathway. BRCA1/2 are functionally important mediators of homologous recombination (HR), a major repair mechanism for double-stranded DNA breaks. Upon pharmacological PARP inhibition, multiple double-stranded DNA breaks are formed during the DNA replication, so that cells with defective BRCA1/2-dependent DNA repair, as is the case for *BRCA* germline mutation carriers, are prone to apoptosis. This rationale supports the development of PARP inhibitors for BRCA-related breast cancer, with multiple clinical trials in development or currently ongoing.

Emerging Molecular Tests in Breast Cancer

Next-Generation Gene Sequencing

The advent of NGS techniques, enabling detailed sequencing of multiple genes in a single experiment, is reshaping our understanding of breast cancer biology (Table 11.4) [11, 13–15, 161, 162]. By elucidating the mutational landscape of breast cancer and thereby enabling us to dissect the intratumoral heterogeneity and clonal evolution governing this common disease in space and time, NGS holds the promise to improve several aspects of personalized breast cancer medicine. This includes identifying new therapeutic targets and predictive biomarkers for molecularly targeted agents under clinical development. Of note, NGS techniques can be applied not only to tumor samples, but to plasma material as well, which could lead to plasma-based prognostic and/or predictive biomarkers. An exciting prospect arising from NGS performed with plasma is the accurate monitoring of the disease, since micro-residual tumor burden could then be assessed with unprecedented accuracy. Circulating cell-free DNA assessment through NGS techniques was recently shown to be closely associated with response to therapy and clinical

Table 11.4 Next-generation sequencing and layers of genomic information it provides

Category	Alteration
Nucleotide sequencing	DNA mutations (whole genome/exome)
	RNA mutations
Structural rearrangements	Intrachromosomal structural rearrangements
	Interchromosomal structural rearrangements
	Fusion transcripts
	Splice variants
Other	Single-cell genome/transcriptome sequencing

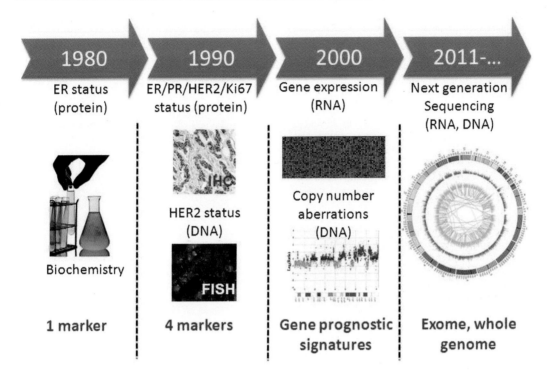

Fig. 11.2 Evolution of molecular testing in breast cancer

outcome in the metastatic setting [163]. Such applications in the adjuvant setting would be even more exciting; however, clinical data are still missing [164].

Conclusions

Breast cancer is a heterogeneous disease encompassing diverse subtypes, with different molecular backgrounds, different sensitivity profiles to various treatment modalities, and different clinical outcomes. Currently, a limited number of molecular tests are routinely applied for the clinical management of these patients with breast cancer, referring mostly to ER, PgR, and HER2 testing and, less frequently, to Ki67 assessment. Several prognostic multigene classifiers of the disease have become commercially available to improve prognostication, but their clinical utility remains to be proven. *BRCA1/2* mutational analysis is restricted to a small subpopulation of patients, and CTCs enu-

meration is mostly relevant in the metastatic setting, the latter still far from being performed on a routine basis. However, clinical investigation of these molecular tests is being undertaken, as is active development of newly emerging technologies. NGS could have great impact on personalized breast cancer medicine in the future; however, it should be still considered experimental. Solid clinical evidence needs to be generated before new molecular tests (Fig. 11.2) can be implemented for the clinical management of breast cancer.

References

1. Sotiriou C, Pusztai L. Gene-expression signatures in breast cancer. N Engl J Med. 2009;360(8):790–800.
2. Perou CM, Sørlie T, Eisen MB, van de Rijn M, Jeffrey SS, Rees CA, et al. Molecular portraits of human breast tumours. Nature. 2000;406(6797): 747–52.
3. Sørlie T, Perou CM, Tibshirani R, Aas T, Geisler S, Johnsen H, et al. Gene expression patterns of breast

carcinomas distinguish tumor subclasses with clinical implications. Proc Natl Acad Sci USA. 2001;98(19):10869–74.

4. Sorlie T, Tibshirani R, Parker J, Hastie T, Marron JS, Nobel A, et al. Repeated observation of breast tumor subtypes in independent gene expression data sets. Proc Natl Acad Sci USA. 2003;100(14):8418–23.

5. Sotiriou C, Neo S-Y, McShane LM, Korn EL, Long PM, Jazaeri A, et al. Breast cancer classification and prognosis based on gene expression profiles from a population-based study. Proc Natl Acad Sci USA. 2003;100(18):10393–8.

6. Prat A, Parker JS, Karginova O, Fan C, Livasy C, Herschkowitz JI, et al. Phenotypic and molecular characterization of the claudin-low intrinsic subtype of breast cancer. Breast Cancer Res. 2010;12(5):R68.

7. Farmer P, Bonnefoi H, Becette V, Tubiana-Hulin M, Fumoleau P, Larsimont D, et al. Identification of molecular apocrine breast tumours by microarray analysis. Oncogene. 2005;24(29):4660–71.

8. Chin K, DeVries S, Fridlyand J, Spellman PT, Roydasgupta R, Kuo W-L, et al. Genomic and transcriptional aberrations linked to breast cancer pathophysiologies. Cancer Cell. 2006;10(6):529–41.

9. Bergamaschi A, Kim YH, Wang P, Sørlie T, Hernandez-Boussard T, Lonning PE, et al. Distinct patterns of DNA copy number alteration are associated with different clinicopathological features and gene-expression subtypes of breast cancer. Genes Chromosom Cancer. 2006;45(11):1033–40.

10. Kan Z, Jaiswal BS, Stinson J, Janakiraman V, Bhatt D, Stern HM, et al. Diverse somatic mutation patterns and pathway alterations in human cancers. Nature. 2010;466(7308):869–73.

11. Koboldt DC, Fulton RS, McLellan MD, Schmidt H, Kalicki-Veizer J, McMichael JF, et al. Comprehensive molecular portraits of human breast tumours. Nature. 2012;490(7418):61–70.

12. Stephens PJ, McBride DJ, Lin M-L, Varela I, Pleasance ED, Simpson JT, et al. Complex landscapes of somatic rearrangement in human breast cancer genomes. Nature. 2009;462(7276):1005–10.

13. Shah SP, Roth A, Goya R, Oloumi A, Ha G, Zhao Y, et al. The clonal and mutational evolution spectrum of primary triple-negative breast cancers. Nature [Internet]. 2012 Apr 4 [cited 2012 Oct 8]. http://www.nature.com/doifinder/10.1038/nature10933

14. Ellis MJ, Ding L, Shen D, Luo J, Suman VJ, Wallis JW, et al. Whole-genome analysis informs breast cancer response to aromatase inhibition. Nature [Internet]. 2012 Jun 10 [cited 2012 Oct 8]. http://www.nature.com/doifinder/10.1038/nature11143

15. Banerji S, Cibulskis K, Rangel-Escareno C, Brown KK, Carter SL, Frederick AM, et al. Sequence analysis of mutations and translocations across breast cancer subtypes. Nature. 2012;486(7403):405–9.

16. Cheang MCU, Chia SK, Voduc D, Gao D, Leung S, Snider J, et al. Ki67 index, HER2 status, and prognosis of patients with luminal B breast cancer. J Natl Cancer Inst. 2009;101(10):736–50.

17. Prat A, Cheang MCU, Martin M, Parker JS, Carrasco E, Caballero R, et al. Prognostic significance of progesterone receptor-positive tumor cells within immunohistochemically defined Luminal A breast cancer. J Clin Oncol. 2012;31(2):203–9.

18. Prat A, Adamo B, Cheang MCU, Anders CK, Carey LA, Perou CM. Molecular characterization of basal-like and non-basal-like triple-negative breast cancer. Oncologist. 2013;18(2):123–33.

19. Zardavas D, Pugliano L, Piccart M. Personalized therapy for breast cancer: a dream or a reality? Future Oncol. 2013;9(8):1105–19.

20. Lemon HM. Abnormal estrogen metabolism and tissue estrogen receptor proteins in breast cancer. Cancer. 1970;25(2):423–35.

21. Nilsson S, Mäkelä S, Treuter E, Tujague M, Thomsen J, Andersson G, et al. Mechanisms of estrogen action. Physiol Rev. 2001;81(4):1535–65.

22. Watanabe T, Inoue S, Ogawa S, Ishii Y, Hiroi H, Ikeda K, et al. Agonistic effect of tamoxifen is dependent on cell type, ERE-promoter context, and estrogen receptor subtype: functional difference between estrogen receptors alpha and beta. Biochem Biophys Res Commun. 1997;236(1):140–5.

23. Barkhem T, Carlsson B, Nilsson Y, Enmark E, Gustafsson J, Nilsson S. Differential response of estrogen receptor alpha and estrogen receptor beta to partial estrogen agonists/antagonists. Mol Pharmacol. 1998;54(1):105–12.

24. Chalbos D, Galtier F. Differential effect of forms A and B of human progesterone receptor on estradiol-dependent transcription. J Biol Chem. 1994;269(37):23007–12.

25. McGuire WL, De La Garza M, Chamness GC. Evaluation of estrogen receptor assays in human breast cancer tissue. Cancer Res. 1977;37(3):637–9.

26. Allred DC, Harvey JM, Berardo M, Clark GM. Prognostic and predictive factors in breast cancer by immunohistochemical analysis. Mod Pathol. 1998;11(2):155–68.

27. Rhodes A, Jasani B, Barnes DM, Bobrow LG, Miller KD. Reliability of immunohistochemical demonstration of oestrogen receptors in routine practice: interlaboratory variance in the sensitivity of detection and evaluation of scoring systems. J Clin Pathol. 2000;53(2):125–30.

28. Rüdiger T, Höfler H, Kreipe H-H, Nizze H, Pfeifer U, Stein H, et al. Quality assurance in immunohistochemistry: results of an interlaboratory trial involving 172 pathologists. Am J Surg Pathol. 2002;26(7):873–82.

29. Hammond MEH, Hayes DF, Dowsett M, Allred DC, Hagerty KL, Badve S, et al. American Society of Clinical Oncology/College Of American Pathologists guideline recommendations for immunohistochemical testing of estrogen and progesterone

receptors in breast cancer. J Clin Oncol. 2010; 28(16):2784–95.

30. Du X, Li X-Q, Li L, Xu Y-Y, Feng Y-M. The detection of ESR1/PGR/ERBB2 mRNA levels by RT-QPCR: a better approach for subtyping breast cancer and predicting prognosis. Breast Cancer Res Treat. 2013;138(1):59–67.

31. Fisher B, Redmond C, Fisher ER, Caplan R. Relative worth of estrogen or progesterone receptor and pathologic characteristics of differentiation as indicators of prognosis in node negative breast cancer patients: findings from National Surgical Adjuvant Breast and Bowel Project Protocol B-06. J Clin Oncol. 1988;6(7):1076–87.

32. Grann VR, Troxel AB, Zojwalla NJ, Jacobson JS, Hershman D, Neugut AI. Hormone receptor status and survival in a population-based cohort of patients with breast carcinoma. Cancer. 2005;103(11):2241–51.

33. Crowe JP, Hubay CA, Pearson OH, Marshall JS, Rosenblatt J, Mansour EG, et al. Estrogen receptor status as a prognostic indicator for stage I breast cancer patients. Breast Cancer Res Treat. 1982;2(2): 171–6.

34. Hilsenbeck SG, Ravdin PM, de Moor CA, Chamness GC, Osborne CK, Clark GM. Time-dependence of hazard ratios for prognostic factors in primary breast cancer. Breast Cancer Res Treat. 1998;52(1–3): 227–37.

35. Schmitt M, Thomssen C, Ulm K, Seiderer A, Harbeck N, Höfler H, et al. Time-varying prognostic impact of tumour biological factors urokinase (uPA), PAI-1 and steroid hormone receptor status in primary breast cancer. Br J Cancer. 1997;76(3): 306–11.

36. Berry DA, Cirrincione C, Henderson IC, Citron ML, Budman DR, Goldstein LJ, et al. Estrogen-receptor status and outcomes of modern chemotherapy for patients with node-positive breast cancer. JAMA. 2006;295(14):1658–67.

37. Clark GM, McGuire WL, Hubay CA, Pearson OH, Marshall JS. Progesterone receptors as a prognostic factor in Stage II breast cancer. N Engl J Med. 1983;309(22):1343–7.

38. Thakkar JP, Mehta DG. A review of an unfavorable subset of breast cancer: estrogen receptor positive progesterone receptor negative. Oncologist. 2011;16(3):276–85.

39. Early Breast Cancer Trialists' Collaborative Group (EBCTCG). Effects of chemotherapy and hormonal therapy for early breast cancer on recurrence and 15-year survival: an overview of the randomised trials. Lancet. 2005;365(9472):1687–717.

40. Howell A, Cuzick J, Baum M, Buzdar A, Dowsett M, Forbes JF, et al. Results of the ATAC (Arimidex, Tamoxifen, Alone or in Combination) trial after completion of 5 years' adjuvant treatment for breast cancer. Lancet. 2005;365(9453):60–2.

41. BIG 1–98 Collaborative Group, Mouridsen H, Giobbie-Hurder A, Goldhirsch A, Thürlimann B, Paridaens R, et al. Letrozole therapy alone or in sequence with tamoxifen in women with breast cancer. N Engl J Med. 2009;361(8):766–76.

42. Boccardo F, Rubagotti A, Guglielmini P, Fini A, Paladini G, Mesiti M, et al. Switching to anastrozole versus continued tamoxifen treatment of early breast cancer. Updated results of the Italian tamoxifen anastrozole (ITA) trial. Ann Oncol. 2006;17 Suppl 7: vii10–4.

43. Coombes RC, Hall E, Gibson LJ, Paridaens R, Jassem J, Delozier T, et al. A randomized trial of exemestane after two to three years of tamoxifen therapy in postmenopausal women with primary breast cancer. N Engl J Med. 2004;350(11): 1081–92.

44. Kaufmann M, Jonat W, Hilfrich J, Eidtmann H, Gademann G, Zuna I, et al. Improved overall survival in postmenopausal women with early breast cancer after anastrozole initiated after treatment with tamoxifen compared with continued tamoxifen: the ARNO 95 Study. J Clin Oncol. 2007;25(19):2664–70.

45. Jakesz R, Jonat W, Gnant M, Mittlboeck M, Greil R, Tausch C, et al. Switching of postmenopausal women with endocrine-responsive early breast cancer to anastrozole after 2 years' adjuvant tamoxifen: combined results of ABCSG trial 8 and ARNO 95 trial. Lancet. 2005;366(9484):455–62.

46. Jonat W, Gnant M, Boccardo F, Kaufmann M, Rubagotti A, Zuna I, et al. Effectiveness of switching from adjuvant tamoxifen to anastrozole in postmenopausal women with hormone-sensitive early-stage breast cancer: a meta-analysis. Lancet Oncol. 2006;7(12):991–6.

47. Van de Velde CJH, Rea D, Seynaeve C, Putter H, Hasenburg A, Vannetzel J-M, et al. Adjuvant tamoxifen and exemestane in early breast cancer (TEAM): a randomised phase 3 trial. Lancet. 2011; 377(9762):321–31.

48. Goss PE, Ingle JN, Martino S, Robert NJ, Muss HB, Piccart MJ, et al. Randomized trial of letrozole following tamoxifen as extended adjuvant therapy in receptor-positive breast cancer: updated findings from NCIC CTG MA.17. J Natl Cancer Inst. 2005;97(17):1262–71.

49. Goss PE, Ingle JN, Martino S, Robert NJ, Muss HB, Piccart MJ, et al. A randomized trial of letrozole in postmenopausal women after five years of tamoxifen therapy for early-stage breast cancer. N Engl J Med. 2003;349(19):1793–802.

50. Goss PE, Ingle JN, Pater JL, Martino S, Robert NJ, Muss HB, et al. Late extended adjuvant treatment with letrozole improves outcome in women with early-stage breast cancer who complete 5 years of tamoxifen. J Clin Oncol. 2008;26(12):1948–55.

51. Ingle JN, Tu D, Pater JL, Muss HB, Martino S, Robert NJ, et al. Intent-to-treat analysis of the placebo-controlled trial of letrozole for extended adjuvant therapy in early breast cancer: NCIC CTG MA.17. Ann Oncol. 2008;19(5):877–82.

52. Pritchard KI. Ovarian suppression/ablation in premenopausal ER-positive breast cancer patients. Issues and recommendations. Oncology (Williston Park, NY). 2009;23(1):27–33.

53. Puhalla S, Brufsky A, Davidson N. Adjuvant endocrine therapy for premenopausal women with breast cancer. Breast. 2009;18 Suppl 3:S122–30.

54. Tan S-H, Wolff AC. The role of ovarian ablation in the adjuvant therapy of breast cancer. Curr Oncol Rep. 2008;10(1):27–37.

55. Paik S, Tang G, Shak S, Kim C, Baker J, Kim W, et al. Gene expression and benefit of chemotherapy in women with node-negative, estrogen receptor-positive breast cancer. J Clin Oncol. 2006;24(23):3726–34.

56. Kim C, Tang G, Pogue-Geile KL, Costantino JP, Baehner FL, Baker J, et al. Estrogen receptor (ESR1) mRNA expression and benefit from tamoxifen in the treatment and prevention of estrogen receptor-positive breast cancer. J Clin Oncol. 2011;29(31):4160–7.

57. Viale G, Regan MM, Maiorano E, Mastropasqua MG, Dell'Orto P, Rasmussen BB, et al. Prognostic and predictive value of centrally reviewed expression of estrogen and progesterone receptors in a randomized trial comparing letrozole and tamoxifen adjuvant therapy for postmenopausal early breast cancer: BIG 1–98. J Clin Oncol. 2007;25(25):3846–52.

58. Albain KS, Paik S, van't Veer L. Prediction of adjuvant chemotherapy benefit in endocrine responsive, early breast cancer using multigene assays. Breast. 2009;18 Suppl 3:S141–5.

59. Colleoni M, Viale G, Zahrieh D, Pruneri G, Gentilini O, Veronesi P, et al. Chemotherapy is more effective in patients with breast cancer not expressing steroid hormone receptors: a study of preoperative treatment. Clin Cancer Res. 2004;10(19):6622–8.

60. Ring AE, Smith IE, Ashley S, Fulford LG, Lakhani SR. Oestrogen receptor status, pathological complete response and prognosis in patients receiving neoadjuvant chemotherapy for early breast cancer. Br J Cancer. 2004;91(12):2012–7.

61. Bonneterre J, Thürlimann B, Robertson JF, Krzakowski M, Mauriac L, Koralewski P, et al. Anastrozole versus tamoxifen as first-line therapy for advanced breast cancer in 668 postmenopausal women: results of the Tamoxifen or Arimidex Randomized Group Efficacy and Tolerability study. J Clin Oncol. 2000;18(22):3748–57.

62. Nabholtz JM, Buzdar A, Pollak M, Harwin W, Burton G, Mangalik A, et al. Anastrozole is superior to tamoxifen as first-line therapy for advanced breast cancer in postmenopausal women: results of a North American multicenter randomized trial. Arimidex Study Group. J Clin Oncol. 2000;18(22):3758–67.

63. Paridaens RJ, Dirix LY, Beex LV, Nooij M, Cameron DA, Cufer T, et al. Phase III study comparing exemestane with tamoxifen as first-line hormonal treatment of metastatic breast cancer in postmenopausal women: the European Organisation for Research and Treatment of Cancer Breast Cancer Cooperative Group. J Clin Oncol. 2008;26(30): 4883–90.

64. Vergote I, Bonneterre J, Thürlimann B, Robertson J, Krzakowski M, Mauriac L, et al. Randomised study of anastrozole versus tamoxifen as first-line therapy for advanced breast cancer in postmenopausal women. Eur J Cancer. 2000;36 Suppl 4:S84–5.

65. Gibson L, Lawrence D, Dawson C, Bliss J. Aromatase inhibitors for treatment of advanced breast cancer in postmenopausal women. Cochrane Database Syst Rev. 2009;(4):CD003370.

66. Dowsett M, Houghton J, Iden C, Salter J, Farndon J, A'Hern R, et al. Benefit from adjuvant tamoxifen therapy in primary breast cancer patients according oestrogen receptor, progesterone receptor, EGF receptor and HER2 status. Ann Oncol. 2006;17(5): 818–26.

67. NCCN Guidelines Breast Cancer Version 3.2013 [Internet]. http://www.NCCN.com

68. Schechter AL, Stern DF, Vaidyanathan L, Decker SJ, Drebin JA, Greene MI, et al. The neu oncogene: an erb-B-related gene encoding a 185,000-Mr tumour antigen. Nature. 1984;312(5994):513–6.

69. Hanna W, Kahn HJ, Trudeau M. Evaluation of HER-2/neu (erbB-2) status in breast cancer: from bench to bedside. Mod Pathol. 1999;12(8):827–34.

70. Slamon DJ, Clark GM, Wong SG, Levin WJ, Ullrich A, McGuire WL. Human breast cancer: correlation of relapse and survival with amplification of the HER-2/neu oncogene. Science. 1987;235(4785):177–82.

71. Slamon DJ, Godolphin W, Jones LA, Holt JA, Wong SG, Keith DE, et al. Studies of the HER-2/neu proto-oncogene in human breast and ovarian cancer. Science. 1989;244(4905):707–12.

72. Press MF, Hung G, Godolphin W, Slamon DJ. Sensitivity of HER-2/neu antibodies in archival tissue samples: potential source of error in immunohistochemical studies of oncogene expression. Cancer Res. 1994;54(10):2771–7.

73. Paik S, Bryant J, Tan-Chiu E, Romond E, Hiller W, Park K, et al. Real-world performance of HER2 testing–National Surgical Adjuvant Breast and Bowel Project experience. J Natl Cancer Inst. 2002; 94(11):852–4.

74. Perez EA, Suman VJ, Davidson NE, Martino S, Kaufman PA, Lingle WL, et al. HER2 testing by local, central, and reference laboratories in specimens from the North Central Cancer Treatment Group N9831 intergroup adjuvant trial. J Clin Oncol. 2006;24(19):3032–8.

75. Press MF, Sauter G, Bernstein L, Villalobos IE, Mirlacher M, Zhou J-Y, et al. Diagnostic evaluation of HER-2 as a molecular target: an assessment of accuracy and reproducibility of laboratory testing in large, prospective, randomized clinical trials. Clin Cancer Res. 2005;11(18):6598–607.

76. Wolff AC, Hammond MEH, Schwartz JN, Hagerty KL, Allred DC, Cote RJ, et al. American Society of Clinical Oncology/College of American Pathologists

guideline recommendations for human epidermal growth factor receptor 2 testing in breast cancer. J Clin Oncol. 2007;25(1):118–45.

77. Paik S, Hazan R, Fisher ER, Sass RE, Fisher B, Redmond C, et al. Pathologic findings from the National Surgical Adjuvant Breast and Bowel Project: prognostic significance of erbB-2 protein overexpression in primary breast cancer. J Clin Oncol. 1990;8(1):103–12.

78. Gilcrease MZ, Woodward WA, Nicolas MM, Corley LJ, Fuller GN, Esteva FJ, et al. Even low-level HER2 expression may be associated with worse outcome in node-positive breast cancer. Am J Surg Pathol. 2009;33(5):759–67.

79. Tandon AK, Clark GM, Chamness GC, Ullrich A, McGuire WL. HER-2/neu oncogene protein and prognosis in breast cancer. J Clin Oncol. 1989; 7(8):1120–8.

80. Chia S, Norris B, Speers C, Cheang M, Gilks B, Gown AM, et al. Human epidermal growth factor receptor 2 overexpression as a prognostic factor in a large tissue microarray series of node-negative breast cancers. J Clin Oncol. 2008;26(35):5697–704.

81. Harris L, Fritsche H, Mennel R, Norton L, Ravdin P, Taube S, et al. American Society of Clinical Oncology 2007 update of recommendations for the use of tumor markers in breast cancer. J Clin Oncol. 2007;25(33):5287–312.

82. Muss HB, Thor AD, Berry DA, Kute T, Liu ET, Koerner F, et al. c-erbB-2 expression and response to adjuvant therapy in women with node-positive early breast cancer. N Engl J Med. 1994;330(18):1260–6.

83. Paik S, Bryant J, Park C, Fisher B, Tan-Chiu E, Hyams D, et al. erbB-2 and response to doxorubicin in patients with axillary lymph node-positive, hormone receptor-negative breast cancer. J Natl Cancer Inst. 1998;90(18):1361–70.

84. Paik S, Bryant J, Tan-Chiu E, Yothers G, Park C, Wickerham DL, et al. HER2 and choice of adjuvant chemotherapy for invasive breast cancer: National Surgical Adjuvant Breast and Bowel Project Protocol B-15. J Natl Cancer Inst. 2000;92(24):1991–8.

85. Pritchard KI, Shepherd LE, O'Malley FP, Andrulis IL, Tu D, Bramwell VH, et al. HER2 and responsiveness of breast cancer to adjuvant chemotherapy. N Engl J Med. 2006;354(20):2103–11.

86. Dressler LG, Berry DA, Broadwater G, Cowan D, Cox K, Griffin S, et al. Comparison of HER2 status by fluorescence in situ hybridization and immunohistochemistry to predict benefit from dose escalation of adjuvant doxorubicin-based therapy in node-positive breast cancer patients. J Clin Oncol. 2005;23(19):4287–97.

87. Gennari A, Sormani MP, Pronzato P, Puntoni M, Colozza M, Pfeffer U, et al. HER2 status and efficacy of adjuvant anthracyclines in early breast cancer: a pooled analysis of randomized trials. J Natl Cancer Inst. 2008;100(1):14–20.

88. Bartlett JMS, Munro AF, Dunn JA, McConkey C, Jordan S, Twelves CJ, et al. Predictive markers of

anthracycline benefit: a prospectively planned analysis of the UK National Epirubicin Adjuvant Trial (NEAT/BR9601). Lancet Oncol. 2010;11(3):266–74.

89. Hayes DF, Thor AD, Dressler LG, Weaver D, Edgerton S, Cowan D, et al. HER2 and response to paclitaxel in node-positive breast cancer. N Engl J Med. 2007;357(15):1496–506.

90. Gusterson BA, Gelber RD, Goldhirsch A, Price KN, Säve-Söderborgh J, Anbazhagan R, et al. Prognostic importance of c-erbB-2 expression in breast cancer. International (Ludwig) Breast Cancer Study Group. J Clin Oncol. 1992;10(7):1049–56.

91. Allred DC, Clark GM, Tandon AK, Molina R, Tormey DC, Osborne CK, et al. HER-2/neu in node-negative breast cancer: prognostic significance of overexpression influenced by the presence of in situ carcinoma. J Clin Oncol. 1992;10(4):599–605.

92. Ménard S, Valagussa P, Pilotti S, Gianni L, Biganzoli E, Boracchi P, et al. Response to cyclophosphamide, methotrexate, and fluorouracil in lymph node-positive breast cancer according to HER2 overexpression and other tumor biologic variables. J Clin Oncol. 2001;19(2):329–35.

93. Cobleigh MA, Vogel CL, Tripathy D, Robert NJ, Scholl S, Fehrenbacher L, et al. Multinational study of the efficacy and safety of humanized anti-HER2 monoclonal antibody in women who have HER2-overexpressing metastatic breast cancer that has progressed after chemotherapy for metastatic disease. J Clin Oncol. 1999;17(9):2639–48.

94. Slamon DJ, Leyland-Jones B, Shak S, Fuchs H, Paton V, Bajamonde A, et al. Use of chemotherapy plus a monoclonal antibody against HER2 for metastatic breast cancer that overexpresses HER2. N Engl J Med. 2001;344(11):783–92.

95. Vogel CL, Cobleigh MA, Tripathy D, Gutheil JC, Harris LN, Fehrenbacher L, et al. Efficacy and safety of trastuzumab as a single agent in first-line treatment of HER2-overexpressing metastatic breast cancer. J Clin Oncol. 2002;20(3):719–26.

96. Joensuu H, Kellokumpu-Lehtinen P-L, Bono P, Alanko T, Kataja V, Asola R, et al. Adjuvant docetaxel or vinorelbine with or without trastuzumab for breast cancer. N Engl J Med. 2006;354(8):809–20.

97. Piccart-Gebhart MJ, Procter M, Leyland-Jones B, Goldhirsch A, Untch M, Smith I, et al. Trastuzumab after adjuvant chemotherapy in HER2-positive breast cancer. N Engl J Med. 2005;353(16):1659–72.

98. Piccart-Gebhart MJ. HERA TRIAL: 2 years versus 1 year of trastuzumab after adjuvant chemotherapy in women with HER2-positive early breast cancer at 8 years of median follow up [Internet]. San Antonio, TX; 2012. http://cancerres.aacrjournals.org/cgi/content/meeting_abstract/72/24_MeetingAbstracts/S5-2

99. Romond EH, Perez EA, Bryant J, Suman VJ, Geyer Jr CE, Davidson NE, et al. Trastuzumab plus adjuvant chemotherapy for operable HER2-positive breast cancer. N Engl J Med. 2005;353(16):1673–84.

100. Romond E. Trastuzumab plus adjuvant chemotherapy for HER2-positive breast cancer: final planned joint

analysis of overall survival (OS) from NSABP B-31 and NCCTG N9831 [Internet]. San Antonio, TX; 2012. http://cancerres.aacrjournals.org/cgi/content/meeting_abstract/72/24_MeetingAbstracts/S5-5

101. Slamon D, Eiermann W, Robert N, Pienkowski T, Martin M, Press M, et al. Adjuvant trastuzumab in HER2-positive breast cancer. N Engl J Med. 2011;365(14):1273–83.

102. Buzdar AU, Ibrahim NK, Francis D, Booser DJ, Thomas ES, Theriault RL, et al. Significantly higher pathologic complete remission rate after neoadjuvant therapy with trastuzumab, paclitaxel, and epirubicin chemotherapy: results of a randomized trial in human epidermal growth factor receptor 2-positive operable breast cancer. J Clin Oncol. 2005;23(16):3676–85.

103. Buzdar AU, Valero V, Ibrahim NK, Francis D, Broglio KR, Theriault RL, et al. Neoadjuvant therapy with paclitaxel followed by 5-fluorouracil, epirubicin, and cyclophosphamide chemotherapy and concurrent trastuzumab in human epidermal growth factor receptor 2-positive operable breast cancer: an update of the initial randomized study population and data of additional patients treated with the same regimen. Clin Cancer Res. 2007;13(1):228–33.

104. Baselga J, Bradbury I, Eidtmann H, Di Cosimo S, de Azambuja E, Aura C, et al. Lapatinib with trastuzumab for HER2-positive early breast cancer (NeoALTTO): a randomised, open-label, multicentre, phase 3 trial. Lancet. 2012;379(9816):633–40.

105. Gianni L, Pienkowski T, Im Y-H, Roman L, Tseng L-M, Liu M-C, et al. Efficacy and safety of neoadjuvant pertuzumab and trastuzumab in women with locally advanced, inflammatory, or early HER2-positive breast cancer (NeoSphere): a randomised multicentre, open-label, phase 2 trial. Lancet Oncol. 2012;13(1):25–32.

106. Zardavas D, Bozovic-Spasojevic I, de Azambuja E. Dual human epidermal growth factor receptor 2 blockade: another step forward in treating patients with human epidermal growth factor receptor 2-positive breast cancer. Curr Opin Oncol. 2012;24(6):612–22.

107. Saini KS, Azim Jr HA, Metzger-Filho O, Loi S, Sotiriou C, de Azambuja E, et al. Beyond trastuzumab: new treatment options for HER2-positive breast cancer. Breast. 2011;20 Suppl 3:S20–7.

108. Scaltriti M, Rojo F, Ocaña A, Anido J, Guzman M, Cortes J, et al. Expression of p95HER2, a truncated form of the HER2 receptor, and response to anti-HER2 therapies in breast cancer. J Natl Cancer Inst. 2007;99(8):628–38.

109. Paik S, Kim C, Wolmark N. HER2 status and benefit from adjuvant trastuzumab in breast cancer. N Engl J Med. 2008;358(13):1409–11.

110. Tuma RS. Inconsistency of HER2 test raises questions. J Natl Cancer Inst. 2007;99(14):1064–5.

111. Perez EA, Reinholz MM, Hillman DW, Tenner KS, Schroeder MJ, Davidson NE, et al. HER2 and chromosome 17 effect on patient outcome in the N9831 adjuvant trastuzumab trial. J Clin Oncol. 2010; 28(28):4307–15.

112. Lam L, McAndrew N, Yee M, Fu T, Tchou JC, Zhang H. Challenges in the clinical utility of the serum test for HER2 ECD. Biochim Biophys Acta. 2012;1826(1):199–208.

113. Gerdes J, Schwab U, Lemke H, Stein H. Production of a mouse monoclonal antibody reactive with a human nuclear antigen associated with cell proliferation. Int J Cancer. 1983;31(1):13–20.

114. Bullwinkel J, Baron-Lühr B, Lüdemann A, Wohlenberg C, Gerdes J, Scholzen T. Ki-67 protein is associated with ribosomal RNA transcription in quiescent and proliferating cells. J Cell Physiol. 2006;206(3):624–35.

115. Rahmanzadeh R, Hüttmann G, Gerdes J, Scholzen T. Chromophore-assisted light inactivation of pKi-67 leads to inhibition of ribosomal RNA synthesis. Cell Prolif. 2007;40(3):422–30.

116. Viale G, Giobbie-Hurder A, Regan MM, Coates AS, Mastropasqua MG, Dell'Orto P, et al. Prognostic and predictive value of centrally reviewed Ki-67 labeling index in postmenopausal women with endocrine-responsive breast cancer: results from Breast International Group Trial 1–98 comparing adjuvant tamoxifen with letrozole. J Clin Oncol. 2008;26(34): 5569–75.

117. Zabaglo L, Ormerod MG, Dowsett M. Measurement of proliferation marker Ki67 in breast tumour FNAs using laser scanning cytometry in comparison to conventional immunocytochemistry. Cytom B Clin Cytom. 2003;56(1):55–61.

118. De Azambuja E, Cardoso F, de Castro G, Jr CM, Mano MS, Durbecq V, et al. Ki-67 as prognostic marker in early breast cancer: a meta-analysis of published studies involving 12,155 patients. Br J Cancer. 2007;96(10):1504–13.

119. Stuart-Harris R, Caldas C, Pinder SE, Pharoah P. Proliferation markers and survival in early breast cancer: a systematic review and meta-analysis of 85 studies in 32,825 patients. Breast. 2008;17(4): 323–34.

120. Hugh J, Hanson J, Cheang MCU, Nielsen TO, Perou CM, Dumontet C, et al. Breast cancer subtypes and response to docetaxel in node-positive breast cancer: use of an immunohistochemical definition in the BCIRG 001 trial. J Clin Oncol. 2009;27(8): 1168–76.

121. Penault-Llorca F, André F, Sagan C, Lacroix-Triki M, Denoux Y, Verriele V, et al. Ki67 expression and docetaxel efficacy in patients with estrogen receptor-positive breast cancer. J Clin Oncol. 2009;27(17):2 809–15.

122. Viale G, Regan MM, Mastropasqua MG, Maffini F, Maiorano E, Colleoni M, et al. Predictive value of tumor Ki-67 expression in two randomized trials of adjuvant chemoendocrine therapy for node-negative breast cancer. J Natl Cancer Inst. 2008;100(3): 207–12.

123. Bottini A, Berruti A, Bersiga A, Brizzi MP, Bruzzi P, Aguggini S, et al. Relationship between tumour shrinkage and reduction in Ki67 expression after primary chemotherapy in human breast cancer. Br J Cancer. 2001;85(8):1106–12.

124. Estévez LG, Cuevas JM, Antón A, Florián J, López-Vega JM, Velasco A, et al. Weekly docetaxel as neoadjuvant chemotherapy for stage II and III breast cancer: efficacy and correlation with biological markers in a phase II, multicenter study. Clin Cancer Res. 2003;9(2):686–92.

125. Chang J, Powles TJ, Allred DC, Ashley SE, Makris A, Gregory RK, et al. Prediction of clinical outcome from primary tamoxifen by expression of biologic markers in breast cancer patients. Clin Cancer Res. 2000;6(2):616–21.

126. Miller WR, White S, Dixon JM, Murray J, Renshaw L, Anderson TJ. Proliferation, steroid receptors and clinical/pathological response in breast cancer treated with letrozole. Br J Cancer. 2006;94(7):1051–6.

127. Yamashita H, Toyama T, Nishio M, Ando Y, Hamaguchi M, Zhang Z, et al. p53 protein accumulation predicts resistance to endocrine therapy and decreased post-relapse survival in metastatic breast cancer. Breast Cancer Res. 2006;8(4):R48.

128. Kai K, Nishimura R, Arima N, Miyayama H, Iwase H. p53 expression status is a significant molecular marker in predicting the time to endocrine therapy failure in recurrent breast cancer: a cohort study. Int J Clin Oncol. 2006;11(6):426–33.

129. Nishimura R, Okumura Y, Arima N. Trastuzumab monotherapy versus combination therapy for treating recurrent breast cancer: time to progression and survival. Breast Cancer. 2008;15(1):57–64.

130. Paik S, Shak S, Tang G, Kim C, Baker J, Cronin M, et al. A multigene assay to predict recurrence of tamoxifen-treated, node-negative breast cancer. N Engl J Med. 2004;351(27):2817–26.

131. Dowsett M, Cuzick J, Wale C, Forbes J, Mallon EA, Salter J, et al. Prediction of risk of distant recurrence using the 21-gene recurrence score in node-negative and node-positive postmenopausal patients with breast cancer treated with anastrozole or tamoxifen: a TransATAC study. J Clin Oncol. 2010;28(11):1829–34.

132. Albain KS, Barlow WE, Shak S, Hortobagyi GN, Livingston RB, Yeh I-T, et al. Prognostic and predictive value of the 21-gene recurrence score assay in postmenopausal women with node-positive, oestrogen-receptor-positive breast cancer on chemotherapy: a retrospective analysis of a randomised trial. Lancet Oncol. 2010;11(1):55–65.

133. Habel LA, Shak S, Jacobs MK, Capra A, Alexander C, Pho M, et al. A population-based study of tumor gene expression and risk of breast cancer death among lymph node-negative patients. Breast Cancer Res. 2006;8(3):R25.

134. Van't Veer LJ, Dai H, van de Vijver MJ, He YD, Hart AAM, Mao M, et al. Gene expression profiling predicts clinical outcome of breast cancer. Nature. 2002;415(6871):530–6.

135. Van de Vijver MJ, He YD, van't Veer LJ, Dai H, Hart AAM, Voskuil DW, et al. A gene-expression signature as a predictor of survival in breast cancer. N Engl J Med. 2002;347(25):1999–2009.

136. Buyse M, Loi S, van't Veer L, Viale G, Delorenzi M, Glas AM, et al. Validation and clinical utility of a 70-gene prognostic signature for women with node-negative breast cancer. J Natl Cancer Inst. 2006; 98(17):1183–92.

137. Sotiriou C, Wirapati P, Loi S, Harris A, Fox S, Smeds J, et al. Gene expression profiling in breast cancer: understanding the molecular basis of histologic grade to improve prognosis. J Natl Cancer Inst. 2006;98(4):262–72.

138. Metzger-Filho O, Michiels S, Bertucci F, Catteau A, Salgado R, Galant C, et al. Genomic grade adds prognostic value in invasive lobular carcinoma. Ann Oncol. 2013;24(2):377–84.

139. Filipits M, Rudas M, Jakesz R, Dubsky P, Fitzal F, Singer CF, et al. A new molecular predictor of distant recurrence in ER-positive, HER2-negative breast cancer adds independent information to conventional clinical risk factors. Clin Cancer Res. 2011;17(18):6012–20.

140. Dubsky P, Filipits M, Jakesz R, Rudas M, Singer CF, Greil R, et al. EndoPredict improves the prognostic classification derived from common clinical guidelines in ER-positive, HER2-negative early breast cancer. Ann Oncol. 2013;24(3):640–7.

141. Varga Z, Sinn P, Fritzsche F, von Hochstetter A, Noske A, Schraml P, et al. Comparison of EndoPredict and Oncotype DX Test Results in Hormone Receptor Positive Invasive Breast Cancer. PLoS ONE. 2013;8(3):e58483.

142. Parker JS, Mullins M, Cheang MCU, Leung S, Voduc D, Vickery T, et al. Supervised risk predictor of breast cancer based on intrinsic subtypes. J Clin Oncol. 2009;27(8):1160–7.

143. Nielsen TO, Parker JS, Leung S, Voduc D, Ebbert M, Vickery T, et al. A comparison of PAM50 intrinsic subtyping with immunohistochemistry and clinical prognostic factors in tamoxifen-treated estrogen receptor-positive breast cancer. Clin Cancer Res. 2010;16(21):5222–32.

144. Chia SK, Bramwell VH, Tu D, Shepherd LE, Jiang S, Vickery T, et al. A 50-gene intrinsic subtype classifier for prognosis and prediction of benefit from adjuvant tamoxifen. Clin Cancer Res. 2012;18(16): 4465–72.

145. Cuzick J, Dowsett M, Pineda S, Wale C, Salter J, Quinn E, et al. Prognostic Value of a Combined Estrogen Receptor, Progesterone Receptor, Ki-67, and Human Epidermal Growth Factor Receptor 2 Immunohistochemical Score and Comparison With the Genomic Health Recurrence Score in Early Breast Cancer. J Clin Oncol. 2011;29(32):4273–8.

146. Zardavas D, Fumagalli D, Loi S. Phosphatidylinositol 3-kinase/AKT/mammalian target of rapamycin pathway inhibition: a breakthrough in the management of luminal (ER+/HER2-) breast cancers? Curr Opin Oncol [Internet]. 2012 Sep 6 [cited 2012 Sep 18]. http://www.ncbi.nlm.nih.gov/pubmed/22960556

147. Loi S, Haibe-Kains B, Majjaj S, Lallemand F, Durbecq V, Larsimont D, et al. PIK3CA mutations associated with gene signature of low mTORC1 signaling and better outcomes in estrogen receptor-positive breast cancer. Proc Natl Acad Sci USA. 2010;107(22):10208–13.

148. Loi S, Michiels S, Baselga J, Bartlett JMS, Singhal SK, Sabine VS, et al. PIK3CA genotype and a PIK3CA mutation-related gene signature and response to everolimus and letrozole in estrogen receptor positive breast cancer. PLoS ONE. 2013;8(1):e53292.

149. Cristofanilli M, Budd GT, Ellis MJ, Stopeck A, Matera J, Miller MC, et al. Circulating tumor cells, disease progression, and survival in metastatic breast cancer. N Engl J Med. 2004;351(8):781–91.

150. Allard WJ, Matera J, Miller MC, Repollet M, Connelly MC, Rao C, et al. Tumor cells circulate in the peripheral blood of all major carcinomas but not in healthy subjects or patients with nonmalignant diseases. Clin Cancer Res. 2004;10(20):6897–904.

151. Budd GT, Cristofanilli M, Ellis MJ, Stopeck A, Borden E, Miller MC, et al. Circulating tumor cells versus imaging–predicting overall survival in metastatic breast cancer. Clin Cancer Res. 2006;12(21):6403–9.

152. De Giorgi U, Valero V, Rohren E, Dawood S, Ueno NT, Miller MC, et al. Circulating tumor cells and [18F]fluorodeoxyglucose positron emission tomography/computed tomography for outcome prediction in metastatic breast cancer. J Clin Oncol. 2009; 27(20):3303–11.

153. Edge SB, Byrd DR, Compton CC, Fritz AG, Greene FL, Trotti A, editors. American joint committee on cancer: breast. AJCC cancer staging manual. 7th ed. New York, NY: Springer; 2010. p. 347–76.

154. Struewing JP, Hartge P, Wacholder S, Baker SM, Berlin M, McAdams M, et al. The risk of cancer associated with specific mutations of BRCA1 and BRCA2 among Ashkenazi Jews. N Engl J Med. 1997;336(20):1401–8.

155. Lee E-H, Park SK, Park B, Kim S-W, Lee MH, Ahn SH, et al. Effect of BRCA1/2 mutation on short-term and long-term breast cancer survival: a systematic review and meta-analysis. Breast Cancer Res Treat. 2010;122(1):11–25.

156. Eccles D, Gerty S, Simmonds P, Hammond V, Ennis S, Altman DG. Prospective study of Outcomes in Sporadic versus Hereditary breast cancer (POSH): study protocol. BMC Cancer. 2007;7:160.

157. Bhattacharyya A, Ear US, Koller BH, Weichselbaum RR, Bishop DK. The breast cancer susceptibility gene BRCA1 is required for subnuclear assembly of Rad51 and survival following treatment with the DNA cross-linking agent cisplatin. J Biol Chem. 2000;275(31):23899–903.

158. Byrski T, Huzarski T, Dent R, Gronwald J, Zuziak D, Cybulski C, et al. Response to neoadjuvant therapy with cisplatin in BRCA1-positive breast cancer patients. Breast Cancer Res Treat. 2009;115(2): 359–63.

159. Kurebayashi J, Yamamoto Y, Kurosumi M, Okubo S, Nomura T, Tanaka K, et al. Loss of BRCA1 expression may predict shorter time-to-progression in metastatic breast cancer patients treated with taxanes. Anticancer Res. 2006;26(1B):695–701.

160. Byrski T, Gronwald J, Huzarski T, Grzybowska E, Budryk M, Stawicka M, et al. Response to neoadjuvant chemotherapy in women with BRCA1-positive breast cancers. Breast Cancer Res Treat. 2008;108(2):289–96.

161. Stephens PJ, Tarpey PS, Davies H, Van Loo P, Greenman C, Wedge DC, et al. The landscape of cancer genes and mutational processes in breast cancer. Nature [Internet]. 2012 May 16 [cited 2012 Oct 8]. http://www.nature.com/doifinder/10.1038/nature11017

162. Nik-Zainal S, Alexandrov LB, Wedge DC, Van Loo P, Greenman CD, Raine K, et al. Mutational Processes Molding the Genomes of 21 Breast Cancers. Cell. 2012;149(5):979–93.

163. Dawson S-J, Tsui DWY, Murtaza M, Biggs H, Rueda OM, Chin S-F, et al. Analysis of circulating tumor DNA to monitor metastatic breast cancer. N Engl J Med. 2013;368(13):1199–209.

164. De Mattos-Arruda L, Cortes J, Santarpia L, Vivancos A, Tabernero J, Reis-Filho JS, et al. Circulating tumour cells and cell-free DNA as tools for managing breast cancer. Nat Rev Clin Oncol. 2013;10(7): 377–89.

Molecular Pathology of Gastrointestinal Tumors

Andrea Grin and Serge Jothy

Hereditary Diffuse Gastric Cancer

The Lauren classification broadly divides gastric cancer into two types: intestinal and diffuse. The diffuse type is also known as "linitis plastica" due to the resemblance of the involved stomach to a leather bottle. Histologically, diffuse gastric cancer is composed of infiltrating individual "signet-ring cells," so named due to the accumulation of cytoplasmic mucin compressing the nucleus to one side. The diffuse type is also known as signet-ring cell carcinoma in the WHO Classification. While most diffuse gastric cancers are sporadic, approximately 1 % are familial.

The original criteria for diagnosis of hereditary diffuse gastric cancer (HDGC) were the following: (1) two or more documented cases of diffuse gastric cancer in first- or second-degree relatives, with at least one diagnosed before the age of 50, or (2) three or more cases of documented diffuse gastric cancer in first- or second-degree relatives, independent of the age of onset [1]. In order to increase detection rates, particularly in low incidence areas, these criteria were revised and expanded by the International Gastric Cancer Linkage Consortium (IGCLC) and now also include: (1) diffuse gastric cancer diagnosed before the age of 40, without requirement of a family history, and (2) personal or family history of diffuse gastric cancer and lobular breast cancer, one diagnosed below the age of 50 [2].

The first genetic susceptibility locus for HDGC was identified in 1998 through study of a large Maori family from New Zealand [3]. Based on the pedigree pattern, the candidate susceptibility gene appeared to follow an autosomal dominant pattern of inheritance with incomplete penetrance. Through linkage analysis using microsatellite markers flanking candidate genes of interest, a significant linkage to the CDH1 gene encoding the E-cadherin protein was identified. E-cadherin is a transmembrane cell-adhesion glycoprotein, whose cytoplasmic domain connects to the actin cytoskeleton through a catenin complex. E-cadherin plays an important role in maintaining cell–cell adhesion and polarity. In the original Maori kindred, sequencing of the CDH1 gene revealed a G to T single nucleotide substitution in exon 7 affecting the splice site and leading to a truncated protein. The role of the E-cadherin gene was further confirmed in two other families. One contained an insertion of an additional cytosine residue, resulting in a frameshift mutation, and the other showed a C to T substitution in exon 13, leading to a premature stop codon. This report was the first to demonstrate the implication of E-cadherin in HDGC.

A. Grin, M.D. • S. Jothy, M.D., Ph.D. (✉)
Department of Laboratory Medicine,
St. Michael's Hospital, University of Toronto,
30 Bond Street, Toronto, ON, Canada M5B 1W8

Department of Laboratory Medicine and
Pathobiology, University of Toronto,
Toronto, ON, Canada
e-mail: jothys@smh.ca

G.M. Yousef and S. Jothy (eds.), *Molecular Testing in Cancer*,
DOI 10.1007/978-1-4899-8050-2_12, © Springer Science+Business Media New York 2014

Since the discovery of the role of E-cadherin, it has been shown that approximately 30–50 % of patients meeting clinical criteria for HDGC have a germline mutation in the CDH1 gene. Germline CDH1 mutations occur throughout the 16 exons with no reported hot spots. Mutations may include insertions, deletions, and point mutations and have variable effects on the protein such as truncation, altered structure, deletion of key domains, or instability of the mRNA. A small proportion (6.5 %) of the so-called CDH1-negative HDGC were found to have large genomic deletions detected by multiplex ligation-dependent probe amplification (MLPA) [4]. As CDH1 is a tumor suppressor gene, both genes must be mutated or inactivated for the development of disease. The second gene may become inactivated by mutation or methylation, the mechanism and trigger of which are yet to be understood.

Patients who fulfill diagnostic criteria for HDGC described above should be referred for genetic testing [2]. Testing may be done on blood leukocytes, mucosal epithelial cells, or paraffin-embedded tissue. As the quality of the DNA may be compromised in formalin-fixed paraffin-embedded tissue, testing living individuals is preferable if possible. Since mutations may occur anywhere in the CDH1 gene, and genetic sequencing has become cost- and time-efficient, sequencing the entire coding portion and intron–exon boundaries is usually performed. Once a mutation is identified within a family, targeted sequencing of the exon involved can be done to identify other individuals at risk.

Individuals with a CDH1 mutation carry an 80 % lifetime risk of diffuse gastric cancer by age 80, for both men and women [2]. The age at onset is variable with an average of 38 years (range 14–85 years). For women, the risk of lobular breast cancer is 60 % by age 80 with an average age of 53 years at the time of diagnosis. In some families, there is also an increased risk of colon cancer with signet-ring cell features [5].

Given the high penetrance of diffuse gastric cancer, individuals who test positive for a CDH1 mutation should be advised to undergo prophylactic gastrectomy [2]. There is no consensus as to the optimal timing for this operation. If prophylactic gastrectomy is not performed, annual endoscopic surveillance should be done. Consensus guidelines advise at least 30 biopsies: six from each of the antrum, transitional zone, body, fundus, and cardia. In Maori families, early invasive tumors tend to cluster in the body-antral transition zone, while in North American and European families, carcinoma was most often found proximally [2, 6]. Negative biopsies however do not exclude the presence of invasive carcinoma. A study of ten prophylactic gastrectomies examined in toto histologically determined that 1,768 biopsies are required to detect at least one cancer focus with a 90 % detection rate [6]. In fact 81–93 % of prophylactic gastrectomies with negative preoperative biopsies contained at least one focus of early invasive signet-ring cell carcinoma [2]. Most cases without invasive carcinoma contained small foci of in situ signet-ring cell carcinoma.

Currently there is limited data to support a particular breast cancer screening strategy for women with CDH1 mutations. Based on recommendations in other hereditary breast cancer syndromes, the consensus guidelines recommend annual screening mammograms and MRI starting at age 35 or 5–10 years prior to earliest breast cancer diagnosis in the family [2, 5]. Prophylactic mastectomy may also be considered, but there is limited data to support this measure as a primary recommendation. Similarly, there is limited data on the risk of signet-ring colon cancer and at this time increased screening is limited to those families with documented cases.

In summary, HDGC is a syndrome of diffuse gastric cancer and lobular breast cancer diagnosed clinically based on consensus criteria. While many of these tumors are due to germline mutations in the CDH1 gene encoding the E-cadherin protein, it is clear that there are still a number of molecular markers yet to be discovered as in many familial cases a CDH1 mutation is not found.

HER2 in Gastric and Gastroesophageal Junction Cancer

HER2 is a transmembrane receptor that is part of the epidermal growth factor receptor family. The HER2 protein is encoded by the ERBB2 gene located on the long arm of chromosome 17 (17q12). Dimerization of HER2 results in phosphorylation of the intracytoplasmic tyrosine kinase residues and triggers a variety of signaling pathways, including MAPK, PI3K/Akt, PKC, and others, resulting in cell proliferation, apoptosis, cell migration, and differentiation. HER2 amplification or overexpression has been implicated in a number of cancers, but has been most well established in breast cancer. Trastuzumab (Herceptin) is a monoclonal antibody that targets the HER2 receptor and inhibits cell growth by inhibiting HER2-mediated signaling and inducing antibody-dependent cellular cytotoxicity [7]. Trastuzumab has proven survival advantage in breast cancer and has become standard of care.

In 2010, treatment of gastric cancer greatly evolved based on the results of the trastuzumab for Gastric Cancer Study (ToGA trial) [8]. Prior to this study, treatment of advanced gastric cancer was limited to fluoropyrimidine-based or platinum-based chemotherapy and despite treatment, overall median survival remained <1 year. This international, randomized, phase III clinical trial demonstrated the survival benefit of trastuzumab in patients with HER2-positive advanced gastric or gastroesophageal junction (GEJ) adenocarcinoma and was the first evidence for molecular targeted therapy in gastric cancer.

HER2 positivity is present in approximately 20–30 % of gastric and GEJ tumors. GEJ tumors are more likely to be HER2 positive as well as tumors of intestinal type, compared to diffuse or mixed types.

Due to the results of this landmark trial, HER2 testing is now performed on all gastric and GEJ tumors in patients being considered for chemotherapy. Testing is performed by immunohistochemistry (IHC) or a combination of IHC and in situ hybridization (ISH). In the ToGA trial, survival benefit was seen in patients who were scored at 3+ by IHC or 2+ with HER2 amplification by fluorescence in situ hybridization (FISH). Patients with a 0 or 1+ score by IHC with FISH amplification did not show significant benefit with the addition of trastuzumab to standard chemotherapy; therefore, high expression of HER2 protein was most predictive of treatment response. While testing methods are similar to breast cancer, gastric and GEJ tumors have some unique challenges and criteria for HER2 positivity differ.

The criteria for scoring HER2 by IHC and ISH differ in gastric/GEJ cancer, as compared to breast. Applying the breast criteria would generate false negative results, thereby eliminating eligible patients who would benefit from trastuzumab therapy. In gastric/GEJ tumors, basolateral or lateral membrane staining is acceptable [8, 9]. The "magnification rule" is a practical method to determine the IHC score [10]. Briefly, the scores are defined as follows: 3+ if strong membranous staining visible at low magnification (×2.5–5) (Fig. 12.1), 2+ for weak to moderate membranous staining visible at ×10–20 magnification, 1+ for faint or barely perceptible membranous staining visible only at ×40 magnification, and score 0 if no membranous staining [10]. Assessment is also different in surgical resection specimens versus biopsies. In surgical resections, a cutoff of ≥10 % of cells is required, whereas in biopsies, reactivity in only ≥5 clustered cells is needed. Differing criteria were established due to the prevalence of tumor heterogeneity in gastric/GEJ tumors. Similar to breast, a score of 3+ is HER2 positive, 0 or 1+ negative, and 2+ equivocal and requires further testing by ISH (Table 12.1).

Tumors that are equivocal by IHC (score 2+) require testing for HER2 amplification by ISH. Both FISH and brightfield ISH methods use probes that hybridize to the HER2 gene on chromosome 17 or to its centromere (CEP17). Signals in individual cells are then counted and the HER2:CEP17 ratio is calculated. A tumor is considered amplified if the ratio of HER2 signals to CEP17 is ≥2.0 or the average copy number of HER2 is >6 [8, 10]. These criteria differ from breast where a ratio of ≥2.2 is needed. Due to the prevalence of tumor heterogeneity, it is recommended that the entire

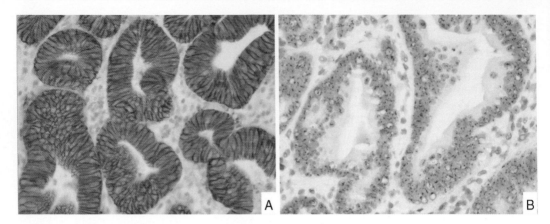

Fig. 12.1 (**a**) HER2 overexpression by immunohistochemistry (IHC) (score 3+). (**b**) HER2 gene amplification by brightfield chromogenic dual color in situ hybridization (**b**). HER2 = *black signal*; centromere of chromosome 17 = *red*

Table 12.1 Immunohistochemistry scoring criteria for HER2 in gastric and gastroesophageal junction tumors [8, 10]

Score	Staining intensity	Magnification rule	Quantification requirement	HER2 assessment
0	No membranous staining	No staining	≥10 % resection specimen; ≥5 cohesive cells in biopsy	Negative
1+	Faint or barely perceptible; staining of only part of the membrane	Staining visible at high power magnification (×40)	≥10 % resection specimen; ≥5 cohesive cells in biopsy	Negative
2+	Weak to moderate complete, basolateral, or lateral membranous staining	Staining visible at ×10–20 magnification	≥10 % resection specimen; ≥5 cohesive cells in biopsy	Equivocal
3+	Strong complete, basolateral, or lateral membranous staining	Staining visible at low magnification (×2.5–5)	≥10 % resection specimen; ≥5 cohesive cells in biopsy	Positive

section be scanned for amplified regions. The IHC slide can also be used as a guide as areas with strong HER2 staining are more likely to show amplification. At least 20 nuclei should be counted and if the HER2:CEP17 ratio falls between 1.8 and 2.2, an additional 20 nuclei should be scored [10]. A number of ISH methods can be used. Traditionally, FISH was performed and is considered by some to be the "gold standard." A number of brightfield methods have been recently developed which prove beneficial in gastric/GEJ tumors due to the preservation of tumor morphology, which is helpful in identifying amplified regions in the case of tumor heterogeneity (Fig. 12.1b) [11].

HER2 testing and treatment with trastuzumab is likely just the beginning in molecular targeted therapy in gastric/GEJ tumors. Studies are currently underway investigating the use of small molecule inhibitors of the HER2 tyrosine kinase domain and therapies targeting downstream-activated pathways.

Gastrointestinal Stromal Tumors

Gastrointestinal stromal tumors (GISTs) are the most common mesenchymal neoplasm in the gastrointestinal tract. They have been reported in

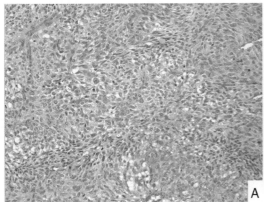
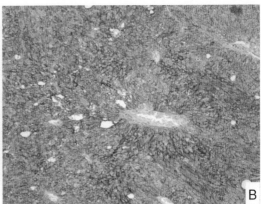
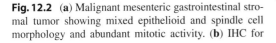

Fig. 12.2 (**a**) Malignant mesenteric gastrointestinal stromal tumor showing mixed epithelioid and spindle cell morphology and abundant mitotic activity. (**b**) IHC for CD117 is positive. The tumor was shown to carry a PDGFRA exon 18 mutation

all age groups, but most commonly present in the 5th to 7th decade of life and show no sex predilection. While GISTs may occur in any location, they are most commonly seen in the stomach (60 %), followed by the jejunum and ileum (30 %). GISTs may also occur in the mesentery, omentum, or retroperitoneum where they are referred to as extraintestinal GIST. Clinically, patients typically present with vague abdominal symptoms or, in approximately 20 % of cases, are asymptomatic and tumors are discovered incidentally by imaging or at the time of endoscopy [12].

GISTs are typically spindle cell neoplasms but may occasionally have an epithelioid morphology, or even mixed (Fig. 12.2a). Their risk for progressive disease is predicted based on tumor location, size, and mitotic rate [13, 14]. Prior to the availability of CD117 IHC, most GISTs were misclassified as leiomyomas or neural tumors. Today, the diagnosis can be made in most cases based on CD117 staining (positive in approximately 95 % of GISTs) and/or DOG1 positivity (approximately 98 % of GISTs) (Fig. 12.2b). DOG1 has been shown to be particularly helpful in KIT-negative tumors [15].

KIT mutations are found in approximately 80 % of GISTs. KIT is located on the long arm of chromosome 4 and encodes a type III receptor tyrosine kinase. The receptor is composed of a ligand-binding extracellular domain, a transmembrane domain, a juxtamembrane domain, and two cytoplasmic tyrosine kinase domains. In the normal condition, binding of a ligand to the extracellular domain triggers dimerization, phosphorylation of the intracytoplasmic tyrosine kinase domains, and activation of intracytoplasmic cascades that results in cell proliferation. In GISTs, mutations lead to constitutional activation of the receptor and unregulated cell growth. Mutations most commonly occur in exon 11, followed by exon 9, both coding for the juxtamembrane domain [16]. Exon 13 and exon 17 mutations are rare. In-frame deletions are the most common type of mutation observed in KIT, followed by single nucleotide substitutions, and duplications. Deletions almost exclusively occur in exon 11. Exon 11 mutations have been associated with a better prognosis and exon 9 a worse prognosis, although some studies contradict this finding [17, 18]. Exon 9 mutations are more commonly found in small intestinal GISTs [13].

Approximately 7 % of GISTs have platelet-derived growth factor receptor alpha (PDGFRA) mutations. Similar to KIT, PDGFRA is also a type III receptor tyrosine kinase and is homologous in structure and function. KIT and PDGFRA mutations are mutually exclusive [19]. Mutations in PDGFR most often occur in exon 18, but may also be seen in exon 16 and exon 14. Single nucleotide substitutions are most common, followed by deletions [20]. GISTs with PDGFRA mutations are strongly associated with gastric or extraintestinal locations, show epithelioid morphology, and may be negative or only weakly positive for CD117.

GISTs that are negative for both KIT and PDGFRA mutations have been referred to as "wild type GISTs." It is now becoming clear that many of these carry mutations in one of the succinate dehydrogenate (SDH) genes and are now known as "SDH-deficient GISTs" [21]. SDH mutations are relatively common, particularly in the stomach, accounting for 5–10 % of all gastric GISTs [22]. SDH-deficient GISTs are distinct from KIT- and PDGFRA-mutant GISTs in many ways. Histologically, they show a distinct multinodular and plexiform growth pattern and are almost always epithelioid in morphology [22]. This pattern was previously observed in children (known as "pediatric-type" GIST) and in patients with Carney triad. We now know that almost all GISTs occurring in children are SDH-deficient [22]. SDH-deficient GISTs predominantly occur in children and young adults and are more likely to be syndromic (Carney triad or Carney–Stratakis syndrome) with associated germline mutations in approximately 30 %. Unlike conventional GISTs, the behavior of SDH-deficient GISTs cannot be predicted based on size and mitotic activity. In addition, tumors are often multifocal, tend to metastasize to lymph nodes, and despite resistance to imatinib therapy, have an indolent clinical course [23].

SDH is an enzyme complex localized to the inner mitochondrial membrane which links the Krebs cycle and electron transport chain. The SDH complex is composed of four subunits: SDHA, SDHB, SDHC, and SDHD. SCHC and D are the hydrophobic membrane anchoring subunits, while SDHA and B are the hydrophilic enzymatic portions. Loss of any member of the SDH complex destabilizes the entire unit and results in degradation of SDHB. Therefore, loss of SDHB expression observed by IHC is a marker of bi-allelic mutation/inactivation of any one of the SDH genes and can be used to identify individuals who should be offered formal genetic testing. Testing for germline mutations in all of the SDH subunit genes can be labor-intensive, particularly for SDHA as it is a large gene with 15 exons

and due to the presence of three confounding pseudogenes, which show homology to SDHA. It has been shown that loss of SDHA by IHC is predictive of a germline mutation in the SDHA gene [24, 25].

Overall, most GISTs are sporadic but some may occur as part of a syndrome. As mentioned above, SDH-deficient GISTs may occur as part of Carney triad or Carney–Stratakis syndrome. Carney–Stratikis syndrome, characterized by multifocal GISTs, paraganglioma, and pheochromocytoma, occurs secondary to a germline mutation in one of the SDH subunits [26]. An underlying genetic cause is unknown for Carney triad. Carney triad typically occurs in young women and is characterized by gastric GISTs, paraganglioma, and pulmonary chondroma [27]. Families with germline mutations in KIT and PDGFRA have also been documented. In addition to GISTs, individuals in these families may also have hyperpigmentation, dysphagia, and urticaria pigmentosa. Syndromic GISTs may also occur in neurofibromatosis type I (NF1). NF1 GISTs are often multiple, tend to be located in the small bowel, and behave in an indolent fashion. NF1-related GISTs are "wild type" in that they do not have KIT, PDGFR, or SDH mutations. The mechanism by which these GISTs develop is not known but it is thought that the neurofibromin protein may activate KIT through the RAS proto-oncogene.

Mutation analysis in GISTs may be helpful in diagnosis, particularly in CD117- and DOG1-negative tumors, but is also used to guide treatment both at the time of diagnosis and in the setting of treatment resistance. Routine mutational analysis is not recommended at this time, but is often done in academic centers and should be considered if treatment will be initiated, in cases with unusual clinical or histologic features, and in small intestinal GISTs due to the prevalence of exon 9 mutations. Tyrosine kinase inhibitors, such as imatinib mesylate and sunitinib malate, inhibit the ATP-binding domain of the KIT and PDGFRA receptor resulting in inactivation and inhibition of phosphorylation and downstream pathways. Variable response to treatment has been documented in various mutations.

GISTs with KIT exon 11 mutations tend to show the best response to imatinib compared to exon 9 mutants and wild type GISTs. However, clinical trials have shown that increased dose (400 vs. 800 mg) significantly improved progression-free survival in those with exon 9 mutations [28]. GISTs with PDGFRA exon 18 Asp842Val have shown primary resistance to both imatinib and sunitinib therapy [29].

Secondary treatment resistance, defined as progression of disease after a 6-month response period on imatinib, occurs in almost 50 % of GISTs and is mostly due to additional mutations. Unlike primary KIT mutations, which occur in the exons coding for the juxtamembrane regions, resistance mutations mainly occur in exons 13 and 14, which encode the ATP-binding pocket and interfere with drug interaction [30]. New mutations in exons 17 and 18 may also be seen, which involve the activating loop domain and lead to intrinsic activation. In some cases, multiple resistance mutations can be seen within one tumor and between multiple tumor sites in one patient.

Peutz–Jeghers Syndrome

Peutz–Jeghers syndrome (PJS) is an autosomal dominant syndrome characterized by multiple hamartomatous polyps located throughout the gastrointestinal tract and mucocutaneous pigmentation. The hamartomatous polyps have a characteristic arborizing ("tree-like") appearance with smooth muscle bands extending throughout the polyp, separating an elongated epithelial component. PJS polyps are most frequent in the small bowel and colon, but may be seen anywhere along the gastrointestinal tract.

PJS is caused by a germline mutation in a serine threonine kinase (LKB1 gene, also known as STK1) located on chromosome 19p13.3. The LKB1 gene is large, measuring 22.6 kb in length and consisting of nine coding and one noncoding exons and functions as a tumor suppressor gene. Its precise actions are complex and not fully understood. The protein is ubiquitously expressed in adult and fetal tissues and has been implicated in regulating G1 cell cycle arrest through induction

of the cyclin-dependent kinase, WAF1. LKB1 has also been shown to play a role in p53-mediated apoptosis, phosphorylation of B-catenin and regulation of the WNT pathway, and regulation of the mammalian target of rapamycin (mTOR) pathway through AMP-activated protein kinase (AMPK) [31]. A germline mutation in the LKB1 gene can be identified in approximately 80 % of patients meeting clinical diagnostic criteria implying that other genes may be involved. Mutations of LKB1 may include deletions, insertions, inversions, or duplications. Most result in a premature stop codon leading to a truncated protein or amino acid changes affecting the catalytic kinase domain [32]. Germline mutations of the STK1 gene in PJS can be found by using a number of techniques, most commonly single-strand conformational electrophoresis, denaturing HPLC, or direct sequencing of the exons [56].

The mechanism by which cancer arises in patients with PJS is poorly understood. There is controversy as to whether cancer arises directly from hamartomatous polyps through a hamartoma–adenoma–carcinoma sequence, or rather that hamartomatous polyps are a marker of mucosal instability at increased risk of carcinogenesis. While the most common malignancy seen in patients with PJS is colorectal cancer (38–66 % lifetime risk) [33], cancers may occur at multiple sites, including sites outside the gastrointestinal tract. The second most common malignancy is breast, followed by small bowel, gastric, and pancreatic cancer. Gynecologic tumors include most notably the ovarian sex cord tumor with annular tubules (SCTAT) and cervical adenoma malignum. In males, large-cell calcifying Sertoli cell tumor of the testis may develop. Due to increased risk of cancer at multiple sites, surveillance recommendations involving a multidisciplinary team have been suggested [33, 34].

Lynch Syndrome

One of the most common genetic forms of colon cancer is Lynch syndrome where colon cancer presents at an average age of 43, but may also be found in patients in their 60s [35]. Lynch syndrome is transmitted with an autosomal dominant pattern and consists of an inherited susceptibility to colorectal cancer in addition to other malignancies which may involve the endometrium, bladder, ureter, renal pelvis, ovary, stomach, small bowel, bile ducts, or pancreas. A variant of Lynch syndrome is Turcot syndrome, characterized by colon cancer and glioblastoma or medulloblastoma, but this association can also be observed in familial adenomatous polyposis (FAP) syndrome with mutations in APC [36]. Another variant of Lynch complex is Muir–Torre syndrome comprising sebaceous tumors or keratoacanthomas of the skin and colon cancer, or other Lynch syndrome-associated tumors [37, 38]. As in most colorectal carcinomas, malignancies arise from the transformation of polyps. However, in the case of Lynch syndrome, the progression from adenomatous polyps to colorectal cancer is much faster than in sporadic adenoma–carcinoma cases.

The molecular defect accounting for Lynch syndrome occurs during DNA replication. Normally, a perfectly complementary copy of the DNA template is expected during DNA replication, based on nucleotide base pairing. However, even in normal proliferating cells, imperfect DNA copies are occasionally made, but they are promptly recognized by a set of proteins collectively called DNA mismatch repair (MMR) proteins. These proteins act as a complex which recognize the mismatched area of the recently replicated double-strand DNA, excise the mismatched area, and repair it by replacing the mismatched with the properly paired nucleotide. In Lynch syndrome, one of these MMR proteins is defective and, therefore, the area of mismatched double-stranded DNA is not repaired. Most defects in MMR proteins are due to mutation in their genes. Mutation in MMR genes accounts for 2–4 % of all colorectal cancers.

Although Lynch syndrome has a relatively low prevalence, distinguishing it from sporadic cases of colon cancer is clinically important for the patient and his or her family. IHC and/or molecular methods are needed to make this distinction as there is a significant overlap in clinical and histopathological features of Lynch syndrome-related and unrelated colon cancer.

Table 12.2 Revised Bethesda criteria for the diagnosis of Lynch syndrome

Tumors should be tested for microsatellite instability in one or more of the following situations:

- **Colorectal cancer** diagnosed in a patient who is **less than 50 years of age**
- Presence of synchronous, metachronous colorectal, or other HNPCC-associated tumors, **regardless of the patient's age**
- Colorectal cancer with the **histologic featuresof microsatellite instability** diagnosed in a patient who is **less than 60** years of age
- Colorectal cancer, or an HNPCC-associated tumor, diagnosed in one or more **first-degree relatives**, with one cancer diagnosed at **less than 50** years of age
- **Colorectal cancer or HNPCC**-associated tumor diagnosed **at any age** in **two first-degree or second-degree relatives**

Clinical and histologic criteria are however used as a trigger for testing. The Revised Bethesda criteria (Table 12.2) outline individuals who should be tested for microsatellite instability based on personal and/or familial history of colon cancer or other Lynch syndrome-associated malignancies, and histologic features of high microsatellite instability (MSI-H) [39].

Histopathological features of MSI-H colorectal tumors include right-sided location, mucinous differentiation, conspicuous lymphocytic infiltrate and lymphoid follicles, pushing margins at the invasion front, and poor differentiation. The presence of intra-tumoral lymphocytes is characteristic of MSI-H tumors and a large proportion of them are cytotoxic T-cells, hence CD8 positive. Besides being associated with Lynch syndrome colorectal tumors, some of these histopathological features can also be observed in sporadic colonic tumors that are MSI-H positive or even microsatellite DNA stable. Nevertheless, when these clinical and/or histopathological features are present, a rational next step is to perform immunohistochemical tests exploring the expression of proteins involved in the repair of mismatched DNA strands, typically MSH2, MLH1, PMS2, and MSH6. In the cell nucleus, MLH1 and PMS2 function as a dimeric molecular complex. MSH2 and MSH6 also function as dimer. This means that the loss of one member of the dimer is often accompanied by the loss of its partner when tested by IHC. In the large majority of Lynch syndrome-associated tumors, but also in a subset of sporadic colonic tumors, there is a decreased expression of one or two of these proteins. The decrease is due to mutations silencing gene expression of MSH2, MSH6, or PMS2, or to methylation of the MLH1 promoter. MSH2 silencing can also be caused by methylation, which is associated with a deletion of EPCAM, a gene adjacent to MSH2 [40].

The molecular testing of Lynch syndrome is based on examining if microsatellite DNA is replicated properly in the tumor cells, as compared to normal cells. Microsatellite DNA is an abundant part of the genome and contains a large number of nucleotide repeats which can be mononucleotides, e.g., GGGGGGG…, or dinucleotides such as GAGAGAGAGAGAGAG. During cell proliferation, the DNA polymerase is sometimes unable to read the exact number of these nucleotide repeats and, consequently, the replicated DNA strand contains a slightly shorter or slightly longer segment of repeats. In this case, the resulting molecular defect is called MicroSatellite DNA Instable (MSI). The difference in the mistakenly duplicated DNA can be as short as one nucleotide base pair as compared to the normal DNA template, and can be recognized by a multiplex PCR method employing primers located on each side of discrete segments of microsatellite DNA where the nucleotide repeats are located. A large majority of MSI cases can be recognized by using the following five molecular markers: BAT-25, BAT-26, MONO-27, NR-21, and NR-24 to which two highly polymorphic pentanucleotide markers can be added: Penta C and Penta D. The BAT-25 and BAT-26 are the most sensitive MSI markers and can be used as a screening approach. The length of the amplified DNA sequences can be visualized by a variety of methods ranging from simple gel electrophoresis to capillary electrophoresis, in the latter case using fluorescent reagents. It is essential to compare DNA extracted from a paraffin block of tumor tissue, with DNA from normal tissue located at a distance from the tumor, most conveniently from a surgical colectomy resection margin. When the paraffin block

of the tumor also contains adjacent normal colonic tissue, it is preferable to microdissect the tumor by scratching away the normal tissue from the unstained slides after localizing the tumor area on an adjacent H&E-stained section. This will facilitate greatly the analysis by minimizing the overlap in the sizing of DNA fragments contributed by normal cells.

When done by electrophoresis, reading of the MSI test is by visual assessment of the profile of separated fragments according to their molecular size and peak height. A profile is said to be MSI positive if there are new species of DNA fragments in the tumor specimen, which are either lighter or heavier than in the normal DNA from the same patient (Fig. 12.3). When comparing the profiles of five molecular markers, a tumor is reported as MSI-H if two or more markers demonstrate MSI. When only 1 out of 5 markers shows MSI, the tumor is reported as MSI-low (MSI-L). When none of the markers show MSI, the tumor is reported as MicroSatellite Stable (MSS), which rules out Lynch syndrome. MSI-L and MSS are thought to belong to the same group from a clinicopathological viewpoint.

Virtually all Lynch syndrome-related colorectal tumors are MSI-H positive. Conversely, not all MSI-positive tumors are related to Lynch syndrome, as 15 % of all sporadic colon cancer cases also have this genotypic alteration in tumor cells [41]. Consequently, it would appear logical to perform germline testing in patients suspected to have Lynch syndrome, searching for mutations and promoter methylation of the MMR genes. However, when present, mutations may occur in different regions of the genes making this type of analysis technically complex.

Because of the complexity in doing germline mutational analysis of the MMR genes, it is more convenient to use an indirect approach helping to resolve the difficulty in distinguishing Lynch syndrome from sporadic colorectal tumors. This is done by analyzing the pattern of immunohistochemical expression of MMR proteins. A number of studies have reported that loss of immunohistochemical expression of MSH2 or MSH6, or both, is a strong indicator of a germline gene mutation and, therefore, represents Lynch syndrome.

Microsatellite stable colon cancer

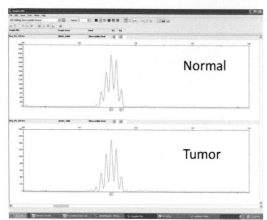

Microsatellite instable colon cancer

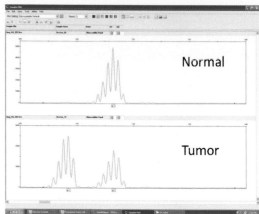

Fig. 12.3 Test for microsatellite instability in two cases of colon carcinoma. The microsatellite stable tumor shows the same pattern and the same molecular size of microsatellite repeats in the normal and tumor areas of the specimen, using the Bat-26 marker (*left two panels*). In the microsatellite instable case, five additional bands with a smaller molecular weight are present in the tumor (*right two panels*)

Loss of immunohistochemical expression of MLH1 is also found in Lynch syndrome and, in fact, loss of MLH1 or MSH2 accounts for 80 % of Lynch syndrome cases. However, immunohistochemical expression of MLH1 can be lost for two reasons: mutation or methylation of its gene promoter. Loss of immunohistochemical expression of MLH1 due to promoter methylation is an indication that the colorectal tumor is sporadic, whereas mutation supports a diagnosis of Lynch syndrome. Methylation of the MLH1 promoter accounts for the majority of MSI-H colorectal cancer cases where there is no familial history of Lynch syndrome. Consequently, loss of immunohistochemical expression of MLH1 in tumor cells alone is not sufficient to diagnose Lynch syndrome.

Another indirect approach in the diagnosis of Lynch syndrome is to test the tumor for the presence of BRAF mutation. BRAF is a cell protein acting distal to, and regulated by, KRAS in the EGFR-driven signal transduction pathway. BRAF is mutated in approximately 13 % of all colorectal cancer cases and in 50 % of MSI high colorectal tumors and when this is observed, it is a strong indication that the tumor is not associated with Lynch syndrome. Testing for BRAF mutation is relatively easy to perform as its gene mutates in most cases at a predictable spot called BRAF^{V600E}, this being at codon 600 where a valine (V) is replaced by glutamic acid (E) in the BRAF protein. PCR followed by single-strand conformation polymorphism electrophoresis is a convenient method to test for BRAF^{V600E} mutation [42]. Overall, the distinction between sporadic and Lynch syndrome-associated colon cancers can be accomplished by following an algorithmic approach combining immunohistochemical, MSI, and germline DNA testing [43]. There is an additional benefit in testing colorectal tumors for MSI as tumors which have an MSI-H genotype are associated with a better prognosis, whether they are sporadic or from a patient with the Lynch syndrome [41]. However, they might not benefit from 5-fluorouracil chemotherapy.

Molecular Pathology Associated with Bi-allelic Mutations in DNA Mismatch Repair Genes

In rare circumstances, patients may inherit two homozygous or heterozygous mutations of the DNA MMR genes: MSH2, MLH1, MSH6, or PMS2. This bi-allelic mutation status results in an accelerated and more widespread phenotype as compared to the usual autosomal dominant form of Lynch syndrome with a single allele mutation [44]. In patients with bi-allelic mutations of the MMR genes, colorectal cancer can appear as early as in the first decade of life. Some of them also have café-au-lait skin lesions, neurofibromas, malignant brain tumors, leukemias and lymphomas. 75 % of colorectal tumors are MSI-H although it was more inconsistent in non-colorectal neoplasms.

Familial Colorectal Cancer Type X

When a large number of families with the typical pattern of inheritance and clinical characteristics of Lynch syndrome were tested for molecular alterations, 44 % did not have evidence of DNA MMR deficiency [45]. In this subset, there was a 2.3× increased risk of colorectal cancer. Colon cancers occurred approximately 10 years earlier than in Lynch syndrome and were often present in the distal colon. Remarkably, there was no increased risk of developing endometrial or other non-colorectal tumors usually associated with Lynch syndrome. Considering that its genetic defect is not definitely identified, this condition is called Familial Colorectal Cancer Type X.

The Molecular Pathology of Familial Adenomatous Polyposis and Its Variants

Familial adenomatous polyposis (FAP) is an autosomal dominant syndrome with a strong predisposition to colon cancer. In its classical form, it is easily recognized at endoscopy by the presence of hundreds of polyps located mostly in the colon of young subjects. Patients with germline mutations of the APC gene also have an increased frequency of duodenal adenomas, duodenal and periampullary cancer, fundic gland polyposis, jejunal polyposis and cancer, pancreatic cancer, papillary carcinoma of the thyroid, hepatoblastoma, hypertrophy of retinal pigmented epithelium, and dental abnormalities. The natural history of FAP is characterized by a 100 % risk

of transformation of some of the colorectal polyps into adenocarcinomas, unless a prophylactic colectomy is done, which is an essential part of current management. The polyps become apparent in the patient's late childhood and the average age of malignant transformation is 39 years. Overall, colorectal cancer arising from FAP accounts for 0.5–1 % of all colorectal cancers. Its early recognition is important as it forms a basis for yearly surveillance and timely colectomy. Most cases have a family history of FAP but 25 % of cases are diagnosed as de novo mutation. The discovery of the gene for FAP represents one of the hallmarks in the history of cancer genetics, and the demonstration, in a human carcinoma, of Knudson's double-hit hypothesis of inherited cancer. It was derived from the cytogenetic investigation of a 42-year-old man with mental retardation, colon carcinoma, horseshoe kidney, the absence of left lobe of the liver, agenesis of the gallbladder, and a clinical variant of FAP, Gardner syndrome [46, 47]. The gene, called APC for *adenomatous polyposis coli*, is located on chromosome 5q and is mutated in the germline DNA of patients with FAP. The second genetic hit occurs somatically and consists of loss or inactivation of APC in the colonic epithelial cells. APC functions as a tumor suppressor gene in normal cells and its double inactivation in intestinal cells of FAP patients is the essential cause of malignant transformation.

The main mechanism by which APC inactivation contributes to malignant transformation involves β-catenin. In normal cells, β-catenin is involved in cell proliferation and migration, regulated by Wnt signaling. When Wnt signaling is activated, β-catenin migrates from the cytoplasm to the nucleus where it stimulates the transcription of genes involved in cell proliferation and migration. The APC protein controls this migration by favoring the sequestration of β-catenin in the cytoplasm and its degradation in the proteosome when Wnt signaling is inactive. Most APC mutations inactivate its sequestrating function, causing inhibition of β-catenin degradation, and increased ability to migrate to the nucleus, resulting in uncontrolled stimulation of cell proliferation and migration.

APC is a large protein with 2,843 amino acids and more than 700 different mutations of the *APC* gene have been described, 98 % of them being frameshift or nonsense mutations resulting in truncation of the protein. Searching for these mutations in germline DNA is an essential part of FAP diagnosis. Of note, testing for somatic mutations of *APC* in colorectal tumors is not a proof of FAP since *APC* is somatically mutated in 70 % of sporadic colon cancers.

The classical form of FAP is associated with discrete mutations spread over 50 % of the *APC* gene length and, furthermore, there is significant overlap in the location of gene mutations in classical FAP and FAP clinical variants. The mutations found in classical FAP are widespread within the APC gene, being found in several regions encompassing 1,086 encoded amino acids. The large number of possible mutation spots complicates the methodology used to locate the *APC* genetic defect mutation when the site is not known from previous study of an affected family member, or when the mutation occurs de novo. In this case, the APC gene can be initially screened for the most common mutations, or analyzed using biochemical assays searching for APC protein truncation. However, the increasing availability of high-throughput methods now allows fast and efficient sequencing of the entire *APC* gene. Once the mutation has been identified in the first patient of an FAP family, the germline DNA of other family members can be tested using methods targeting the mutated gene region of the proband.

In addition to its classical form, there are variants of FAP where intestinal polyposis is associated with extraintestinal lesions. Gardner's syndrome is such a variant and its disease complex includes desmoid tumors, osteomas, and epidermal cysts. Interestingly, in Gardner's syndrome, most germline mutations are located within a 133-amino-acid-encoding region, which is much shorter than the 1,086 amino acid regions mutated in classical FAP. Another variant is Turcot's syndrome, which combines colon cancer with medulloblastoma or glioblastoma. Of note, Turcot's syndrome can also be part of Lynch syndrome, which is due to germline mutations in MMR genes, rather than mutations of APC. There is also a form of FAP, called attenuated FAP, where the number of colonic polyps is less than 100, as compared to the classical FAP form where the colonic mucosa is carpeted with hundreds of polyps. There is significant genotype–phenotype association in the classical and attenuated forms of FAP as most of the *APC* mutations which are associated with attenuated FAP are located in gene regions that are distinct from those of classical FAP, typically the 5′ gene region. Genotypic overlaps exist and it is remarkable that the same APC mutation can lead to two different FAP-related phenotypes; for instance, with or without Gardner's syndrome features.

Molecular Pathology of the Hyperplastic Polyposis and Serrated Pathway Syndromes

The presence of more than 5 large hyperplastic polyps proximal to the sigmoid colon is one indication that the patient might be affected by Serrated Polyposis syndrome (formerly known as Hyperplastic Polyposis syndrome). Serrated polyposis syndrome is typically identified during the 6th decade of life. Patients may have up to approximately 100 hyperplastic or serrated (Fig. 12.4) polyps or sessile adenomas. The inheritance pattern of the Serrated Polyposis syndrome has not been uniformly defined. A study was compatible

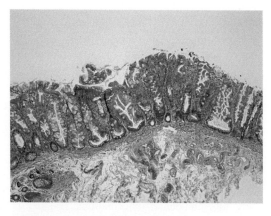

Fig. 12.4 Histology of sessile serrated adenoma

with an autosomal recessive mode of transmission [48]. Depending on the studies the risk of developing colon cancer ranges from 37 to 69 %. Some cases have personal and familial clinical features usually associated with Lynch syndrome. Up to 70 % colonic neoplasms in the Serrated Polyposis syndrome have a BRAF mutation. By comparison, BRAF mutation is extremely rare in Lynch syndrome, and is found in only 15 % of unselected colorectal carcinomas. Another molecular trait of patients with the Serrated Polyposis syndrome is the presence of numerous sites of DNA methylation, including methylation of MLH1, in the polyps and in carcinomas.

Juvenile Polyposis Syndrome

Juvenile polyposis syndrome (JPS) is defined by the presence of more than 5, but up to hundreds of, smooth surface polyps in the colorectum with a histology characterized by cystically dilated glands filled with mucus and inflammatory cells, and an inflamed lamina propria, in the context of a family history with an autosomal mode of transmission. In addition to the colorectum, polyps can also be found in the stomach, duodenum, jejunum, and ileum. Other clinical criteria helping to identify JPS cases are the presence of juvenile polyps in several segments of the gastrointestinal tract, or any number of juvenile polyps in patients with a family history of JPS [49].

The generalized form of JPS can be diagnosed in infancy or in adults. The infantile form is accompanied by intussusception and macrocephaly and leads to early death. In up to 60 % of the JPS cases, the genetic defect consists of a germline mutation in the SMAD4 or BMPR1A genes. The genetic alteration often consists of large deletions affecting SMAD4 or BMPR1A, or mutations in the BMPR1A promoter or in PTEN. A functional feature common to these two genes is their direct involvement in the TGFβ signal transduction pathway. Patients with SMAD4 mutations have more severe clinical course as compared to patients with BMPR1A mutations. Up to 40 % of JPS patients have no known germline mutation. A subset of JPS patients with SMAD4 mutations also has the arteriovenous malformations of hereditary hemorrhagic telangiectasia. Patients with JPS have an increased risk of developing cancer and in particular, 39 % of them have a lifetime risk of being affected with colorectal cancer [50, 51].

The molecular diagnostic methods suited to investigate JPS and document alterations in the SMAD4, BMPR1A or PTEN genes are based on the MLPA assay, or full-length sequencing of the genes [50]. The result of the molecular tests help to document relationships between genotype and disease manifestations.

Sporadic Colorectal Cancer

Presently, more than 75 % of colorectal cancer cases are not known to be associated with an inherited susceptibility to develop cancer. However, research studies derived from inherited forms have shed light on the molecular mechanisms of sporadic colon cancer. Most cases are diagnosed on the basis of histopathology alone; therefore, in most cases, molecular methods are not necessary for diagnosis. However, immunohistochemical and molecular methods are required in the following three circumstances: firstly, to confirm cases as being truly sporadic; secondly, to explore molecular markers predictive of response to targeted therapies; and thirdly, to define prognostic features based on molecular markers.

As in most forms of cancer, the pathogenesis of neoplastic transformation in colorectal cancer is closely related to the emergence of genomic instability in mucosal epithelial cells. Three main mechanisms account for this genomic instability: structural instability of the chromosomes, defects in DNA repair, and abnormal DNA methylation. In the pathway driven by structural instability, chromosomes are altered by deletions or mutations. Significant for colon cancer, chromosome instability causes somatic loss of tumor suppressor genes such as APC or p53. Somatic APC inactivation is an early event in the adenoma–carcinoma transformation sequence and is found in 75 % of sporadic colorectal cancers. Defects in DNA repair result mostly from epigenetic alterations, such as inactivation of the MLH1 gene which occurs in up to 15 % of sporadic colorectal cancers.

The MLH1 gene alteration is, in fact, caused by the third pathway of colorectal pathogenesis, abnormal DNA methylation of CpG islands of DNA, whereby hypermethylation of the MLH1 gene promoter and other genes leads to their functional inactivation. Besides MLH1, three other genes of the MINT family, MINT1, MINT2, and MINT3, as well as p16, are also inactivated epigenetically through methylation in up to 37 % of sporadic colorectal cancer cases. This group of tumors is classified under the name CpG island methylator phenotype (CIMP). Because these colorectal cancer-associated genes are modified by epigenetic changes rather than mutations or gene deletions, it is reasonable to hypothesize that mutagens, dietary habits, or chemopreventive drugs have the potential to impact them.

The function of the APC gene and the consequences of its inactivation are discussed in the section dealing with FAP. In sporadic colorectal cancer, there is no germline mutation of APC but gene inactivation is observed somatically in 75 % of tumors and occurs early during the transition from adenoma to cancer. Another commonly found chromosomal loss in colorectal cancer occurs for p53, affecting 65 % of sporadic tumors. Considering that the main function of p53 is to arrest the cell cycle and induce apoptosis in cells which have undergone genetic injuries, its inactivation creates favorable conditions for uncontrolled proliferation of abnormal cells.

The availability of high-throughput genetic analyses allows comparisons of the full genome of large cohorts of colorectal cancers. Such an approach has shown that the number of somatic mutations and other genetic alterations in sporadic colorectal cancer is quite large, with a median of 76 mutations per tumor [52]. The most common genetic alterations found in sporadic colorectal cancers are listed in Table 12.3. There is no reason to assume that in a given tumor all mutations are obligate determinants of tumorigenesis and, instead, it is important to distinguish "driver" mutations from "passenger" mutations. Based on the frequency of mutations and knowledge of gene function, it appears that commonly observed mutations, such as p53, APC, KRAS, and PIK3CA, can be considered "drivers" of malignant transformation. However,

Table 12.3 Genetic alterations found in sporadic colon cancer at frequency of 5 % or higher

Gene	Frequency of alterations (%)	Type of alteration
APC	75	Mutation, deletion, allele loss
p53	65	Mutation, allele loss
KRAS	40	Mutation
PIK3CA	20	Mutation
FBXW7	20	Mutation
CDK8	13	Gene amplification
SMAD4	13	Mutation, allele loss
PTEN	10	Mutation
ACVR2	10	Mutation
BRAF	8	Mutation
EGFR	8	Gene amplification
CMYC	8	Gene amplification
SMAD2	8	Mutation, allele loss
TGFβIIR	8	Mutation
CCNE1	5	Gene amplification
SMAD3	5	Mutation
TCF7L2	5	Mutation
BAX	5	Mutation

this approach also identified mutations in other genes, such as CSMD3, FBXW7, and NAV3, with a high cancer mutation prevalence score. Their assignment to an unambiguous "driver" or "passenger" status needs to be established. Globally, it appears that malignant transformation of the colorectal epithelium is more the result of changes converging on cellular pathways caused by multiple gene mutations, rather than the dominant role played by an individual mutation [52]. This means that the use of predictive and prognostic molecular markers, and personalized therapy, needs to consider sets of genetic changes altering cellular transduction pathways in tumors, rather than a single genetic change as discussed below with two members of the MAPK/ERK kinase pathway, KRAS and BRAF.

Testing for KRAS in Targeted Therapy of Colorectal Cancer

The introduction of therapies targeting EGFR-driven signal transduction pathways in the treatment of colon cancer led to asking which biomarker should be tested to predict a therapeutic response. Based on the knowledge gained in targeted therapy of breast cancer, and considering that HER2-neu is a member of the EGFR family of receptors, attempts were made to relate therapeutic responses in colorectal cancer to EGFR gene amplification or expression. Because the anti-EGFR drugs such as cetuximab and panitumumab are monoclonal antibodies to EGFR present on the surface of colorectal cancer cells, it was first anticipated that EGFR protein expression would relate it to therapeutic response. However, no consistent association between EGFR expression and therapeutic response was observed [53].

KRAS is an important intermediate in the MAPK/ERK signal transduction pathway driven by EGFR and Lievre et al. were able to demonstrate that the presence of wild type KRAS, which is controlled by EGFR, is a factor predicting a favorable therapeutic response [54]. This discovery led to the widely accepted use of searching for KRAS mutations before treating patients with anti-EGFR antibody infusions.

In normal cells, KRAS cycles from an inactive form, Ras-GDP, to an active molecule, Ras-GTP, under the control of EGFR stimulation. This transition is made possible by the activation of three cytoplasmic proteins binding to the cytoplasmic tail of EGFR: Shc, Grb2, and Sos, which, in turn, stimulate KRAS. When KRAS is mutated, it becomes constitutively activated and no upstream control by EGFR and intermediate molecules are required for its activation. Consequently, when mutated KRAS mutation is present in tumor cells, the blockage of EGFR by anti-EGFR antibodies ceases to be therapeutically effective. Indeed, retrospective analysis of colorectal cancer tumors showed that no consistent response to anti-EGFR antibodies could be observed in patients who had a mutation of KRAS in the tumor cells.

The frequency of KRAS mutation in colorectal cancer is 37 %, combining the results of several studies. Patients with mutated KRAS colorectal cancer are not offered anti-EGFR therapy. Conversely, in the remaining subset of tumors with wild type KRAS, up to 60 % of cases are predicted to respond to anti-EGFR antibody

therapy and approximately 40 % are poor responders. The heterogeneity in the response rate of patients with wild type KRAS is due to other factors downstream of EGFR signaling, including BRAF, as discussed below.

Testing for KRAS mutation in colorectal cancer is performed for patients who have progressed to the stage of distant metastases after failing to respond to conventional chemotherapies. The test is generally performed on the surgical resection specimen, or a biopsy of the primary tumor. In less common circumstances, the KRAS test is performed on a biopsy of a metastatic site. The rate of concordance in KRAS status is 95 % between primary and metastatic sites.

KRAS mutations associated with colon cancer are point mutations found in three codons: 12, 13, and 61. Most laboratories test only codons 12 and 13 as they represent 98.5 % of KRAS mutations found in colorectal cancer. The test is generally performed on formalin-fixed paraffin-embedded tissue sections of tumor and several methods can be used, the most common being real-time PCR and pyrosequencing. The allele-specific real-time PCR method based on ARMS® and Scorpions® technologies is particularly sensitive (Fig. 12.5). Quality assurance is commonly performed by PCR, followed by Sanger sequencing. For each test, circling of adjacent H&E-stained sections by a pathologist is required when a substantial amount of normal colorectal mucosa is present in the paraffin block. To avoid confusion, the result of the KRAS mutation assay is being reported either as "mutated KRAS" or as "wild type KRAS," rather than "positive" or "negative," since having a "positive" (mutated KRAS) test has a negative impact on selecting patients eligible to receive the anti-EGFR antibody.

In one study, 72 % of patients, who had wild type KRAS in their colorectal tumor, still did not respond to anti-EGFR therapy [55]. Searches were made for genetic changes affecting proteins involved in EGFR signaling. It was found that the gene encoding BRAF, the protein directly controlled by and distal to KRAS in the signaling pathway, is mutated in 14 % of patients who have a wild type KRAS in their tumor [55]. None of the patients who have a BRAF mutation responded to

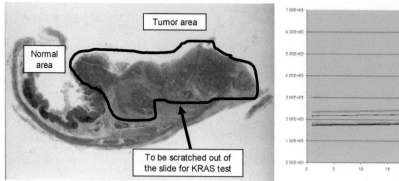
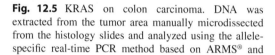
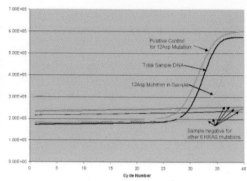

Fig. 12.5 KRAS on colon carcinoma. DNA was extracted from the tumor area manually microdissected from the histology slides and analyzed using the allele-specific real-time PCR method based on ARMS® and

Scorpions® designs. Out of the seven real-time PCRs, only the primers locating the 12ASP mutation allowed amplification of a detectable product

the anti-EGFR antibody treatment. Conversely, in this study 32 % of the patients who had a wild type genotype for both KRAS and BRAF had a positive therapeutic response, as compared to 28 % of favorable responses for the whole group of wild type KRAS patients.

Colorectal Cancer Arising from Inflammatory Bowel Disease: Molecular Markers

Both forms of inflammatory bowel diseases (IBD), ulcerative colitis and Crohn's disease, are associated with an increased risk of colorectal cancer. The overall risk of malignancy is 1 % per year, 10 years after the clinical onset of severe IBD. Although the relationship between IBD and colorectal cancer has been known epidemiologically for many years, it is only recently that the cellular and molecular mechanisms have started to be established. Overall, the presence in the inflamed intestinal mucosa of activated leucocytes, stromal cells, and remodeled extracellular matrix exerts a pro-tumoral effect involving a number of extracellular cytokines and intracellular mediators, NF-κB being a central component of the latter group [56]. Of particular importance is the recent discovery that regulatory T-cells and CTLA-4, a protein present in T-lymphocytes, inhibit the immune response against tumor cells;

both regulatory T-cells and CTLA-4 are increased in IBD lesions [57, 58], therefore allowing the non-elimination of epithelial cells undergoing malignant transformation in IBD intestinal lesions.

The molecular changes involved in malignant transformation of the colonic epithelium in IBD and non-IBD-related colorectal cancer are otherwise similar. However, somatic mutations of *APC* occur late and p53 mutations occur early in IBD, as compared to sporadic cases. Microsatellite DNA instability is also present in IBD-related colorectal cancer, although less frequently than chromosomal instability. The most common cause of microsatellite instability in IBD-related colorectal cancer is caused by methylation of the MLH1 promoter [59]. The promoter of p16INK4a is also hypermethylated in the dysplastic and cancerous mucosa of IBD patients.

Presently, the risk of progression from inflammatory changes to malignant transformation is assessed by histopathology of colorectal biopsies performed at surveillance time points, searching for high-grade dysplasia. However, current investigations aimed at documenting by molecular methods the risk of this transformation have led to the observation of significant changes in the methylation of RUNX3, MINT1, and COX-2 genes in the nonneoplastic mucosa of ulcerative colitis patients who have progressed, versus not progressed, to malignant transformation [59].

Whether these molecular changes in nonneoplastic mucosa precede synchronous colorectal cancer remains to be demonstrated.

MYH Polyposis and Inherited Colon Cancer Due to MYH Inactivation

Another genetic type of colorectal cancer was discovered when a family with multiple adenomas and colon cancer, but with no germline mutation of APC, was reported [60]. Instead, a germline mutation was found in a gene located on the short arm of chromosome 1, called MUTYH glycosylase. More commonly, the gene is referred to as MYH. The normal function of the gene is to repair DNA damage occurring as a result of oxidation; in particular, oxidative damage caused by an oxidized form of guanine which acts as a mutagen. The repair performed by MYH consists of removing adenine when it inappropriately pairs with the oxidized form of guanine, or guanine itself. If not repaired by MYH, oxidized guanine is recognized as thymine during DNA replication and, therefore, aberrantly pairs with adenine. The function of the wild type MYH-encoded protein is to recognize this mispaired adenine and excise the mispair. When MYH is mutated, this repair function is lost and C:G to T:A transversion persists, and may involve several important genes, such as KRAS, which is often mutated in this condition. Most mutations of MYH are located at Y165C and G382D, and are found in up to 2 % of the general population, although different mutation sites are found in different ethnic groups. Unlike FAP, which is transmitted as an autosomal dominant syndrome, MYH polyposis has an autosomal recessive mode of transmission.

Clinically, patients are typically identified by the age of 50 by the presence of polyposis. The clinical phenotype of MYH polyposis is quite variable and can range from finding five polyps to the thousands of polyps typically observed in FAP. There is an association between MYH mutation and colorectal cancer risk [61–65]. In approximately 50 % of patients, carcinoma is already present at the time of diagnosis.

Overall, the incidence of cancers associated with germline MYH bi-allelic mutations is low, at 0.7 % of all colorectal cancers. Patients with heterozygous MYH mutations in their germline DNA have a 1.3-fold increased risk of developing colorectal cancer, compared to a 177-fold increase in subjects with bi-allelic mutations. Colorectal cancers associated with germline bi-allelic mutations of MYH are more likely to be low grade as compared to sporadic carcinomas, or in cancers found in carriers of mono-allelic MYH mutations [66]. Hyperplastic and serrated polyps are present in MYH-associated polyposis and, characteristically they contain G:C to T:A transversions in the KRAS gene [67]. Although the frequency of synchronous or metachronous polyps is higher in colorectal cancer patients with germline mutation of MYH as compared to sporadic cancers, up to 72 % of cases in the former group have no polyps. Overall, the pathological changes of colorectal cancers associated with MYH bi-allelic mutations do not have sharply defined features as compared to nongenetic forms of cancer. MYH-associated polyposis is associated with extra-colonic manifestations, with duodenal adenomas or carcinomas found in up to 17 % of patients [68]. Also, ovarian, bladder, and skin cancers are found at higher frequency, compared to sporadic colorectal cancer cases.

Due to the clinical and histologic overlap between MYH polyposis and classical FAP, attempts have been made to identify distinguishing features. Although inconstant, it was found that the presence of multiple hyperplastic polyps in the context of adenomatous polyposis is an indication that the polyposis could be due to an MYH genetic alteration [69].

Unlike HNPCC-related colorectal cancers where IHC is a useful screening test, immunostaining using anti-MYH antibodies does not help in associating colorectal cancers to germline mutations of MYH. Therefore, molecular methods, such as PCR followed by denaturing high pressure liquid chromatography (dHPLC), are required to test germline DNA [70].

Recently, a set of criteria have been proposed to guide molecular testing for MYH polyposis [71].

These criteria include the presence of ten or more polyps, the absence of APC mutations, the absence of MSI-H molecular changes, young age, and non-autosomal dominant inheritance pattern. However, it is accepted that the clinical and pathologic features of MYH-associated neoplasia can imitate many other genetic forms of colorectal polyposis and cancer. Family history can be misleading as some cases have a history resembling the Lynch syndrome, whereas other cases have no family history, and some cases represent new mutations.

Patients with documented polyps and biallelic mutations of MYH should be offered surveillance colonoscopy and duodenoscopy every 3–5 years. Their siblings should be tested in their early 20s and offered genetic counseling.

Summary

Molecular alterations are the root of a variety of gastrointestinal malignancies. Herein, the molecular basis of upper and lower gastrointestinal tumors is presented, along with pertinent clinical and pathologic features. Adenocarcinomas of the upper and lower gastrointestinal tract may present as part of a variety of inherited syndromes. HDGC, FAP, Lynch syndrome, and MYH polyposis are discussed. Polyposis syndromes, such as juvenile polyposis and PJS, also put patients at increased risk of malignancy. Mesenchymal tumors, particularly GISTs, have well-established and emerging molecular abnormalities. Treatment of GIST targets the underlying molecular abnormality. Molecular targeted therapy is also being used in the treatment of HER2-positive GEJ and gastric adenocarcinoma. HER2 testing methods in gastric and GEJ tumors are discussed. DNA microsatellite instability is a typical feature of Lynch syndrome, and also a prognostic factor in a subset of sporadic colorectal cancer. In the case of sporadic tumors, investigations of discrete molecular alterations are required for the use of some targeted therapies, such as anti-EGFR antibody in the treatment of colorectal cancer harboring a wild type KRAS genotype.

References

1. Caldas C, Carneiro F, Lynch HT, Yokota J, Wiesner GL, Powell SM, et al. Familial gastric cancer: overview and guidelines for management. J Med Genet. 1999;36:873–80.
2. Fitzgerald RC, Hardwick R, Huntsman D, Carneiro F, Guilford P, Blair V, et al. Hereditary diffuse gastric cancer: updated consensus guidelines for clinical management and directions for future research. J Med Genet. 2010;47:436–44.
3. Guilford P, Hopkins J, Harraway J, McLeod M, McLeod N, Harawira P, et al. E-cadherin germline mutations in familial gastric cancer. Nature. 1998;392:402–5.
4. Oliveira C, Senz J, Kaurah P, Pinheiro H, Sanges R, Haegert A, et al. Germline CDH1 deletions in hereditary diffuse gastric cancer families. Hum Mol Genet. 2009;18:1545–55.
5. Schrader K, Huntsman D. Hereditary diffuse gastric cancer. Cancer Treat Res. 2010;155:33–63.
6. Fujita H, Lennerz JK, Chung DC, Patel D, Deshpande V, Yoon SS, et al. Endoscopic surveillance of patients with hereditary diffuse gastric cancer: biopsy recommendations after topographic distribution of cancer foci in a series of 10 CDH1-mutated gastrectomies. Am J Surg Pathol. 2012;36:1709–17.
7. Hudis CA. Trastuzumab—mechanism of action and use in clinical practice. N Engl J Med. 2007;357:39–51.
8. Bang YJ, Van Cutsem E, Feyereislova A, Chung HC, Shen L, Sawaki A, et al. Trastuzumab in combination with chemotherapy versus chemotherapy alone for treatment of HER2-positive advanced gastric or gastro-oesophageal junction cancer (ToGA): a phase 3, open-label, randomised controlled trial. Lancet. 2010;376:687–97.
9. Hofmann M, Stoss O, Shi D, Buttner R, van de Vijver M, Kim W, et al. Assessment of a HER2 scoring system for gastric cancer: results from a validation study. Histopathology. 2008;52:797–805.
10. Ruschoff J, Hanna W, Bilous M, Hofmann M, Osamura RY, Penault-Llorca F, et al. HER2 testing in gastric cancer: a practical approach. Mod Pathol. 2012;25:637–50.
11. Grin A, Brezden-Masley C, Bauer S, Streutker CJ. HER2 in situ hybridization in gastric and gastroesophageal adenocarcinoma: comparison of automated dual ISH to FISH. Appl Immunohistochem Mol Morphol. 2013;21(6):561–6.
12. Nilsson B, Bumming P, Meis-Kindblom JM, Oden A, Dortok A, Gustavsson B, et al. Gastrointestinal stromal tumors: the incidence, prevalence, clinical course, and prognostication in the preimatinib mesylate era—a population-based study in western Sweden. Cancer. 2005;103:821–9.
13. Miettinen M, Makhlouf H, Sobin LH, Lasota J. Gastrointestinal stromal tumors of the jejunum and

ileum: a clinicopathologic, immunohistochemical, and molecular genetic study of 906 cases before imatinib with long-term follow-up. Am J Surg Pathol. 2006;30:477–89.

14. Miettinen M, Sobin LH, Lasota J. Gastrointestinal stromal tumors of the stomach: a clinicopathologic, immunohistochemical, and molecular genetic study of 1765 cases with long-term follow-up. Am J Surg Pathol. 2005;29:52–68.

15. Liegl B, Hornick JL, Corless CL, Fletcher CD. Monoclonal antibody DOG1.1 shows higher sensitivity than KIT in the diagnosis of gastrointestinal stromal tumors, including unusual subtypes. Am J Surg Pathol. 2009;33:437–46.

16. Lasota J, Miettinen M. Clinical significance of oncogenic KIT and PDGFRA mutations in gastrointestinal stromal tumours. Histopathology. 2008;53:245–66.

17. Lasota J, Jasinski M, Sarlomo-Rikala M, Miettinen M. Mutations in exon 11 of c-Kit occur preferentially in malignant versus benign gastrointestinal stromal tumors and do not occur in leiomyomas or leiomyosarcomas. Am J Pathol. 1999;154:53–60.

18. Steigen SE, Eide TJ, Wasag B, Lasota J, Miettinen M. Mutations in gastrointestinal stromal tumors—a population-based study from Northern Norway. APMIS. 2007;115:289–98.

19. Heinrich MC, Corless CL, Duensing A, McGreevey L, Chen CJ, Joseph N, et al. PDGFRA activating mutations in gastrointestinal stromal tumors. Science. 2003;299:708–10.

20. Lasota J, Dansonka-Mieszkowska A, Sobin LH, Miettinen M. A great majority of GISTs with PDGFRA mutations represent gastric tumors of low or no malignant potential. Lab Invest. 2004;84:874–83.

21. Janeway KA, Kim SY, Lodish M, Nose V, Rustin P, Gaal J, et al. Defects in succinate dehydrogenase in gastrointestinal stromal tumors lacking KIT and PDGFRA mutations. Proc Natl Acad Sci U S A. 2011;108:314–8.

22. Miettinen M, Wang ZF, Sarlomo-Rikala M, Osuch C, Rutkowski P, Lasota J. Succinate dehydrogenase-deficient GISTs: a clinicopathologic, immunohistochemical, and molecular genetic study of 66 gastric GISTs with predilection to young age. Am J Surg Pathol. 2011;35:1712–21.

23. Janeway KA, Albritton KH, Van Den Abbeele AD, D'Amato GZ, Pedrazzoli P, Siena S, et al. Sunitinib treatment in pediatric patients with advanced GIST following failure of imatinib. Pediatr Blood Cancer. 2009;52:767–71.

24. Dwight T, Benn DE, Clarkson A, Vilain R, Lipton L, Robinson BG, et al. Loss of SDHA expression identifies SDHA mutations in succinate dehydrogenase-deficient gastrointestinal stromal tumors. Am J Surg Pathol. 2013;37:226–33.

25. Wagner AJ, Remillard SP, Zhang YX, Doyle LA, George S, Hornick JL. Loss of expression of SDHA predicts SDHA mutations in gastrointestinal stromal tumors. Mod Pathol. 2013;26:289–94.

26. Pasini B, McWhinney SR, Bei T, Matyakhina L, Stergiopoulos S, Muchow M, et al. Clinical and molecular genetics of patients with the Carney-Stratakis syndrome and germline mutations of the genes coding for the succinate dehydrogenase subunits SDHB, SDHC, and SDHD. Eur J Hum Genet. 2008;16:79–88.

27. Carney JA, Stratakis CA. Familial paraganglioma and gastric stromal sarcoma: a new syndrome distinct from the Carney triad. Am J Med Genet. 2002;108:132–9.

28. Debiec-Rychter M, Sciot R, Le Cesne A, Schlemmer M, Hohenberger P, van Oosterom AT, et al. KIT mutations and dose selection for imatinib in patients with advanced gastrointestinal stromal tumours. Eur J Cancer. 2006;42:1093–103.

29. Heinrich MC, Marino-Enriquez A, Presnell A, Donsky RS, Griffith DJ, McKinley A, et al. Sorafenib inhibits many kinase mutations associated with drug-resistant gastrointestinal stromal tumors. Mol Cancer Ther. 2012;11:1770–80.

30. Corless CL, Barnett CM, Heinrich MC. Gastrointestinal stromal tumours: origin and molecular oncology. Nat Rev Cancer. 2011;11:865–78.

31. McGarrity TJ, Amos C. Peutz-Jeghers syndrome: clinicopathology and molecular alterations. Cell Mol Life Sci. 2006;63:2135–44.

32. Launonen V. Mutations in the human LKB1/STK11 gene. Hum Mutat. 2005;26:291–7.

33. van Lier MG, Wagner A, Mathus-Vliegen EM, Kuipers EJ, Steyerberg EW, van Leerdam ME. High cancer risk in Peutz-Jeghers syndrome: a systematic review and surveillance recommendations. Am J Gastroenterol. 2010;105:1258–64; author reply 65.

34. Beggs AD, Latchford AR, Vasen HF, Moslein G, Alonso A, Aretz S, et al. Peutz-Jeghers syndrome: a systematic review and recommendations for management. Gut. 2010;59:975–86.

35. van Lier MG, Wagner A, van Leerdam ME, Biermann K, Kuipers EJ, Steyerberg EW, et al. A review on the molecular diagnostics of Lynch syndrome: a central role for the pathology laboratory. J Cell Mol Med. 2010;14:181–97.

36. Paraf F, Jothy S, Van Meir EG. Brain tumor-polyposis syndrome: two genetic diseases? J Clin Oncol. 1997;15:2744–58.

37. Paraf F, Sasseville D, Watters AK, Narod S, Ginsburg O, Shibata H, et al. Clinicopathological relevance of the association between gastrointestinal and sebaceous neoplasms: the Muir-Torre syndrome. Hum Pathol. 1995;26:422–7.

38. Entius MM, Keller JJ, Drillenburg P, Kuypers KC, Giardiello FM, Offerhaus GJ. Microsatellite instability and expression of hMLH-1 and hMSH-2 in sebaceous gland carcinomas as markers for Muir-Torre syndrome. Clin Cancer Res. 2000;6:1784–9.

39. Umar A, Boland CR, Terdiman JP, Syngal S, de la Chapelle A, Ruschoff J, et al. Revised Bethesda Guidelines for hereditary nonpolyposis colorectal

cancer (Lynch syndrome) and microsatellite instability. J Natl Cancer Inst. 2004;96:261–8.

40. Huth C, Kloor M, Voigt AY, Bozukova G, Evers C, Gaspar H, et al. The molecular basis of EPCAM expression loss in Lynch syndrome-associated tumors. Mod Pathol. 2012;25:911–6.

41. Vilar E, Gruber SB. Microsatellite instability in colorectal cancer-the stable evidence. Nat Rev Clin Oncol. 2010;7:153–62.

42. Adeniran AJ, Theoharis C, Hui P, Prasad ML, Hammers L, Carling T, et al. Reflex BRAF testing in thyroid fine-needle aspiration biopsy with equivocal and positive interpretation: a prospective study. Thyroid. 2011;21:717–23.

43. Lindor NM, Petersen GM, Hadley DW, Kinney AY, Miesfeldt S, Lu KH, et al. Recommendations for the care of individuals with an inherited predisposition to Lynch syndrome: a systematic review. JAMA. 2006; 296:1507–17.

44. Felton KEA, Gilchrist DM, Andrew SE. Constitutive deficiency in DNA mismatch repair. Clin Genet. 2007;71:483–98.

45. Lindor NM, Rabe K, Petersen GM, Haile R, Casey G, Baron J, et al. Lower cancer incidence in Amsterdam-I criteria families without mismatch repair deficiency: familial colorectal cancer type X. JAMA. 2005;293: 1979–85.

46. Herrera L, Kakati S, Gibas L, Pietrzak E, Sandberg AA. Gardner syndrome in a man with an interstitial deletion of 5q. Am J Med Genet. 1986;25:473–6.

47. Solomon E, Voss R, Hall V, Bodmer WF, Jass JR, Jeffreys AJ, et al. Chromosome 5 allele loss in human colorectal carcinomas. Nature. 1987;328:616–9.

48. Young J, Jass JR. The case for a genetic predisposition to serrated neoplasia in the colorectum: hypothesis and review of the literature. Cancer Epidemiol Biomarkers Prev. 2006;15:1778–84.

49. Jass JR, Williams CB, Bussey HJ, Morson BC. Juvenile polyposis—a precancerous condition. Histopathology. 1988;13:619–30.

50. Aretz S, Stienen D, Uhlhaas S, Stolte M, Entius MM, Loff S, et al. High proportion of large genomic deletions and a genotype phenotype update in 80 unrelated families with juvenile polyposis syndrome. J Med Genet. 2007;44:702–9.

51. Brosens LA, Langeveld D, van Hattem WA, Giardiello FM, Offerhaus GJ. Juvenile polyposis syndrome. World J Gastroenterol. 2011;17:4839–44.

52. Wood LD, Parsons DW, Jones S, Lin J, Sjoblom T, Leary RJ, et al. The genomic landscapes of human breast and colorectal cancers. Science. 2007;318:1108–13.

53. Cunningham D, Humblet Y, Siena S, Khayat D, Bleiberg H, Santoro A, et al. Cetuximab monotherapy and cetuximab plus irinotecan in irinotecan-refractory metastatic colorectal cancer. N Engl J Med. 2004;351: 337–45.

54. Lievre A, Bachet JB, Boige V, Cayre A, Le Corre D, Buc E, et al. KRAS mutations as an independent

prognostic factor in patients with advanced colorectal cancer treated with cetuximab. J Clin Oncol. 2008;26: 374–9.

55. Di Nicolantonio F, Martini M, Molinari F, Sartore-Bianchi A, Arena S, Saletti P, et al. Wild-type BRAF is required for response to panitumumab or cetuximab in metastatic colorectal cancer. J Clin Oncol. 2008;26: 5705–12.

56. Danese S, Mantovani A. Inflammatory bowel disease and intestinal cancer: a paradigm of the Yin-Yang interplay between inflammation and cancer. Oncogene. 2010;29:3313–23.

57. Reikvam DH, Perminow G, Lyckander LG, Gran JM, Brandtzaeg P, Vatn M, et al. Increase of regulatory T cells in ileal mucosa of untreated pediatric Crohn's disease patients. Scand J Gastroenterol. 2011;46: 550–60.

58. Chen Z, Zhou F, Huang S, Jiang T, Chen L, Ge L, et al. Association of cytotoxic T lymphocyte associated antigen-4 gene (rs60872763) polymorphism with Crohn's disease and high levels of serum sCTLA-4 in Crohn's disease. J Gastroenterol Hepatol. 2011;26: 924–30.

59. Garrity-Park MM, Loftus Jr EV, Sandborn WJ, Bryant SC, Smyrk TC. Methylation status of genes in non-neoplastic mucosa from patients with ulcerative colitis-associated colorectal cancer. Am J Gastroenterol. 2010;105:1610–9.

60. Al-Tassan N, Chmiel NH, Maynard J, Fleming N, Livingston AL, Williams GT, et al. Inherited variants of MYH associated with somatic G:C→T:A mutations in colorectal tumors. Nat Genet. 2002;30: 227–32.

61. Croitoru ME, Cleary SP, Di Nicola N, Manno M, Selander T, Aronson M, et al. Association between biallelic and monoallelic germline MYH gene mutations and colorectal cancer risk. J Natl Cancer Inst. 2004;96:1631–4.

62. Win AK, Hopper JL, Jenkins MA. Association between monoallelic MUTYH mutation and colorectal cancer risk: a meta-regression analysis. Fam Cancer. 2011;10:1–9.

63. Lindor NM. Hereditary colorectal cancer: MYH-associated polyposis and other newly identified disorders. Best Pract Res Clin Gastroenterol. 2009;23: 75–87.

64. Cleary SP, Cotterchio M, Jenkins MA, Kim H, Bristow R, Green R, et al. Germline MutY human homologue mutations and colorectal cancer: a multi-site case-control study. Gastroenterology. 2009;136: 1251–60.

65. Tenesa A, Campbell H, Barnetson R, Porteous M, Dunlop M, Farrington SM. Association of MUTYH and colorectal cancer. Br J Cancer. 2006;95:239–42.

66. O'Shea AM, Cleary SP, Croitoru MA, Kim H, Berk T, Monga N, et al. Pathological features of colorectal carcinomas in MYH-associated polyposis. Histopathology. 2008;53:184–94.

67. Boparai KS, Dekker E, Van ES, Polak MM, Bartelsman JF, Mathus-Vliegen EM, et al. Hyperplastic polyps and sessile serrated adenomas as a phenotypic expression of MYH-associated polyposis. Gastroenterology. 2008;135:2014–8.

68. Vogt S, Jones N, Christian D, Engel C, Nielsen M, Kaufmann A, et al. Expanded extracolonic tumor spectrum in MUTYH-associated polyposis. Gastroenterology. 2009;137:1976–85.e1–10.

69. Jass JR. Colorectal polyposes: from phenotype to diagnosis. Pathol Res Pract. 2008;204:431–47.

70. Croitoru ME, Cleary SP, Berk T, Di NN, Kopolovic I, Bapat B, et al. Germline MYH mutations in a clinic-based series of Canadian multiple colorectal adenoma patients. J Surg Oncol. 2007;95:499–506.

71. Church J, Heald B, Burke C, Kalady M. Understanding MYH-associated neoplasia. Dis Colon Rectum. 2012; 55:359–62.

Molecular Testing in Pulmonary Tumors

13

Jeffrey J. Tanguay, Shirin Karimi, David M. Hwang, and Ming-Sound Tsao

Introduction

Lung cancer remains the leading cause of cancer deaths worldwide, claiming more than one million lives annually [1]. In North America, lung cancer was responsible for more deaths in 2012 than breast, colon, and prostate cancers combined [2]. While there have been advances in the management of many other types of cancer resulting in significantly improved survival rates over the past 40 years, the mortality associated with lung cancer remains stubbornly high, due in large part to the advanced stage at which patients typically present and to the limited effectiveness of current therapeutic options. The response rate for standard platinum-based chemotherapy in patients with advanced disease is 30–40 %, and the development of resistance to chemotherapy limits the median survival to 8–10 months in these patients. Even in early-stage patients who are treated primarily by surgical resection with curative intent, the rate of recurrence is estimated to be as high as 30–60 % [3].

The past decade, however, has seen a dramatic revolution in the treatment of lung cancer, resulting in large part from the discovery of specific molecular alterations that render tumors with these alterations amenable to targeted therapies (Fig. 13.1, Table 13.1). In particular, the discovery of activating epidermal growth factor receptor (EGFR) gene mutations in the tyrosine kinase domain and rearrangements of the anaplastic lymphoma kinase-1 (ALK) gene that render these tumors sensitive to their respective small-molecule kinase inhibitors have rapidly been translated from bench to bedside with dramatic effects [4–6]. As a result, an increasing array of molecular tests is now being implemented as part of routine diagnostic algorithms for personalizing the treatment of lung cancers. Here, we review the molecular alterations that are commonly present in lung cancers and discuss tests for these alterations currently in clinical use, with an emphasis on EGFR mutations and ALK rearrangements.

Molecular Alterations in Lung Cancer Subtypes

Historically, primary lung cancers have been categorized broadly into two major clinically relevant subtypes: small cell lung cancer (SCLC) and non-small cell lung cancer (NSCLC). While division along these two lines has traditionally been acceptable for deciding treatment options, more precise subclassification of the NSCLC into its

J.J. Tanguay, M.D. • S. Karimi, M.D.
D.M. Hwang, M.D., Ph.D.
M.-S. Tsao, M.D. (✉)
Department of Pathology, University Health Network,
Toronto General Hospital, 200 Elizabeth Street,
11E424, Toronto, ON, Canada M5G 2C4

Department of Laboratory Medicine
and Pathobiology, University of Toronto,
Toronto, ON, Canada
e-mail: ming.tsao@uhn.ca

G.M. Yousef and S. Jothy (eds.), *Molecular Testing in Cancer*,
DOI 10.1007/978-1-4899-8050-2_13, © Springer Science+Business Media New York 2014

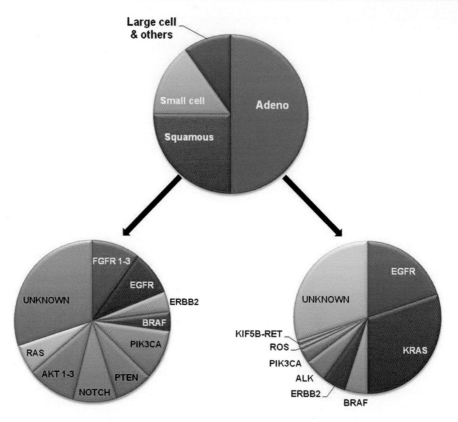

Fig. 13.1 Approximate distribution of lung cancer according to histology and putative "driver" genetic aberrations. Note that epidermal growth factor receptor (EGFR) gene aberrations in adenocarcinoma are mainly represented by kinase domain mutations and in squamous cell carcinoma by gene amplification

Table 13.1 Currently available targeted therapies and patient selection markers in advanced non-small cell lung carcinoma

Agent	Molecular marker selection	Histology selection
Bevacizumab	None	Non-squamous NSCLC
Pemetrexed		
Gefitinib/ Erlotinib/ Afatinib	EGFR kinase domain mutation (first line)	NSCLC with adenocarcinoma component
Crizotinib	ALK/ROS gene rearrangement	

NSCLC non-small cell lung carcinoma, *EGFR* epidermal growth factor receptor

major histologic subtypes—adenocarcinoma, squamous cell carcinoma, and large cell carcinoma—has assumed growing clinical importance in recent years. This has been in part due to the findings of increased incidence of potentially life-threatening hemorrhage in squamous cell carcinomas treated with bevacizumab [7] and efficacy of pemetrexed in the treatment of non-squamous NSCLC [8]. At the same time, however, it has been increasingly recognized that the different histologic subtypes of NSCLC are associated with specific molecular alterations that are, by and large, relatively unique to each subset. Therefore, the need for more precise delineation of NSCLC subtypes by the pathologist is being increasingly driven by the need to triage samples for appropriate molecular testing (Fig. 13.1). This recognition in part provided the impetus for the recent recommendation for the revision of lung adenocarcinoma classification by the International Association for the Study of Lung Cancer (IASLC), the American Thoracic Society (ATS), and the European Respiratory Society (ERS) [9], as well as for the recent guidelines on molecular testing in lung cancer by the College of American Pathologists (CAP), IASLC, and the Association for Molecular Pathology (AMP) [10]. In this chapter, we provide an overview of molecular alterations associated with the major subtypes of lung cancer and review the current state of testing for such alterations.

Molecular Pathology of Pulmonary Adenocarcinoma

EGFR

EGFR was first discovered several decades ago [11, 12], and its overexpression has been reported in many human cancers including lung, breast, head and neck, colorectal, pancreatic, and bladder cancers [13]. The EGFR gene is located on the short arm of chromosome 7 (7p11.2). The EGFR or human epidermal growth factor receptor 1 (HER1/erbB1) is a transmembrane tyrosine kinase (TK) receptor. When EGFR is bound by its ligands to the extracellular domain, it forms homodimers or heterodimers with other members of the EGFR family (HER 1–4). Activation of the intracellular TK results in phosphorylation of various intracellular proteins, especially the

RAS-RAF1-MAP2K1/MAPK1 and PI3K/AKT/mTOR signaling pathways [14]. Activation of these pathways promotes cellular proliferation, angiogenesis, mobility, and metastasis and decreases apoptosis. The constitutive activation of EGFR TK results in increased autophosphorylation and may promote carcinogenesis. Most EGFR mutations in the kinase domain alter the adenosine triphosphate (ATP) binding cleft which is the site where most TK inhibitors (TKIs) compete for binding [15].

EGFR Mutations

The majority of mutations involve exons 18–21 [16–19] and are grouped into three major categories: in-frame deletions of exon 19, insertion mutations in exon 20, and missense mutations in exons 18–21. The vast majority of mutations, approximately 85–90 %, involve exon 19 deletions (of which there are over 20) and the exon 21 L858R substitution (Fig. 13.2). About 5 % of mutations are due to substitutions in exon 18 (E709 and G719), and there are additional substitutions in exon 21 (L861) accounting for about 3 % of mutations [20]. Mutations in exon 20 are frequently associated with either primary (P772 to V774) or acquired resistance (T790M) to EGFR TKIs and will be further discussed below.

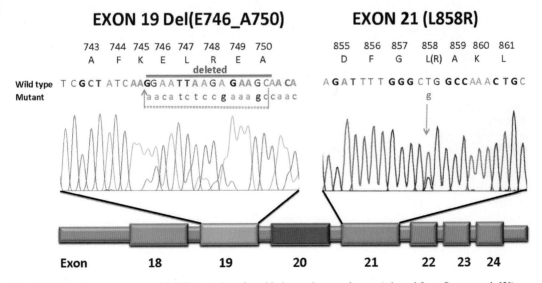

Fig. 13.2 Most common types of EGFR mutations found in lung adenocarcinoma (adapted from Santos et al. [3])

EGFR mutations tend to have greater association with certain patient characteristics, including East Asian ethnicity, females, and never smokers. The frequency of EGFR mutations in East Asians is approximately 32 %, and in the NSCLC of East Asian never smokers, it can approach to as high as 50 % [21]. By far, the vast majority of EGFR mutations are associated with adenocarcinoma histology, in particular well-differentiated adeno-carcinomas with lepidic, papillary, or acinar growth patterns [4, 5, 22, 23].

EGFR Inhibitors

There are currently two major classes of EGFR inhibitors: anti-EGFR monoclonal antibodies and small-molecule TKIs [2]. Anti-EGFR anti-bodies which include cetuximab and panitu-mumab are monoclonal antibodies directed at the extracellular ligand binding domain. These act as competitive antagonists and can promote inter-nalization and breakdown of the EGFR receptor [24]. These types of agents reportedly inhibit ligand-dependant activation of EGFR receptors without preventing autophosphorylation that can result from TK mutations [20]. Small-molecule TKIs such as gefitinib or erlotinib reversibly bind the ATP-binding site of the TK domain and pre-vent downstream signaling [15].

EGFR Mutations as a Predictive Marker

The most important factor in predicting response to anti-EGFR therapies is whether an activating mutation is present in the TK. Earlier work focused on EGFR protein overexpression and increased EGFR gene copy number, but these have been found to be less relevant [25, 26]. Mutations in the EGFR receptor TK were ini-tially reported in three landmark studies in 2004 [4, 5, 27] and were the first to discover that muta-tions in the TK domain correlated with sensitivity to the EGFR TKIs gefitinib or erlotinib. Prior to that, it was known that some patients with meta-static non-small cell carcinoma responded to TKIs but the mechanism was unknown [25]. In 2009, the phase 3 IRESSA Pan-Asia Study (IPASS) [28] trial demonstrated that patients with EGFR muta-tions had significantly greater response rate and longer progression-free survival with gefitinib

treatment compared to conventional chemotherapy. Most importantly, patients with EGFR mutation-negative tumors had a better response rate and progression-free survival with standard chemo-therapy over the TKI. Similar findings have been found in the WJTOG3405 [29] and NEJ002 [30] trials with gefitinib and the OPTIMAL [31] and EURTAC [32] trials with erlotinib.

EGFR Resistance

Many patients with specific activating mutations in EGFR show very promising initial responses to targeted treatments. Unfortunately, most will eventually relapse in 10–14 months [28, 31] as they develop resistance to the drug. The clinical definition of acquired resistance is as follows: a lung cancer patient on a single-agent TKI, who has either a TKI-sensitive EGFR mutation or observed clinical benefit from treatment while on a TKI, who undergoes disease progression while on continuous treatment with a TKI within the last 30 days, and who has no intervening sys-temic treatment between stopping a TKI and starting the new therapy [33]. The most estab-lished mechanisms of secondary resistance are due to additional mutation in the EGFR gene arising during treatment and amplification of other oncogenic intracellular signaling pathways [20]. Occasionally, resistance in NSCLC can be attributed to histologic transformation into small cell carcinoma or through epithelial to mesen-chymal transformation [34].

Repeat biopsies of tumors from patients that initially responded to TKI treatment but subse-quently relapsed led to the discovery of many secondary mutations [35]. The most common mechanism of secondary resistance involves the T790M substitution mutation on exon 20 of the EGFR gene [35, 36]. This substitution is present in about 50 % of cases of acquired resistance to EGFR TKIs [37–40]. This mutation results in increased affinity of the EGFR receptor TK for ATP making it more difficult for first-generation TKIs to inhibit the kinase activity [41]. The T790M mutation is uncommonly (<5 %) identi-fied in TKI treatment-naïve tumors [28, 42], sug-gesting that it is present as a minor subclone in pretreatment tumors and becomes enriched during

TKI treatment that causes massive apoptosis of tumor cells without this resistant mutation.

Another mechanism of resistance to TKIs results from amplification of other signaling pathways that promote oncogenesis. One of the most common is due to activation of the MET pathway which is believed to arise through a "kinase switch" mechanism [43]. This occurs when, for example, a cancer dependent on an EGFR-mediated kinase signaling pathway overcomes TKI-mediated inhibition by switching dependency to another tyrosine kinase-mediated signaling pathway [44]. The MET gene encodes the hepatocyte growth factor (HGF) receptor which is also a transmembrane TK receptor. The MET receptor couples with other ErbB receptors and activates PI3K-AKT signaling [45], promoting cell proliferation and inhibiting apoptosis. Amplification of this gene or its ligand, HGF, is associated with approximately 20 % of secondary resistance to EGFR TKIs [45–47]. Patients with surgically resected NSCLC with MET amplifications have a poorer prognosis [48].

Testing for EGFR Mutations
Pre-analytic Considerations

The CAP/IASLC/AMP molecular testing guidelines for lung cancer recommend that EGFR testing be initiated at the time of diagnosis for patients with advanced (stage IV) disease or at time of recurrence or progression for earlier-stage patients who would benefit from EGFR TKI therapy. As staging information may not always be available to the pathologist, close collaboration with the treating physician or oncologist is needed to facilitate timely testing. Reflex testing of early-stage tumors at time of resection may be advantageous in terms of eliminating time for testing if the patient later develops metastatic recurrence and is encouraged by the CAP/IASLC/AMP guidelines, but the decision whether to do so is left to individual laboratories, in collaboration with their oncology teams [10].

EGFR testing may be performed on a wide range of specimen types including both cytology and surgical pathology specimens and including fresh, frozen, formalin-fixed, paraffin-embedded, and alcohol-fixed material. However, samples treated with acid decalcification or fixed with heavy metal ion-containing fixatives may be suboptimal for testing due to degradation of DNA and/or inhibition of the PCR reaction [49, 50]. Formalin fixation also results in degradation and cross-linking of DNA, as well as nucleotide alterations. Hence, while specimens fixed in formalin for standard durations are in general suitable for EGFR mutation and other DNA-based molecular tests, prolonged fixation times may diminish suitability for such tests.

Beyond these considerations, probably the single most important determinant of success or failure of EGFR testing is the tumor content in the specimen being tested, in terms of both the absolute number of tumor cells present and the proportion of tumor cells present relative to total cellularity in the sample. Thus, as a general principle, during the diagnostic process, as much tissue as possible should be conserved for molecular testing, with only a minimal immunohistochemical panel (e.g., TTF-1, P63 or P40, ± mucin) performed if necessary to differentiate between squamous and adeno differentiation in small biopsy specimens [9, 51]. Specimens available for testing should be reviewed by a pathologist familiar with the molecular testing protocols being used, to assess for adequacy based on the performance characteristics of the particular test being used (see below). Areas of higher tumor cellularity should be marked in histologic sections by the reviewing pathologist, for tumor enrichment by micro- or macrodissection. When multiple specimens are available, the pathologist should select the one most likely to yield interpretable results (usually the one with the greatest tumor cellularity, without decalcification or heavy metal fixatives). Either primary tumor or metastatic tumor samples may be tested, given the high rate of concordance of mutations between primary and metastatic lesions in NSCLC [52].

Molecular Testing for EGFR Mutations

Many different platforms for EGFR mutation testing exist, none of which are specifically endorsed by the CAP/IASLC/AMP guidelines, which state that "Laboratories may use any validated EGFR testing method with sufficient performance characteristics" [10]. Historically,

EGFR testing relied on Sanger sequencing, typically of the exon 18–21 region that harbors the vast majority of EGFR mutations known to occur in lung cancer. While Sanger sequencing has the advantage of being able, at least theoretically, to detect all mutations present in the sequenced region, it has the disadvantage of relatively low analytic sensitivity, requiring up to 50 % tumor cellularity in a sample for reliable detection of EGFR mutations that are not simultaneously amplified. This degree of tumor cellularity may be difficult to achieve in many tumor samples, in which there is frequently admixture with nonneoplastic cells that may exceed tumor cells in number. A host of other molecular strategies for EGFR mutation testing have since arisen that detect specific mutations by a range of strategies, including among others, size fractionation, restriction fragment length polymorphism (RFLP) analysis, allele-specific PCR, and mass spectrometry-based genotyping [3, 53]. While these approaches are limited to detection of specific, previously known mutations and therefore typically do not identify new mutations, they also generally have higher analytic sensitivity than Sanger sequencing, with some methods requiring 10 % or less tumor cellularity for reliable mutation detection, at a lower cost per mutation tested. Some of these methods (e.g., mass spectrometry-based approaches such as the Sequenom MassArray technology [54]) are also amenable to a high degree of multiplexing, permitting even rare mutations to be assayed while containing costs. Next-generation sequencing (NGS) platforms have also started finding their way into clinical applications in more recent years. While the costs associated with NGS technologies are as yet prohibitive for widespread routine clinical use, these powerful platforms allow for detection of both known and previously unknown genomic alterations in large numbers of genes simultaneously [55].

Whereas many laboratories have been limiting EGFR mutation testing to the most common activating mutations conferring sensitivity to EGFR TKIs (exon 19 deletions and exon 21 L858R mutation), there is growing consensus that mutations comprising >1 % of known EGFR muta-

tions, including both activating mutations and those conferring resistance to TKIs, should also be routinely tested [10].

EGFR Copy Number Assessment

Increased copy numbers of the EGFR gene, whether by amplification or polysomy, has been associated with response to EGFR TKIs in various studies [56–58]. However, this effect is thought to be driven primarily by the coexistence of EGFR mutant alleles (which are frequently amplified), rather than by the effects of increased copy number itself [26, 59, 60]. Thus, EGFR copy number analysis, whether by FISH or by chromogenic in situ hybridization (CISH), is not recommended as a predictor of tumor response to TKI therapy [10].

EGFR Immunohistochemistry

Immunohistochemical staining for total EGFR may be associated to an extent with copy number increases, but correlates poorly with the presence of EGFR mutations [59–61] and is therefore not recommended for selection of patients for TKI therapy [10]. However, high expression of EGFR by immunohistochemistry may have a role in selecting patients for treatment with the monoclonal anti-EGFR antibody cetuximab [62].

Mutation-specific anti-EGFR antibodies targeting both exon 19 deletions and the exon 21 L858R mutation have also been developed and tested. These typically demonstrate excellent specificity for detecting the mutations by IHC, but their sensitivity in multiple studies has been too low to permit their use as a stand-alone test for selection of TKI therapy [63–68]. Nevertheless, with proper validation, their use as a screen for positive cases, limiting further molecular testing for IHC-negative cases, may be warranted, particularly in populations with higher frequencies of EGFR mutations.

ALK

ALK Gene Fusions in NSCLC

The anaplastic lymphoma kinase (ALK) gene was originally identified as part of a translocation in anaplastic large cell lymphoma. In 2007, Soda et al. described a small inversion in the short arm of chromosome 2 resulting in a fusion between the echinoderm microtubule-like (EML)-4 gene and the ALK gene, in 5 of 75 (6.7 %) NSCLC cases [6]. Multiple variant fusion products differing in translocation sites in the EML4 and ALK genes have been identified, as have translocations involving other chromosomes and fusion partners with the ALK gene, namely, KIF5B and TFG [6, 69–72]. The NPM-ALK translocation present in anaplastic large cell lymphoma has not been reported in lung cancers. Subsequent studies have confirmed the presence of EML4-ALK translocations in a relatively small subset of pulmonary adenocarcinomas (3–13 %) [73–77] or approximately 5 % of NSCLC in a recent large clinical series [69]. The EML4-ALK fusion is present more frequently in lung adenocarcinomas from younger patients with either never- or light-smoking history [69, 75–79]. Some studies have reported associations with solid, mucinous cribriform, and/or signet ring histology [75, 78, 80]. The translocation is infrequent in pure squamous cell carcinoma, but has been reported in adenosquamous carcinoma [81].

The EML4-ALK fusion results in constitutive activation of ALK tyrosine kinase activity that is amenable to inhibition by the ALK tyrosine kinase inhibitor (TKI), crizotinib. Early studies of crizotinib in patients with ALK-rearranged NSCLC demonstrate striking antitumor activity, with ≥ 60 % of patients demonstrating at least partial response and median progression-free survival of approximately 10 months [69, 82]. Overall survival is also improved in crizotinib-treated patients compared with crizotinib-naive controls (70 % vs. 44 %, respectively, at 1 year and 55 % vs. 12 %, respectively, at 2 years) [83]. More recently, crizotinib was demonstrated in a phase 3 clinical trial to be superior to standard chemotherapy in previously treated, advanced stage ALK-rearranged NSCLC, with the crizotinib-treated group showing both higher overall response rate than the standard chemotherapy group (65 % vs. 20 %, respectively) and longer progression-free survival (7.7 vs. 3.0

months, respectively) [84]. However, as also occurs in treatments with EGFR TKIs, several ALK gene mutations resulting in acquired resistance to crizotinib have been described [85, 86].

Testing for ALK Gene Rearrangement
FISH

A number of methods for detecting ALK rearrangements have been developed, including FISH, RT-PCR, and immunohistochemistry. Of these, FISH has been the gold standard and, in the USA, is the basis of the companion diagnostic approved by the FDA for selection of patients who would benefit from treatment with crizotinib. This commercially available FISH assay (Abbott Molecular probes) utilizes a "break-apart" strategy in which the ALK gene is labeled with a green fluorescent probe hybridizing to the 5' end of the gene and a red probe hybridizing to the 3' end of the gene, resulting in a yellow fusion signal in the setting of a normal (non-rearranged) ALK gene. In the presence of translocations involving the ALK gene, there is loss of either green signals or distinct red and green signals (separated by >2 signal diameters) (Fig. 13.3a). Extra ALK signals may also often be seen, resulting from polysomies or alterations in tumor ploidy, the significance of which is presently uncertain.

As is the case with any FISH-based test, proper interpretation by a skilled interpreter is of paramount importance to avoid false positives and negatives, and thresholds for assessing test results as either positive or negative need to be established by each lab, using appropriate controls [10].

RT-PCR

Reverse-transcriptase PCR for detection of ALK fusion transcripts, while theoretically possible, has been recommended against in the CAP/IASLC/AMP guidelines, given the growing number of variant translocations that may result in an EML4-ALK fusion transcript, each requiring a different pair of PCR primers, and given concerns about the generally suboptimal performance of RT-PCR in FFPE tissue [10].

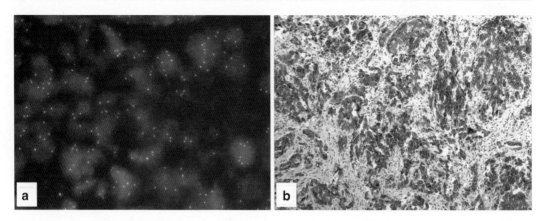

Fig. 13.3 ALK gene aberration in lung cancer. (**a**) ALK gene rearrangement detected by fluorescence in situ hybridization using the ALK break-apart probe. (**b**) ALK protein overexpression detected by immunohistochemistry

Immunohistochemistry

Given the cost and complexity of FISH analysis, there has been significant interest in the use of immunohistochemical staining for ALK overexpression as an alternative to FISH testing. In this regard, the anti-ALK1 mouse monoclonal antibody (anti-human CD246 clone ALK1, Dako) may demonstrate positive staining in some cases, but may fail to identify a significant proportion of ALK-rearranged lung cancers especially when a signal amplification step is not applied [78, 79, 87, 88]. However, another mouse monoclonal anti-ALK antibody (5A4, Novocastra) and two rabbit monoclonal antibodies (D5F3 and D9E4 from Cell Signaling Technology) have demonstrated high sensitivity and specificity compared to FISH for the detection of ALK-rearranged tumors [87, 89] (Fig. 13.3b). In our opinion, with proper validation and appropriate positive and negative controls, non-reactivity for ALK using the 5A4 antibody eliminates the need for FISH testing for ALK rearrangements, significantly reducing the number of FISH tests and limiting FISH testing to cases with equivocal IHC staining and to confirmation ALK gene rearrangements in IHC-positive cases.

KRAS

Kirsten rat sarcoma (KRAS) viral oncogene homologue is one of the RAS oncogenes (in addition to HRAS and NRAS) and accounts for most of the RAS mutations in cancer. RAS functions in intracellular signal transduction downstream of transmembrane receptor TKs such as EGFR. RAS is activated by binding guanosine triphosphate (GTP) which enables signaling via several pathways most notably the Raf/Mek/Erk pathway [25]. Activation of this pathway promotes mitosis and cell survival. Normally functioning KRAS has intrinsic GTPase activity to catalyze GTP breakdown and stop downstream signaling. Mutations in KRAS result in continuous binding of GTP causing constitutive activation of the receptor and its downstream pathways, thereby promoting oncogenesis [90].

In 1984, an activating mutation in KRAS was first identified in a human lung cancer [91]. Since then it has been determined that most KRAS mutations occur in codon 12 or 13 of exon 2 [92] and are found in approximately 25–35 % of pulmonary adenocarcinomas [93]. KRAS mutations are more commonly associated with mucinous morphology including mucinous areas within mixed adenocarcinomas and mucinous bronchioloalveolar carcinoma [93]. Unlike EGFR, KRAS mutations are more likely to be seen in tumors from smokers. They are also associated with a more aggressive clinical course and decreased patient survival [94–96].

There is currently no effective therapy targeting KRAS. A great majority of KRAS mutant lung cancers do not respond to EGFR, ALK, and ROS1 (discussed below) targeted therapies, but the presence of KRAS mutations should not be used to exclude patients from receiving EGFR TKI therapy, as differential survival benefit between KRAS wild-type and mutant patients treated by TKI has not been demonstrated [3, 97]. It is worth noting that these driver oncogenic mutations tend to occur mutually exclusive of each other, supporting further the need of mutation profiling for personalizing targeted therapies.

ROS1

The ROS1 gene is located on chromosome 6 and encodes a receptor tyrosine kinase [98]. Although an extracellular ligand has yet to be identified, it is known that ROS1 is involved in various signaling pathways including the MAPK pathway through phosphorylation of RAS [99]. Dysregulated ROS1 activity results in continuous downstream signaling of pathways promoting cell survival.

ROS1 rearrangements were first discovered in NSCLC in 2007 [71]. Currently, nine ROS1 fusion partners have been identified, and the most common is with CD74 located on chromosome 5 t(5;6)(q32;q22). ROS1 fusions are believed to result in constitutive activation of the receptor TK to promote oncogenesis [71]. ROS1 rearrangements in NSCLC are rare and have an estimated prevalence of 1–2.5 % [100–104]. Patients with ROS1 rearrangements tend to have similar demographics to patients with ALK gene rearrangements including younger age, never-smoking history, Asian ethnicity, and adenocarcinoma morphology [100], often with high-grade areas. ROS1 and ALK rearrangements appear to be mutually exclusive [100].

Although rare, ROS1 rearrangements are becoming increasingly important clinically as patients with these alterations appear to be sensitive to crizotinib [100, 103, 105]. This is currently being further evaluated in clinical trials. Similar to ALK rearrangements, a mechanism for secondary resistance to crizotinib has also been recently discovered by Awad et al. [106]. This group identified an acquired substitution muta-tion (G2032R) in a tumor with a CD74-ROS1 fusion. This was felt to be responsible for the development of resistance after a successful treatment response to crizotinib.

BRAF

BRAF is a non-receptor serine/threonine kinase that works downstream from KRAS in the MAPK signaling pathway [99]. Mutations in BRAF are believed to result in constitutive activation of the kinase to promote oncogenesis via downstream signaling [107]. Two recent studies identified that the most common BRAF mutation in pulmonary adenocarcinoma is the V600E substitution muta-tion which accounts for approximately 50 % of mutations [108, 109]. Other mutations include G469A and D594G. These studies found BRAF mutations in 3 % [108] and 4.9 % [109] of adeno-carcinomas. BRAF mutations are strongly asso-ciated with a history of smoking [108, 109]. Marchetti et al. reported an association of BRAF mutation with a micropapillary component of the tumor morphology and poorer prognosis [109]. Currently, multiple BRAF inhibitors are under development, and clinical trials are underway to assess for BRAF mutations as clinically relevant targets [17, 99].

HER-2

Similar to EGFR, the HER2 (ERBB2) protein is a tyrosine kinase receptor that is part of the HER family of receptors and is activated by homodi-merization or heterodimerization with other receptors, in particular EGFR and HER3 [93]. Activation of signaling pathways including the PI3K/AKT/mTOR and RAS/RAF/MEK path-ways promotes cellular proliferation [93], and dysregulation of HER2 signaling results in onco-genesis. Less than 5 % of NSCLC demonstrate amplifications of HER2 [110, 111] or mutations [112–114] and tend to be associated with never-smoking females with adenocarcinomas [114]. Several therapeutic agents targeting HER2 are currently under investigation.

Other Genetic Alterations in Lung Adenocarcinoma

Numerous studies characterizing mutations and other genomic alterations in pulmonary adenocarcinoma have been published in recent years. In a genome-wide analysis of copy number alterations in 371 pulmonary adenocarcinomas, Weir et al. identified 57 recurrent copy number alterations (gains or losses) involving 26 of 39 autosomal chromosome arms, with the most frequent being an amplification of chromosome 14q13.3, the region containing the Nkx2-1 gene (also known as TTF-1), present in 12 % of cases [115]. In a parallel study sequencing coding exons and splice sites of 623 candidate genes in 188 lung adenocarcinomas, Ding et al. found over 1,000 somatic mutations across the samples, with 26 genes that were mutated at high frequencies, suggesting their involvement in carcinogenesis. These include known oncogenes (e.g., KRAS, NRAS), tumor suppressor genes (e.g., P53, NF1, APC, RB1), and tyrosine kinases (e.g., EGFR, FGFR4, NTRK1, NTRK3, PDGFRA), as well as several genes with yet unknown function [116]. An ever-growing number of studies using a range of large-scale characterization approaches including high-resolution comparative genomic hybridization (CGH), exome and whole-genome sequencing, and RNA/transcriptome sequencing continue to add to the list of potential driver mutations and other genetic alterations in lung adenocarcinomas [117–123]. While there is presently insufficient evidence to warrant routine testing for these alterations, technologies such as mass spectrometry-based genotyping and NGS that permit simultaneous analysis of large numbers of target genes are likely to move increasingly into clinical use, as more of these alterations are validated and demonstrated to be of potential prognostic or predictive significance [124].

Squamous Cell Carcinoma

Squamous cell carcinomas comprise approximately 20 % of all lung cancer in the North America [125]. Relatively little was known until the past decade regarding the important molecular and genomic alterations in squamous cell carcinomas of the lung, and only more recently have potentially targetable alterations been identified in pulmonary squamous cell carcinomas. While various studies have suggested that the EGFR and KRAS mutations present in pulmonary adenocarcinomas (see above) are also present in pulmonary squamous cell carcinomas, these mutations are now thought to be rare in pure squamous cell carcinomas, with reports of their presence likely representing detection in undersampled adenosquamous carcinomas, which are known to harbor these mutations [126]. However, type III EGFR mutations (resulting from deletion of exons 2–7) have been described in up to 8 % of pulmonary squamous cell carcinomas [127, 128]. These mutations are not thought to be associated with sensitivity to gefitinib or erlotinib, but may be sensitive to some irreversible EGFR inhibitors [127].

A number of studies assessing genomic alterations in pulmonary squamous cell carcinoma have identified recurrent amplifications or losses in a number of chromosomal regions, including 2p, 3q, 5p, 7, 8p, 8q, 11q, 12q, 13q, 14q, 17q, 19p, 19q, and 20q [129–135], which appear to accumulate though the metaplasia-dysplasia-carcinoma sequence [136]. One amplified region of particular interest has been 3q, which harbors the SOX2 gene, amplified in approximately 20 % of lung squamous cell carcinomas [132, 134]; TP63, which is amplified in up to 88 % of lung squamous cell carcinomas [129]; and PIK3CA, which is amplified in approximately 40 % of these tumors [137, 138]. PIK3CA mutations have also been found in 3.6–6.5 % of squamous carcinomas [126, 139, 140]. The PIK3CA gene is part of the phosphatidylinositol-3-kinase (PI3K) pathway, which is a signal transduction pathway critical to, among other things, cell survival. Mutations involving other genes encoding proteins in this pathway have also been demonstrated in pulmonary squamous carcinoma, including PTEN (10 % of tumors) [141] and AKT1 (up to 7 % of tumors) [126, 142, 143]. Given that alterations in multiple members of this pathway have been identified, various inhibitors targeting this pathway (e.g., mTOR inhibitors such as sirolimus and everolimus) are being evaluated for potential role in the treatment of pulmonary squamous cell carcinomas.

Other recurrent, potentially targetable genetic alterations that have been identified in squamous cell carcinomas of the lung include FGFR1 amplification and DDR2 mutation. Fibroblast growth factor receptor (FGFR) is receptor tyrosine kinase with four isoforms. FGFR1 amplification in pulmonary squamous cell carcinomas, first reported in 2010 by Weiss et al. [144], is present in approximately 22 % of pulmonary squamous cell carcinomas and a smaller proportion (1–3 %) of pulmonary adenocarcinomas [144, 145]. Lung cancer cells harboring FGFR1 amplifications show growth inhibition and increased apoptosis when exposed to FGFR1 inhibitors [144, 145]. Several small-molecule inhibitors of FGFR1 are presently undergoing testing for potential clinical use [99].

The discoidin domain receptor (DDR) is a transmembrane receptor tyrosine kinase for interstitial collagen, with roles in regulating cell adhesion, proliferation, and migration. Upregulation of DDR1 expression has been reported to be associated with improved survival in NSCLC [146]. Several mutations in DDR2 have also been identified in 4 % of pulmonary squamous cell carcinomas [147]. Tumor xenografts established from DDR2-mutant lung cancer cell lines were sensitive to the multi-targeted kinase inhibitor dasatinib [147], and several clinical trials investigating dasatinib in the treatment of pulmonary squamous cell carcinoma are under way [99]. Several other small-molecule inhibitors currently in use for chronic myelogenous leukemia have also been found to demonstrate activity against DDR1 and DDR2 [148], suggesting their potential utility in the treatment of DDR2-mutated lung tumors.

In addition to the mutations and genomic alterations discussed above, recent comprehensive profiling of 178 pulmonary squamous carcinomas as part of The Cancer Genome Atlas (TCGA) project has identified recurrent mutations in at least 11 genes, with significant alterations affecting multiple different pathways and potentially targetable alterations in the most tumors [149].

At present, there is insufficient evidence to recommend routine testing for mutations or other genetic alterations in pulmonary squamous carcinomas outside of research settings, although this will no doubt change in coming years, as results of clinical trials targeting some of these alterations become available.

Small Cell Carcinoma

Small cell carcinoma comprises approximately 15 % of lung cancers worldwide and is associated with dismal prognosis [150]. However, characterization of genomic alterations in SCLC has been hindered in part by the relative paucity of material available for testing compared with non-small cell carcinomas, due to the fact that SCLC is not often treated by surgical resection. In an array CGH study that included 33 SCLC tumors and 13 SCLC cell lines, Voortman et al. found that SCLC demonstrates markedly aberrant karyotypes. Multiple recurrent copy number alterations were identified, including loss of the retinoblastoma (RB1) and TP53 genes and high copy number gains of MYC family member genes [151]; findings are also noted in a report of whole-genome sequencing of a single case of SCLC [152]. Peifer et al. likewise identified evidence of RB1 and TP53 inactivation in all cases and MYC family amplifications in 16 % of cases. They also found a very high rate of non-synonymous coding region mutations in these tumors (average of 7.4 per one million base pairs), including recurrent mutations of PTEN and of multiple histone modifier genes and focal amplifications of the FGFR1 gene (6 % of cases) [153]. In another large study of SCLC tumors and SCLC cell lines, Rudin et al. found at least 22 significantly mutated genes, including RB1, TP53, PIK3CA, and PTEN. Mutations clustering in several gene families and pathways were also noted, including the PI3K pathway, previously discussed in relation to squamous cell carcinoma. Of interest, high-level amplification of SOX2 was also found to be present in 27 % of samples, and treatment of cell lines harboring SOX2 amplifications with an anti-SOX2 short hairpin RNA (shRNA) resulted in decreased cell proliferation [154].

Various preclinical and early clinical studies assessing the role of targeted therapies (e.g., FGFR, PI3K pathway) are ongoing [155], but at present, there remains insufficient evidence to warrant routine clinical testing for these and other genetic alterations in SCLC.

Conclusion

The discovery only a decade ago of EGFR mutations with important predictive and prognostic implications for NSCLC has very rapidly resulted in significant paradigm shifts in the diagnosis and management of lung cancer. As growing numbers of targetable genetic alterations are discovered and validated across the spectrum of lung cancers, pathologists will be called upon not only to provide accurate histologic classification of tumors but increasingly also to provide and interpret concurrent molecular profiling data to help refine diagnosis and guide treatment of patients with lung cancer.

Acknowledgments This work is supported by the Ontario Ministry of Health and Long Term Care. Dr. Tsao is the M. Qasim Choksi Chair in Lung Cancer Translational Research.

References

1. Cagle TP, Allen TC, Dacic S, Beasley MB, Borczuk AC, Chirieac LR, et al. Revolution in lung cancer: new challenges for the surgical pathologist. Arch Pathol Lab Med. 2011;135:110–6.
2. Cagle PT, Myers J. Precision medicine for lung cancer: role of the surgical pathologist. Arch Pathol Lab Med. 2012;136:1186–9.
3. da Cunha Santos G, Shepherd FA, Tsao MS. EGFR mutations and lung cancer. Annu Rev Pathol. 2011; 6:49–69.
4. Lynch TJ, Bell DW, Sordella R, Gurubhagavatula S, Okimoto RA, Brannigan BW, et al. Activating mutations in the epidermal growth factor receptor underlying responsiveness of non-small-cell lung cancer to gefitinib. N Engl J Med. 2004;350:2129–39.
5. Paez TJ, Janne PA, Lee JC, Tracy S, Greulich H, Gabriel S, et al. EGFR mutations in lung cancer: correlation with clinical response to gefitinib therapy. Science. 2004;304:1497–500.

6. Soda M, Choi YL, Enomoto M, Takada S, Yamashita Y, Ishikawa S, et al. Identification of the transforming EML4-ALK fusion gene in non-small-cell lung cancer. Nature. 2007;448:561–6.
7. Johnson DH, Fehrenbacher L, Novotny WF, Herbst RS, Nemunaitis JJ, Jablons DM, et al. Randomized phase II trial comparing bevacizumab plus carboplatin and paclitaxel with carboplatin and paclitaxel alone in previously untreated locally advanced or metastatic non-small-cell lung cancer. J Clin Oncol. 2004;22:2184–91.
8. Scagliotti G, Brodowicz T, Shepherd FA, Zielinski C, Vansteenkiste J, Manegold C, et al. Treatment-by-histology interaction analyses in three phase III trials show superiority of pemetrexed in nonsquamous non-small cell lung cancer. J Thorac Oncol. 2011; 6:64–70.
9. Travis WD, Brambilla E, Noguchi M, Nicholson AG, Geisinger KR, Yatabe Y, et al. International Association for the Study of Lung Cancer/American Thoracic Society/European Respiratory Society international multidisciplinary classification of lung adenocarcinoma. J Thorac Oncol. 2011;6:244–85.
10. Lindeman NI, Cagle PT, Beasley MB, Chitale DA, Dacic S, Giaccone G, et al. Molecular testing guideline for selection of lung cancer patients for EGFR and ALK tyrosine kinase inhibitors: guideline from the College of American Pathologists, International Association for the Study of Lung Cancer, and Association for Molecular Pathology. Arch Pathol Lab Med. 2013;137:828–60.
11. Hollenberg MD, Cuatrecasas P. Epidermal growth factor: receptors in human fibroblasts and modulation of action by cholera toxin. Proc Natl Acad Sci USA. 1973;70:2964–8.
12. Wrann MM, Fox CF. Identification of epidermal growth factor receptors in a hyperproducing human epidermoid carcinoma cell line. J Biol Chem. 1979; 254:8083–6.
13. Hembrough T, Thyparambil S, Liao WL, Darfler MM, Abdo J, Bengali KM, et al. Selected reaction monitoring (SRM) analysis of epidermal growth factor receptor (EGFR) in formalin fixed tumor tissue. Clin Proteomics. 2012;9:5.
14. Hynes NE, Lane HA. ERBB receptors and cancer: the complexity of targeted inhibitors. Nat Rev Cancer. 2005;5:341–54.
15. Sordella R, Bell DW, Haber DA, Settleman J. Gefitinib-sensitizing EGFR mutations in lung cancer activate anti-apoptotic pathways. Science. 2004; 305:1163–7.
16. Zhou W, Ercan D, Janne PA, Gray NS. Discovery of selective irreversible inhibitors for EGFR-T790M. Bioorg Med Chem Lett. 2011;21:638–43.
17. Pao W, Girard N. New driver mutations in non-small-cell lung cancer. Lancet Oncol. 2011;12:175–80.
18. Penzel R, Sers C, Chen Y, Lehmann-Muhlenhoff U, Merkelbach-Bruse S, Jung A, et al. EGFR mutation detection in NSCLC—assessment of diagnostic application and recommendations of the German

Panel for Mutation Testing in NSCLC. Virchows Arch. 2011;458:95–8.

19. Sakurada A, Shepherd FA, Tsao MS. Epidermal growth factor receptor tyrosine kinase inhibitors in lung cancer: impact of primary or secondary mutations. Clin Lung Cancer. 2006;7 Suppl 4:S138–44.

20. Cheng L, Alexander RE, Maclennan GT, Cummings OW, Montironi R, Lopez-Beltran A, et al. Molecular pathology of lung cancer: key to personalized medicine. Mod Pathol. 2012;25:347–69.

21. Cagle PT, Allen TC. Lung cancer genotype-based therapy and predictive biomarkers. Present and future. Arch Pathol Lab Med. 2012;136:1482–91.

22. Ciardiello F, Tortora G. EGFR antagonists in cancer treatment. N Engl J Med. 2008;358:1160–74.

23. Pao W, Wang TY, Riely GJ, Miller VA, Pan Q, Ladanyi M, et al. KRAS mutations and primary resistance of lung adenocarcinomas to gefitinib or erlotinib. PLoS Med. 2005;2:e17.

24. Wheeler DL, Dunn EF, Harari PM. Understanding resistance to EGFR inhibitors- impact on future treatment strategies. Nat Rev Clin Oncol. 2010;7:493–501.

25. Vincent MD, Kuruvilla MS, Leighl NB, Kamel-Reid S. Biomarkers that currently affect clinical practice: EGFR, ALK, MET, KRAS. Curr Oncol. 2012;19:S33–44.

26. Fukuoka M, Wu YL, Thongprasert S, Sunpaweravong P, Leong SS, Sriuranpong V, et al. Biomarker analyses and final overall survival results from a phase III, randomized, open-label, first-line study of gefitinib versus carboplatin/paclitaxel in clinically selected patients with advanced non-small-cell lung cancer in Asia (IPASS). J Clin Oncol. 2011;29:2866–74.

27. Pao W, Miller V, Zakowski M, Doherty J, Politi K, Sarkari I, et al. EGF receptor gene mutations are common in lung cancers from "never smokers" and are associated with sensitivity of tumors to gefitinib and erlotinib. Proc Natl Acad Sci USA. 2004;101:13306–11.

28. Mok TS, Wu YL, Thongprasert S, Yang CH, Chu DT, Saijo N. Gefitinib or carboplatin-paclitaxel in pulmonary adenocarcinoma. N Engl J Med. 2009;361:947–57.

29. Mitsudomi T, Morita S, Yatabe Y, Negoro S, Okamoto I, Tsurutani J, et al. Gefitinib versus cisplatin plus docetaxel in patients with non-small-cell lung cancer harbouring mutations of the epidermal growth factor receptor (WJTOG3405): an open label, randomized phase 3 trial. Lancet Oncol. 2010;11:121–8.

30. Maemondo M, Inoue A, Kobayashi K, Sugawara S, Oizumi S, Isobe H, et al. Gefitinib or chemotherapy for non-small-cell lung cancer with mutated EGFR. N Engl J Med. 2010;362:2380–8.

31. Zhou C, Wu YL, Chen G, Feng J, Liu XQ, Wang C, et al. Erlotinib versus chemotherapy as first-line treatment for patients with advanced EGFR mutation-positive non-small-cell lung cancer (OPTIMAL, CTONG-0802): a multicentre, open-label, ran-

domised, phase 3 study. Lancet Oncol. 2011;12:735–42.

32. Rosell R, Carcereny E, Gervais R, Vergnenegre A, Massuti B, Felip E, et al. Erlotinib versus standard chemotherapy as first-line treatment for European patients with advanced EGFR mutation-positive non-small-cell lung cancer (EURTAC): a multicentre, open-label, randomised phase 3 trial. Lancet Oncol. 2012;13:239–46.

33. Jackman D, Pao W, Riely GJ, Engelman JA, Kris MG, Jänne PA, et al. Clinical definition of acquired resistance to epidermal growth factor receptor tyrosine kinase inhibitors in non-small-cell lung cancer. J Clin Oncol. 2010;28:357–60.

34. Sequist LV, Waltman BA, Dias-Santagata D, Digumarthy S, Turke AB, Fidias P, et al. Genotypic and histological evolution of lung cancers acquiring resistance to EGFR inhibitors. Sci Transl Med. 2011;3:75ra26.

35. Pao W, Miller VA, Politi KA, Riely GJ, Somwar R, Zakowski MF, et al. Acquired resistance of lung adenocarcinomas to gefitinib or erlotinib is associated with a second mutation in the EGFR kinase domain. PLoS Med. 2005;2:e73.

36. Kobayashi S, Boggon TJ, Dayaram T, Jänne PA, Kocher O, Meyerson M, et al. EGFR mutation and resistance of non-small-cell lung cancer to gefitinib. N Engl J Med. 2005;352:786–92.

37. Engleman JA, Janne PA. Mechanisms of acquired resistance to epidermal growth factor receptor tyrosine kinase inhibitors in non-small cell lung cancer. Clin Cancer Res. 2008;12:2895–9.

38. Balak MN, Gong Y, Riely GJ, Somwar R, Li AR, Zakowski MF, et al. Novel D761Y and common secondary T790M mutations in epidermal growth factor receptor-mutant lung adenocarcinomas with acquired resistance to kinase inhibitors. Clin Cancer Res. 2006;12:6494–501.

39. Chen HJ, Mok TS, Chen ZH, Guo AL, Zhang XC, Su J, et al. Clinicopathologic and molecular features of epidermal growth factor receptor T790M mutation and c-MET amplification in tyrosine kinase inhibitor-resistant Chinese non-small cell lung cancer. Pathol Oncol Res. 2009;15:651–8.

40. Costa DB, Schumer ST, Tenen DG, Kobayashi S. Differential responses to erlotinib in epidermal growth factor receptor (EGFR)-mutated lung cancers with acquired resistance to gefitinib carrying the L747S or T790M secondary mutations. J Clin Oncol. 2008;26:1182–4.

41. Yun CH, Mengwasser KE, Toms AV, Woo MS, Greulich H, Wong KK, et al. The T790M mutation in EGFR kinase causes drug resistance by increasing the affinity for ATP. Proc Natl Acad Sci USA. 2008;105:2070–5.

42. Bell DW, Gore I, Okimoto RA, Godin-Heymann N, Sordella R, Mulloy R, et al. Inherited susceptibility to lung cancer may be associated with the T790M drug resistance mutation in EGFR. Nat Genet. 2005;37:1315–6.

43. Nguyen KS, Kobayashi S, Costa DB. Acquired resistance to epidermal growth factor receptor tyrosine kinase inhibitors in non-small-cell lung cancers dependent on the epidermal growth factor receptor pathway. Clin Lung Cancer. 2009;10:281–9.

44. Mahadevan D, Cooke L, Riley C, Swart R, Simons B, Della Croce K, et al. A novel tyrosine kinase switch is a mechanism of imatinib resistance in gastrointestinal stromal tumors. Oncogene. 2007; 26:3909–19.

45. Engelman JA, Zejnullahu K, Mitsudomi T, Song Y, Hyland C, Park JO, et al. MET amplification leads to gefitinib resistance in lung cancer by activating ERBB3 signaling. Science. 2007;316:1039–43.

46. Bean J, Brennan C, Shih JY, Riely G, Viale A, Wang L, et al. MET amplification occurs with or without T790M mutations in EGFR mutant lung tumors with acquired resistance to gefitinib or erlotinib. Proc Natl Acad Sci USA. 2007;104:20932–7.

47. Yano S, Wang W, Li Q, Matsumoto K, Sakurama H, Nakamura T, et al. Hepatocyte growth factor induces gefitinib resistance of lung adenocarcinoma with epidermal growth factor receptor activating mutations. Cancer Res. 2008;68:9479–87.

48. Cappuzzo F, Marchetti A, Skokan M, Rossi E, Gajapathy S, Felicioni L, et al. Increased MET gene copy number negatively affects survival of surgically resected non-small-cell lung cancer patients. J Clin Oncol. 2009;27:1667–74.

49. Wilson IG. Inhibition and facilitation of nucleic acid amplification. Appl Environ Microbiol. 1997;63: 3741–51.

50. Baloglu G, Haholu A, Kucukodaci Z, Yilmaz I, Yildirim S, Baloglu H. The effects of tissue fixation alternatives on DNA content: a study on normal colon tissue. Appl Immunohistochem Mol Morphol. 2008;16:485–92.

51. Ellis PM, Blais N, Soulieres D, Ionescu DN, Kashyap M, Liu G, et al. A systematic review and Canadian consensus recommendations on the use of biomarkers in the treatment of non-small cell lung cancer. J Thorac Oncol. 2011;6:1379–91.

52. Vignot S, Frampton GM, Soria JC, Yelensky R, Commo F, Brambilla C, et al. Next-generation sequencing reveals high concordance of recurrent somatic alterations between primary tumor and metastases from patients with non-small-cell lung cancer. J Clin Oncol. 2013;31:2167–72.

53. Pao W, Ladanyi M. Epidermal growth factor receptor mutation testing in lung cancer: searching for the ideal method. Clin Cancer Res. 2007;13:4954–5.

54. Leushner J, Chiu NH. Automated mass spectrometry: a revolutionary technology for clinical diagnostics. Mol Diagn. 2000;5:341–8.

55. Tuononen K, Mäki-Nevala S, Sarhadi VK, Wirtanen A, Rönty M, Salmenkivi K, et al. Comparison of targeted next-generation sequencing (NGS) and real-time PCR in the detection of EGFR, KRAS, and BRAF mutations on formalin-fixed, paraffin-embedded tumor material of non-small cell lung

carcinoma-superiority of NGS. Genes Chromosomes Cancer. 2013;52:503–11.

56. Hirsch FR, Varella-Garcia M, McCoy J, West H, Xavier AC, Gumerlock P, et al. Increased epidermal growth factor receptor gene copy number detected by fluorescence in situ hybridization associates with increased sensitivity to gefitinib in patients with bronchioloalveolar carcinoma subtypes: a Southwest Oncology Group Study. J Clin Oncol. 2005;23:6838–45.

57. Takano T, Ohe Y, Sakamoto H, Tsuta K, Matsuno Y, Tateishi U, et al. Epidermal growth factor receptor gene mutations and increased copy numbers predict gefitinib sensitivity in patients with recurrent non-small-cell lung cancer. J Clin Oncol. 2005;23:6829–37.

58. Zhu CQ, da Cunha SG, Ding K, Sakurada A, Cutz JC, Liu N, et al. Role of KRAS and EGFR as biomarkers of response to erlotinib in National Cancer Institute of Canada Clinical Trials Group Study BR.21. J Clin Oncol. 2008;26:4268–75.

59. Miller VA, Riely GJ, Zakowski MF, Li AR, Patel JD, Heelan RT, et al. Molecular characteristics of bronchioloalveolar carcinoma and adenocarcinoma, bronchioloalveolar carcinoma subtype, predict response to erlotinib. J Clin Oncol. 2008;26:1472–8.

60. Sholl LM, Xiao Y, Joshi V, Yeap BY, Cioffredi LA, Jackman DM, et al. EGFR mutation is a better predictor of response to tyrosine kinase inhibitors in non-small cell lung carcinoma than FISH, CISH, and immunohistochemistry. Am J Clin Pathol. 2010; 133:922–34.

61. Li AR, Chitale D, Riely GJ, Pao W, Miller VA, Zakowski MF, et al. EGFR mutations in lung adenocarcinomas: clinical testing experience and relationship to EGFR gene copy number and immunohistochemical expression. J Mol Diagn. 2008;10:242–8.

62. Pirker R, Pereira JR, von Pawel J, Krzakowski M, Ramlau R, Park K, et al. EGFR expression as a predictor of survival for first-line chemotherapy plus cetuximab in patients with advanced non-small-cell lung cancer: analysis of data from the phase 3 FLEX study. Lancet Oncol. 2012;13:33–42.

63. Brevet M, Arcila M, Ladanyi M. Assessment of EGFR mutation status in lung adenocarcinoma by immunohistochemistry using antibodies specific to the two major forms of mutant EGFR. J Mol Diagn. 2010;12:169–76.

64. Yu J, Kane S, Wu J, Benedettini E, Li D, Reeves C, et al. Mutation-specific antibodies for the detection of EGFR mutations in non-small-cell lung cancer. Clin Cancer Res. 2009;15:3023–8.

65. Kato Y, Peled N, Wynes MW, Yoshida K, Pardo M, Mascaux C, et al. Novel epidermal growth factor receptor mutation-specific antibodies for non-small cell lung cancer: immunohistochemistry as a possible screening method for epidermal growth factor receptor mutations. J Thorac Oncol. 2010;5:1551–8.

66. Kawahara A, Yamamoto C, Nakashima K, Azuma K, Hattori S, Kashihara M, et al. Molecular diagnosis of activating EGFR mutations in non-small cell lung cancer using mutation-specific antibodies for

immunohistochemical analysis. Clin Cancer Res. 2010;16:3163–70.

67. Kitamura A, Hosoda W, Sasaki E, Mitsudomi T, Yatabe Y. Immunohistochemical detection of EGFR mutation using mutation-specific antibodies in lung cancer. Clin Cancer Res. 2010;16:3349–55.

68. Kozu Y, Tsuta K, Kohno T, Sekine I, Yoshida A, Watanabe S, et al. The usefulness of mutation-specific antibodies in detecting epidermal growth factor receptor mutations and in predicting response to tyrosine kinase inhibitor therapy in lung adenocarcinoma. Lung Cancer. 2011;73:45–50.

69. Kwak EL, Bang YJ, Camidge DR, Shaw AT, Solomon B, Maki RG, et al. Anaplastic lymphoma kinase inhibition in non-small-cell lung cancer. N Engl J Med. 2010;363:1693–703.

70. Horn L, Pao W. EML4-ALK: honing in on a new target in non-small-cell lung cancer. J Clin Oncol. 2009;27:4232–5.

71. Rikova K, Guo A, Zeng Q, Possemato A, Yu J, Haack H, et al. Global survey of phosphotyrosine signaling identifies oncogenic kinases in lung cancer. Cell. 2007;131:1190–203.

72. Takeuchi K, Choi YL, Togashi Y, Soda M, Hatano S, Inamura K, et al. KIF5B-ALK, a novel fusion onco-kinase identified by an immunohistochemistry-based diagnostic system for ALK-positive lung cancer. Clin Cancer Res. 2009;15:3143–9.

73. Boland JM, Erdogan S, Vasmatzis G, Yang P, Tillmans LS, Johnson MR, et al. Anaplastic lymphoma kinase immunoreactivity correlates with ALK gene rearrangement and transcriptional up-regulation in non-small cell lung carcinomas. Hum Pathol. 2009;40:1152–8.

74. Sasaki T, Rodig SJ, Chirieac LR, Jänne PA. The biology and treatment of EML4-ALK non-small cell lung cancer. Eur J Cancer. 2010;46:1773–80.

75. Shaw AT, Yeap BY, Mino-Kenudson M, Digumarthy SR, Costa DB, Heist RS, et al. Clinical features and outcome of patients with non-small-cell lung cancer who harbor EML4-ALK. J Clin Oncol. 2009; 27:4247–53.

76. Wong DW, Leung EL, So KK, Tam IY, Sihoe AD, Cheng LC, et al. The EML4-ALK fusion gene is involved in various histologic types of lung cancers from nonsmokers with wild-type EGFR and KRAS. Cancer. 2009;115:1723–33.

77. Inamura K, Takeuchi K, Togashi Y, Nomura K, Ninomiya H, Okui M, et al. EML4-ALK fusion is linked to histological characteristics in a subset of lung cancers. J Thorac Oncol. 2008;3:13–7.

78. Rodig SJ, Mino-Kenudson M, Dacic S, Yeap BY, Shaw A, Barletta JA, et al. Unique clinicopathologic features characterize ALK-rearranged lung adenocarcinoma in the western population. Clin Cancer Res. 2009;15:5216–23.

79. Inamura K, Takeuchi K, Togashi Y, Hatano S, Ninomiya H, Motoi N, et al. EML4-ALK lung cancers are characterized by rare other mutations, a TTF-1 cell lineage, an acinar histology, and young onset. Mod Pathol. 2009;22:508–15.

80. Yoshida A, Tsuta K, Nakamura H, Kohno T, Takahashi F, Asamura H, et al. Comprehensive histologic analysis of ALK-rearranged lung carcinomas. Am J Surg Pathol. 2011;35:1226–34.

81. Chaft JE, Rekhtman N, Ladanyi M, Riely GJ. ALK-rearranged lung cancer: adenosquamous lung cancer masquerading as pure squamous carcinoma. J Thorac Oncol. 2012;7:768–9.

82. Camidge DR, Bang YJ, Kwak EL, Iafrate AJ, Varella-Garcia M, Fox SB, et al. Activity and safety of crizotinib in patients with ALK-positive non-small-cell lung cancer: updated results from a phase 1 study. Lancet Oncol. 2012;13:1011–9.

83. Shaw AT, Yeap BY, Solomon BJ, Riely GJ, Gainor J, Engelman JA, et al. Effect of crizotinib on overall survival in patients with advanced non-small-cell lung cancer harbouring ALK gene rearrangement: a retrospective analysis. Lancet Oncol. 2011;12:1004–12.

84. Shaw AT, Kim DW, Nakagawa K, Seto T, Crinó L, Ahn MJ, et al. Crizotinib versus chemotherapy in advanced ALK-positive lung cancer. N Engl J Med. 2013;368:2385–94.

85. Choi YL, Soda M, Yamashita Y, Ueno T, Takashima J, Nakajima T, et al. EML4-ALK mutations in lung cancer that confer resistance to ALK inhibitors. N Engl J Med. 2010;363:1734–9.

86. Heuckmann JM, Hölzel M, Sos ML, Heynck S, Balke-Want H, Koker M, et al. ALK mutations conferring differential resistance to structurally diverse ALK inhibitors. Clin Cancer Res. 2011;17:7394–401.

87. Mino-Kenudson M, Chirieac LR, Law K, Hornick JL, Lindeman N, Mark EJ, et al. A novel, highly sensitive antibody allows for the routine detection of ALK-rearranged lung adenocarcinomas by standard immunohistochemistry. Clin Cancer Res. 2010; 16:1561–71.

88. Yi ES, Boland JM, Maleszewski JJ, Roden AC, Oliveira AM, Aubry MC, et al. Correlation of IHC and FISH for ALK gene rearrangement in non-small cell lung carcinoma: IHC score algorithm for FISH. J Thorac Oncol. 2011;6:459–65.

89. Paik JH, Choe G, Kim H, Choe JY, Lee HJ, Lee CT, et al. Screening of anaplastic lymphoma kinase rearrangement by immunohistochemistry in non-small cell lung cancer: correlation with fluorescence in situ hybridization. J Thorac Oncol. 2011;6:466–72.

90. Roberts PJ, Stinchcombe TE. KRAS mutation: should we test for it, and does it matter? J Clin Oncol. 2013;31:1112–21.

91. Santos E, Martin-Zanca D, Reddy EP, Pierotti MA, Della Porta G, Barbacid M. Malignant activation of a K-ras oncogene in lung carcinoma but not in normal tissue of the same patient. Science. 1984; 223:661–4.

92. Forbes S, Clements J, Dawson E, Bamford S, Webb T, Dogan A, et al. COSMIC 2005. Br J Cancer. 2006; 94:318–22.

93. Raparia K, Villa C, DeCamp MM, Patel JD, Mehta MP. Molecular profiling in non-small cell lung cancer—a step toward personalized medicine. Arch Pathol Lab Med. 2013;137:481–91.

94. Cho JY, Kim JH, Lee YH, Chung KY, Kim SK, Gong SJ, et al. Correlation between K-ras gene mutation and prognosis of patients with non small cell lung carcinoma. Cancer. 1997;79:462–7.

95. Slebos RJ, Kibbelaar RE, Dalesio O, Kooistra A, Stam J, Meijer CJ, et al. K-ras oncogene activation as a prognostic marker in adenocarcinoma of the lung. N Engl J Med. 1990;323:561–5.

96. Keohavong P, DeMichele MA, Melacrinos AC, Landreneau RJ, Weyant RJ, Siegfried JM. Detection of K-ras mutations in lung carcinomas: relationship to prognosis. Clin Cancer Res. 1996;2:411–8.

97. John T, Liu G, Tsao MS. Overview of molecular testing in non-small-cell lung cancer: mutational analysis, gene copy number, protein expression and other biomarkers of EGFR for the prediction of response to tyrosine kinase inhibitors. Oncogene. 2009;28 Suppl 1:S14–23.

98. Nagarajan L, Louie E, Tsujimoto Y, Balduzzi PC, Huebner K, Croce CM. The human c-ros gene (ROS) is located at chromosome 6q16-6q22. Proc Natl Acad Sci USA. 1986;83:6568–72.

99. Oxnard GR, Binder A, Janne PA. New targetable oncogenes in non-small cell lung cancer. J Clin Oncol. 2013;31:1097–104.

100. Bergethon K, Shaw AT, Ou SH, Katayama R, Lovly CM, McDonald NT, et al. ROS1 rearrangements define a unique molecular class of lung cancers. J Clin Oncol. 2012;30:863–70.

101. Rimkunas VM, Crosby KE, Li D, Hu Y, Kelly ME, Gu TL, et al. Analysis of receptor tyrosine kinase ROS1-positive tumors in non-small cell lung cancer: identification of a FIG-ROS1 fusion. Clin Cancer Res. 2012;18:4449–57.

102. Stumpfova M, Janne PA. Zeroing in on ROS1 rearrangements in non-small cell lung cancer. Clin Cancer Res. 2012;18:4222–4.

103. Davies KD, Le AT, Theodoro MF, Skokan MC, Aisner DL, Berge EM, et al. Identifying and targeting ROS1 gene fusions in non-small cell lung cancer. Clin Cancer Res. 2012;18:4570–9.

104. Yoshida A, Kohno T, Tsuta K, Wakai S, Arai Y, Shimada Y, et al. ROS1-rearranged lung cancer: a clinicopathologic and molecular study of 15 surgical cases. Am J Surg Pathol. 2013;37:554–62.

105. Shaw AT, Camidge DR, Engelman JA, Solomon BJ, Kwak EL, Clark JW, et al. Clinical activity of crizotinib in advanced non-small cell lung cancer harboring ROS1 gene rearrangement. J Clin Oncol. 2012;30(Suppl):7508.

106. Awad MM, Katayama R, McTigue M, Liu W, Deng YL, Brooun A, et al. Acquired resistance to crizotinib from a mutation in CD74-ROS1. N Engl J Med. 2013;368:2395–401.

107. Wan PT, Garnett MJ, Roe SM, Lee S, Niculescu-Duvaz D, Good VM, et al. Mechanism of activation of the RAF-ERK signaling pathway by oncogenic mutations of B-RAF. Cell. 2004;116:855–67.

108. Paik PK, Arcila ME, Fara M, Sima CS, Miller VA, Kris MG, et al. Clinical characteristics of patients with lung adenocarcinoma harboring BRAF mutations. J Clin Oncol. 2011;29:2046–51.

109. Marchetti A, Felicioni L, Malatesta S, Grazia Sciarrotta M, Guetti L, Chella A, et al. Clinical features and outcome of patients with non-small-cell lung cancer harboring BRAF mutations. J Clin Oncol. 2011;29:3574–9.

110. Junker K, Stachetzki U, Rademacher D, Linder A, Macha HN, Heinecke A, et al. HER2/neu expression and amplification in non-small cell lung cancer prior to and after neoadjuvant therapy. Lung Cancer. 2005;48:59–67.

111. Ramieri MT, Murari R, Botti C, Pica E, Zotti G, Alo PL. Detection of HER2 amplification using the SISH technique in breast, colon, prostate, lung and ovarian carcinoma. Anticancer Res. 2010;20:1287–92.

112. Shigematsu H, Takahashi T, Nomura M, Majmudar K, Suzuki M, Lee H, et al. Somatic mutations of the HER2 kinase domain in lung adenocarcinomas. Cancer Res. 2005;65:1642–6.

113. Tomizawa K, Suda K, Onozato R, Kosaka T, Endoh H, Sekido Y, et al. Prognostic and predictive implications of HER2/ERBB2/neu gene mutations in lung cancers. Lung Cancer. 2011;74:139–44.

114. Li C, Sun Y, Fang R, Han X, Luo X, Wang R, et al. Lung adenocarcinomas with HER2-activating mutations are associated with distinct clinical features and HER2/EGFR copy number gains. J Thorac Oncol. 2012;7:85–9.

115. Weir BA, Woo MS, Getz G, Perner S, Ding L, Beroukhim R, et al. Characterizing the cancer genome in lung adenocarcinoma. Nature. 2007;450:893–8.

116. Ding L, Getz G, Wheeler DA, Mardis ER, McLellan MD, Cibulskis K, et al. Somatic mutations affect key pathways in lung adenocarcinoma. Nature. 2008;455:1069–75.

117. Job B, Bernheim A, Beau-Faller M, Camilleri-Broet S, Girard P, Hofman P, et al. Genomic aberrations in lung adenocarcinoma in never smokers. PLoS One. 2010;5:e15145.

118. Govindan R, Ding L, Griffith M, Subramanian J, Dees ND, Kanchi KL, et al. Genomic landscape of non-small cell lung cancer in smokers and never-smokers. Cell. 2012;150:1121–34.

119. Imielinski M, Berger AH, Hammerman PS, Hernandez B, Pugh TJ, Hodis E, et al. Mapping the hallmarks of lung adenocarcinoma with massively parallel sequencing. Cell. 2012;150:1107–20.

120. Kohno T, Ichikawa H, Totoki Y, Yasuda K, Hiramoto M, Nammo T, et al. KIF5B-RET fusions in lung adenocarcinoma. Nat Med. 2012;18:375–7.

121. Lipson D, Capelletti M, Yelensky R, Otto G, Parker A, Jarosz M, et al. Identification of new ALK and RET gene fusions from colorectal and lung cancer biopsies. Nat Med. 2012;18:382–4.

122. Seo JS, Ju YS, Lee WC, Shin JY, Lee JK, Bleazard T, et al. The transcriptional landscape and mutational profile of lung adenocarcinoma. Genome Res. 2012;22:2109–19.

123. Kim SC, Jung Y, Park J, Cho S, Seo C, Kim J, et al. A high-dimensional, deep-sequencing study of lung adenocarcinoma in female never-smokers. PLoS One. 2013;8:e55596.

124. Li T, Kung HJ, Mack PC, Gandara DR. Genotyping and genomic profiling of non-small-cell lung cancer: implications for current and future therapies. J Clin Oncol. 2013;31:1039–49.

125. Travis WD. Pathology of lung cancer. Clin Chest Med. 2011;32:669–92.

126. Rekhtman N, Paik PK, Arcila ME, Tafe LJ, Oxnard GR, Moreira AL, et al. Clarifying the spectrum of driver oncogene mutations in biomarker-verified squamous carcinoma of lung: lack of EGFR/KRAS and presence of PIK3CA/AKT1 mutations. Clin Cancer Res. 2012;18:1167–76.

127. Ji H, Zhao X, Yuza Y, Shimamura T, Li D, Protopopov A, et al. Epidermal growth factor receptor variant III mutations in lung tumorigenesis and sensitivity to tyrosine kinase inhibitors. Proc Natl Acad Sci USA. 2006;103:7817–22.

128. Sasaki H, Kawano O, Endo K, Yukiue H, Yano M, Fujii Y. EGFRvIII mutation in lung cancer correlates with increased EGFR copy number. Oncol Rep. 2007;17:319–23.

129. Massion PP, Kuo WL, Stokoe D, Olshen AB, Treseler PA, Chin K, et al. Genomic copy number analysis of non-small cell lung cancer using array comparative genomic hybridization: implications of the phosphatidylinositol 3-kinase pathway. Cancer Res. 2002;62:3636–40.

130. Garnis C, Lockwood WW, Vucic E, Ge Y, Girard L, Minna JD, et al. High resolution analysis of non-small cell lung cancer cell lines by whole genome tiling path array CGH. Int J Cancer. 2006;118:1556–64.

131. Garnis C, Davies JJ, Buys TP, Tsao MS, MacAulay C, Lam S, et al. Chromosome 5p aberrations are early events in lung cancer: implication of glial cell line-derived neurotrophic factor in disease progression. Oncogene. 2005;24:4806–12.

132. Bass AJ, Watanabe H, Mermel CH, Yu S, Perner S, Verhaak RG, et al. SOX2 is an amplified lineage-survival oncogene in lung and esophageal squamous cell carcinomas. Nat Genet. 2009;41:1238–42.

133. Boelens MC, Kok K, van der Vlies P, van der Vries G, Sietsma H, Timens W, et al. Genomic aberrations in squamous cell lung carcinoma related to lymph node or distant metastasis. Lung Cancer. 2009; 66:372–8.

134. Hussenet T, Dali S, Exinger J, Monga B, Jost B, Dembele D, et al. SOX2 is an oncogene activated by recurrent 3q26.3 amplifications in human lung squamous cell carcinomas. PLoS One. 2010;5:e8960.

135. Craddock KJ, Lam WL, Tsao MS. Applications of array-CGH for lung cancer. Methods Mol Biol. 2013;973:297–324.

136. Wistuba II, Behrens C, Milchgrub S, Bryant D, Hung J, Minna JD, et al. Sequential molecular abnormalities are involved in the multistage devel-opment of squamous cell lung carcinoma. Oncogene. 1999;18:643–50.

137. Okudela K, Suzuki M, Kageyama S, Bunai T, Nagura K, Igarashi H, et al. PIK3CA mutation and amplification in human lung cancer. Pathol Int. 2007;57:664–71.

138. Ji M, Guan H, Gao C, Shi B, Hou P. Highly frequent promoter methylation and PIK3CA amplification in non-small cell lung cancer (NSCLC). BMC Cancer. 2011;11:147.

139. Kawano O, Sasaki H, Endo K, Suzuki E, Haneda H, Yukiue H, et al. PIK3CA mutation status in Japanese lung cancer patients. Lung Cancer. 2006;54:209–15.

140. Yamamoto H, Shigematsu H, Nomura M, Lockwood WW, Sato M, Okumura N, et al. PIK3CA mutations and copy number gains in human lung cancers. Cancer Res. 2008;68:6913–21.

141. Jin G, Kim MJ, Jeon HS, Choi JE, Kim DS, Lee EB, et al. PTEN mutations and relationship to EGFR, ERBB2, KRAS, and TP53 mutations in non-small cell lung cancers. Lung Cancer. 2010;69:279–83.

142. Do H, Solomon B, Mitchell PL, Fox SB, Dobrovic A. Detection of the transforming AKT1 mutation E17K in non-small cell lung cancer by high resolution melting. BMC Res Notes. 2008;1:14.

143. Malanga D, Scrima M, De Marco C, Fabiani F, De Rosa N, De Gisi S, et al. Activating E17K mutation in the gene encoding the protein kinase AKT1 in a subset of squamous cell carcinoma of the lung. Cell Cycle. 2008;7:665–9.

144. Weiss J, Sos ML, Seidel D, Peifer M, Zander T, Heuckmann JM, et al. Frequent and focal FGFR1 amplification associates with therapeutically tracta-ble FGFR1 dependency in squamous cell lung can-cer. Sci Transl Med. 2010;2:62ra93.

145. Dutt A, Ramos AH, Hammerman PS, Mermel C, Cho J, Sharifnia T, et al. Inhibitor-sensitive FGFR1 amplification in human non-small cell lung cancer. PLoS One. 2011;6:e20351.

146. Ford CE, Lau SK, Zhu CQ, Andersson T, Tsao MS, Vogel WF. Expression and mutation analysis of the discoidin domain receptors 1 and 2 in non-small cell lung carcinoma. Br J Cancer. 2007;96:808–14.

147. Hammerman PS, Sos ML, Ramos AH, Xu C, Dutt A, Zhou W, et al. Mutations in the DDR2 kinase gene identify a novel therapeutic target in squamous cell lung cancer. Cancer Discov. 2011;1:78–89.

148. Day E, Waters B, Spiegel K, Alnadaf T, Manley PW, Buchdunger E, et al. Inhibition of collagen-induced discoidin domain receptor 1 and 2 activation by ima-tinib, nilotinib and dasatinib. Eur J Pharmacol. 2008; 599:44–53.

149. Cancer Genome Atlas Research Network. Comprehensive genomic characterization of squa-mous cell lung cancers. Nature. 2012;489:519–25.

150. Travis WD. Update on small cell carcinoma and its differentiation from squamous cell carcinoma and other non-small cell carcinomas. Mod Pathol. 2012;25 Suppl 1:S18–30.

151. Voortman J, Lee JH, Killian JK, Suuriniemi M, Wang Y, Lucchi M, et al. Array comparative genomic hybridization-based characterization of genetic alterations in pulmonary neuroendocrine tumors. Proc Natl Acad Sci USA. 2010;107:13040–5.

152. Pleasance ED, Stephens PJ, O'Meara S, McBride DJ, Meynert A, Jones D, et al. A small-cell lung cancer genome with complex signatures of tobacco exposure. Nature. 2010;463:184–90.

153. Peifer M, Fernandez-Cuesta L, Sos ML, George J, Seidel D, Kasper LH, et al. Integrative genome analyses identify key somatic driver mutations of small-cell lung cancer. Nat Genet. 2012;44:1104–10.

154. Rudin CM, Durinck S, Stawiski EW, Poirier JT, Modrusan Z, Shames DS, et al. Comprehensive genomic analysis identifies SOX2 as a frequently amplified gene in small-cell lung cancer. Nat Genet. 2012;44:1111–6.

155. Pietanza MC, Ladanyi M. Bringing the genomic landscape of small-cell lung cancer into focus. Nat Genet. 2012;44:1074–5.

Molecular testing in Gynecological Malignancies

14

Pamela M. Ward and Louis Dubeau

Gynecological Tumors of Epithelial Origin

Current FDA-approved molecular tests for gynecological malignancies apply exclusively to epithelial tumors, which are the main focus of this chapter. We grouped these tumors into those derived from the lower and upper reproductive tract because such classification is convenient for a discussion of molecular tests relevant to their clinical management. Carcinomas of the upper reproductive tract should be further subdivided into those of uterine versus extrauterine origin because of differences in their clinicopathological parameters, such as approach to staging and others, but are indistinguishable from a molecular pathological viewpoint.

Embryological Concepts Relevant to Understanding Epithelial Tumor Development in Gynecological Organs

Epithelial tumors of the female reproductive organs can be grouped into those from the upper reproductive tract embryologically derived from

the Müllerian ducts and those from the lower reproductive tract that can be regarded as extensions of the perineal integument. A brief review of their embryological development is relevant in our understanding of their molecular, etiological, and morphological differences. The upper reproductive tract is almost entirely derived from the Müllerian ducts, which first appear as two distinct tubular structures closely related to the fetal kidneys that eventually fuse in their most distal portion, initially giving rise to the upper third of the vagina, cervix, and uterus. The most proximal portions remain unfused and give rise to the fallopian tubes. The lower portion of the vagina is the result of an invagination of the perineal skin that later connects to the Müllerian duct derivatives. The boundary between the stratified squamous epithelium derived from the skin and the columnar epithelium derived from the Müllerian ducts, first located in the upper vagina, migrates to the cervix at later stages of development, giving rise to the squamocolumnar junction delineating the exocervix from the endocervix. This boundary, often referred to as the transformation zone, is the site of origin of most cervical carcinomas. It is not static, as it shifts upwards towards the uterus or downwards towards the vagina during the reproductive years, resulting in fluctuations in the nature of the lining epithelia immediately adjacent to the transition zone.

Not only does the epithelial lining of the lower and upper reproductive tract show fundamental differences at the morphological and functional levels, but also the mechanisms of tumor

P.M. Ward, Ph.D. • L. Dubeau, M.D., Ph.D. (✉)
USC/Norris Comprehensive Cancer Center,
Keck School of Medicine of University of Southern California, 1441 Eastlake Avenue, Los Angeles, CA 90089, USA
e-mail: ldubeau@usc.edu

G.M. Yousef and S. Jothy (eds.), *Molecular Testing in Cancer*,
DOI 10.1007/978-1-4899-8050-2_14, © Springer Science+Business Media New York 2014

229

development from these sites and, therefore, of molecular changes targeted by molecular pathological tests relevant to the management of these tumors are different. For example, organs from the lower reproductive tract, which include vulva, vagina, and exocervix lined by stratified squamous epithelium, give rise to tumors driven by infections with human papillomaviruses (HPV). The upper reproductive tract, which includes endocervix, uterus, fallopian tube, and extrauterine Müllerian duct derivatives, is lined by various types of columnar epithelium that give rise to tumors driven primarily by reproductive hormones. A notable exception to this concept is the frequent presence of human papillomavirus infections in endocervical adenocarcinomas [3]. This may be due not only to the vicinity of this organ to the exocervix, a frequent site of infection by these viruses, but also to the mobility of the transformation zone. There is no evidence that mucinous tumors of the upper reproductive tract, which are morphologically indistinguishable from those arising within the endocervix, are associated with such infections and the exact role of human papillomavirus in the development of endocervical adenocarcinomas is currently unclear.

The ovary, which until recently was thought to be the site of origin of most extrauterine serous, endometrioid, clear cell, and mucinous carcinomas, is not derived from the Müllerian ducts. The fact that these epithelial tumors historically considered to be of primary ovarian origin are morphologically identical to tumors arising in Müllerian duct derivatives [4] has intrigued pathologists over much of the last century, leading to the formulation of a theory based on Müllerian metaplasia of the ovarian surface epithelium, the merit of which continues to be debated [1].

Epithelial Tumors of the Lower Reproductive Tract

This group comprises tumors arising in the stratified squamous epithelium of the vulva, vagina, and exocervix. Embryologically, these epithelia are extensions of the epithelial lining of the skin. They are almost always associated with prior infection with HPV, a non-enveloped, double-stranded DNA virus with a genome of approximately 8 kb [5–9].

Table 14.1 Human papillomavirus subtypes commonly found in the lower reproductive tract

Oncogenic risk classification	Human papillomavirus subtypes
High risk (HR)	16, 18, 31, 33, 35, 39, 45, 51, 52, 56, 58, 59, 68, 73, 82
Probable HR	26, 53, 66
Low risk (LR)	6, 11, 40, 42, 43, 44, 54, 61, 72, 81, CP6108

Mechanism of infection with human papillomaviruses. The genome of HPV, first sequenced in 1982 [10, 11], consists of (1) two major oncogenes, E6 and E7, which bind and inactivate the P53 and RB proteins, respectively; (2) two regulatory proteins, E1 and E2, involved in transcription and replication; and (3) two structural proteins, L1 and L2, which comprise the viral capsid. Over 200 human papillomavirus subtypes have been described, approximately 40 of which are known to infect the human genital mucosa. Of these, only a subset has carcinogenic potential [6, 7, 9]. The International Agency for Research on Cancer classifies these viruses based on such potential [8], which is primarily determined by the affinity of viral E6 and E7 proteins to P53 and RB. Most of the experimental data on viruses associated with high carcinogenic risk comes from work with HPV-16 and HPV-18, so the classification into high- versus low-risk groups is often based on epidemiologic evidence. All human papillomavirus subtypes that belong to a few genetically similar species in the α genus of the evolutionary tree are cervical carcinogens [12]. All others are not carcinogenic and are associated with the development of benign genital warts [7, 12]. Based on prevalence, the subtypes included in screening tests are generally from those listed in Table 14.1.

Approximately 90 % of human papillomavirus infections are resolved by cell-mediated immunity within 1–2 years of exposure, which also obviates the risk of disease progression. While all of the high-risk subtypes have varying degrees of oncogenic potential, HPV-16 and HPV-18 alone are respectively responsible for approximately 55–60 % and 10–15 % of all squamous cell carcinomas of the vulva, vagina, and cervix. HPV-18 infection is found to be more closely associated with cervical adenocarcinomas than with squamous cell carcinomas [5, 6, 8, 9, 13, 14].

Upon infection of the cervical epithelium, the circular viral DNA first remains episomal and carries a low risk of transformation of the host cell. The viral DNA eventually integrates into the host genome, at which time the viral E2 gene is commonly lost leading to constitutive expression of the oncoproteins E6 and E7. These two proteins bind to and cause degradation of the p53 and RB proteins, respectively, resulting in constitutive activation of the cell cycle and disruption of important cell cycle checkpoints, both of which predispose the host cell to malignant transformation. Such transformation is usually preceded by cervical intraepithelial neoplasia, the precursor lesion targeted by early detection screening programs based on the Papanicolaou test. It is the differences in affinity of the viral E6 and E7 proteins to P53 and RB that distinguishes viral subtypes associated with high versus low risk of malignant transformation [5, 6, 8, 9].

Detection of human papillomavirus DNA. Molecular tests used in the clinical management of tumors of the lower reproductive tract and of their precursor lesions focus on the demonstration of the presence of human papillomavirus DNA in surgical or cytological specimens and on the subtyping of such viruses based on their oncogenic potential. Most of the data comes from studies of squamous cell carcinoma of the cervix and of cervical intraepithelial neoplasia as the exocervix is by far the most common site of origin of these lesions. In spite of more than 10 years of testing, there are still 12,000 new cases of cervical cancer each year in the USA and a further 500,000 women are diagnosed with moderate- or high-grade cervical intraepithelial neoplasia grade 2 and 3 [15, 16], underscoring the need for improved diagnostic algorithms and testing availability. The exclusivity of human papillomavirus infections as the single cause of cervical cancer should theoretically allow for near eradication of this disease.

Most tests for HPV target the genotype-specific differences of the well-conserved *L1* locus in the late gene region of the viral genome.

Table 14.2 FDA-approved liquid cytology-based assays for human papillomavirus

Name	Manufacturer	FDA approval date
Aptima HPV-16 18/45 genotype assay	Gen-Probe, Inc.	10/12/2012
Aptima HPV assay	Gen-Probe, Inc.	10/28/2011
COBAS HPV test	Roche molecular systems, Inc.	4/19/2011
Cervista HPV-16/18	Hologic, Inc.	3/12/2009
Cervista HPV HR and Genfind DNA extraction kit	Hologic, Inc.	3/12/2009
Digene hybrid capture (HC2) high-risk HPV DNA test	Digene Corporation (acquired by Qiagen)	12/14/2004

The L1 protein is a major viral capsid protein that is the antigen against which both current vaccines, Gardasil and Cervarix, were raised. In contrast to infections with high-risk subtypes, the viral DNA remains episomal in infections with low-risk subtypes.

The first commercially available assay for HPV was the Roche Linear Array assay that came to the market in 2003. This assay, which is no longer available, allowed detection of high- and low-risk subtypes but did not distinguish between these two groups. Liquid cytology-based tests currently approved by the FDA are listed in Table 14.2. High-risk human papillomavirus subtypes identified in different FDA-approved assays are listed in Table 14.3. The Digene Hybrid Capture 2 test, which became available in 2004, was the first to distinguish high- from low-risk groups and rapidly became the established standard as a versatile platform allowing for either low-volume, manual, or large-scale automated approaches.

The ATHENA (Addressing the Need for Advanced HPV Diagnostics) trial. The single most important issue is the ability to detect infections with viruses associated with the highest risk of progression to carcinoma, 70 % of which involve either HPV-16 or HPV-18. The importance of identifying these subtypes is also evidenced in the 2012 revised guidelines for the prevention and early detection of cervical cancer [14]. A clinical trial named "Addressing the Need for Advanced HPV

Table 14.3 High-risk human papillomavirus subtypes identified in FDA-approved assays

Name	Detection target	High-risk human papillomavirus subtypes detected
COBAS HPV	Viral DNA	Individual: 16,18
		Pooled: 31, 33, 35, 39, 45, 51, 52, 56, 58, 59, 66, and 68
Aptima HPV-16 18/45 genotype	E6 and E7 RNA	16
		18/45
Aptima HPV	E6 and E7 RNA	Pooled: 16, 18, 31, 33, 35, 39, 45, 51, 52, 56, 58, 66, and 68
Cervista HPV-16/18	Viral DNA	Pooled: 16 and 18
Cervista HPV HR	Viral DNA	16, 18, 31, 33, 35, 39, 45, 51, 52, 56, 58, 59, and 68
Digene HC2 HPV HR/LR	Viral DNA	Pooled high risk: 16, 18, 31, 33, 35, 39, 45, 51, 52, 56, 58, 59, and 68
		Pooled low risk: 6, 11, 42, 43, and 44

Diagnostics" (ATHENA) was initiated to provide new diagnostic algorithms to improve patient outcome [16, 17]. The main objectives were (1) to evaluate performance of the COBAS HPV test for triage of women with abnormal cytology and (2) to provide an adjunctive test for guidance in the clinical management in women with no cytological evidence of intraepithelial lesions or carcinoma. The trial evaluated the clinical performance of a new COBAS test (Table 14.3) that individually reports on HPV-16 and HPV-18 subtypes within a pool of an additional 12 high-risk subtypes. For the first time, this test platform enabled stratification of women into those infected with HPV-16/18 versus those infected with high-risk groups other than HPV-16/18 without the need of a secondary test.

The ATHENA trial enrolled 46,887 women between 21 and 93 years of age. Cytological abnormalities were found in 6.9, 6.2, and 4.1 % of women aged 30–39, 40–49, and 50–59 years, respectively. High-risk infections were found in 25 % of women aged 21–29 and declined with increasing age, affecting only 5.0 % of women infected after the age of 70 (Fig. 14.1). The trial also confirmed a low overall prevalence of HPV-16 in women older

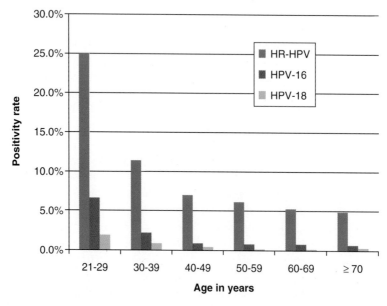

Fig. 14.1 Age distribution of high-risk human papillomavirus infections from ATHENA trial. Adapted from Wright et al. [16]

than 30 years (2.3–0.7 % depending on age group) compared to 6.8 % in the 21–29-year age group; a similar pattern was seen for HPV-18 but with much lower prevalences (2.0–0.2 %) (Fig. 14.1).

The sensitivity of the COBAS test to detect high-grade cervical intraepithelial neoplasia in women with atypical squamous cells in their cytological specimen was 90 %, which compared well to the performance of the established standard, the Digene HC2 test with a sensitivity of 87.2 %. The COBAS and HC2 tests have similar specificity metrics of 70.5 % and 71.1 %, respectively. Importantly, the COBAS test allows for patient stratification by identifying those women harboring HPV-16 and HPV-18 infections. Women who were HPV-16 positive were more than twice as likely to have moderate- to high-grade cervical intraepithelial neoplasia as those with high-risk infections not involving HPV-16 or HPV-18 [16, 17]. Persistence of infection increases the risk of developing a precancerous lesion; women infected with HPV-16 for 3–5 years have a 40 % risk of developing high-grade cervical intraepithelial neoplasia, which in turn carries a 30 % risk of progression to invasive carcinoma in 30 years compared to 1 % if treated.

Other competing tests. Kinney et al. [18] compared the Cervista package insert to that of published data for the HC2 test. They concluded that the Cervista test detected 2- to 4-fold more human papillomavirus infections than the HC2 test in women older than 30 years and with normal cytology. True performance metrics for the Cervista test were subsequently published that do not support these initial findings. Quigley et al. [19] found no significant differences between the percent positive cases detected by Cervista versus HC2 in women with no evidence of intraepithelial lesion or malignancy and in women aged 30 years or more with atypical squamous cells of unknown significance tested at three different sites. Similar results were obtained by Chateau et al. [20] and Kurian et al. [21].

The Aptima test stands apart from the other tests in that it targets the detection of E6/E7 mRNA, which is associated with integration of the virus into the host cell genome and malignant transformation [22]. It therefore probes the most clinically relevant infections. L1/L2 deletion sometimes occurs in addition to loss of E1/E2 following integration, leading to potential false-negative results with L1-based detection assays [23]. However, E6/E7 is only transcriptionally active once the virus has integrated so false-negative results are primarily seen with early high-risk infections when episomal virus is present. While Gen-Probe does offer two Aptima tests, the latter allowing detection of either pooled high-risk virions or HPV-16/18/45 versus HPV-18 and HPV-45, this assay is unable to distinguish between HPV-18 and HPV-45 subtypes, which does not meet the revised screening guidelines. Interestingly, HPV-18 and HPV-45 are very closely related subtypes belonging to the α7 HPV species while HPV-16 belongs to the more distal α9 HPV species [12].

Szarewski et al. [24] used liquid-based cytology samples from 1,099 women referred to colposcopy to compare the HC2, COBAS and APTIMA tests, and three other tests from the European market (Abbott real-time HR-HPV, BD real-time HPV, and NORCHIP *PreTect* HPV-Proofer NASBA based). With the exception of the *PreTect* assay, all platforms had similar detection rates of reporting either HPV-16 infections or all high-risk infections considered as a group (Fig. 14.2). All tests showed similar sensitivities between 93.3 and 96.3 % and specificities between 19.5 and 28.8 % for detection of moderate (Fig. 14.2) and high-grade cervical intraepithelial neoplasia. The HC2 test was the least specific while the APTIMA test was the most specific for the detection of moderate- and high-grade intraepithelial neoplasia. There was generally high sensitivity for detection of high-grade lesions (Fig. 14.2). The *PreTect* NASBA-based assay also targets E6/E7 expression and shows increased specificity compared to the APTIMA test but was less sensitive, diminishing its clinical utility (Fig. 14.2).

Alternative testing platforms. Cervical biopsies can be screened by in situ hybridization, which has the advantage of detecting the virus in morphologically preserved tissue. Although this approach

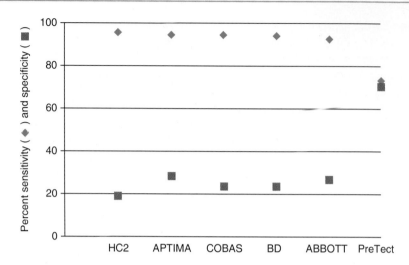

Fig. 14.2 Performance of commonly used tests for human papillomavirus infection in detecting moderate cervical intraepithelial neoplasia (CIN2). Adapted from Szarewski et al. [24]

has historically been associated with poor sensitivity, improved signal-detection methods are now obtainable [25] allowing routine detection of 50–100 copies per cell. The College of American Pathologists concluded in a recent survey (CAP ISH Survey Summary 2010B) that the test by Ventana, Inc. is the preferred source of HPV in situ hybridization probes. The Ventana INFORM HPV III Family 16 Probe (B) contains a mixture of viral genomic probes targeting a number of high-risk subtypes (16, 18, 31, 33, 35, 39, 45, 51, 52, 56, 58, and 66) that can detect as few as 1–2 integrated HPV-16 copies per cell. In situ hybridization also allows evaluation of infection progression, as early infections are characterized by episomal virus presenting with globular-like staining patterns while integration, seen at later stages of disease progression, is characterized by a dot-like signal.

Current testing guidelines for the prevention of cervical carcinoma. The 2012 revised screening recommendations for the prevention and early detection of cervical cancer [14] introduced a new diagnostic algorithm, to simultaneously perform cytological examination and test for human papillomavirus infection in all women 30–65 years old. Women who test positive for

the HPV-16 and HPV-18 and those infected with other high-risk viruses are stratified into different diagnostic algorithms. The goal is to identify infections that are most likely to progress to invasive cancer while minimizing the detection of false-positive results given that 90 % of HPV infections are known to resolve spontaneously.

Identification of infections associated with low-risk of progression to carcinoma, which is of little diagnostic value, is no longer included in the newer generations of tests for human papillomavirus.

Testing for human papillomavirus in a screening setting will allow comparing the performance metrics of the various assays that are as yet untested. Data from the ATHENA trial in which samples were collected from women aged 21 years and older during routine screening included results from both liquid-based cytology and COBAS HPV testing. As expected, the prevalence of high-risk infection declined with increasing age as did the incidence of abnormal cytology [16, 17]. Likewise, the disparity between the presence of infection and abnormal cytology lessened with increasing age. More specifically, the incidence of HPV-16/18 infection in women aged 40 years or more aligns closely to that of low-grade squamous intraepithelial lesions.

Already, the ATHENA data supports the new algorithm for co-testing and stratification of women with HPV-16/18 infections irrespective of the cytology results.

Endocervical adenocarcinoma. Although there has been a steady decline in the incidence of invasive cervical cancer since the implementation of cervical screening, this mostly benefited the incidence of squamous cell carcinoma. In fact, the incidence of cervical adenocarcinoma is rising [8, 26]. While it is expected that cervical screening is not as sensitive to detect cervical adenocarcinoma compared to squamous lesions due to their relative decreased accessibility, this cannot account for the observed increase in adenocarcinoma. Although an underlying infection with human papillomavirus is invariably present in essentially all squamous cell carcinomas of the cervix, such infections are absent in a significant proportion of adenocarcinomas [3]. Thus, the exact role of this virus in the development of endocervical tumors is still unclear. The spectrum of human papillomavirus subtypes associated with endocervical adenocarcinoma is slightly different than that associated with squamous cell carcinoma of the exocervix, with HPV-18 infections being slightly more prevalent in adenocarcinomas [13, 14].

Prevention of cervical carcinoma by vaccination against human papillomaviruses. It is hoped that the development of vaccines against the human papillomavirus will significantly decrease the incidence of cervical carcinoma. Such vaccines are not effective once integration of the viral genome into that of the host has occurred. Thus, current vaccines can only be effective in preventing future infections in unexposed individuals and, at least based on current technology, cannot be used to treat existing infections. The *Gardasil* (Merck, NJ) and *Cervarix* (GlaxoSmithKline, London, UK) vaccines exploit the HPV L1 protein as the antigen. *Gardasil* was approved in 2006 and targets HPV-6, 11, 16, and 18, while *Cervarix* was approved in 2009 and targets HPV-16 and HPV-18. Vaccination is approved for women between the ages approximately 10–25 years.

Epithelial Tumors of Müllerian Origin

This group includes serous, endometrioid, clear cell and mucinous tumors either of endocervical, endometrial, or extrauterine origin. The latter category includes tumors historically classified as of primary ovarian and peritoneal origins as well as carcinomas arising in the fallopian tube fimbriae [2]. Currently, all molecular tests applicable to epithelial tumors of Müllerian origin are performed in the context of specific familial predisposition syndromes, namely, the hereditary breast and ovarian cancer syndrome and Lynch syndrome [27–29].

Hereditary Breast and Extrauterine Müllerian (Ovarian) Cancer

Almost all individuals with hereditary breast and extrauterine Müllerian (ovarian) cancer syndromes harbor germline mutations in either BRCA1 or BRCA2. Such mutations are associated with increased risk of serous carcinoma of the fallopian tube fimbriae and of other extrauterine Müllerian structures historically classified as of primary ovarian or peritoneal origin. Whether BRCA1/2 mutation carriers are also at increased risk of developing serous carcinoma of the endometrium is still unclear. Although BRCA1/2 mutations have been reported in serous endometrial carcinomas [30], there is a debate as to whether or not tamoxifen therapy is the main driver of endometrial carcinoma in BRCA1/2 mutation carriers [31, 32].

Role of BRCA1/2 in cancer development. In the general population, BRCA1 mutations carry a 39 % risk of developing ovarian cancer by age 70 years and an 11 % risk for BRCA2 mutations. While pathogenic mutations are distributed across the entire genes, some regions are more closely associated with ovarian cancer. Exon 11 of the BRCA2 gene constitutes the Ovarian Cancer Cluster Region. Families with mutations in this region are more likely to develop ovarian cancer than breast cancer. The cluster region contains conserved BRC motifs (so named from BRCA2 gene) that interact with Rad51 recombinase, the critical component driving homologous recombination to repair DNA double-stranded breaks [29]. Other mechanisms of DNA repair include mismatch repair, nucleotide excision repair, transcription-coupled repair, and nonhomologous end joining. While the role of BRCA2 in DNA repair is more closely associated with homologous recombination, that of BRCA1 is associated with multiple mechanisms. BRCA1 is also involved in cell cycle checkpoints including the mitotic checkpoint at the anaphase-promoting complex and in the control of cytokinesis, failure of which leads to polyploidy, a precursor to aneuploidy [33]. Thus, with BRCA1/2 protein loss of function, normal DNA repair mechanisms and other important cellular regulatory mechanisms are disrupted. When these are superimposed on a p53 mutation, which is present in essentially all high-grade serous gynecological tumors, the genomic abnormalities that result from loss of functional BRCA1 or BRCA2 proteins are unchecked, increasing the risk of malignant transformation. Although the fact that most tumors that arise in BRCA mutation carriers show loss of heterozygosity affecting the wild-type allele suggests that these two proteins are classical tumor suppressors, this does not account for their site specificity. Indeed, although tumors arising in *BRCA2* mutation carriers show a less restricted organ distribution, those arising in *BRCA1* mutation carriers develop almost exclusively in breast and gynecological organs. It has been suggested that BRCA1 mutations are associated with cancer predisposition via a cell-nonautonomous mechanism driven by consequences of such mutations on the menstrual cycle, which in turn is the greatest risk factor for epithelial tumors of the female upper reproductive tract [33–35].

Screening for BRCA1 and BRCA2 mutations. The lifetime risk of extrauterine Müllerian (ovarian) cancer in the US general population is 1.4 %, which dramatically increases to 15–40 % in women who carry germline mutations in *BRCA1* or *BRCA2*. Overall, the incidence of *BRCA1/2* mutations in the US population is 0.2 % and includes numerous sequence variants of unknown significance. Screening is not recommended for

Table 14.4 Founder BRCA1/2 mutations in Ashkenazi Jews

Gene	Mutation	Incidence (%)
BRCA1	187delAG (formerly 185delAG)	1.1
	5385insC	0.15
BRCA2	6174delT	1.5

the general population, but should be considered for those women with close relatives diagnosed with breast and ovarian cancer, especially if the relative is less than 50 years old. A person is also strongly recommended to consider testing if a BRCA1/2 mutation has been found in a family member, or if a male family member develops breast cancer.

Many BRCA1/2 sequence variants have been detected. As of September 2012, 1,484 of such variants are listed for *BRCA1* and 1,886 for *BRCA2* on the Universal Mutation Database website (www.umd.be). Most are rare or have not been associated with an increased cancer risk, implying that they may represent inconsequential polymorphisms. Frequency of individual mutations associated with increased cancer risk differs by ethnicity [36]. For example, Ashkenazi Jews, who have substantially elevated risk for breast and extrauterine serous cancers, have three well-described founder mutations (Table 14.4) with a combined frequency of 1:40.

Myriad Genetics, Inc. is the owner of patents relating to the genetic testing of BRCA1 and BRCA2 with the right to sublicense. This has created a testing landscape where the majority of the testing is performed by this organization, with some laboratories around the USA performing limited mutations panels (e.g., Ashkenazi Jewish panels) under sublicensed agreements. Myriad Genetics offers three different levels of testing: (1) comprehensive analysis for full sequencing of the BRCA genes, (2) multisite panels for specific founder mutations, and (3) single site analysis for those families in which a specific mutation has already been described. This monopoly of BRCA testing at a single commercial site has been at the center of legal debate for some time.

Recently, DNA patent laws have been successfully challenged (*Assoc. for Mol. Path. v. Myriad*: Isolated Human DNA is Not Patent-Eligible Subject Matter 2013) in that the US Supreme Court invalidated several BRCA-1/-2 patents. However, legal hurdles around methodology patents remain, which will continue to limit wide spread adoption of testing across the US.

Lynch Syndrome

Lynch syndrome is an autosomal dominant disorder that increases the risk of affected families for a broad spectrum of malignancies. This syndrome has historically been called hereditary nonpolyposis colorectal cancer (HNPCC) to distinguish it from familial polyposis coli, another syndrome associated with increased predisposition to colorectal cancer, the malignancy most frequently associated with Lynch syndrome. In the general population, the incidence of Lynch syndrome is estimated to be between 1:2,000 and 1:660 with a 25–60 % lifetime risk of developing endometrioid cancers of either uterine or extrauterine origin, the latter typically associated with endometriosis. Approximately 50,000 new cases of such cancers are diagnosed each year, of which 5 % are attributed to Lynch syndrome. This syndrome is caused by mutations in the mismatch repair enzymes *MLH1, MSH2, MSH6*, and *PSM2* that catalyze the repair of small base-pair substitutions and insertion/deletion errors that arise during DNA replication [37]. It is thought that loss of function of these enzymes leads to an increased rate of mutations that in turn predispose to malignant transformation. Overall, 90 % of germline mutations in mismatch repair genes are found in MLH1 and MSH2, with 7–10 % involvement of MSH6 and less than 5 % in PSM2. However, most endometrioid gynecological cancers are associated with MSH6 mutations [38, 39].

Microsatellite DNA. The accumulation of DNA replication errors is the hallmark of Lynch syndrome. While such errors are evidenced across the entire genome, microsatellite sequences, which are tandem repeats of short sequences ranging from one to six nucleotides in length widely distributed throughout the genome, are

particularly sensitive. In addition, they are readily amenable to molecular testing in clinical settings. The length of the repeated monomeric sequence in microsatellites is inversely proportional to the frequency of base mismatch occurring during DNA replication, implying that single-nucleotide repeats are more prone to replication errors than longer repeats. These single-nucleotide repeats are also the most abundant in the human genome, with poly(A) and poly(T) being more frequent than poly(C) and poly(G).

Microsatellite instability (MSI). Although DNA sequencing of genes encoding mismatch repair enzymes is the most definitive test for Lynch syndrome, documentation of microsatellite instability, often evaluated together with immunohistochemistry for mismatch repair enzymes, is a widely used and much more economical approach. This approach entails enzymatic amplification of a panel of microsatellite sequences in paired samples from normal and cancerous tissues from the same individuals, followed by electrophoresis of the PCR product in order to separate them based on their size. The number of repeated units within a microsatellite locus is maintained when normal mismatch repair mechanisms are intact so that the overall length of any given microsatellite in cancerous tissues is not different from that in normal cells from the same individuals (microsatellite stable). Frequent shifts in the electrophoretic mobility of amplicons from microsatellites isolated from cancerous tissues (Fig. 14.3) are the diagnostic hallmark of microsatellite instability, which is frequently seen with defective mismatch repair mechanisms such as in individuals with Lynch syndrome.

The use of this approach in the diagnosis of Lynch syndrome is based on a statistical argument demonstrating that the frequency of microsatellite instability is higher in cancerous tissues than in normal tissues from the same individual. Such frequency can vary depending on the nature and number of the microsatellite sequences examined. Thus, there is a need for standardization of these parameters in order to ensure reproducibility among different laboratories. To this end, a panel of microsatellite loci was established by the

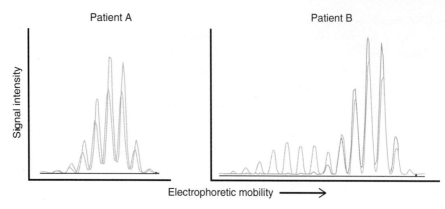

Fig. 14.3 Example of microsatellite instability detected by capillary electrophoresis. DNA samples isolated from matched normal and cancerous tissues from two different patients were amplified enzymatically using primers for a monomeric microsatellite locus (NR-21). The PCR products were subjected to capillary electrophoresis. The electrophoretic mobility tracings of the products obtained with the normal tissue samples (*blue*) and those obtained from the cancerous tissues (*orange*) are superimposed in order to allow for better comparison. Identical patterns are seen for the normal and cancerous tissues in patient A, indicating microsatellite stability in this patient's tumor at this locus. Although the mobility tracings from the cancerous tissue completely overlap those from the normal tissue sample in patient B, additional signals of lower electrophoretic mobility are also present in the cancerous sample that are not seen with the normal tissue sample indicating microsatellite instability

Table 14.5 Microsatellite markers from the original and revised Bethesda guidelines

Original Bethesda panel	GenBank no.	Revised Bethesda panel marketed by Promega	GenBank no.
Bat-25 $(A)_{25}$	L04143	Bat-25 $(A)_{25}$	L04143
Bat-26 $(A)_{26}$	U41210	Bat-26 $(A)_{26}$	U41210
D2S123 $(CA)_n$	Z16551	NR-21 $(A)_{21}$	XM_033393
D5S346 $(CA)_n$	NM_005669	NR-24 $(A)_{24}$	X60152
D17S250 $(CA)_n$	NT_010783.15	Mono-27 $(A)_{27}$	AC007684
		Penta C $(AAAAG)_{3-15}$	AL138752
		Penta D $(AAAAG)_{2-17}$	AC000014

Bethesda guidelines in 1996 [40] (Table 14.5). The original panel consisted of two mononucleotide and three dinucleotide repeats. Revised guidelines from 2004 [41] recommended emphasis on the more sensitive mononucleotide repeats (Table 14.5). Also recommended is inclusion of penta-nucleotide repeats to verify that the matched normal and tumor samples used are indeed from the same patient. The finding of microsatellite instability in more than one third of microsatellite sequences examined (MSI-High) is regarded as indicative of an abnormality in a mismatch repair enzyme.

Many laboratories offer testing for microsatellite instability in formalin-fixed paraffin-embedded tissues. A 2012 proficiency survey by the College of American Pathologists revealed that 63 % of laboratories use the kit marketed by Promega Corporation, which was specifically designed to meet the recommendations in the revised Bethesda guidelines.

Issues related to gynecological tumors specifically. Most of the work on microsatellite instability has been carried out on colorectal carcinomas and is discussed in a separate chapter. It is estimated that Lynch syndrome accounts for 5 % of endometrioid carcinomas of either the endometrium or extrauterine endometrial tissues, the latter usually associated with endometriosis [2].

Although microsatellite instability can also be seen in endometrioid tumors not associated with Lynch syndrome such as those with methylation of the promoter region of genes encoding mismatch repair enzymes, it still needs to be determined whether or not these are associated with a different prognosis, as is the case for colorectal carcinomas. Another issue is whether the fact that mutations in MSH6 are more frequent in these tumors than in colorectal tumors among individuals affected by Lynch syndrome has any consequences on the type of microsatellite sequences more prone to show instability. Should this be the case, there will be a need for tumor type-specific microsatellite panels applicable to some, but not all cancers associated with Lynch syndrome.

Other Gynecological Cancers That May Benefit from Molecular Tests

There are currently no established molecular pathological tests commonly used in the management of other epithelial tumors of Müllerian origin or in gynecological tumors of stromal or germ cell origins. This is likely to change with the development of novel targeted therapies, many of which are currently under investigation [42, 43]. Additionally, data from next generation sequencing will provide a clearer understanding of the molecular basis of these tumors that will drive the exploitation of such therapies. This effort contributes to the increasing list of mutations associated with specific tumor types that may become the target of clinically useful molecular tests in the near future [44–48] (Table 14.6). For example, serous carcinomas arising either in the endometrium or in extrauterine Müllerian epithelium generally lack microsatellite instability but are associated with mutations in P53. In contrast, endometrioid tumors often show microsatellite instability and are also associated with mutations in PTEN but lack P53 mutations. These differences could provide means of distinguishing the clinically more aggressive high-grade serous tumors from the less aggressive endometrioid tumors, an important clinical problem. Mutations

Table 14.6 Genetic alterations commonly associated with gynecological tumors of the upper reproductive tract

Origin	Histological subtype	Genetic anomalies
Epithelial	Low-grade serous	BRAF/KRAS
		IGF receptor
	High-grade serous	p53
		PI3K/AKT
		BRCA1/2
	Endometrioid	PTEN
		Microsatellite instability
		β-catenin
		ARID1A
	Mucinous	K-RAS
	Clear cell	PTEN
		Microsatellite instability
		TMS-1/ASC
		ARID1A
Stromal	Granulosa cell	FOXL2

in ARID1A, which are associated with non-serous endometrial tumors [49], could provide the basis for another molecular test allowing distinction between these tumors and the less aggressive endometrioid and clear cell tumors.

Although the PI3K/AKT/mTOR signaling pathway is often altered in both serous and endometrioid tumors, documentation of such activity is becoming relevant given that new mTOR inhibitors are currently in clinical trials that have shown some efficacy against endometrioid cancers [50, 51]. Likewise, the PI3K/AKT pathway is frequently deregulated in high-grade serous ovarian cancer, while activation of the KRAS/BRAF/MEK/MAPK signaling pathway is primarily seen in low-grade serous (and mucinous) tumors, providing a potential molecular diagnostic tool to complement morphological criteria in distinguishing between these histological subtypes associated with significant differences in prognosis and therapeutic management.

Additional examples include the association between clear cell carcinomas and TMS-1-/ASC-targeted methylation [48]. FOXL2 C134W mutation is seen in 97 % of granulosa cell tumors [52]. These alterations restricted to specific tumor types could become useful in confirming these diagnoses.

Another important diagnostic problem is in evaluating the malignant potential of stromal tumors such as smooth muscle tumors of the myometrium or the various mixed Müllerian stromal tumors. It is hoped that molecular tests will complement morphological criteria to assist pathologists in making such clinically important distinctions in the foreseeable future.

References

1. Dubeau L, Drapkin R. Coming into focus: the non-ovarian origins of ovarian cancer. Ann Oncol. 2013; 24:viii28–35.
2. Dubeau L. The cell of origin of ovarian epithelial tumours. Lancet Oncol. 2008;9:1191–7.
3. Ferguson AW, Svoboda-Newman SM, Frank TS. Analysis of human papillomavirus infection and molecular alterations in adenocarcinoma of the cervix. Mod Pathol. 1998;11:11–8.
4. Dubeau L. The cell of origin of ovarian epithelial tumors and the ovarian surface epithelium dogma: does the emperor have no clothes? Gynecol Oncol. 1999;72:437–42.
5. Bosch FX, Lorincz A, Munoz N, et al. The causal relation between human papillomavirus and cervical cancer. J Clin Pathol. 2002;55:244–65.
6. Burd EM. Human papilloma virus and cervical cancer. Clin Microbiol Rev. 2003;16:1–17.
7. de Villiers EM, Fauquet C, Broker TR, et al. Classification of papillomaviruses. Virology. 2004;324: 17–27.
8. Schiffman M, Castle PE, Jeronimo J, et al. Human papillomavirus and cervical cancer. Lancet. 2007;370: 890–907.
9. Zheng Z-M, Baker CC. Papillomavirus structure, expression, and post-transcriptional regulation. Front Biosci. 2006;11:2286–302.
10. Chen EY, Howley PM, Levinson AD, Seeburg PH. The primary structure and genetic organization of the bovine papillomavirus type 1 genome. Nature. 1982; 299:529–34.
11. Danos O, Katinka M, Yaniv M. Human papillomavirus 1a complete DNA sequence: a novel type of genome organization among papovaviridae. EMBO J. 1982;1: 231–6.
12. Schiffman M, Clifford G, Buonaguro FM. Classification of weakly carcinogeneic papillomavirus types: addressing the limits of epidemiology at the borderline. Infect Agent Cancer. 2009;4:8.
13. Dunne EF, Unger ER, Sternberg M, et al. Prevalence of HPV infection among females in the United States. JAMA. 2007;297:813–9.
14. Saslow D, Solomon D, Lawson HW, et al. American Cancer Society, American Society for Colposcopy

and Cervical Pathology, and American Society for Clinical Pathology screening guidelines for the prevention and early detection of cervical cancer. Am J Clin Pathol. 2012;137:516–42.
15. Hariri S, Unger ER, Powell SE, et al. Human papillomavirus genotypes in high-grade cervical lesions in the United States. J Infect Dis. 2012;206:1878–86.
16. Wright Jr TC, Stoler MH, Behrens CM, et al. The ATHENA human papillomavirus study: design, methods, and baseline results. Am J Obstet Gynecol. 2012;206:46.e1–46.e11.
17. Stoler MH, Wright Jr TC, Sharma A, et al. High-risk human papillomavirus testing in women with ASC-US cytology: results from the ATHENA HPV study. Am J Clin Pathol. 2011;135:468–75.
18. Kinney W, Stoler MH, Castle PE. Special commentary: patient safety and the next generation of HPV DNA tests. Am J Clin Pathol. 2010;134:193–9.
19. Quigley NB, Potter NT, Chivukula M, et al. Rate of detection of high-risk HPV with two assays in women >/= 30 years of age. J Clin Virol. 2011;52:23–7.
20. du Chateau BK, Schroeder ER, Munson E. Clinical laboratory experience with CERvista HPV HR as a function of cytological classification: comparison with retrospective digene HC@ high-risk HPV DNA test data. J Clin Microbiol. 2013;51:1057–62.
21. Kurian EM, Caporelli M-L, Baker S, et al. Cervista HR and HPV16/18 Assays vs hybrid capture: outcome comparison in women with negative cytology. Am J Clin Pathol. 2011;136:808–16.
22. Morris BJ. Cervical human papillomavirus screening by PCR: advantages of targeting the E6/E7 region. Clin Chem Lab Med. 2005;43:1171–7.
23. Karlsen F, Kalantari M, Jenkins A, et al. Use of multiple PCR primer sets for optimal detection of human papillomavirus. J Clin Microbiol. 1996;34:2095–100.
24. Szarewski A, Mesher D, Cadman L, et al. Comparison of seven tests for high-grade cervical intraepithelial neoplasia in women with abnormal smears: the Predictors 2 study. J Clin Microbiol. 2012;50: 1867–73.
25. Kelesidis T, Aish L, Steller MA, et al. Human papillomavirus (HPV) detection using in situ hybridization in histologic samples: correlations with cytologic changes and polymerase chain reaction HPV detection. Am J Clin Pathol. 2011;136:119–27.
26. Seoud M, Tjalma WA, Ronsse V. Cervical adenocarcinoma: moving towards better prevention. Vaccine. 2011;29:9148–58.
27. Folkins AK, Longacre TA. Hereditary gynaecological malignancies: advances in screening and treatment. Histopathology. 2013;62:2–30.
28. Smith JA. Gynecologic cancers. In Pharmacotherapy Self-Assessment Program-VII Book 6 (Oncology), Edition 7. American College of Clinical Pharmacy; 2011. p. 129–143.
29. Sowter HM, Ashworth A. BRCA1 and BRCA2 as ovarian cancer susceptibility genes. Carcinogenesis. 2005;26:1651–6.

30. Pennington KP, Walsh T, Lee M, et al. BRCA1, TP53, and CHEK2 germline mutations in uterine serous carcinoma. Cancer. 2013;119:332–8.

31. Beiner ME, Finch A, Rosen B, et al. The risk of endometrial cancer in women with BRCA1 and BRCA2 mutations. A prospective study. Gynecol Oncol. 2007; 104:7–10.

32. Duffy DL, Antill YC, Stewart CJ, et al. Report of endometrial cancer in Australian BRCA1 and BRCA2 mutation-positive families. Twin Res Hum Genet. 2011;14:111–8.

33. Yu VM, Marion CM, Austria TM, et al. Role of BRCA1 in controlling mitotic arrest in ovarian cystadenoma cells. Int J Cancer. 2011;130:2495–504.

34. Chodankar R, Kwang S, Sangiorgi F, et al. Cell-nonautonomous induction of ovarian and uterine serous cystadenomas in mice lacking a functional Brca1 in ovarian granulosa cells. Curr Biol. 2005;15: 561–5.

35. Hong H, Yen H-Y, Brockmeyer A, et al. Changes in the mouse estrus cycle in response to Brca1 inactivation suggest a potential link between risk factors for familial and sporadic ovarian cancer. Cancer Res. 2010;70:221–8.

36. Janavicius R. Founder BRCA1/2 mutations in the Europe: implications for hereditary breast-ovarian cancer prevention and control. EPMA J. 2010;1:397–412.

37. Meyer LA, Broaddus RR, Lu KH. Endometrial cancer and Lynch syndrome: clinical and pathologic considerations. Cancer Control. 2009;16:14–22.

38. Goodfellow PJ, Buttin PM, Herzog TJ, et al. Prevalence of defective DNA mismatch repair and MSH6 mutation in an unselected series of endometrial cancers. Proc Natl Acad Sci U S A. 2009;100: 5908–13.

39. Ramsoekh D, Wagner A, van Leerdam EV, et al. Cancer risk in MLH1, MSH2, and MSH6 mutation carriers; different risk profiles may influence clinical management. Hered Cancer Clin Pract. 2009;7:17.

40. Rodriguez-Bigas MA, Boland CR, Hamilton SR, et al. A national cancer institute workshop on hereditary nonpolyposis colorectal cancer syndrome: meeting highlights and Bethesda guidelines. J Natl Cancer Inst. 1997;89:1758–60.

41. Umar A, Boland CR, Terdiman JP, et al. Revised Bethesda guidelines for hereditary nonpolyposis colorectal cancer (Lynch syndrome) and microsatellite instability. J Natl Cancer Inst. 2004;96:261–8.

42. Banerjee S, Kaye SB. New strategies in the treatment of ovarian cancer: current clinical perspectives and future potential. Clin Cancer Res. 2013;19:961–8.

43. Modugno F, Edwards RP. Ovarian cancer: prevention, detection, and treatment of the disease and its recurrence. Molecular mechanisms and personalized medicine meeting report. Int J Gynecol Cancer. 2012;22: S45–57.

44. Ketabi Z, Bartuma K, Bernstein I, et al. Ovarian cancer linked to Lynch syndrome typically presents as early-onset, non-serous epithelial tumors. Gynecol Oncol. 2011;121:462–5.

45. Nout RA, Bosse T, Creutzberg CL, et al. Improved risk assessment of endometrial cancer by combined analysis of MSI, PI3K-AKT, Wnt/beta-catenin and P53 pathway activation. Gynecol Oncol. 2012;126: 466–73.

46. Peterson LM, Kipp BR, Halling KC, et al. Molecular characterization of endometrial cancer: a correlative study assessing microsatellite instability, MLH1 hypermethylation, DNA mismatch repair protein expression, and PTEN, PIK3CA, KRAS, and BRAF mutation analysis. Int J Gynecol Pathol. 2012;31: 195–205.

47. Romero I, Bast Jr RC. Minireview: human ovarian cancer: biology, current management, and paths to personalizing therapy. Endocrinology. 2012;153: 1593–602.

48. Rosen DG, Yang G, Liu G, et al. Ovarian cancer: pathology, biology, and disease models. Front Biosci. 2009;14:2089–102.

49. Wiegand KC, Shah SP, Al-Agha OM, et al. ARID1A mutations in endometriosis-associated ovarian carcinomas. N Engl J Med. 2010;363:1532–43.

50. Diaz-Padilla I, Duran I, Clarke BA, Oza AM. Biologic rationale and clinical activity of mTOR inhibitors in gynecological cancer. Cancer Treat Rev. 2012;38: 767–75.

51. Suh DH, Kim JW, Kim K, et al. Major clinical research advances in gynecologic cancer in 2012. J Gynecol Oncol. 2013;24:66–82.

52. Shah SP, Kobel M, Senz J, et al. Mutation of FOXL2 in granulosa-cell tumors of the ovary. N Engl J Med. 2009;360:2719–29.

Jason Karamchandani

Introduction

The advancing molecular era has fundamentally reshaped the landscape of neuro-oncologic neuropathology. The ever-increasing interest in molecular-based classification algorithms will fundamentally change the way that pathologists classify and surgeons and oncologists treat brain tumors [1]. Recent clinical trials have identified clear differences in prognosis and therapeutic selection for primary brain tumors on the basis of genetic and epigenetic changes, and members of the neuro-oncologic community have called for the assessment of molecular alterations with treatment implications as standard of care [2]. Molecular neuropathology is in rapid transition from the esoteric to the exoteric.

Molecular Alterations in Glioma and Glioneuronal Tumors

Isocitrate Dehydrogenase

The characterization of isocitrate dehydrogenase (IDH) mutations has unquestionably altered our understanding of the biology of adult gliomas.

J. Karamchandani, M.D. (✉)
Department of Laboratory Medicine and Pathobiology,
St. Michael's Hospital, University of Toronto,
30 Bond Street, CC Wing, Room 2-013, Toronto, ON,
Canada M5B 1W8
e-mail: karamchandaj@smh.ca

In their landmark paper on the integrated genomic analysis of glioblastoma, Parsons et al. identified a subpopulation of glioblastomas featuring somatic mutations of IDH1 [3]. In the majority of cases, the alteration involved the R132 amino acid. Even in this initial study, the prognostic benefit and lower age of the afflicted patient population was noted as well as the association with secondary glioblastomas. A year later the prognostic difference between IDH-mutated (IDH2 mutations were also characterized in gliomas) and IDH wild-type tumors was confirmed on a larger data set [4], with the patients with IDH mutations having better outcomes. Mutation of IDH was also characterized in the majority of low-grade astrocytomas and the vast majority of oligodendrogliomas (irrespective of grade). IDH mutation was also identified as a marker of positive prognosis and response to temozolomide in low-grade gliomas [5]. The discovery of IDH mutations in low-grade gliomas also provided insight into the biology of pediatric diffuse astrocytomas, as IDH1 mutations are absent in pediatric cases of infiltrating gliomas [6, 7]. This significant difference in the molecular alterations driving these tumors provides evidence to support what many neuropathologists had suspected for decades—that the biology of pediatric and adult low-grade astrocytoma is different, despite similar morphologic appearance.

Given that the R132H alteration accounted for 90 % of IDH mutations in glioma, a monoclonal antibody directed against the mutant protein was generated and characterized [8–10].

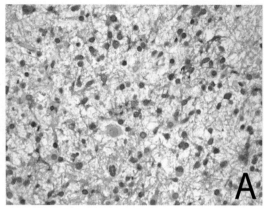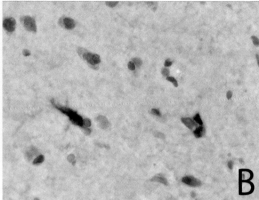

Fig. 15.1 (**a**) IDH1R132H mutant-specific antibody shows diffuse staining in an anaplastic astrocytoma (×400 magnification). (**b**) The mutant-specific antibody can be of considerable diagnostic utility in cases of infiltrating low-grade glioma (especially in needle biopsies) where the stain can highlight rare infiltrating neoplastic cells (×630 magnification)

This antibody has excellent sensitivity and is entirely specific for the mutant protein. This breakthrough has granted neuropathologists the ability to permit directed molecular characterization of brain tumors using brightfield microscopy (Fig. 15.1). The uses of this mutant-specific antibody are manifold. The ability to identify infiltrating tumor cells in a background of predominantly nonneoplastic glial tissue has vastly improved diagnosis of subtle low-grade gliomas. The often morphologically challenging distinction between reactive gliosis and tumor is also markedly improved with the use of IDH1 mutant-specific antibody [8]. The immunohistochemical test for mutant-specific IDH1 has largely supplanted assessment with PCR, though several centers still offer this test. For practicing pathologists, it is worth noting in patient reports that absence of R132H mutant IDH expression does not preclude other mutations of IDH1 or IDH2.

MGMT

O-6-methylguanine-DNA methyltransferase (official symbol MGMT) is a DNA repair gene located on chromosome 10q26. The MGMT gene codes for a DNA repair protein that transfers the alkyl group at the O-6 position (an important site of DNA alkylation) to a cysteine residue within the catalytic site of the enzyme, consequently consuming the MGMT protein. The ability of MGMT to repair the DNA damage caused by alkylating agents renders tumor cells with high levels of MGMT less susceptible to the therapeutic effects of this chemotherapeutic class. Methylation of the MGMT promoter silences the gene and renders cells more susceptible to irreparable DNA damage. Promoter methylation and consequent epigenetic silencing of MGMT associated with longer survival in patients with glioblastoma who receive alkylating agents [11, 12]. This benefit is particularly pronounced in patients of advanced age, as these patients may benefit from temozolomide therapy alone (typical therapy combines chemotherapy with radiotherapy) [13, 14].

Several methods are currently employed to evaluate the methylation status of the MGMT promoter region [15, 16].

MGMT methylation status can be measured in many ways, including assessment of DNA, RNA, or protein expression. With regard to DNA, most of the techniques employed in assessing MGMT promoter methylation status rely upon the differential behavior of 5-methylcytosine and cytosine following treatment with bisulfite: unmethylated

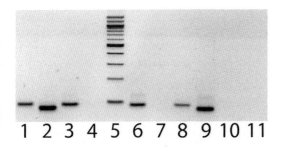

Fig. 15.2 Nested methylation-specific PCR for the MGMT promoter. Lane 1: MGMT promoter methylated sample (Sample 1) with unmethylated primers. Lane 2: Sample 1 with methylation-specific primers (showing methylation of the MGMT promoter). Lane 3: MGMT promoter non-methylated sample (Sample 2) with unmethylated primers. Lane 4: Sample 2 with methylation-specific primers (showing no evidence of methylation of the MGMT promoter). Lane 5: 100 base-pair ladder. Lane 6: Unmethylated MGMT promoter control DNA with unmethylated primers. Lane 7: Unmethylated MGMT promoter control DNA with methylated primers (showing no reaction product). Lane 8: Methylated MGMT promoter control DNA with unmethylated primers (admixed normal tissue shows amplification product). Lane 9: Methylated MGMT promoter control DNA with methylated primers (showing amplification product). Lane 10: Water control with unmethylated primers. Lane 11: Water control with methylated primers. Image courtesy of Catherine Fen Li, M.D., Ph.D. and Sharon Bauer, M.Sc.

cytosine is converted to uracil, while methylated cytosine is not. Methylation sites typically involve CpG dinucleotides or CpG islands (CPI). Unmethylated cytosines consequently appear as T and methylated cytosines as C in the consequent sequences. Methylation-specific PCR (MSP) is currently the most commonly employed method to determine MGMT promoter methylation status and was the method employed in the original study which established the survival benefit associated with this alteration [11] (Fig. 15.2). This study and several subsequent reports have described the difficulties encountered when using MSP in formalin-fixed paraffin-embedded (FFPE) materials [17], though nested PCR methods have improved the sensitivity [12]. The subjectivity of reading the gel has also been cited as a limitation of this technique [18]. Manifold other bisulfite-dependent methods have been characterized and published:

- MethyLight is a fluorescence-based real-time PCR assay that does not require visualization on a gel [19]; while RT-PCR-based methods have been shown to have high concordance with MSP [20], recent studies have shown lower sensitivity than MSP in some cases of glioblastoma [18].
- Pyrosequencing offers the advantage of providing information about individual CpG positions and is a robust method of assessing MGMT status [15, 18]; however, the technology is not currently available in most laboratories.
- Combined bisulfite restriction analysis (COBRA) employs restriction endonucleases to cut genomic DNA to produce different fragment lengths based on the methylation status, and robust techniques have been developed to employ this technique [15].
- Methylation-sensitive high-resolution melting protocols, relying on the different melting points of methylated and non-methylated PCR bisulfite-modified PCR products, has also been shown to be a specific test for MGMT promoter methylation status, though the sensitivity may be lower than MSP and other methods [18].
- A method employing primer extension and high-performance liquid chromatography (SIRPH) [15] has also been developed, though this method ends up basing the assessment of promoter methylation on the basis of only one CpG position.

Methylation-specific multiplex ligation-dependent probe amplification (MS-MLPA) is somewhat unique in that it avoids the bisulfite conversion step. In this method, the methylation-specific probe contains a methylation-sensitive restriction site. The sample is split and one-half is subjected to a single ligation step, while the second is also subjected to the methylation-specific digestion. Both samples are amplified with PCR, and comparing the subsequent peak ratios of the fragment analysis generates the methylation ratio [21].

Bead methylation arrays (Illumina), also a bisulfite-dependent method, have been used to determine the methylation status of up to several thousand CpG sites in brain tumors (including assessment of the MGMT promoter). Studies employing this technique have also demonstrated the expected correlation between MGMT methylation status and outcome [22].

The reliability of immunohistochemical staining for MGMT is controversial, and while some studies have shown association between protein expression and survival [23], several studies have not shown concordance between protein expression and methylation studies, while other studies have shown no association between survival and MGMT protein expression. Many groups consider immunohistochemistry unsuitable for clinical use at this time [16, 21]. As with any immunohistochemical test, difficulties include standardization of antibodies and protocols, as well as interobserver variability and establishing cutoff values.

1p/19q

The discovery of the co-deletion of chromosomes 1p and 19q [24–26] in oligodendrogliomas could perhaps be credited with ushering oncologic neuropathology into the molecular era. The loss of 1p/19q occurs as the consequence of an unbalanced translocation between chromosome 1 and chromosome 19 [t(1;19)(q10;p10)] [27]. More recently, next-generation sequencing studies have identified concurrent mutations on the remaining 19q in the CIC gene and FUBP1 on the remaining 1p [28, 29]. Nearly all 1p/19q co-deleted oligodendrogliomas are also mutated on IDH1 or IDH2 [30].

The survival benefit associated with this genetic alteration [31] made the molecular testing of oligodendrogliomas of unquestionable importance, and this testing became the first widely adopted molecular assay in a primary brain tumor. Recently, the European Organisation for Research and Treatment of Cancer 26951 trial also established a clinical survival benefit for patients treated with radiation specifically in patients with 1p/19q co-deletion [32].

Given the importance of assessing the 1p/19q status of a tumor, as is the case with regard to MGMT, many methods of assessing for this signature chromosomal alteration have been developed. Fluorescence in situ hybridization is the most commonly employed of these methods as most laboratories have the equipment necessary to perform this assay. Protocols to evaluate for 1p/19q co-deletion (including reliable probes) are well established and widely used [33–35] (Fig. 15.3).

Several PCR-based methods for testing for loss of heterozygosity (LOH) have been described which work with FFPE material [36, 37].

Comparative genomic hybridization, a technique particularly well suited to evaluate for chromosomal alterations, was originally used in the research setting [38] but was quickly validated in the clinical setting in FFPE material [39].

Multiplex ligation-dependent probe amplification is a comparatively newer technique in which as many as 40 loci can be evaluated. This method has also been established as a reliable and sensitive method to evaluate for 1p19q co-deletion [40].

Many other existing molecular techniques can be adapted to assess for copy number alterations, notably SNP chip arrays [41] and next-generation sequencing [42].

BRAF

BRAF (official name: v-raf murine sarcoma viral oncogene homolog B1) is located on chromosome 7q34. This gene belongs to the raf family of serine/threonine kinases and plays a role in modulating MAP kinase and extracellular signal-related kinases and plays a role in cell division and differentiation.

BRAF plays a role in multiple tumors of the central nervous system (CNS) but does so in two distinct and mutually exclusive fashions: V600E mutation and tandem duplication resulting in a novel fusion product.

BRAF Mutation

BRAF mutations have been implicated in many types of neoplasms including non-Hodgkin lymphoma, colorectal cancer, thyroid carcinoma, pulmonary adenocarcinoma, and notably malignant cutaneous melanoma, in which BRAF is mutated in approximately 50 % of cases. The V600E mutation involves the substitution of glutamic acid for valine at amino acid 600. This particular mutation is responsible for the vast majority of oncogenic BRAF mutations and to

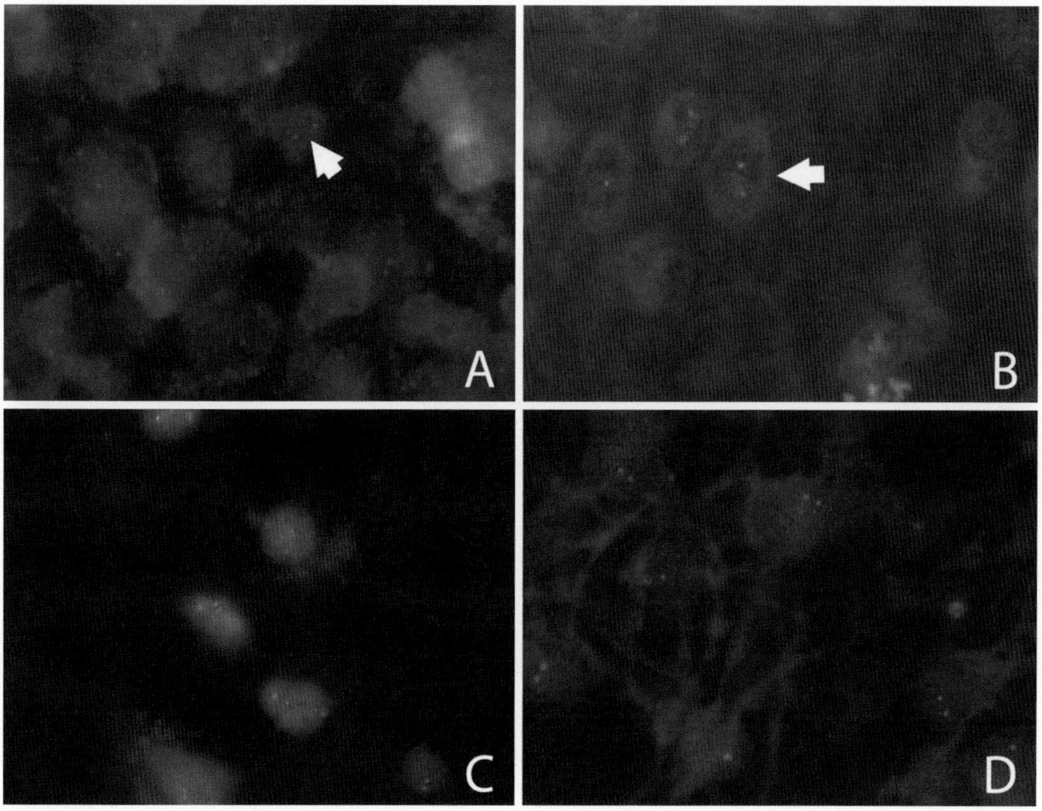

Fig. 15.3 Fluorescence in situ hybridization performed on an oligodendroglioma shows (**a**) only one *orange signal* for 1p36 and two *green signals* for 1q25 (*arrowhead*) and (**b**) one *orange signal* for 19q13 and two *green signals* for 19p13 (*arrowhead*). The same test on a glioma with no evidence of co-deletion for 1p (**c**) or 19q (**d**). All images at ×1,000 magnification. Image courtesy of Catherine Fen Li, M.D., Ph.D. and Sharon Bauer, M.Sc.

date is the only BRAF mutation known as an agent of CNS tumor genesis.

A large study of 1,320 brain tumors identified a subset of tumors with high BRAF mutation frequency, notably pleomorphic xanthoastrocytoma (PXA), ganglioglioma, extra-cerebellar pilocytic astrocytoma [43], and pediatric low-grade astrocytoma [44].

PXA and ganglioglioma are both malignancies more frequent in younger patients with peak incidence in the second and third decades of life [45]. The morphology of these tumors frequently overlaps, and indeed the composite PXA-ganglioglioma is well described [46]. The study also took care to note that the BRAF-mutated pilocytic astrocytomas typically occurred in the diencephalon and were seen in only 1/53 (2 %) of cerebellar cases.

As noted in the section devoted to IDH mutation, pediatric low-grade astrocytomas appear to be distinct from their adult counterparts at the molecular level. IDH mutations, common in adult low-grade astrocytomas, are not present in pediatric low-grade astrocytoma. Conversely, BRAF mutation is frequently seen in pediatric astrocytomas [44].

Testing for the BRAFV600E mutation has traditionally been carried out with PCR and Sanger sequencing, but recently a monoclonal antibody has been developed against the V600E mutant protein [47]. Published reports suggest this antibody is both sensitive and specific with high concordance when compared to sequencing results (97.1 %) [48]. It is expected that this antibody will be made widely available by the time this chapter is published.

Our understanding of BRAF V600E mutation is perhaps made more important by vemurafenib (brand name: Zelboraf). This oral medication is a potent BRAF kinase inhibitor that inhibits tumor growth by inhibiting kinase activity of mutated forms of BRAF, including the V600E mutation. The drug does not have activity against cells with wild-type BRAF. This drug is currently employed in the treatment of patients with malignant melanoma with BRAF mutation. It is already being employed in patients with metastatic melanoma to the CNS. It is likely that the number of metastatic lesions with BRAF mutations treated with vemurafenib will expand in the coming years. The effectiveness of this treatment in primary neoplasms of the CNS has yet to be characterized, though trials in pediatric glioma are under way [49].

BRAF Tandem Duplication/Fusion

BRAF has also been implicated in the pathogenesis of pilocytic astrocytoma. Pilocytic astrocytomas are associated with neurofibromatosis type 1 (and associated loss of the NF1 gene neurofibromin 1, 17q11.2). In patients with NF1, these tumors frequently involve the optic nerve. The majority of pilocytic astrocytomas involving the posterior fossa show no evidence of NF1 alterations [50]. More sensitive methods identified gains of chromosome 17q34 involving the BRAF gene [51]. This alteration was accompanied by increased MEK-ERK signaling. The specific rearrangement involves a tandem duplication of the BRAF gene with an in-frame fusion with KIAA1549 resulting in a novel fusion gene [52]. This rearrangement is most common in pilocytic astrocytomas arising in the posterior fossa [53]. The BRAF status does not appear to alter the behavior of pilocytic astrocytomas when adjusted with the site of origin, with cerebellar and superficial cortical tumors behaving more favorably (likely due to comparative facility of surgical resection) [54].

Several methods are employed to assess for the BRAF tandem duplication/fusion product. Fluorescence in situ hybridization using a fusion probe is a sensitive and specific method for evaluating for this genetic alteration (Fig. 15.3) [55].

A robust RT-PCR-based method suitable for use in FFPE tissue has also been described [56]. The presence of this fusion is highly specific for a diagnosis of pilocytic astrocytoma.

EGFR

Epidermal growth factor receptor is a cell surface protein kinase that binds epidermal growth factor. Mutations in EGFR are well characterized and are covered in the chapter on molecular oncology of pulmonary neoplasms. EGFR is the most commonly amplified gene in glioblastoma and occurs in more than a third of cases of glioblastoma [57]. EGFR amplification, which typically occurs as double-minute extrachromosomal elements, is more common in primary glioblastoma as opposed to secondary tumors [58]. EGFR participates in the phosphatase and tensin homologue (PTEN)/Akt/MTOR pathway—an important driver of glioma-genesis. The small cell variant of glioblastoma in particular has a high frequency of EGFR amplification [59]. Given the diagnostic challenge occasionally posed by this unusual morphologic variant (notably with anaplastic oligodendroglioma), assessing EGFR amplification status may serve a role in diagnostic classification. EGFR amplification is easily assessed by fluorescence in situ hybridization. Roche has recently released a probe for EGFR and chromosome 7 suitable for evaluation for EGFR amplification by dual in situ hybridization (DISH) suitable for interpretation with brightfield microscopy [60]. The expected result should appear similar to the Her2/neu chromosome 17 assay which is FDA and Health Canada approved for the evaluation of Her2/neu amplification (Fig. 15.4).

EGFR vIII is the most common mutant variant of EGFR in glioblastoma, and more than half of EGFR amplified tumors show amplification of this variant [61], which is marked by an in-frame deletion of amino acid residues 6 through 273 of the extracellular domain of the EGFR protein [62]. This variant protein presents a unique opportunity for targeted immunotherapy, and an antibody was developed against the mutant protein [62, 63]. A variant-specific peptide vaccine

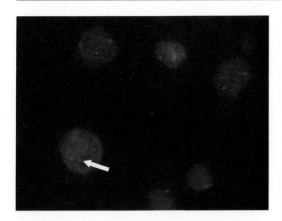

Fig. 15.4 Fluorescence in situ hybridization on a case of pilocytic astrocytoma showing duplication of BRAF with fusion with KIAA1549 resulting in a *yellow signal* [*arrow*] (×1,000 magnification). Image courtesy of Catherine Fen Li, M.D., Ph.D. and Sharon Bauer, M.Sc.

was also developed, and phase I and phase II trials were completed with positive results [64]. Recently, an EGFRvIII-specific recombinant antibody has been developed which, in addition to possibly having therapeutic uses, is suitable for diagnostic use in FFPE tissue [65].

TP53

TP53 is a tumor suppressor protein of crucial importance. As in so many other organ systems, mutations of the TP53 are well characterized in tumors of the CNS. In astrocytic tumors, mutations in TP53 occur more frequently in low-grade astrocytomas and secondary glioblastoma (>60 %) than in primary glioblastoma (<30 %) [66]. Mutations in TP53 are particularly common in the gemistocytic variant of diffuse astrocytoma (which also carries comparatively increased risk for progression to anaplastic astrocytoma and secondary glioblastoma) [45]. The giant-cell variant of glioblastoma, characterized by an abundance of large, multinucleated cells, is also characterized by frequent TP53 mutations in as many as 90 % of cases.

The determination of a tumor's p53 status is most commonly assessed with immunohistochemistry. This technique is easy and inexpensive, but the testing conditions as well as the interpretation of this test can vary from laboratory to laboratory [67]. Varying methods have

been proposed for interpreting p53 immunostains [68]. Some laboratories employ a four-category semiquantitative scale: no staining, 0; strong focal staining in <10 % of cells, 1+; strong staining in 10–50 % of cells or weak staining of >50 % of cells, 2+; and strong staining in >50 % of cells, 3+ [69]. Strong arguments have been suggesting a three-category scoring system: abnormal, no staining; abnormal, moderate to strong staining in >50 % of tumor cells; and normal, moderate to strong staining in <50 % of tumor cells [70]. This scoring system has the added advantage of identifying tumors with a homozygous deletion or null mutations.

MDM2

MDM2 participates in the p53 pathway. p53 induces MDM2 expression which in turn inhibits p53 transcriptional activity. MDM2 also oligomerizes with MDMX and acts as an E3 ubiquitin ligase complex, targeting MDM2 and p53 for proteasome degradation [71]. Several studies have used immunohistochemistry to evaluate for possible MDM2 amplification [72]. Fluorescence in situ hybridization is more specific and more sensitive for MDM2 amplification [73], and Health Canada-approved probes have been released for assessment with brightfield in situ hybridization [74]. Nonetheless, while such testing is commonly employed for soft-tissue tumors [75], this testing is not routinely performed in glioblastoma. A DISH probe is also available for use with brightfield microscopy.

Other Chromosomal Alterations in Glioblastoma

Several other chromosomal alterations are well documented in glioblastoma. Loss of chromosome 10q is the most common of these alterations, present in more than 60 % of glioblastoma cases [66, 76]. Isolated LOH of 22q, 1p, and 19q is also well described—the awareness of the latter is important as these deletions can be identified as a consequence of FISH analysis for 1p/19q co-deletion in oligodendroglioma.

PTEN

PTEN suppresses the PI3K-AKT-mTOR pathway resulting in cell proliferation and survival [77]. Patients with germline mutations of PTEN are at increased risk for developing breast, thyroid, and endometrial cancer. PTEN is mutated in approximately 25 % of glioblastomas with the vast majority of cases consisting of secondary rather than primary glioblastomas [78]. PTEN has also been implicated in adult-onset Lhermitte-Duclos (dysplastic gangliocytoma of the cerebellum) [79]. The assessment of PTEN mutational status is typically performed with traditional sequencing. The mechanism in Lhermitte-Duclos disease is typically LOH for the non-mutated allele.

MYC/MYCN

A variant of malignant glioma with areas resembling primitive neuroectodermal tumors (PNETs) has recently been identified [80]. These tumors frequently show MYC or MYCN amplification in the PNET component. Amplification for MYC/MYCN can be performed in most laboratories by FISH (Fig. 15.5), but probes for dual-ISH are also available [81].

Fig. 15.5 Fluorescence in situ hybridization on a glioblastoma with primitive neuroectodermal tumor (PNET) component. In the areas with the PNET morphology, there is amplification of MYC (*red signals*) (×1,000 magnification). Image courtesy of Catherine Fen Li, M.D., Ph.D. and Sharon Bauer, M.Sc.

Molecular Alterations in Embryonal Tumors of the CNS

Medulloblastoma

Medulloblastoma is the most common malignant primary brain tumor in children [82]. The 2007 WHO classified medulloblastoma into classical medulloblastoma and four morphologic variants. Two of these variants, desmoplastic/nodular and medulloblastoma with excessive nodularity, are associated with a favorable prognosis, while the other two variants, anaplastic and large cell, were associated with poorer outcomes [45]. Some of the well-characterized genetic alterations were known to be enriched in the morphologic variants. Notably, tumors with amplification of MYC and MYCN were associated with the anaplastic and large-cell variants and poor outcomes [83]. Alterations in the PTCH gene, with consequent dysregulation of the Hedgehog/Sonic Hedgehog (SHH) pathway, were enriched in cases of desmoplastic/nodular variant [84]. Turcot syndrome describes patients with familial adenomatous polyposis syndrome who also develop medulloblastoma. The APC/CTNNB1 (β-catenin)/AXINI1/2 mutations in these patients disrupt the Wnt pathway and allow for nuclear localization of β-catenin with subsequent altered regulation of downstream targets. Consequently, immunohistochemistry for β-catenin (CTNNB1) can be used to identify some of the tumors driven by Wnt pathway signaling alterations [85].

Children diagnosed with brain tumors in infancy are at risk for developing delays in skills related to daily living, socialization, and cognition [86]. Given the heterogenous outcomes for patients diagnosed with medulloblastoma, recent studies have aimed to identify an outcome-based classification scheme that may permit oncologist to use aggressive therapy only in cases of biologically aggressive tumors. Several large studies evaluating gene expression and copy number alterations have suggested revising the classification into four categories based on the molecular signature of the tumor [87, 88].

These studies identified four distinct groups of medulloblastoma that relate in part to the afore-mentioned subgroups: Wnt, SHH, group 3, and group 4. Mutations in exon 3 of CTNNB1 were identified in 89 % of Wnt pathway tumors. Amplifications of GLI2 and deletions of PTCH1 were common in SHH tumors. MYCN was fre-quently amplified in SHH tumors, but this amplifi-cation was also seen in non-SHH tumors. Group 3 was marked most significantly by amplifications in MYC and group 4 by MYCN amplification. Several papers have advanced immunohistochem-ical methods for classifying FFPE material of medulloblastoma into this recently proposed molecular classification, with β-catenin and DKK1 for Wnt tumors, GAB1 and SFRP1 for SHH tumors, negative staining for YAP1 and filamin A in non-SSH/Wnt tumors, or alternately positive staining for NPR3 in group 3 tumors/positive staining for KCNA1 in group 4 tumors [87, 89].

SMARCB1 (INI-1)

SMARCB1 (also widely known in the pathology community as INI1 and BAF47) is a tumor sup-pressor gene located on chromosome 22. Germline mutations in SMARCB1 have been identified in nearly one-third of patients diag-nosed with atypical teratoid rhabdoid tumors (ATRT) [45]. The loss of nuclear labeling for SMARCB1 by immunohistochemistry is extremely helpful in the diagnosis of ATRT, which previously required staining for EMA, GFAP, and smooth muscle actin [90]. The preser-vation in blood vessels and normal tissue nuclei serves as a valuable internal control when evalu-ating this immunohistochemical stain.

Though initially thought to be specific for ATRT in the CNS, SMARCB1 loss has been described in several entities. The recently described cribriform neuroepithelial tumor (CRINET) also features a loss of nuclear expression for SMARCB1. Unlike ATRT, CRINET is associated with a favorable prognosis [91]. FISH can also be employed to show LOH for SMARCB1 [92]. There is some controversy over whether choroid plexus carcinomas can lose SMARCB1 expression, but some authors suggest that SMARCB1 expres-sion loss in tumors that resemble choroid plexus carcinoma should be classified as ATRT [93]. Other tumors known to lack SMARCB1 nuclear positivity include poorly differentiated chordomas [94] and epithelioid malignant peripheral nerve sheath tumors [95]. Mutations in SMARCB1 have also been identified in familial schwannomatosis [96]; a mosaic pattern of SMARCB1 expression has also been identified in the schwannomas of these patients [97].

Paradigm Shift in Diagnostic Neuropathology

The reigning dogma in neuropathology has been to privilege morphology above molecular informa-tion about a tumor. The importance of morphologic assessment cannot be underestimated, as (discussed earlier in this chapter) identical molec-ular alterations (e.g., BRAFV600E mutation) can be seen in tumors with distinct morphology and clinical behavior. The current era has afforded neuropathologists the opportunity to debate the meaning (or even existence) of tumors such as the p53 mutant 1p19q wild-type oligoastrocy-toma. Nonetheless, the neuro-oncologic neuro-pathologic community may have reached a tipping point in which the molecular information about a neoplasm is considered of parallel impor-tance. The identification of a NAB2-STAT6 fusion in solitary fibrous tumor (SFT) [98] led within only months to the verification of similar fusion products in hemangiopericytoma of the CNS [99] (which, unlike in the soft-tissue oncol-ogy community, was considered by many neuro-pathologists to be distinct from SFT). These recent discoveries have provided insight into the relationship between these entities and have immediately suggested a reevaluation of prior classifications. With the pace of discoveries quickening, the current era may be one in which the molecular alterations of a tumor are consid-ered of tantamount importance to the histoge-netic morphologic information.

References

1. Louis DN. The next step in brain tumor classification: "Let us now praise famous men"... or molecules? Acta Neuropathol. 2012;124:761–2.
2. Weller M, Stupp R, Hegi ME, van den Bent M, Tonn JC, Sanson M, et al. Personalized care in neuro-oncology coming of age: why we need MGMT and 1p/19q testing for malignant glioma patients in clinical practice. Neuro Oncol. 2012;14 Suppl 4:iv100–8.
3. Parsons DW, Jones S, Zhang X, Lin JC, Leary RJ, Angenendt P, et al. An integrated genomic analysis of human glioblastoma multiforme. Science. 2008;321:1807–12.
4. Yan H, Parsons DW, Jin G, McLendon R, Rasheed BA, Yuan W, et al. IDH1 and IDH2 mutations in gliomas. N Engl J Med. 2009;360:765–73.
5. Houillier C, Wang X, Kaloshi G, Mokhtari K, Guillevin R, Laffaire J, et al. IDH1 or IDH2 mutations predict longer survival and response to temozolomide in low-grade gliomas. Neurology. 2010;75:1560–6.
6. Antonelli M, Buttarelli FR, Arcella A, Nobusawa S, Donofrio V, Oghaki H, et al. Prognostic significance of histological grading, p53 status, YKL-40 expression, and IDH1 mutations in pediatric high-grade gliomas. J Neuro-Oncol. 2010;99:209–15.
7. Paugh BS, Qu C, Jones C, Liu Z, Adamowicz-Brice M, Zhang J, et al. Integrated molecular genetic profiling of pediatric high-grade gliomas reveals key differences with the adult disease. J Clin Oncol. 2010; 28:3061–8.
8. Capper D, Sahm F, Hartmann C, Meyermann R, von Deimling A, Schittenhelm J. Application of mutant IDH1 antibody to differentiate diffuse glioma from nonneoplastic central nervous system lesions and therapy-induced changes. Am J Surg Pathol. 2010; 34:1199–204.
9. Capper D, Weissert S, Balss J, Habel A, Meyer J, Jager D, et al. Characterization of R132H mutation-specific IDH1 antibody binding in brain tumors. Brain Pathol. 2010;20:245–54.
10. Capper D, Zentgraf H, Balss J, Hartmann C, von Deimling A. Monoclonal antibody specific for IDH1 R132H mutation. Acta Neuropathol. 2009;118: 599–601.
11. Esteller M, Garcia-Foncillas J, Andion E, Goodman SN, Hidalgo OF, Vanaclocha V, et al. Inactivation of the DNA-repair gene MGMT and the clinical response of gliomas to alkylating agents. N Engl J Med. 2000;343:1350–4.
12. Hegi ME, Diserens AC, Gorlia T, Hamou MF, de Tribolet N, Weller M, et al. MGMT gene silencing and benefit from temozolomide in glioblastoma. N Engl J Med. 2005;352:997–1003.
13. Wick W, Platten M, Meisner C, Felsberg J, Tabatabai G, Simon M, et al. Temozolomide chemotherapy alone versus radiotherapy alone for malignant astrocytoma in the elderly: the NOA-08 randomised, phase 3 trial. Lancet Oncol. 2012;13:707–15.
14. Malmstrom A, Gronberg BH, Marosi C, Stupp R, Frappaz D, Schultz H, et al. Temozolomide versus standard 6-week radiotherapy versus hypofractionated radiotherapy in patients older than 60 years with glioblastoma: the Nordic randomised, phase 3 trial. Lancet Oncol. 2012;13:916–26.
15. Mikeska T, Bock C, El-Maarri O, Hubner A, Ehrentraut D, Schramm J, et al. Optimization of quantitative MGMT promoter methylation analysis using pyrosequencing and combined bisulfite restriction analysis. J Mol Diagn. 2007;9:368–81.
16. Mason S, McDonald K. MGMT testing for glioma in clinical laboratories: discordance with methylation analyses prevents the implementation of routine immunohistochemistry. J Cancer Res Clin Oncol. 2012;138:1789–97.
17. Preusser M, Elezi L, Hainfellner JA. Reliability and reproducibility of PCR-based testing of O6-methylguanine-DNA methyltransferase gene (MGMT) promoter methylation status in formalin-fixed and paraffin-embedded neurosurgical biopsy specimens. Clin Neuropathol. 2008;27:388–90.
18. Quillien V, Lavenu A, Karayan-Tapon L, Carpentier C, Labussiere M, Lesimple T, et al. Comparative assessment of 5 methods (methylation-specific polymerase chain reaction, MethyLight, pyrosequencing, methylation-sensitive high-resolution melting, and immunohistochemistry) to analyze O6-methylguanine-DNA-methyltranferase in a series of 100 glioblastoma patients. Cancer. 2012;118: 4201–11.
19. Eads CA, Danenberg KD, Kawakami K, Saltz LB, Blake C, Shibata D, et al. MethyLight: a high-throughput assay to measure DNA methylation. Nucleic Acids Res. 2000;28:E32.
20. Vlassenbroeck I, Califice S, Diserens AC, Migliavacca E, Straub J, Di Stefano I, et al. Validation of real-time methylation-specific PCR to determine O6-methylguanine-DNA methyltransferase gene promoter methylation in glioma. J Mol Diagn. 2008;10: 332–7.
21. Jeuken JW, Cornelissen SJ, Vriezen M, Dekkers MM, Errami A, Sijben A, et al. MS-MLPA: an attractive alternative laboratory assay for robust, reliable, and semiquantitative detection of MGMT promoter hypermethylation in gliomas. Lab Invest. 2007;87: 1055–65.
22. Bady P, Sciuscio D, Diserens AC, Bloch J, van den Bent MJ, Marosi C, et al. MGMT methylation analysis of glioblastoma on the Infinium methylation BeadChip identifies two distinct CpG regions associated with gene silencing and outcome, yielding a prediction model for comparisons across datasets, tumor grades, and CIMP-status. Acta Neuropathol. 2012;124:547–60.
23. Hsu CY, Lin SC, Ho HL, Chang-Chien YC, Hsu SP, Yen YS, et al. Exclusion of histiocytes/endothelial

cells and using endothelial cells as internal reference are crucial for interpretation of MGMT immunohisto-chemistry in glioblastoma. Am J Surg Pathol. 2013;37:264–71.

24. Louis DN, Gusella JF. A tiger behind many doors: multiple genetic pathways to malignant glioma. Trends Genet. 1995;11:412–5.

25. Reifenberger J, Reifenberger G, Liu L, James CD, Wechsler W, Collins VP. Molecular genetic analysis of oligodendroglial tumors shows preferential allelic deletions on 19q and 1p. Am J Pathol. 1994;145:1175–90.

26. von Deimling A, Louis DN, von Ammon K, Petersen I, Wiestler OD, Seizinger BR. Evidence for a tumor suppressor gene on chromosome 19q associated with human astrocytomas, oligodendrogliomas, and mixed gliomas. Cancer Res. 1992;52:4277–9.

27. Griffin CA, Burger P, Morsberger L, Yonescu R, Swierczynski S, Weingart JD, et al. Identification of der(1;19)(q10;p10) in five oligodendrogliomas suggests mechanism of concurrent 1p and 19q loss. J Neuropathol Exp Neurol. 2006;65:988–94.

28. Bettegowda C, Agrawal N, Jiao Y, Sausen M, Wood LD, Hruban RH, et al. Mutations in CIC and FUBP1 contribute to human oligodendroglioma. Science. 2011;333:1453–5.

29. Sahm F, Koelsche C, Meyer J, Pusch S, Lindenberg K, Mueller W, et al. CIC and FUBP1 mutations in oligodendrogliomas, oligoastrocytomas and astrocytomas. Acta Neuropathol. 2012;123:853–60.

30. Labussiere M, Idbaih A, Wang XW, Marie Y, Boisselier B, Falet C, et al. All the 1p19q codeleted gliomas are mutated on IDH1 or IDH2. Neurology. 2010;74:1886–90.

31. Cairncross JG, Ueki K, Zlatescu MC, Lisle DK, Finkelstein DM, Hammond RR, et al. Specific genetic predictors of chemotherapeutic response and survival in patients with anaplastic oligodendrogliomas. J Natl Cancer Inst. 1998;90:1473–9.

32. Kouwenhoven MC, Gorlia T, Kros JM, Ibdaih A, Brandes AA, Bromberg JE, et al. Molecular analysis of anaplastic oligodendroglial tumors in a prospective randomized study: a report from EORTC study 26951. Neuro Oncol. 2009;11:737–46.

33. Woehrer A, Sander P, Haberler C, Kern S, Maier H, Preusser M, et al. FISH-based detection of 1p 19q codeletion in oligodendroglial tumors: procedures and protocols for neuropathological practice—a publication under the auspices of the Research Committee of the European Confederation of Neuropathological Societies (Euro-CNS). Clin Neuropathol. 2011;30:47–55.

34. Smith JS, Alderete B, Minn Y, Borell TJ, Perry A, Mohapatra G, et al. Localization of common deletion regions on 1p and 19q in human gliomas and their association with histological subtype. Oncogene. 1999;18:4144–52.

35. Reddy KS. Assessment of 1p/19q deletions by fluorescence in situ hybridization in gliomas. Cancer Genet Cytogenet. 2008;184:77–86.

36. Hatanpaa KJ, Burger PC, Eshleman JR, Murphy KM, Berg KD. Molecular diagnosis of oligodendroglioma in paraffin sections. Lab Invest. 2003;83:419–28.

37. Nigro JM, Takahashi MA, Ginzinger DG, Law M, Passe S, Jenkins RB, et al. Detection of 1p and 19q loss in oligodendroglioma by quantitative microsatellite analysis, a real-time quantitative polymerase chain reaction assay. Am J Pathol. 2001;158:1253–62.

38. Kros JM, van Run PR, Alers JC, Beverloo HB, van den Bent MJ, Avezaat CJ, et al. Genetic aberrations in oligodendroglial tumours: an analysis using comparative genomic hybridization (CGH). J Pathol. 1999;188:282–8.

39. Burger PC, Minn AY, Smith JS, Borell TJ, Jedlicka AE, Huntley BK, et al. Losses of chromosomal arms 1p and 19q in the diagnosis of oligodendroglioma. A study of paraffin-embedded sections. Mod Pathol. 2001;14:842–53.

40. Natte R, van Eijk R, Eilers P, Cleton-Jansen AM, Oosting J, Kouwenhove M, et al. Multiplex ligation-dependent probe amplification for the detection of 1p and 19q chromosomal loss in oligodendroglial tumors. Brain Pathol. 2005;15:192–7.

41. Bengtsson H, Wirapati P, Speed TP. A single-array pre-processing method for estimating full-resolution raw copy numbers from all Affymetrix genotyping arrays including GenomeWideSNP 5 & 6. Bioinformatics. 2009;25:2149–56.

42. Xie C, Tammi MT. CNV-seq, a new method to detect copy number variation using high-throughput sequencing. BMC Bioinformatics. 2009;10:80.

43. Schindler G, Capper D, Meyer J, Janzarik W, Omran H, Herold-Mende C, et al. Analysis of BRAF V600E mutation in 1,320 nervous system tumors reveals high mutation frequencies in pleomorphic xanthoastrocytoma, ganglioglioma and extra-cerebellar pilocytic astrocytoma. Acta Neuropathol. 2011;121:397–405.

44. Schiffman JD, Hodgson JG, VandenBerg SR, Flaherty P, Polley MY, Yu M, et al. Oncogenic BRAF mutation with CDKN2A inactivation is characteristic of a subset of pediatric malignant astrocytomas. Cancer Res. 2010;70:512–9.

45. Louis DN. International Agency for Research on Cancer, World Health Organization. WHO classification of tumours of the central nervous system. 4th ed. Lyon: International Agency for Research on Cancer; 2007.

46. Perry A, Giannini C, Scheithauer BW, Rojiani AM, Yachnis AT, Seo IS, et al. Composite pleomorphic xanthoastrocytoma and ganglioglioma: report of four cases and review of the literature. Am J Surg Pathol. 1997;21:763–71.

47. Capper D, Preusser M, Habel A, Sahm F, Ackermann U, Schindler G, et al. Assessment of BRAF V600E mutation status by immunohistochemistry with a mutation-specific monoclonal antibody. Acta Neuropathol. 2011;122:11–9.

48. Capper D, Berghoff AS, Magerle M, Ilhan A, Wohrer A, Hackl M, et al. Immunohistochemical testing of

BRAF V600E status in 1,120 tumor tissue samples of patients with brain metastases. Acta Neuropathol. 2012;123:223–33.

49. Horbinski C. To BRAF or not to BRAF: is that even a question anymore? J Neuropathol Exp Neurol. 2013;72:2–7.

50. Sanoudou D, Tingby O, Ferguson-Smith MA, Collins VP, Coleman N. Analysis of pilocytic astrocytoma by comparative genomic hybridization. Br J Cancer. 2000;82:1218–22.

51. Bar EE, Lin A, Tihan T, Burger PC, Eberhart CG. Frequent gains at chromosome 7q34 involving BRAF in pilocytic astrocytoma. J Neuropathol Exp Neurol. 2008;67:878–87.

52. Jones DT, Kocialkowski S, Liu L, Pearson DM, Backlund LM, Ichimura K, et al. Tandem duplication producing a novel oncogenic BRAF fusion gene defines the majority of pilocytic astrocytomas. Cancer Res. 2008;68:8673–7.

53. Forshew T, Tatevossian RG, Lawson AR, Ma J, Neale G, Ogunkolade BW, et al. Activation of the ERK/MAPK pathway: a signature genetic defect in posterior fossa pilocytic astrocytomas. J Pathol. 2009;218: 172–81.

54. Horbinski C, Hamilton RL, Nikiforov Y, Pollack IF. Association of molecular alterations, including BRAF, with biology and outcome in pilocytic astrocytomas. Acta Neuropathol. 2010;119:641–9.

55. Korshunov A, Meyer J, Capper D, Christians A, Remke M, Witt H, et al. Combined molecular analysis of BRAF and IDH1 distinguishes pilocytic astrocytoma from diffuse astrocytoma. Acta Neuropathol. 2009;118:401–5.

56. Tian Y, Rich BE, Vena N, Craig JM, Macconaill LE, Rajaram V, et al. Detection of KIAA1549-BRAF fusion transcripts in formalin-fixed paraffin-embedded pediatric low-grade gliomas. J Mol Diagn. 2011; 13:669–77.

57. Ohgaki H, Dessen P, Jourde B, Horstmann S, Nishikawa T, Di Patre PL, et al. Genetic pathways to glioblastoma: a population-based study. Cancer Res. 2004;64:6892–9.

58. Watanabe K, Tachibana O, Sata K, Yonekawa Y, Kleihues P, Ohgaki H. Overexpression of the EGF receptor and p53 mutations are mutually exclusive in the evolution of primary and secondary glioblastomas. Brain Pathol. 1996;6:217–23; discussion 23–4.

59. Burger PC, Pearl DK, Aldape K, Yates AJ, Scheithauer BW, Passe SM, et al. Small cell architecture—a histological equivalent of EGFR amplification in glioblastoma multiforme? J Neuropathol Exp Neurol. 2001;60:1099–104.

60. Gaiser T, Waha A, Moessler F, Bruckner T, Pietsch T, von Deimling A. Comparison of automated silver enhanced in situ hybridization and fluorescence in situ hybridization for evaluation of epidermal growth factor receptor status in human glioblastomas. Mod Pathol. 2009;22:1263–71.

61. Kuan CT, Wikstrand CJ, Bigner DD. EGFRvIII as a promising target for antibody-based brain tumor therapy. Brain Tumor Pathol. 2000;17:71–8.

62. Wikstrand CJ, Hale LP, Batra SK, Hill ML, Humphrey PA, Kurpad SN, et al. Monoclonal antibodies against EGFRvIII are tumor specific and react with breast and lung carcinomas and malignant gliomas. Cancer Res. 1995;55:3140–8.

63. Moscatello DK, Ramirez G, Wong AJ. A naturally occurring mutant human epidermal growth factor receptor as a target for peptide vaccine immunotherapy of tumors. Cancer Res. 1997;57:1419–24.

64. Li G, Mitra S, Wong AJ. The epidermal growth factor variant III peptide vaccine for treatment of malignant gliomas. Neurosurg Clin N Am. 2010;21:87–93.

65. Gupta P, Han SY, Holgado-Madruga M, Mitra SS, Li G, Nitta RT, et al. Development of an EGFRvIII specific recombinant antibody. BMC Biotechnol. 2010;10:72.

66. Ohgaki H, Kleihues P. Genetic pathways to primary and secondary glioblastoma. Am J Pathol. 2007;170:1445–53.

67. Adams EJ, Green JA, Clark AH, Youngson JH. Comparison of different scoring systems for immunohistochemical staining. J Clin Pathol. 1999;52:75–7.

68. Zlobec I, Steele R, Michel RP, Compton CC, Lugli A, Jass JR. Scoring of p53, VEGF, Bcl-2 and APAF-1 immunohistochemistry and interobserver reliability in colorectal cancer. Mod Pathol. 2006;19:1236–42.

69. Giannini C, Hebrink D, Scheithauer BW, Dei Tos AP, James CD. Analysis of p53 mutation and expression in pleomorphic xanthoastrocytoma. Neurogenetics. 2001;3:159–62.

70. Lassus H, Butzow R. The classification of p53 immunohistochemical staining results and patient outcome in ovarian cancer. Br J Cancer. 2007;96:1621–2; author reply 3–4.

71. Wade M, Li YC, Wahl GM. MDM2, MDMX and p53 in oncogenesis and cancer therapy. Nat Rev Cancer. 2013;13:83–96.

72. Biernat W, Kleihues P, Yonekawa Y, Ohgaki H. Amplification and overexpression of MDM2 in primary (de novo) glioblastomas. J Neuropathol Exp Neurol. 1997;56:180–5.

73. Weaver J, Downs-Kelly E, Goldblum JR, Turner S, Kulkarni S, Tubbs RR, et al. Fluorescence in situ hybridization for MDM2 gene amplification as a diagnostic tool in lipomatous neoplasms. Mod Pathol. 2008;21:943–9.

74. Zhang W, McElhinny A, Nielsen A, Wang M, Miller M, Singh S, et al. Automated brightfield dual-color in situ hybridization for detection of mouse double minute 2 gene amplification in sarcomas. Appl Immunohistochem Mol Morphol. 2011;19:54–61.

75. Nishio J. Contributions of cytogenetics and molecular cytogenetics to the diagnosis of adipocytic tumors. J Biomed Biotechnol. 2011;2011:524067.

76. Karlbom AE, James CD, Boethius J, Cavenee WK, Collins VP, Nordenskjold M, et al. Loss of

heterozygosity in malignant gliomas involves at least three distinct regions on chromosome 10. Hum Genet. 1993;92:169–74.

77. Song MS, Salmena L, Pandolfi PP. The functions and regulation of the PTEN tumour suppressor. Nat Rev Mol Cell Biol. 2012;13:283–96.

78. Duerr EM, Rollbrocker B, Hayashi Y, Peters N, Meyer-Puttlitz B, Louis DN, et al. PTEN mutations in gliomas and glioneuronal tumors. Oncogene. 1998;16:2259–64.

79. Zhou XP, Marsh DJ, Morrison CD, Chaudhury AR, Maxwell M, Reifenberger G, et al. Germline inactivation of PTEN and dysregulation of the phosphoinositol-3-kinase/Akt pathway cause human Lhermitte-Duclos disease in adults. Am J Hum Genet. 2003;73:1191–8.

80. Perry A, Miller CR, Gujrati M, Scheithauer BW, Zambrano SC, Jost SC, et al. Malignant gliomas with primitive neuroectodermal tumor-like components: a clinicopathologic and genetic study of 53 cases. Brain Pathol. 2009;19:81–90.

81. Valentino C, Kendrick S, Johnson N, Gascoyne R, Chan WC, Weisenburger D, et al. Colorimetric in situ hybridization identifies MYC gene signal clusters correlating with increased copy number, mRNA, and protein in diffuse large B-cell lymphoma. Am J Clin Pathol. 2013;139:242–54.

82. Dolecek TA, Propp JM, Stroup NE, Kruchko C. CBTRUS statistical report: primary brain and central nervous system tumors diagnosed in the United States in 2005–2009. Neuro Oncol. 2012;14 Suppl 5:v1–49.

83. Aldosari N, Bigner SH, Burger PC, Becker L, Kepner JL, Friedman HS, et al. MYCC and MYCN oncogene amplification in medulloblastoma. A fluorescence in situ hybridization study on paraffin sections from the Children's Oncology Group. Arch Pathol Lab Med. 2002;126:540–4.

84. Pomeroy SL, Tamayo P, Gaasenbeek M, Sturla LM, Angelo M, McLaughlin ME, et al. Prediction of central nervous system embryonal tumour outcome based on gene expression. Nature. 2002;415:436–42.

85. Eberhart CG, Tihan T, Burger PC. Nuclear localization and mutation of beta-catenin in medulloblastomas. J Neuropathol Exp Neurol. 2000;59:333–7.

86. Stargatt R, Rosenfeld JV, Anderson V, Hassall T, Maixner W, Ashley D. Intelligence and adaptive function in children diagnosed with brain tumour during infancy. J Neurooncol. 2006;80:295–303.

87. Northcott PA, Korshunov A, Witt H, Hielscher T, Eberhart CG, Mack S, et al. Medulloblastoma comprises four distinct molecular variants. J Clin Oncol. 2011;29:1408–14.

88. Northcott PA, Shih DJ, Peacock J, Garzia L, Morrissy AS, Zichner T, et al. Subgroup-specific structural variation across 1,000 medulloblastoma genomes. Nature. 2012;488:49–56.

89. Ellison DW, Dalton J, Kocak M, Nicholson SL, Fraga C, Neale G, et al. Medulloblastoma: clinicopathological correlates of SHH, WNT, and non-SHH/WNT molecular subgroups. Acta Neuropathol. 2011;121:381–96.

90. Greenfield JG, Love S, Louis DN, Ellison D. Greenfield's neuropathology. 8th ed. London: Hodder Arnold; 2008.

91. Hasselblatt M, Oyen F, Gesk S, Kordes U, Wrede B, Bergmann M, et al. Cribriform neuroepithelial tumor (CRINET): a nonrhabdoid ventricular tumor with INI1 loss and relatively favorable prognosis. J Neuropathol Exp Neurol. 2009;68:1249–55.

92. Ibrahim GM, Huang A, Halliday W, Dirks PB, Malkin D, Baskin B, et al. Cribriform neuroepithelial tumour: novel clinicopathological, ultrastructural and cytogenetic findings. Acta Neuropathol. 2011;122:511–4.

93. Judkins AR, Burger PC, Hamilton RL, Kleinschmidt-DeMasters B, Perry A, Pomeroy SL, et al. INI1 protein expression distinguishes atypical teratoid/rhabdoid tumor from choroid plexus carcinoma. J Neuropathol Exp Neurol. 2005;64:391–7.

94. Mobley BC, McKenney JK, Bangs CD, Callahan K, Yeom KW, Schneppenheim R, et al. Loss of SMARCB1/INI1 expression in poorly differentiated chordomas. Acta Neuropathol. 2010;120:745–53.

95. Hollmann TJ, Hornick JL. INI1-deficient tumors: diagnostic features and molecular genetics. Am J Surg Pathol. 2011;35:e47–63.

96. Hulsebos TJ, Plomp AS, Wolterman RA, Robanus-Maandag EC, Baas F, Wesseling P. Germline mutation of INI1/SMARCB1 in familial schwannomatosis. Am J Hum Genet. 2007;80:805–10.

97. Patil S, Perry A, Maccollin M, Dong S, Betensky RA, Yeh TH, et al. Immunohistochemical analysis supports a role for INI1/SMARCB1 in hereditary forms of schwannomas, but not in solitary, sporadic schwannomas. Brain Pathol. 2008;18:517–9.

98. Chmielecki J, Crago AM, Rosenberg M, O'Connor R, Walker SR, Ambrogio L, et al. Whole-exome sequencing identifies a recurrent NAB2-STAT6 fusion in solitary fibrous tumors. Nat Genet. 2013;45:131–2.

99. Schweizer L, Koelsche C, Sahm F, Piro RM, Capper D, Reuss DE, et al. Meningeal hemangiopericytoma and solitary fibrous tumors carry the NAB2-STAT6 fusion and can be diagnosed by nuclear expression of STAT6 protein. Acta Neuropathol. 2013;125:651–8.

Molecular Testing in Adult Kidney Tumors

16

Manal Y. Gabril and George M. Yousef

Renal cell carcinoma (RCC) is the most common neoplasm of the adult kidney. It is a heterogenous disease of multiple subtypes. Clear cell renal cell carcinoma (ccRCC) is the most common subtype which accounts for approximately 80 % of all adult renal cancers followed by the papillary subtype (pRCC, 10–15 %) and less common subtypes including chromophobe RCC (chRCC, 5 %), medullary RCC, collecting duct carcinoma (CDC), and translocation carcinomas, among others.

Familial Kidney Cancer Syndromes

1. von Hippel-Lindau (VHL) Disease

VHL disease is characterized by autosomal dominant germ-line mutations of the *VHL* tumor suppressor gene on 3p25. It is most frequently associated with retinal and central nervous system haemangioblastomas, ccRCC, pheochromocytoma, and pancreatic islet tumors [1]. Approximately 75 % of patients with VHL disease

M.Y. Gabril, M.D.
Department of Pathology and Laboratory Medicine, University Hospital, 339 Windermere Road, London, ON, Canada N6A 5A5
e-mail: manal.gabril@lhsc.on.ca

G.M. Yousef, M.D., Ph.D. (✉)
Department of Laboratory Medicine and Pathobiology, University of Toronto, Medical Sciences Building, 1 King's College Circle, Toronto, ON, Canada M5S 1A8
e-mail: yousefg@smh.ca

develop ccRCC by age 60, which is a leading cause of death among these patients [2].

Distinct genotype-phenotype correlations have allowed for the classification of two clinical types of VHL disease based on the absence (type 1) or presence (type 2) of pheochromocytoma. Type 1 is more common (30–40 %) and is associated with *VHL* germ-line exon deletions or truncating mutations and the risk of developing RCC. Type 2 patients, on the other hand, harbor missense mutations of *VHL* which range from having no effect to complete functional loss of VHL protein (pVHL) [3]. There is also evidence to suggest that a specific subgroup of type 1 patients who have a contiguous deletion of all or part of *VHL* and the adjacent *C3orf10* (*HSPC300*) gene have lower risk of RCC (proposed type 1B) [4–6]. Type 2 disease is further subdivided into three subtypes: type 2A (low risk of RCC), type 2B (high risk of RCC), and type 2C (pheochromocytoma only) [3]. Type 2A patients are associated with missense mutations that impact pVHL target interactions with hypoxia-inducible factor (HIF), elongin B, and elongin C. Type 2B patients are associated with missense mutations that lead to severe destabilization of pVHL. Type 2C patients are associated with *VHL* missense mutations that retain comparable wild-type pVHL function [3, 7, 8]. There was no significant association between *VHL* mutation type and prognosis [7, 9].

2. Hereditary Papillary RCC

Hereditary papillary RCC is characterized by autosomal dominant germ-line activating mutations of the *MET* proto-oncogene, located on 7q31. Individuals with this syndrome are at risk of developing bilateral, multifocal, type 1 pRCC. Approximately 30 % of *MET* carriers develop renal cancer by age 50 [10].

3. Birt-Hogg-Dubé (BHD) Syndrome

BHD syndrome is characterized by autosomal dominant germ-line mutations of the *BHD* tumor suppressor gene, also known as folliculin (*FLCN*), located on 17p11.2. *BHD* plays a role in the 5′ AMP-activated protein kinase (AMPK) and mammalian target of rapamycin (mTOR) signaling pathways. The syndrome is associated with high risk of developing cutaneous fibrofolliculomas, pulmonary cysts, spontaneous pneumothorax, and bilateral, multifocal RCC [11]. Chromophobe and hybrid oncocytic RCCs are more commonly associated with BHD syndrome patients [12].

4. Hereditary Leiomyomatosis/RCC (HLRCC) Syndrome

This syndrome is characterized by autosomal dominant germ-line mutations of the fumarate hydratase (*FH*) tumor suppressor gene, located on 1q42.1. It is characterized by cutaneous leiomyoma, uterine fibroid, and/or kidney cancer manifestations [13]. Renal tumors have been observed in approximately one third of HLRCC families and tend to manifest as solitary renal lesions; however, bilateral and multifocal RCC cases have been reported [14].

5. Tuberous Sclerosis Complex (TSC)

TSC has been linked to germ-line inactivating mutations of either of *TSC1* (9q34) encoding hamartin or *TSC2* (16p13.3) encoding tuberin, and affected patients have an increased risk of developing renal tumors including clear cell RCC, papillary RCC, and chromophobe RCC [15].

Genetic Alteration in Renal Cell Carcinoma

Chromosomal Aberrations

Benign Kidney Tumors

Renal oncocytomas have been reported to have either rearrangements or translocations involving chromosome 11q13 or partial or complete losses of chromosomes 1 and 14 and/or a sex chromosome. Chromosome 3p loss is not detectable in oncocytoma. Because of the frequent association between oncocytomas and chromosome 1p alterations, the loss of a tumor suppressor gene residing on chromosome 1p has been proposed as an early genetic event associated with the development of renal oncocytoma. Oncocytomas have also been shown to exhibit microsatellite instabilities and alterations in mitochondrial DNA.

In angiomyolipoma, frequent imbalances are losses on chromosomes 19, 16p, 17p, 1p, and 18p and gains on chromosomes X, 12q, 3q, 5, and 2q. The frequent deletion of 16p in which TSC2 gene is located indicates the oncogenetic relationship of PEComas with angiomyolipoma as a TSC2-linked neoplasm [16].

Malignant Tumors

Chromophobe cell carcinoma: Frequent losses of chromosomes 1, 2, Y, 6, 10, 13, 17, and 21 and gains of chromosomes 4, 7, 11, 12, 14q, and 18q are observed. At the molecular level, the association between loss of chromosome 17 and mutation of the p53 tumor suppressor gene is reported in 27 % of cases [17]. It is noteworthy that there are no apparent overlapping genetic alterations shared by eosinophilic chromophobe RCC and oncocytoma, despite their morphologic similarities. Other genetic alterations include −5q22, −8p, −9p23, and −18q22.

Clear cell renal cell carcinoma: 3p deletion (LOH 3p) is the most typical genetic abnormality of ccRCC. In addition to VHL, recent data suggest the presence of other putative tumor suppressor genes at the 3p region, such as *RASSF1A* and *SETD2* located on 3p21 and *NRC-1* on 3p12 [18, 19]. Recent analyses have revealed peak deletions, specifically targeting *VHL* (3p25) and CDKN2A and CDKN2B (9p21), and peak amplifications of MYC (8q24) in subsets of ccRCC [20]. Studies suggested the accumulation of additional genetic alterations during the process of tumor progression and metastasis [21–25]. Metastasis was found to be associated with losses of 3p, 8p, 9p, and 13q and gains of 17q and Xq. Also, a correlation was observed between metastasis and increase in the copy number of genes located at 1q [22].

Other genetic alterations include +5q22, −6q, −8p12, −9p21, −9q22, −10q, and −14q.

Papillary renal cell carcinoma: This subtype is not commonly associated with 3p deletions but rather with trisomies of chromosomes 7, 8, 12, 16, 17, and 20 and loss of Y. These most consistent genetic abnormalities are present in both solitary and multifocal papillary RCCs, and they occur early in the evolution of this neoplasm [26, 27]. Some authors have suggested genetic differences between types; type 1 papillary RCC cases seem to have a significantly higher frequency of allelic imbalance on 17q than type 2 cases, and type 2 cases have a higher frequency of allelic imbalance on 9p than type 1 cases [28, 29]. Other genetic alterations include +3q, +8, −921, +12, −14q, +16, +17q21, and +20.

Translocation carcinomas: A breakpoint at Xp11, which harbors the transcription factor E3 (*TFE3*) gene, can result in subsequent fusion of *TFE3* with several partners depending on the exact translocation. Four distinct recipients have been identified: *PRCC* (1q21), *PSF* (1p34), *ASPL* (17q25), and *NonO* (Xq12) [30–33].

Other subtypes: The most constant change in collecting duct carcinoma (CDC) is 1q32 deletion. Loss of chromosome 3p including the *VHL* gene is not common in CDC. Some studies have described that activation of vascular endothelial growth factor (VEGF) signaling, which is analogous to the clear cell RCC hypoxia pathway, may be related to renal medullary carcinoma. Mucinous tubular and spindle cell carcinoma shows genetic alterations including −8p, −9p, −11q, +12q, +16q, +17, and +20q [34].

Genome-Wide Association Studies (GWAS) and Susceptibility to RCC

Three genetic susceptibility loci have been found to be associated with the risk of RCC [35, 36]. In individuals of European descent, genetic loci on 2p21, 11q13.3, and 12p11.23 were identified. Three variants map to the endothelial PAS domain protein 1 (EPAS1) gene on 2p21, which encodes hypoxia-inducible factor-2a (HIF2α).

Two of these variants were also associated with former and current smokers, but not in never smokers, suggesting the effect of EPAS1 is dependent on tobacco smoking [35, 36]. The third variant is associated with VHL [35].

The locus on 11q13.3 is significantly associated with reduced risk of RCC, especially among normal-weight never smokers and nondrinkers in the Chinese population [37]. Two variants on 12p11.23 map to the ITPR2 gene [36]; one of them is also associated with waist-hip ratio phenotype, suggesting a genetic link between obesity and RCC risk [38]. A recent study [39] observed VHL germline variants were associated with a higher risk of VHL inactivation via promoter hypermethylation compared to VHL mutation in sporadic ccRCC, suggesting the utility of genetic polymorphisms as indicators of increased risk of epigenetic alterations and cancer susceptibility [39].

Exome Sequencing Identifies Novel Mutations in RCC

The Cancer Genome Project (CGP) recently conducted exome sequencing of ccRCC that revealed novel recurrent mutations of the SWI/SNF chromatin remodeling complex gene, PBRM1 (41 %), and of genes encoding enzymes that methylate (SETD2, 3 %) or demethylate (JARID1C and UTX, 3 %) key lysine residues of histone H3 [18, 40]. The CGP also identified mutations of the tumor suppressor neurofibromin 2 (NF2) in non-VHL mutated ccRCCs [18, 40].

In addition to VHL, the PBRM1 and SETD2 genes map to the frequently deleted 3p21 region, suggesting a link between frequent overlapping biallelic inactivation of these genes and ccRCC tumorigenesis [41]. An independent exome sequencing study confirmed several mutations cataloged by the CGP and also identified 12 additional mutations [42].

Epigenetics Changes

Recent data from the Cancer Genome Atlas (TCGA) showed a widespread DNA hypomethylation in ccRCC that is associated with mutation of the H3K36 methyltransferase SETD2, and integrative analysis suggested that mutations involving the SWI/SNF chromatin remodeling complex (PBRM1, ARID1A, SMARCA4) could have far-reaching effects on other pathways [43].

CDKN2A and *THBS-1* genes seem to be hot spots of regional DNA hypermethylation during renal tumorigenesis. Other epigenetic changes include HAT hMOF which belongs to the MYST family and is believed to be responsible for histone H4 acetylation. hMOF expression was frequently downregulated in human RCC (>90 %) [44]. Downregulation of hMOF was detected in all types of RCCs, suggesting that hMOF might be a new common diagnostic marker for human different RCC.

Several classic tumor suppressor genes can be inactivated by hypermethylation as an alternative mechanism of silencing including VHL that hypermethylated in 10–15 % of ccRCC [45]. Promoter hypermethylation of p16INK4a is present in 5–10 % of primary RCC [46]. Another candidate tumor suppressor gene is the Ras association domain family 1 gene (RASSF1A) which is methylated in 28–91 % of primary renal tumors [47, 48]. Two studies reported that the frequency of RASSF1A methylation is higher in papillary compared to ccRCC and is also found in chromophobe tumors [48]. FHIT hypermethylation has also been reported in 54 % of ccRCC [49]. This gene encompasses the common fragile site FRA3B on chromosome 3p, where carcinogen-induced damage can lead to translocations and aberrant transcripts of this gene. HAI-2/SPINT2 encodes Kunitz-type protease inhibitor, which functions as a regulator of hepatocyte growth factor (HGF) activity. Tumor suppressor activity as well as inactivation by hypermethylation of SPINT2 has been identified in both the clear cell (30 %) and papillary (40 %) subtypes of RCC [50].

miRNAs: A New Dimension in the Pathogenesis of RCC

Recently, a number of studies documented the differential expression of miRNAs in kidney cancer [51–55]. White et al. [52] identified 166 miRNAs that were significantly dysregulated in ccRCC compared to normal kidney tissue. miR-122, miR-155, and miR-210 had the highest overexpression, while miR-200c, miRA-141, miR-335, and miR-218 were the most downregulated. Evidence is accumulating regarding the involvement of miRNAs in RCC pathogenesis. A recent study showed an effect of the oncogenic miRNA cluster miR-17-92 on tumor cell proliferation [56], and preliminary evidence showed that miRNAs can affect key molecules in the VHL-HIF-hypoxia pathway [57, 58]. miRNAs have also been shown to be epigenetically regulated in ccRCC. Vogt et al. [59] found that miR-34 was methylated in 58 % cases while miR-34b/c was methylated in 100 % cases. The inactivation of miR-34a and miR-34b/c were concomitant in most cases. The proposed mechanisms of miRNA involvement in RCC pathogenesis have been recently reviewed [60]. Recent evidence showed the diverse clinical uses of miRNAs in cancer as diagnostic, prognostic, and predictive markers [61].

Molecular Pathways of Renal Cell Carcinoma

1. *The VHL-HIF hypoxia pathway*

VHL is a classic two-hit tumor suppressor gene. It has been shown that inactivation of the VHL gene is an early step in the development of ccRCC. The majority of ccRCC demonstrate either a mutation of the VHL gene or a downregulation of its protein product. The VHL protein product (pVHL) has an important role in cellular response to hypoxia. VHL inactivation leads to the stabilization of the hypoxia-inducible factors (HIFs) with subsequent activation of a number of downstream target proteins such as VEGF, platelet-derived growth factor (PDGF), transforming growth factor-alpha (TGFα), and transforming growth factor-beta (TGFB) [62, 63]. A simplified overview of the main events in ccRCC pathogenesis is shown in Fig. 16.1.

2. *The VEGFR pathway*

Biallelic loss of VHL leads to upregulated transcription of growth factors such as VEGF, PDGF, and TGF-α. These factors bind to their respective tyrosine kinase receptors (VEGFR,

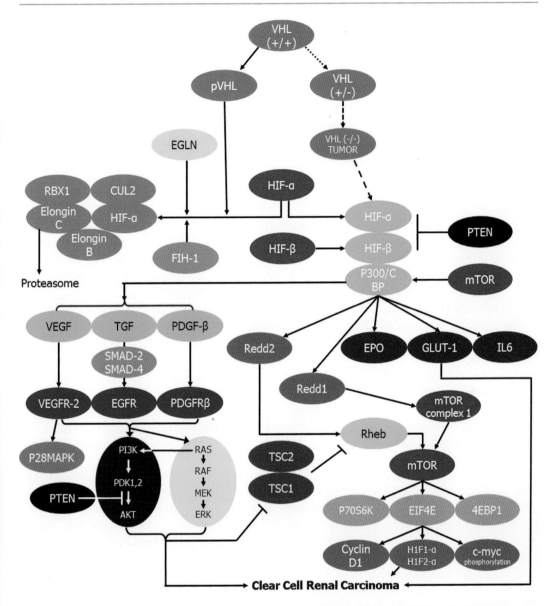

Fig. 16.1 A schematic outline of the pathogenesis of ccRCC. Inactivation of the VHL tumor suppressor gene plays a central role. While the functional VHL protein directs HIF-1α to the proteosome for degradation through hydroxylation, the inactive product allows HIF-1α dimerization with HIF-1β, leading to the activation of multiple downstream pathways which promote cell growth and division, including VEGF, PI3K, MAPK, and mTOR pathways

PDGFR, and EGFR) leading to downstream signaling that results in increased cell proliferation, upregulated angiogenesis, and decreased apoptosis. Induction of the HIF pathway results in production of VEGF, which is a key regulator of angiogenesis in vascular endothelial cells. VEGF initially interacts with VEGFR2 to promote endothelial cell proliferation, migration, and vascular permeability and subsequently activates VEGFR1 to assist in the organization of new capillaries [3, 64, 65].

3. *The Phosphatidylinositol-3-Kinase/Akt/mTOR pathway*

Recent large-scale analysis from The Cancer Genome Atlas (TCGA) showed that the PI(3)K/AKT pathway was recurrently mutated, suggesting this pathway as a potential therapeutic target [43]. mTOR is an important component of the phosphoinositide 3-kinase (PI3K)/Akt signaling pathway. PI3K/Akt/mTOR signaling activation has been suggested to correlate with aggressive behavior and poor prognosis in RCC. Hyperactivity of mTOR signaling can occur via a number of mechanisms, including overexpression or activation of growth factor receptors, activating mutations in PI3K/Akt, or decreased expression of tuberous sclerosis (TSC1/2), PTEN, or VHL tumor suppressor genes. Overproduction of growth factors such as VEGF in tumor cells can result in activation of mTOR signaling in neighboring endothelial cells, leading to increased angiogenesis. mTOR also regulates HIF-1α and HIF-2α, as well as p70S6 kinase, in cancer cells [66].

4. *The Metabolic pathways in ccRCC*

Several studies have shown a diverse range of dysplastic metabolic processes, including mutations in genes encoding tricarboxylic acid (TCA) cycle enzymes, defects in hypoxic and antioxidant signaling, and abnormalities in nutrient-sensing phosphorylation cascades [67, 68]. Recent data from TCGA showed also that aggressive cancers demonstrated evidence of a metabolic shift, involving downregulation of genes involved in the TCA cycle, decreased AMPK and PTEN protein levels, upregulation of the pentose phosphate pathway and the glutamine transporter genes, and increased acetyl-CoA carboxylase protein [43].

The Molecular Classification of RCC

RCC is a group of heterogeneous subtypes, each with distinct morphology, prognosis, and response to therapy [69]. Distinguishing between subtypes relies on histomorphology. There are, however, a significant number of cases where morphology is not conclusive. Moreover, some subtypes have overlapping features, and some of the newly recognized entities, like translocation carcinomas, have histological patterns that are overlapping with other subtypes.

Using different platforms, several groups have shown that gene expression profiling can be used for a more precise renal tumor classification [70–74]. Yang et al. [75] demonstrated the viability of using molecular signatures for the accurate classification of renal tumors. Gene expression analyses showed that oncocytoma and chRCC are also closely related at the molecular level. A distinct pattern of gene expression can, however, separate these two tumors. Another study used mRNA expression profiles to properly distinguish between ccRCC and chRCC [76].

Also, specific miRNA signatures have shown to be able to accurately distinguish between kidney cancer subtypes. Youssef et al. [77] developed a unique classification system that can accurately distinguish between the RCC subtypes with high precision (Fig. 16.2). Similar findings were reported by other groups [78–80]. Recently, a genome-wide DNA methylation study was able to accurately distinguish between type 1 and type 2 pRCCs and discriminate chRCCs from oncocytomas [81].

Recent reports also suggest that even tumors with the same subtype (e.g., ccRCC) can be further subclassified based on their molecular signature. This can have a great impact on patient management, since these "biological" subtypes can have different prognosis and may be subject to different types of targeted therapy.

ccRCC can be classified into two distinct biological subgroups based on gene expression profile. Under normal conditions, VHL is the recognition component of a complex that is responsible for the degradation of HIF1α and HIF2α [82]. When VHL is inactivated, the HIFs become constitutively activated and can induce a number of genes that promote tumor growth by enhancing cell proliferation and angiogenesis [83]. Although HIF1α and HIF2α have been both shown to play significant roles in ccRCC pathogenesis, recently, it has been shown that they can have different effects [84]. Gordan et al. [85] classified VHL-deficient tumors into two groups based on their HIF expression; one subtype expressed both HIF1α and HIF2α (H1H2), while the other expressed HIF2α only (H2) (Fig. 16.3).

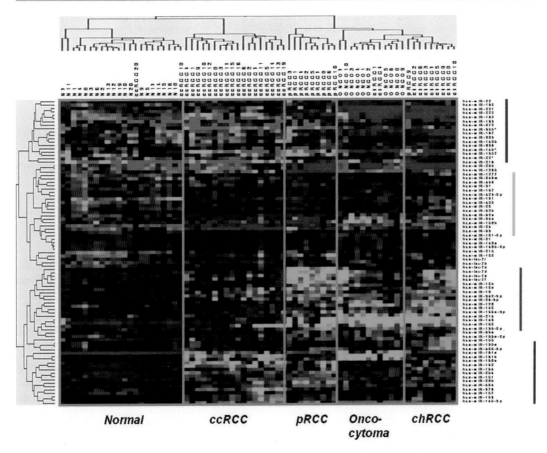

Normal   ccRCC   pRCC   Onco-   chRCC
                                          cytoma

Fig. 16.2 A hierarchic cluster heat map showing differential microRNA (miRNA) expression in normal kidney, oncocytoma, and different renal cell carcinoma (RCC) subtypes. The bars on the *right* indicate miRNA clusters among subtypes that appear highly dysregulated across the samples. miRNA expression profiles can distinguish between the subtypes with high accuracy. *ccRCC* clear cell renal cell carcinoma, *chRCC* chromophobe renal cell carcinoma, *pRCC* papillary renal cell carcinoma (figure obtained with permission from [77])

Interestingly, distinct pathways were shown to be significantly dysregulated in each of these groups. The H1H2 tumors showed increased MAPK and mTOR signaling, while the H2 group showed increased c-Myc activity. More recently, distinct chromosomal aberrations were identified in each of these subtypes, adding to the growing evidence that these two subgroups are distinct [86]. Another study identified two distinct biological subtypes of ccRCC based on gene expression signatures [87]. These two subtypes also showed significant differences in disease-free survival.

Klatte et al. [88] showed that there are distinct cytogenetic aberrations associated with type 1 and type 2 pRCCs. Type 1 tumors frequently had trisomy 17, while type 2 tumors were associated with loss of chromosomes 1p and 3p and gain of 5q. Type 2 was also associated with worse overall survival than type 1 but was not retained as an independent prognostic factor.

Molecular Markers for Kidney Cancer

There are currently no established tumor markers for RCC in clinical practice. Diagnosis of kidney cancer relies on imaging studies [89]. The most commonly used prognostic model for patients with metastatic disease is based on a multivariate

CLEAR CELL RENAL CARCINOMA

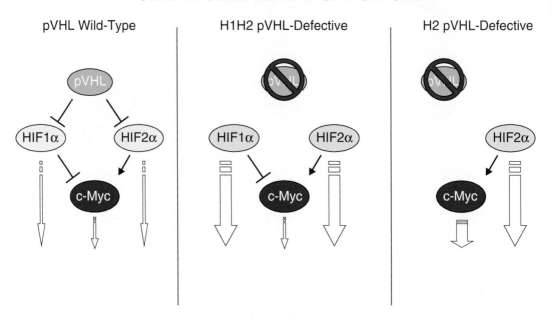

Fig. 16.3 Clear cell renal carcinoma subtypes. pVHL targets HIF-α for proteasomal degradation. Accordingly, tumors with wild-type pVHL have low levels of HIF-α. pVHL-defective tumors can be subdivided based on whether they accumulate both HIF-1α and HIF-2α (H1H2) or HIF-2α alone (H2). In the former, HIF-1α antagonizes c-Myc. In the latter, this antagonism is lost and c-Myc activity is therefore increased (figure obtained with permission from: Kaelin WG Jr. Kidney cancer: now available in a new flavor. Cancer Cell. 2008, 14(6):423–4)

analysis of clinical parameters that was developed at Memorial Sloan-Kettering [90] and later validated and enhanced based on data from the Cleveland Clinic [91]. A number of molecular markers have been investigated, and although many show clinical potential, none have gained approved clinical application [92]

Molecular Diagnostic Markers

Molecular profiling has been used to determine the presence of a "signature expression profile" in RCC that can accurately distinguish between cancerous and normal kidney tissues. A number of studies have analyzed differential gene expressions in RCC at the mRNA [76, 93–95] and the protein levels [96, 97]. The differentially expressed genes and proteins are candidate diagnostic markers that await validation as tissue markers or as noninvasive serum and/or urine markers for early detection of RCC. miRNAs

have also been recently shown to have great diagnostic potential in RCC. A number of miRNAs have been identified that can distinguish between normal and cancerous tissues with high accuracy. These might be particularly important in small biopsy specimens when the available material is not enough for histological evaluation [52, 98].

Molecular Diagnostic Biomarkers of Renal Tumors in Urine and Serum

14-3-3-beta/alpha is higher in urine samples from patients with RCC than healthy volunteers [99]. Methylation-specific PCR showed that hypermethylation of VHL was only found in ccRCC urine samples but not in normal. Hypermethylation of p14ARF, APC, and RASSF1A were more frequent in non-ccRCC and none of these genes were methylated in normal urine controls [100]. Two novel urine biomarkers, aquaporin 1 and adipophilin, were found to be highly expressed in RCCs that originate from the proximal tubules (ccRCC and pRCC) [101, 102].

Urinary nuclear matrix protein 22 (NMP 22) is the only FDA-approved screening marker. It is known to be specific for urothelial carcinoma of renal pelvis, and it is available as a flow-through rapid diagnostic test. In a study on 41 patients, 60 % of the RCC patients had a positive urinary NMP 22 test, compared with only 13 % of the control group [103].

To screen for specific markers in the urine of RCCs patients, surface-enhanced laser desorption and ionization time of flight mass spectrometry (SELDI-TOF-MS) was used and coupled with a tree analysis pattern to develop SELDI protein profiling of urine and serum. Four differentially expressed potential biomarkers from urine were identified. A sensitivity of 67.8 % (19/28) and a specificity of 81.4 % (35/43) for the blinded test were obtained when comparing the RCC versus non-RCC [104].

Reports also suggest that miRNAs are present in stable form in body fluids, and as such, they can be useful as noninvasive diagnostic tests. In addition to distinguishing normal from cancerous tissues, molecular markers can also be used to determine the tissue of origin in tumors of unknown primary [61].

Molecular Prognostic Markers

Recent evidence shows that the integration of molecular markers can lead to significant improvement in the accuracy of the available clinical parameters that are currently used to assess prognosis in RCC [105].

Chromosomal Prognostic Markers

A growing body of evidence has shown copy number aberrations in ccRCC to be dynamically related to patient prognosis and suggest the utility of chromosomal aberrations as prognostic markers in RCC. Apart from gain of chromosome 5q which was associated with a better overall survival [106], most chromosomal aberrations are related to worse prognosis, such as associations of the loss of 4p, 9p, and 14q and gains of 7q, 8q, and 20q, with higher TNM stages, higher grade, and/or worse prognosis [107–112]. 9p loss

has been observed in association with poor outcome in several studies [18, 113]. In locally advanced ccRCC, the loss of heterozygosity (LOH) of 8p and 9p were found to be strong predictors of recurrence post-nephrectomy [114]. It was also observed that LOH of 8p was a better predictor of recurrence compared to tumor grade [114]. Moreover, copy-number alterations in chromosomes 1q, 12q, and 20q have been associated with metastatic ccRCC [111].

In pRCC, 1q gain was shown to be a marker of poor prognosis [115]. In addition, loss of 1p, 3p, or 9p and the absence of trisomy 17 were all associated with poor prognosis [88]. Also, amplifications of 8q were associated with MYC oncogene activation and overexpression in high-grade and aggressive type 2 pRCC [116].

mRNA Prognostic Markers

Earlier reports identified a number of potential prognostic markers for RCC. Lower *PTEN*, *EPCAM*, and higher carbonic anhydrase IX (*CAIX*), *VEGF-R2*, and *VEGF-R3* were all associated with poor prognosis in papillary RCC [88]. A number of potential prognostic markers have been identified in ccRCC, as discussed below.

Carbonic anhydrase IX: CAIX is gaining attention as a potential prognostic biomarker for RCC. CAIX is a HIF-1α-regulated transmembrane protein associated with neoplastic growth, aggressive tumor phenotype, and poor prognosis in a large spectrum of human tumors. A number of studies showed that high CAIX expression is associated with favorable prognosis in localized and metastatic RCC [117–119]. In metastatic RCC, CAIX staining levels have been shown to be inversely related to metastatic spread, and high CAIX expression predicted better survival, even after adjusting for the effects of T stage, Fuhrman grade, nodal status, and performance status. Low CAIX staining (≤85 %) predicted a worse outcome in patients with metastatic RCC. These findings were, however, not reproducible in other studies [120]. Besides prognostic value, the tumor-specific and high prevalence of CAIX in RCC makes it a great target for imaging and therapy using monoclonal antibodies such as

G250. CAIX was also proposed as diagnostic marker (when incorporated into imaging studies) and a predictor of treatment efficiency [121].

VEGF: VEGF expression correlates with tumor size, Fuhrman grade, tumor necrosis, tumor stage, microvessel invasion, RCC progression rate, and RCC-specific survival. Despite its promising characteristics, VEGF awaits validation studies.

Survivin: It is expressed in all RCC variants. High survivin expression is associated with poor differentiation, more aggressive behavior, and lower survival in clear cell RCC. In localized RCC, high survivin expression predicted disease progression [122, 123].

p53: p53 overexpression in papillary, chromophobe, and clear cell RCC was recorded in 70 %, 27 %, and 12 % of tumors, respectively [124]. p53 overexpression was an independent predictor of metastasis-free survival in patients with localized ccRCC. The prognostic role of p53 in RCC remains controversial with studies failing to show any independent prognostic value for survival [124]. In other studies, its prognostic significance was limited to patients with localized disease. Earlier reports have shown that p53 overexpression is associated with sarcomatoid differentiation and poor prognosis [125].

Matrix metalloproteinases: MMP-2 and MMP-9 were found to be overexpressed in 67–76 % and 43 % of tumors, respectively. In addition, overexpression of MMP-2 and MMP-9 was more common in non-ccRCC tumors. MMP-2 and MMP-9 overexpression was associated with aggressive behavior, tumor grade, and survival [126, 127].

Insulin-like growth factor II mRNA-binding protein 3: IMP3 is associated with higher RCC stage, grade, sarcomatoid differentiation, and cancer-specific mortality. In a cohort of 371 patients with localized clear cell, papillary, chromophobe, and unclassified RCC, Jiang et al. reported that tumor cell IMP3 expression was significantly associated with progression to distant metastases

and death [128]. The prognostic value of IMP3 was externally validated in 716 clear cell RCC tumors [129] .

Ki-67: It is associated with an aggressive phenotype in ccRCC. High Ki-67 expression predicts higher recurrence rates and worse survival, and interestingly, the combination of Ki-67 and CAIX surpassed the prognostic ability of nuclear grade in cancer-specific mortality analyses [130, 131].

Caveolin-1: It is a structural component of caveolae. These are plasma membrane microdomains involved in the intracellular signaling pathways that regulate cell adhesion, growth, and survival [132]. Membranous caveolin-1 is expressed in 86 % of ccRCC and <5 % of chromophobe or papillary RCC. Caveolin-1 co-expression with Akt/mTOR pathway components portended worse survival [133].

Vimentin: Vimentin expression is common in clear cell (26–51 %) and papillary RCCs (61 %). Vimentin overexpression (30–53 %) predicted poor prognosis, independent of the effect of stage and grade [134].

Fascin: High fascin expression correlated with sarcomatoid transformation, high tumor stage, high tumor grade, tumor size, and metastatic progression [135].

Other potential markers: B7H1 overexpression was found to be associated with poor survival [136]. Rini et al. showed that 60 % of metastatic RCC patients had VHL mutations and that 48 % of those patients achieved an objective response to targeted therapy versus 35 % for patients with no VHL mutation or methylation [137]. The prognostic significance of HIF-α levels was reported only in patients with ccRCC but not in pRCC.

miRNA Prognostic Markers

miRNA signatures associated with tumor progression and metastasis have been recently reported. Heinzelmann et al. [138] defined an miRNA signature of 33 differentially expressed miRNAs distinguishing between metastatic and non-metastatic ccRCCs. These include miR-451, miR-221, miR-30a, miR-10b, and miR-29a. A number of these miRNAs were associated with progression-free and overall survival. White et al. [139] identified 65 miRNAs that were significantly altered in metastatic ccRCC compared to primary ccRCC. Another study reported miR-155 expression to correlate with tumor size [52]. A study suggested the utility of miR-106b under expression as an indicator of early metastasis in ccRCC patients post-nephrectomy [140]. miR-215 was also reported as prognostic marker in ccRCC [141].

Lin et al. [142] identified seven SNPs in miRNA and miRNA-related genes that are associated with survival and five SNPs associated with recurrence. These SNPs were linked to genes involved in pre-mRNA splicing, ribonucleoprotein assembly, and miRNA processing. They also observed associated haplotypes of *DICER* and *DROSHA* (proteins involved in miRNA processing) with survival and recurrence.

Proteomic Prognostic Markers

A study found that high caveolin-1 (CAV1) protein expression level in the tumor cell cytoplasm may be an independent poor prognostic marker of both overall and tumor-specific survival in ccRCC patients [143]. In addition, increased levels of HIF-1α and phosphorylated ribosomal protein S6 kinase (Phos-S6) were associated with disease-specific survival and tumor progression [144]. The chromatin remodeling gene ARID1a and its protein product BAF250a were recently shown to have prognostic significance in ccRCC [145]. Recent molecular profiling analysis using mass spectrometry identified a number of potential proteins that are differentially expressed between primary and metastatic tumors and can serve as prognostic markers [68]

Epigenetic Prognostic Markers

Arai et al. [146] identified two methylation subclasses for both tumor and nonmalignant tissues that were associated with significantly different survival. Another study demonstrated global hypermethylation as an independent indicator of aggressiveness in early-stage confined ccRCC [147]. Methylation status of the *DLEC1* tumor suppressor was associated with more advanced stages and grades [148]. *GREM1* methylation was associated with increased Fuhrman grade and decreased overall survival in ccRCC [149]. Several hypermethylated genes and miRNAs show promise as independent markers of poor prognosis in RCC such as gamma-catenin, *RASSF1A*, *BNC1*, collagen, type XIV, *COL14A1*, *UCHL1*, *APAF-1*, *DAPK1*, *miR-9-1*, and *miR-9-3* [150–154].

There is evidence to support global histone modification levels as prognostic markers in RCC. Rogenhofer et al. [155] demonstrated lower levels of H3K27me1, H3K27me2, and H3K27me3 in RCC with tumor relapse compared to benign renal tissue. Lower levels of H3K27me1 and H3K27me3 were also associated with shorter progression-free survival. Ellinger et al. [156] observed lower levels of H3K4 in correlation with Fuhrman grading, staging, lymph node, and distant metastasis. Lower levels of H3K4 were also associated with shorter progression-free and cancer-specific survival. Mosashvilli et al. [157] observed an inverse correlation between histone H3 acetylation levels and stage, distant metastasis, Fuhrman grade, and RCC progression.

Molecular Profiling and Integrated Genomics

Molecular profiling is the global analysis at the DNA, gene, or protein levels, to obtain a more comprehensive understanding of a specific pattern or signatures in cancer. A wide spectrum of clinical applications is gradually evolving from molecular profiling of RCC [158, 159], including diagnosis, accurate subclassification, prognosis, and prediction of treatment response. Molecular signatures were shown to supersede conventional staging in predicting outcome.

The use of microarray analysis led to the identification of batches of genes, or gene signatures, which can be of prognostic significance.

Takahashi et al. [101] showed that a group of 40 genes could accurately distinguish between patients who died of cancer and those who did not developed metastasis. Another study identified a 45-gene signature that was associated with poor prognosis [160]. Kosari et al. [161] identified a 35-gene signature that is associated with tumor aggressiveness.

Interestingly, Jones et al. [162] identified a metastatic 155-gene signature in primary tumors that can be used to differentiate ccRCC patient with distant metastasis at the time of surgery from patients with localized disease, suggesting that patients presenting with distant metastasis represent a biologically distinct subgroup. Sultmann et al. [163] independently validated this gene set on a different platform. This concept was further supported by a study that examined a metastatic signature across a number of tumor types and found that solid tumors carrying the gene expression signature were more likely to be associated with metastasis and poor clinical outcome [164].

A recent microarray analysis identified two subgroups within ccRCC, based on gene expression profiling, that differ in biological behavior despite similarity in histology, as described above.

Studies have also shown that the integration of expression profiling data with standard clinical parameters can enhance the assessment of prognosis in RCC [101]. One predictive model for survival included CAIX, p53, and vimentin in addition to standard biomarkers like metastasis status, tumor stage, and the Eastern Cooperative Oncology Group performance status [91]. The combination of biomarkers in a biomarker panel can also enhance the biomarker efficiency. For example, the dual expression of survivin and B7-H1 was shown to be a better predictor of ccRCC tumor aggressiveness [165]. Another study showed that increased expression of p53, gelsolin, and Ki-67 and decreased expression of carbonic anhydrases 9 and 12 correlated better with unfavorable prognosis.

The concept of "integrated genomics" is also very promising. By simultaneously analyzing different molecular levels of changes in the cancer genomes, we can obtain a better understanding of the overall changes of biological processes. Employing this approach overcomes to a large extent the limitation of overlooking critical genes that are disrupted at low frequencies [166, 167]. It also facilitates the discovery of tumor suppressor genes exhibiting multiple concerted disruptions, where each allele may be disrupted by a different mechanism. Also, an oncogene could be activated by two separate mechanisms such as DNA amplification with a simultaneous activating mutation and DNA hypomethylation. In addition to enhancing the ability to detect candidate driver genes, this integrative approach is useful for detecting deregulated pathways [166, 168]. Integrative software for integration of genomic and epigenetic data to decipher their effect on gene expression and disease phenotype is emerging.

The Role of Genomics in RCC Therapy

Molecular Predictive Markers

Managing advanced metastatic RCC is a clinical challenge. New targeted therapies have led to improvements in survival over traditional treatments; however, most patients ultimately develop resistance. Response rates vary among patients and the optimal combination and sequence of therapy is yet to be defined. There are currently no validated biomarkers that can predict treatment outcome in metastatic RCC.

Genetic polymorphisms in key genes associated with sunitinib response and/or toxicity have been recently reviewed [169]. A study found that genetic polymorphisms in three genes involved in sunitinib pharmacokinetics are associated with progression-free survival in mRCC patients treated with this drug [170]. Likewise, in a phase III clinical trial of pazopanib in RCC, three polymorphisms in *IL8* and *HIF1α* and five polymorphisms in *HIF1α*, *NR1I2*, and *VEGFA* showed a significant association with PFS and response rate, respectively [171].

Serum/plasma levels of VEGF, soluble VEGFR-2, CAIX, TIMP-1, and Ras p21 have shown prognostic value in sorafenib-treated RCC patients [172]. Also, TIMP-1 was demonstrated as an independent poor prognostic marker in sorafenib-treated patients [172]. miRNAs represent another class of predictive markers for treatment outcome with successful potential use in other cancers [173–175]. Recent reports provide preliminary encouraging results about the potential role of miRNAs as predictive markers for response to targeted therapy [176, 177]

Molecular Therapeutic Targets

Currently, anti-angiogenic therapies and mTOR inhibitors are the first-line treatment for metastatic cancer but their response rates are in the moderate range. More in-depth understanding of the pathways affected in RCC will allow for the introduction of new more effective targeted therapies [178]. Interestingly, targeted therapies that are used for other cancers might be also applicable to RCC if the same pathway is affected. Molecular profiling analysis has a potential promise in modifying the eligibility of patients for clinical trials, to be based on their biological behavior rather than the anatomical site of their tumors. Recently, initial data showed the feasibility of using genomic and transcriptomic data from integrative sequencing of tumors as a means to identify the most suitable clinical trial for each individual patient [179]. If this is validated on large-scale studies, it will represent a revolutionary improvement in personalized medicine. Finally, miRNAs represent new potential therapies with the unique advantage of controlling the expression of multiple targets by altering the level of a single miRNA [180].

References

1. Maher ER, Neumann HP, Richard S. von Hippel-Lindau disease: a clinical and scientific review. Eur J Hum Genet. 2011;19(6):617–23.
2. Richard S, Lidereau R, Giraud S. The growing family of hereditary renal cell carcinoma. Nephrol Dial Transplant. 2004;19(12):2954–8.
3. Kim WY, Kaelin WG. Role of VHL gene mutation in human cancer. J Clin Oncol. 2004;22(24):4991–5004.
4. Franke G, Bausch B, Hoffmann MM, et al. Alu-alu recombination underlies the vast majority of large VHL germline deletions: molecular characterization and genotype-phenotype correlations in VHL patients. Hum Mutat. 2009;30(5):776–86.
5. Cascon A, Escobar B, Montero-Conde C, et al. Loss of the actin regulator HSPC300 results in clear cell renal cell carcinoma protection in von Hippel-Lindau patients. Hum Mutat. 2007;28(6):613–21.
6. McNeill A, Rattenberry E, Barber R, Killick P, MacDonald F, Maher ER. Genotype-phenotype correlations in VHL exon deletions. Am J Med Genet A. 2009;149A(10):2147–51.
7. Rechsteiner MP, von Teichman A, Nowicka A, Sulser T, Schraml P, Moch H. VHL gene mutations and their effects on hypoxia inducible factor HIFalpha: identification of potential driver and passenger mutations. Cancer Res. 2011;71(16):5500–11.
8. Li L, Zhang L, Zhang X, et al. Hypoxia-inducible factor linked to differential kidney cancer risk seen with type 2A and type 2B VHL mutations. Mol Cell Biol. 2007;27(15):5381–92.
9. Banks RE, Tirukonda P, Taylor C, et al. Genetic and epigenetic analysis of von Hippel-Lindau (VHL) gene alterations and relationship with clinical variables in sporadic renal cancer. Cancer Res. 2006;66(4):2000–11.
10. Choyke PL, Walther MM, Glenn GM, et al. Imaging features of hereditary papillary renal cancers. J Comput Assist Tomogr. 1997;21(5):737–41.
11. Linehan WM, Pinto PA, Bratslavsky G, et al. Hereditary kidney cancer: unique opportunity for disease-based therapy. Cancer. 2009;115(10 Suppl):2252–61.
12. Woodward ER, Ricketts C, Killick P, et al. Familial non-VHL clear cell (conventional) renal cell carcinoma: clinical features, segregation analysis, and mutation analysis of FLCN. Clin Cancer Res. 2008;14(18):5925–30.
13. Launonen V, Vierimaa O, Kiuru M, et al. Inherited susceptibility to uterine leiomyomas and renal cell cancer. Proc Natl Acad Sci USA. 2001;98(6):3387–92.
14. Sudarshan S, Pinto PA, Neckers L, Linehan WM. Mechanisms of disease: hereditary leiomyomatosis and renal cell cancer—a distinct form of hereditary kidney cancer. Nat Clin Pract Urol. 2007;4(2):104–10.
15. Baldewijns MM, van Vlodrop IJ, Schouten LJ, Soetekouw PM, de Bruine AP, van Engeland M. Genetics and epigenetics of renal cell cancer. Biochim Biophys Acta. 2008;1785(2):133–55.
16. Pan CC, Jong YJ, Chai CY, Huang SH, Chen YJ. Comparative genomic hybridization study of perivascular epithelioid cell tumor: molecular genetic evidence of perivascular epithelioid cell tumor as a distinct neoplasm. Hum Pathol. 2006;37(5):606–12.
17. Schwerdtle RF, Storkel S, Neuhaus C, et al. Allelic losses at chromosomes 1p, 2p, 6p, 10p, 13q, 17p, and 21q significantly correlate with the chromophobe

subtype of renal cell carcinoma. Cancer Res. 1996;56(13):2927–30.

18. Dalgliesh GL, Furge K, Greenman C, et al. Systematic sequencing of renal carcinoma reveals inactivation of histone modifying genes. Nature. 2010;463(7279):360–3.

19. Duns G, van den Berg E, van Duivenbode I, et al. Histone methyltransferase gene SETD2 is a novel tumor suppressor gene in clear cell renal cell carcinoma. Cancer Res. 2010;70(11):4287–91.

20. Beroukhim R, Brunet JP, Di Napoli A, et al. Patterns of gene expression and copy-number alterations in von-Hippel Lindau disease-associated and sporadic clear cell carcinoma of the kidney. Cancer Res. 2009;69(11):4674–81.

21. Bissig H, Richter J, Desper R, et al. Evaluation of the clonal relationship between primary and metastatic renal cell carcinoma by comparative genomic hybridization. Am J Pathol. 1999;155(1):267–74.

22. Gronwald J, Storkel S, Holtgreve-Grez H, et al. Comparison of DNA gains and losses in primary renal clear cell carcinomas and metastatic sites: importance of 1q and 3p copy number changes in metastatic events. Cancer Res. 1997;57(3):481–7.

23. Jiang F, Desper R, Papadimitriou CH, et al. Construction of evolutionary tree models for renal cell carcinoma from comparative genomic hybridization data. Cancer Res. 2000;60(22):6503–9.

24. Moch H, Presti Jr JC, Sauter G, et al. Genetic aberrations detected by comparative genomic hybridization are associated with clinical outcome in renal cell carcinoma. Cancer Res. 1996;56(1):27–30.

25. Schullerus D, Herbers J, Chudek J, Kanamaru H, Kovacs G. Loss of heterozygosity at chromosomes 8p, 9p, and 14q is associated with stage and grade of non-papillary renal cell carcinomas. J Pathol. 1997;183(2):151–5.

26. Hes O, Brunelli M, Michal M, et al. Oncocytic papillary renal cell carcinoma: a clinicopathologic, immunohistochemical, ultrastructural, and interphase cytogenetic study of 12 cases. Ann Diagn Pathol. 2006;10(3):133–9.

27. Argani P, Netto GJ, Parwani AV. Papillary renal cell carcinoma with low-grade spindle cell foci: a mimic of mucinous tubular and spindle cell carcinoma. Am J Surg Pathol. 2008;32(9):1353–9.

28. Jiang F, Richter J, Schraml P, Bubendorf L, Gasser T, Sauter G, Mihatsch MJ, Moch H. Chromosomal imbalances in papillary renal cell carcinoma: genetic differences between histological subtypes. Am J Pathol. 1998;153(5):1467–73.

29. Yang XJ, Tan MH, Kim HL, et al. A molecular classification of papillary renal cell carcinoma. Cancer Res. 2005;65(13):5628–37.

30. Argani P, Antonescu CR, Couturier J, et al. PRCC-TFE3 renal carcinomas: morphologic, immunohistochemical, ultrastructural, and molecular analysis of an entity associated with the t(X;1)(p11.2;q21). Am J Surg Pathol. 2002;26(12):1553–66.

31. Clark J, Lu YJ, Sidhar SK, et al. Fusion of splicing factor genes PSF and NonO (p54nrb) to the TFE3 gene in papillary renal cell carcinoma. Oncogene. 1997;15(18):2233–9.

32. Weterman MA, Wilbrink M, Geurts van Kessel A. Fusion of the transcription factor TFE3 gene to a novel gene, PRCC, in t(X;1)(p11;q21)-positive papillary renal cell carcinoma. Proc Natl Acad Sci USA. 1996;93(26):15294–8.

33. Argani P, Antonescu CR, Illei PB, et al. Primary renal neoplasms with the ASPL-TFE3 gene fusion of alveolar soft part sarcoma: a distinctive tumor entity previously included among renal cell carcinomas of children and adolescents. Am J Pathol. 2001;159(1):179–92.

34. Gregori-Romero MA, Morell-Quadreny L, Llombart-Bosch A. Cytogenetic analysis of three primary bellini duct carcinomas. Genes Chromosomes Cancer. 1996;15(3):170–2.

35. Han SS, Yeager M, Moore LE, et al. The chromosome 2p21 region harbors a complex genetic architecture for association with risk for renal cell carcinoma. Hum Mol Genet. 2012;21(5):1190–200.

36. Wu X, Scelo G, Purdue MP, et al. A genome-wide association study identifies a novel susceptibility locus for renal cell carcinoma on 12p11.23. Hum Mol Genet. 2012;21(2):456–62.

37. Cao Q, Qin C, Ju X, et al. Chromosome 11q13.3 variant modifies renal cell cancer risk in a Chinese population. Mutagenesis. 2012;27(3):345–50.

38. Chow WH, Dong LM, Devesa SS. Epidemiology and risk factors for kidney cancer. Nat Rev Urol. 2010;7(5):245–57.

39. Moore LE, Nickerson ML, Brennan P, et al. von Hippel-Lindau (VHL) inactivation in sporadic clear cell renal cancer: associations with germline VHL polymorphisms and etiologic risk factors. PLoS Genet. 2011;7(10):e1002312.

40. Varela I, Tarpey P, Raine K, et al. Exome sequencing identifies frequent mutation of the SWI/SNF complex gene PBRM1 in renal carcinoma. Nature. 2011;469(7331):539–42.

41. New gene mutation implicated in renal cancer. Study findings could shed light on the intricate biology of kidney cancer. Duke Med Health News. 2011;17(4):6–7.

42. Guo G, Gui Y, Gao S, et al. Frequent mutations of genes encoding ubiquitin-mediated proteolysis pathway components in clear cell renal cell carcinoma. Nat Genet. 2011;44(1):17–9.

43. Cancer Genome Atlas Research Network. Comprehensive molecular characterization of clear cell renal cell carcinoma. Nature. 2013;499(7456):43–9.

44. Wang Y, Zhang R, Wu D, et al. Epigenetic change in kidney tumor: downregulation of histone acetyltransferase MYST1 in human renal cell carcinoma. J Exp Clin Cancer Res. 2013;32:8. doi:10.1186/1756-9966-32-8.

45. Herman JG, Latif F, Weng Y, et al. Silencing of the VHL tumor-suppressor gene by DNA methylation in

renal carcinoma. Proc Natl Acad Sci USA. 1994;91(21):9700–4.

46. Dulaimi E, Uzzo RG, Greenberg RE, Al-Saleem T, Cairns P. Detection of bladder cancer in urine by a tumor suppressor gene hypermethylation panel. Clin Cancer Res. 2004;10(6):1887–93.

47. Dreijerink K, Braga E, Kuzmin I, et al. The candidate tumor suppressor gene, RASSF1A, from human chromosome 3p21.3 is involved in kidney tumorigenesis. Proc Natl Acad Sci USA. 2001;98(13):7504–9.

48. Morrissey C, Martinez A, Zatyka M, et al. Epigenetic inactivation of the RASSF1A 3p21.3 tumor suppressor gene in both clear cell and papillary renal cell carcinoma. Cancer Res. 2001;61(19):7277–81.

49. Kvasha S, Gordiyuk V, Kondratov A, et al. Hypermethylation of the 5′CpG island of the FHIT gene in clear cell renal carcinomas. Cancer Lett. 2008;265(2):250–7.

50. Morris MR, Gentle D, Abdulrahman M, et al. Tumor suppressor activity and epigenetic inactivation of hepatocyte growth factor activator inhibitor type 2/SPINT2 in papillary and clear cell renal cell carcinoma. Cancer Res. 2005;65(11):4598–606.

51. Gottardo F, Liu CG, Ferracin M, et al. Micro-RNA profiling in kidney and bladder cancers. Urol Oncol. 2007;25(5):387–92.

52. White NM, Bao TT, Grigull J, et al. miRNA profiling for clear cell renal cell carcinoma: biomarker discovery and identification of potential controls and consequences of miRNA dysregulation. J Urol. 2011;186(3):1077–83.

53. Chow TF, Youssef YM, Lianidou E, et al. Differential expression profiling of microRNAs and their potential involvement in renal cell carcinoma pathogenesis. Clin Biochem. 2010;43(1–2):150–8.

54. Huang Y, Dai Y, Yang J, et al. Microarray analysis of microRNA expression in renal clear cell carcinoma. Eur J Surg Oncol. 2009;35(10):1119–23.

55. Yi Z, Fu Y, Zhao S, Zhang X, Ma C. Differential expression of miRNA patterns in renal cell carcinoma and nontumorous tissues. J Cancer Res Clin Oncol. 2010;136(6):855–62.

56. Chow TF, Mankaruos M, Scorilas A, et al. The miR-17-92 cluster is over expressed in and has an oncogenic effect on renal cell carcinoma. J Urol. 2010;183(2):743–51.

57. Ghosh AK, Shanafelt TD, Cimmino A, et al. Aberrant regulation of pVHL levels by microRNA promotes the HIF/VEGF axis in CLL B cells. Blood. 2009;113(22):5568–74.

58. Lichner Z, Mejia-Guerrero S, Ignacak M, et al. Pleiotropic action of renal cell carcinoma-dysregulated miRNAs on hypoxia-related signaling pathways. Am J Pathol. 2012;180(4):1675–87.

59. Vogt M, Munding J, Gruner M, et al. Frequent concomitant inactivation of miR-34a and miR-34b/c by CpG methylation in colorectal, pancreatic, mammary, ovarian, urothelial, and renal cell carcinomas and soft tissue sarcomas. Virchows Arch. 2011;458(3):313–22.

60. White NM, Yousef GM. MicroRNAs: exploring a new dimension in the pathogenesis of kidney cancer. BMC Med. 2010;8:65. doi:10.1186/1741-7015-8-65.

61. Lu J, Getz G, Miska EA, et al. MicroRNA expression profiles classify human cancers. Nature. 2005;435(7043):834–8.

62. Mena AC, Pulido EG, Guillen-Ponce C. Understanding the molecular-based mechanism of action of the tyrosine kinase inhibitor: sunitinib. Anticancer Drugs. 2010;21 Suppl 1:S3–11.

63. Pfaffenroth EC, Linehan WM. Genetic basis for kidney cancer: opportunity for disease-specific approaches to therapy. Expert Opin Biol Ther. 2008;8(6):779–90.

64. Cheng L, Zhang S, MacLennan GT, Lopez-Beltran A, Montironi R. Molecular and cytogenetic insights into the pathogenesis, classification, differential diagnosis, and prognosis of renal epithelial neoplasms. Hum Pathol. 2009;40(1):10–29.

65. Kim WY, Kaelin Jr WG. Molecular pathways in renal cell carcinoma—rationale for targeted treatment. Semin Oncol. 2006;33(5):588–95.

66. Pal SK, Quinn DI. Differentiating mTOR inhibitors in renal cell carcinoma. Cancer Treat Rev. 2013;39(7):709–19.

67. Yang OC, Maxwell PH, Pollard PJ. Renal cell carcinoma: translational aspects of metabolism and therapeutic consequences. Kidney Int. 2013;84(4): 667–81.

68. Masui O, White NM, DeSouza LV, et al. Quantitative proteomic analysis in metastatic renal cell carcinoma reveals a unique set of proteins with potential prognostic significance. Mol Cell Proteomics. 2013;12(1):132–44.

69. Bex A, Larkin J, Blank C. Non-clear cell renal cell carcinoma: how new biological insight may lead to new therapeutic modalities. Curr Oncol Rep. 2011;13(3):240–8.

70. Higgins JP, Shinghal R, Gill H, et al. Gene expression patterns in renal cell carcinoma assessed by complementary DNA microarray. Am J Pathol. 2003;162(3):925–32.

71. Takahashi M, Rhodes DR, Furge KA, et al. Gene expression profiling of clear cell renal cell carcinoma: gene identification and prognostic classification. Proc Natl Acad Sci USA. 2001;98(17): 9754–9.

72. Yao M, Tabuchi H, Nagashima Y, et al. Gene expression analysis of renal carcinoma: adipose differentiation-related protein as a potential diagnostic and prognostic biomarker for clear-cell renal carcinoma. J Pathol. 2005;205(3):377–87.

73. Young AN, Amin MB, Moreno CS, et al. Expression profiling of renal epithelial neoplasms: a method for tumor classification and discovery of diagnostic molecular markers. Am J Pathol. 2001;158(5): 1639–51.

74. Chuang ST, Chu P, Sugimura J, et al. Overexpression of glutathione s-transferase alpha in clear cell renal cell carcinoma. Am J Clin Pathol. 2005;123(3):421–9.

75. Yang XJ, Sugimura J, Schafernak KT, et al. Classification of renal neoplasms based on molecular signatures. J Urol. 2006;175(6):2302–6.

76. Gieseg MA, Cody T, Man MZ, Madore SJ, Rubin MA, Kaldjian EP. Expression profiling of human renal carcinomas with functional taxonomic analysis. BMC Bioinforma. 2002;3:26.

77. Youssef YM, White NM, Grigull J, et al. Accurate molecular classification of kidney cancer subtypes using microRNA signature. Eur Urol. 2011;59(5): 721–30.

78. Fridman E, Dotan Z, Barshack I, et al. Accurate molecular classification of renal tumors using microRNA expression. J Mol Diagn. 2010;12(5): 687–96.

79. Petillo D, Kort EJ, Anema J, Furge KA, Yang XJ, Teh BT. MicroRNA profiling of human kidney cancer subtypes. Int J Oncol. 2009;35(1):109–14.

80. Powers MP, Alvarez K, Kim HJ, Monzon FA. Molecular classification of adult renal epithelial neoplasms using microRNA expression and virtual karyotyping. Diagn Mol Pathol. 2011;20(2):63–70.

81. Arai E, Wakai-Ushijima S, Fujimoto H, et al. Genome-wide DNA methylation profiles in renal tumors of various histological subtypes and nontumorous renal tissues. Pathobiology. 2011; 78(1):1–9.

82. Arjumand W, Sultana S. Role of VHL gene mutation in human renal cell carcinoma. Tumour Biol. 2012;33(1):9–16.

83. Turner KJ, Moore JW, Jones A, et al. Expression of hypoxia-inducible factors in human renal cancer: relationship to angiogenesis and to the von Hippel-Lindau gene mutation. Cancer Res. 2002;62(10):2957–61.

84. Biswas S, Troy H, Leek R, et al. Effects of HIF-1alpha and HIF2alpha on growth and metabolism of clear-cell renal cell carcinoma 786–0 xenografts. J Oncol. 2010;2010:757908.

85. Gordan JD, Lal P, Dondeti VR, et al. HIF-alpha effects on c-myc distinguish two subtypes of sporadic VHL-deficient clear cell renal carcinoma. Cancer Cell. 2008;14(6):435–46.

86. Dondeti VR, Wubbenhorst B, Lal P, et al. Integrative genomic analyses of sporadic clear cell renal cell carcinoma define disease subtypes and potential new therapeutic targets. Cancer Res. 2012;72(1):112–21.

87. Brannon AR, Reddy A, Seiler M, et al. Molecular stratification of clear cell renal cell carcinoma by consensus clustering reveals distinct subtypes and survival patterns. Genes Cancer. 2010;1(2):152–63.

88. Klatte T, Pantuck AJ, Said JW, et al. Cytogenetic and molecular tumor profiling for type 1 and type 2 papillary renal cell carcinoma. Clin Cancer Res. 2009;15(4):1162–9.

89. Metias SM, Lianidou E, Yousef GM. MicroRNAs in clinical oncology: at the crossroads between promises and problems. J Clin Pathol. 2009;62(9):771–6.

90. Motzer RJ, Mazumdar M, Bacik J, Berg W, Amsterdam A, Ferrara J. Survival and prognostic stratification of 670 patients with advanced renal cell carcinoma. J Clin Oncol. 1999;17(8):2530–40.

91. Mekhail TM, Abou-Jawde RM, Boumerhi G, et al. Validation and extension of the memorial sloan-kettering prognostic factors model for survival in patients with previously untreated metastatic renal cell carcinoma. J Clin Oncol. 2005;23(4):832–41.

92. Lam JS, Pantuck AJ, Belldegrun AS, Figlin RA. Protein expression profiles in renal cell carcinoma: staging, prognosis, and patient selection for clinical trials. Clin Cancer Res. 2007;13(2 Pt 2):703s–8.

93. Boer JM, Huber WK, Sultmann H, et al. Identification and classification of differentially expressed genes in renal cell carcinoma by expression profiling on a global human 31,500-element cDNA array. Genome Res. 2001;11(11):1861–70.

94. Lenburg ME, Liou LS, Gerry NP, Frampton GM, Cohen HT, Christman MF. Previously unidentified changes in renal cell carcinoma gene expression identified by parametric analysis of microarray data. BMC Cancer. 2003;3:31.

95. Rae FK, Stephenson SA, Nicol DL, Clements JA. Novel association of a diverse range of genes with renal cell carcinoma as identified by differential display. Int J Cancer. 2000;88(5):726–32.

96. Han WK, Alinani A, Wu CL, et al. Human kidney injury molecule-1 is a tissue and urinary tumor marker of renal cell carcinoma. J Am Soc Nephrol. 2005;16(4):1126–34.

97. Hwa JS, Kim HJ, Goo BM, et al. The expression of ketohexokinase is diminished in human clear cell type of renal cell carcinoma. Proteomics. 2006;6(3):1077–84.

98. Jung M, Mollenkopf HJ, Grimm C, et al. MicroRNA profiling of clear cell renal cell cancer identifies a robust signature to define renal malignancy. J Cell Mol Med. 2009;13(9B):3918–28.

99. Minamida S, Iwamura M, Kodera Y, et al. 14-3-3 protein Beta/alpha as a urinary biomarker for renal cell carcinoma: proteomic analysis of cyst fluid. Anal Bioanal Chem. 2011;401(1):245–52.

100. Battagli C, Uzzo RG, Dulaimi E, et al. Promoter hypermethylation of tumor suppressor genes in urine from kidney cancer patients. Cancer Res. 2003;63(24):8695–9.

101. Takahashi M, Rhodes DR, Furge KA, et al. Gene expression profiling of clear cell renal cell carcinoma: gene identification and prognostic classification. Proc Natl Acad Sci USA. 2001;98(17):9754–9.

102. Yao M, Huang Y, Shioi K, et al. Expression of adipose differentiation-related protein: a predictor of cancer-specific survival in clear cell renal carcinoma. Clin Cancer Res. 2007;13(1):152–60.

103. Kaya K, Ayan S, Gokce G, Kilicarslan H, Yildiz E, Gultekin EY. Urinary nuclear matrix protein 22 for diagnosis of renal cell carcinoma. Scand J Urol Nephrol. 2005;39(1):25–9.

104. Wu DL, Zhang WH, Wang WJ, Jing SB, Xu YM. Proteomic evaluation of urine from renal cell carcinoma using SELDI-TOF-MS and tree analysis pattern. Technol Cancer Res Treat. 2008;7(3):155–60.

105. Kopper L, Timar J. Genomics of renal cell cancer—does it provide breakthrough? Pathol Oncol Res. 2006;12(1):5–11.

106. Gunawan B, Huber W, Holtrup M, et al. Prognostic impacts of cytogenetic findings in clear cell renal cell carcinoma: gain of 5q31-qter predicts a distinct clinical phenotype with favorable prognosis. Cancer Res. 2001;61(21):7731–8.

107. Chen M, Ye Y, Yang H, et al. Genome-wide profiling of chromosomal alterations in renal cell carcinoma using high-density single nucleotide polymorphism arrays. Int J Cancer. 2009;125(10):2342–8.

108. Klatte T, Rao PN, de Martino M, et al. Cytogenetic profile predicts prognosis of patients with clear cell renal cell carcinoma. J Clin Oncol. 2009;27(5):746–53.

109. La Rochelle J, Klatte T, Dastane A, et al. Chromosome 9p deletions identify an aggressive phenotype of clear cell renal cell carcinoma. Cancer. 2010;116(20):4696–702.

110. Monzon FA, Alvarez K, Peterson L, et al. Chromosome 14q loss defines a molecular subtype of clear-cell renal cell carcinoma associated with poor prognosis. Mod Pathol. 2011;24(11):1470–9.

111. Sanjmyatav J, Junker K, Matthes S, et al. Identification of genomic alterations associated with metastasis and cancer specific survival in clear cell renal cell carcinoma. J Urol. 2011;186(5):2078–83.

112. Yoshimoto T, Matsuura K, Karnan S, et al. High-resolution analysis of DNA copy number alterations and gene expression in renal clear cell carcinoma. J Pathol. 2007;213(4):392–401.

113. Hagenkord JM, Gatalica Z, Jonasch E, Monzon FA. Clinical genomics of renal epithelial tumors. Cancer Genet. 2011;204(6):285–97.

114. Presti Jr JC, Wilhelm M, Reuter V, Russo P, Motzer R, Waldman F. Allelic loss on chromosomes 8 and 9 correlates with clinical outcome in locally advanced clear cell carcinoma of the kidney. J Urol. 2002;167(3):1464–8.

115. Szponar A, Zubakov D, Pawlak J, Jauch A, Kovacs G. Three genetic developmental stages of papillary renal cell tumors: duplication of chromosome 1q marks fatal progression. Int J Cancer. 2009;124(9):2071–6.

116. Furge KA, Chen J, Koeman J, et al. Detection of DNA copy number changes and oncogenic signaling abnormalities from gene expression data reveals MYC activation in high-grade papillary renal cell carcinoma. Cancer Res. 2007;67(7):3171–6.

117. Bui MH, Seligson D, Han KR, et al. Carbonic anhydrase IX is an independent predictor of survival in advanced renal clear cell carcinoma: implications for prognosis and therapy. Clin Cancer Res. 2003;9(2):802–11.

118. Sandlund J, Oosterwijk E, Grankvist K, Oosterwijk-Wakka J, Ljungberg B, Rasmuson T. Prognostic impact of carbonic anhydrase IX expression in human renal cell carcinoma. BJU Int. 2007;100(3):556–60.

119. Patard JJ, Fergelot P, Karakiewicz PI, et al. Low CAIX expression and absence of VHL gene mutation are associated with tumor aggressiveness and poor survival of clear cell renal cell carcinoma. Int J Cancer. 2008;123(2):395–400.

120. Leibovich BC, Sheinin Y, Lohse CM, et al. Carbonic anhydrase IX is not an independent predictor of outcome for patients with clear cell renal cell carcinoma. J Clin Oncol. 2007;25(30):4757–64.

121. Stillebroer AB, Mulders PF, Boerman OC, Oyen WJ, Oosterwijk E. Carbonic anhydrase IX in renal cell carcinoma: implications for prognosis, diagnosis, and therapy. Eur Urol. 2010;58(1):75–83.

122. Zamparese R, Pannone G, Santoro A, et al. Survivin expression in renal cell carcinoma. Cancer Invest. 2008;26(9):929–35.

123. Parker AS, Kosari F, Lohse CM, et al. High expression levels of survivin protein independently predict a poor outcome for patients who undergo surgery for clear cell renal cell carcinoma. Cancer. 2006;107(1):37–45.

124. Zigeuner R, Ratschek M, Rehak P, Schips L, Langner C. Value of p53 as a prognostic marker in histologic subtypes of renal cell carcinoma: a systematic analysis of primary and metastatic tumor tissue. Urology. 2004;63(4):651–5.

125. Oda H, Nakatsuru Y, Ishikawa T. Mutations of the p53 gene and p53 protein overexpression are associated with sarcomatoid transformation in renal cell carcinomas. Cancer Res. 1995;55(3):658–62.

126. Kallakury BV, Karikehalli S, Haholu A, Sheehan CE, Azumi N, Ross JS. Increased expression of matrix metalloproteinases 2 and 9 and tissue inhibitors of metalloproteinases 1 and 2 correlate with poor prognostic variables in renal cell carcinoma. Clin Cancer Res. 2001;7(10):3113–9.

127. Kawata N, Nagane Y, Igarashi T, et al. Strong significant correlation between MMP-9 and systemic symptoms in patients with localized renal cell carcinoma. Urology. 2006;68(3):523–7.

128. Jiang Z, Chu PG, Woda BA, et al. Analysis of RNA-binding protein IMP3 to predict metastasis and prognosis of renal-cell carcinoma: a retrospective study. Lancet Oncol. 2006;7(7):556–64.

129. Hoffmann NE, Sheinin Y, Lohse CM, et al. External validation of IMP3 expression as an independent prognostic marker for metastatic progression and death for patients with clear cell renal cell carcinoma. Cancer. 2008;112(7):1471–9.

130. Klatte T, Seligson DB, LaRochelle J, et al. Molecular signatures of localized clear cell renal cell carcinoma to predict disease-free survival after nephrectomy. Cancer Epidemiol Biomarkers Prev. 2009;18(3):894–900.

131. Visapaa H, Bui M, Huang Y, et al. Correlation of ki-67 and gelsolin expression to clinical outcome in renal clear cell carcinoma. Urology. 2003; 61(4):845–50.

132. Anderson RG. The caveolae membrane system. Annu Rev Biochem. 1998;67:199–225.

133. Campbell L, Jasani B, Edwards K, Gumbleton M, Griffiths DF. Combined expression of caveolin-1 and an activated AKT/mTOR pathway predicts reduced disease-free survival in clinically confined renal cell carcinoma. Br J Cancer. 2008;98(5): 931–40.

134. Moch H, Schraml P, Bubendorf L, et al. High-throughput tissue microarray analysis to evaluate genes uncovered by cDNA microarray screening in renal cell carcinoma. Am J Pathol. 1999;154(4): 981–6.

135. Zigeuner R, Droschl N, Tauber V, Rehak P, Langner C. Biologic significance of fascin expression in clear cell renal cell carcinoma: systematic analysis of primary and metastatic tumor tissues using a tissue microarray technique. Urology. 2006;68(3):518–22.

136. Thompson RH, Kwon ED. Significance of B7-H1 overexpression in kidney cancer. Clin Genitourin Cancer. 2006;5(3):206–11.

137. Rini BI, Jaeger E, Weinberg V, et al. Clinical response to therapy targeted at vascular endothelial growth factor in metastatic renal cell carcinoma: impact of patient characteristics and von Hippel-Lindau gene status. BJU Int. 2006;98(4):756–62.

138. Heinzelmann J, Henning B, Sanjmyatav J, et al. Specific miRNA signatures are associated with metastasis and poor prognosis in clear cell renal cell carcinoma. World J Urol. 2011;29(3):367–73.

139. White NM, Khella HW, Grigull J, et al. miRNA profiling in metastatic renal cell carcinoma reveals a tumour-suppressor effect for miR-215. Br J Cancer. 2011;105(11):1741–9.

140. Slaby O, Redova M, Poprach A, et al. Identification of MicroRNAs associated with early relapse after nephrectomy in renal cell carcinoma patients. Genes Chromosomes Cancer. 2012;51(7):707–16.

141. Khella HW, Bakhet M, Allo G, Jewett MA, Girgis AH, Latif A, Girgis H, Von Both I, Bjarnason GA, Yousef GM. miR-192, miR-194 and miR-215: a convergent microRNA network suppressing tumor progression in renal cell carcinoma. Carcinogenesis. 2013;34(10):2231–9.

142. Lin J, Horikawa Y, Tamboli P, Clague J, Wood CG, Wu X. Genetic variations in microRNA-related genes are associated with survival and recurrence in patients with renal cell carcinoma. Carcinogenesis. 2010;31(10):1805–12.

143. Steffens S, Schrader AJ, Blasig H, et al. Caveolin 1 protein expression in renal cell carcinoma predicts survival. BMC Urol. 2011;11:25. doi:10.1186/ 1471-2490-11-25.

144. Schultz L, Chaux A, Albadine R, et al. Immunoexpression status and prognostic value of mTOR and hypoxia-induced pathway members in primary and metastatic clear cell renal cell carcinomas. Am J Surg Pathol. 2011;35(10):1549–56.

145. Lichner Z, Scorilas A, White NM, et al. The chromatin remodeling gene ARID1A is a new prognostic marker in clear cell renal cell carcinoma. Am J Pathol. 2013;182(4):1163–70.

146. Arai E, Ushijima S, Fujimoto H, et al. Genome-wide DNA methylation profiles in both precancerous conditions and clear cell renal cell carcinomas are correlated with malignant potential and patient outcome. Carcinogenesis. 2009;30(2):214–21.

147. Minardi D, Lucarini G, Filosa A, et al. Prognostic role of global DNA-methylation and histone acetylation in pT1a clear cell renal carcinoma in partial nephrectomy specimens. J Cell Mol Med. 2009;13(8B):2115–21.

148. Zhang Q, Ying J, Li J, et al. Aberrant promoter methylation of DLEC1, a critical 3p22 tumor suppressor for renal cell carcinoma, is associated with more advanced tumor stage. J Urol. 2010;184(2):731–7.

149. van Vlodrop IJ, Baldewijns MM, Smits KM, et al. Prognostic significance of Gremlin1 (GREM1) promoter CpG island hypermethylation in clear cell renal cell carcinoma. Am J Pathol. 2010;176(2): 575–84.

150. Kagara I, Enokida H, Kawakami K, et al. CpG hypermethylation of the UCHL1 gene promoter is associated with pathogenesis and poor prognosis in renal cell carcinoma. J Urol. 2008;180(1):343–51.

151. Breault JE, Shiina H, Igawa M, et al. Methylation of the gamma-catenin gene is associated with poor prognosis of renal cell carcinoma. Clin Cancer Res. 2005;11(2 Pt 1):557–64.

152. Kawai Y, Sakano S, Suehiro Y, et al. Methylation level of the RASSF1A promoter is an independent prognostic factor for clear-cell renal cell carcinoma. Ann Oncol. 2010;21(8):1612–7.

153. Morris MR, Ricketts C, Gentle D, et al. Identification of candidate tumour suppressor genes frequently methylated in renal cell carcinoma. Oncogene. 2010;29(14):2104–17.

154. Hildebrandt MA, Gu J, Lin J, et al. Hsa-miR-9 methylation status is associated with cancer development and metastatic recurrence in patients with clear cell renal cell carcinoma. Oncogene. 2010;29(42): 5724–8.

155. Rogenhofer S, Kahl P, Mertens C, et al. Global histone H3 lysine 27 (H3K27) methylation levels and their prognostic relevance in renal cell carcinoma. BJU Int. 2012;109(3):459–65.

156. Ellinger J, Kahl P, Mertens C, et al. Prognostic relevance of global histone H3 lysine 4 (H3K4) methylation in renal cell carcinoma. Int J Cancer. 2010;127(10):2360–6.

157. Mosashvilli D, Kahl P, Mertens C, et al. Global histone acetylation levels: prognostic relevance in patients with renal cell carcinoma. Cancer Sci. 2010;101(12):2664–9.

158. Arsanious A, Bjarnason GA, Yousef GM. From bench to bedside: current and future applications of

molecular profiling in renal cell carcinoma. Mol Cancer. 2009;8:20. doi:10.1186/1476-4598-8-20.

159. Brannon AR, Rathmell WK. Renal cell carcinoma: where will the state-of-the-art lead us? Curr Oncol Rep. 2010;12(3):193–201.

160. Vasselli JR, Shih JH, Iyengar SR, et al. Predicting survival in patients with metastatic kidney cancer by gene-expression profiling in the primary tumor. Proc Natl Acad Sci USA. 2003;100(12):6958–63.

161. Kosari F, Parker AS, Kube DM, et al. Clear cell renal cell carcinoma: gene expression analyses identify a potential signature for tumor aggressiveness. Clin Cancer Res. 2005;11(14):5128–39.

162. Jones J, Otu H, Spentzos D, et al. Gene signatures of progression and metastasis in renal cell cancer. Clin Cancer Res. 2005;11(16):5730–9.

163. Sultmann H, von Heydebreck A, Huber W, et al. Gene expression in kidney cancer is associated with cytogenetic abnormalities, metastasis formation, and patient survival. Clin Cancer Res. 2005;11(2 Pt 1):646–55.

164. Ramaswamy S, Ross KN, Lander ES, Golub TR. A molecular signature of metastasis in primary solid tumors. Nat Genet. 2003;33(1):49–54.

165. Crispen PL, Boorjian SA, Lohse CM, Leibovich BC, Kwon ED. Predicting disease progression after nephrectomy for localized renal cell carcinoma: the utility of prognostic models and molecular biomarkers. Cancer. 2008;113(3):450–60.

166. Chari R, Thu KL, Wilson IM, et al. Integrating the multiple dimensions of genomic and epigenomic landscapes of cancer. Cancer Metastasis Rev. 2010;29(1):73–93.

167. Cancer Genome Atlas Research Network. Comprehensive genomic characterization defines human glioblastoma genes and core pathways. Nature. 2008;455(7216):1061–8.

168. Chari R, Coe BP, Vucic EA, Lockwood WW, Lam WL. An integrative multi-dimensional genetic and epigenetic strategy to identify aberrant genes and pathways in cancer. BMC Syst Biol. 2010;4:67. doi:10.1186/1752-0509-4-67.

169. Yuasa T, Takahashi S, Hatake K, Yonese J, Fukui I. Biomarkers to predict response to sunitinib therapy and prognosis in metastatic renal cell cancer. Cancer Sci. 2011;102(11):1949–57.

170. van der Veldt AA, Eechoute K, Gelderblom H, et al. Genetic polymorphisms associated with a prolonged progression-free survival in patients with metastatic renal cell cancer treated with sunitinib. Clin Cancer Res. 2011;17(3):620–9.

171. Xu CF, Bing NX, Ball HA, et al. Pazopanib efficacy in renal cell carcinoma: evidence for predictive genetic markers in angiogenesis-related and exposure-related genes. J Clin Oncol. 2011;29(18):2557–64.

172. Pena C, Lathia C, Shan M, Escudier B, Bukowski RM. Biomarkers predicting outcome in patients with advanced renal cell carcinoma: results from sorafenib phase III treatment approaches in renal cancer global evaluation trial. Clin Cancer Res. 2010;16(19):4853–63.

173. Wu WY, Xue XY, Chen ZJ, et al. Potentially predictive microRNAs of gastric cancer with metastasis to lymph node. World J Gastroenterol. 2011;17(31): 3645–51.

174. Teo MT, Landi D, Taylor CF, et al. The role of microRNA-binding site polymorphisms in DNA repair genes as risk factors for bladder cancer and breast cancer and their impact on radiotherapy outcomes. Carcinogenesis. 2012;33(3):581–6.

175. Gao W, Lu X, Liu L, Xu J, Feng D, Shu Y. MiRNA-21: a biomarker predictive for platinum-based adjuvant chemotherapy response in patients with non-small cell lung cancer. Cancer Biol Ther. 2012;13(5):330–40.

176. Gamez-Pozo A, Anton-Aparicio LM, Bayona C, et al. MicroRNA expression profiling of peripheral blood samples predicts resistance to first-line sunitinib in advanced renal cell carcinoma patients. Neoplasia. 2012;14(12):1144–52.

177. Berkers J, Govaere O, Wolter P, et al. A possible role for microRNA-141 down-regulation in sunitinib resistant metastatic clear cell renal cell carcinoma through induction of epithelial-to-mesenchymal transition and hypoxia resistance. J Urol. 2013; 189(5):1930–8.

178. White NM, Yousef GM. Translating molecular signatures of renal cell carcinoma into clinical practice. J Urol. 2011;186(1):9–11.

179. Roychowdhury S, Iyer MK, Robinson DR, et al. Personalized oncology through integrative high-throughput sequencing: a pilot study. Sci Transl Med. 2011;3(111):111ra121.

180. Lundstrom K. Micro-RNA in disease and gene therapy. Curr Drug Discov Technol. 2011;8(2):76–86.

Manal Y. Gabril and George M. Yousef

Prostate cancer (PCa) is the most common malignancy and the second most common cancer-related cause of death among men in North America. It is a heterogeneous disease with frequent multifocality and morphological variability. The majority of PCa patients are diagnosed with curable, organ-confined disease. Accurate identification of patients with an increased risk of postsurgical recurrence is of major importance for personalizing patient management plan.

The Genomics of Prostate Cancer

Germline Genetic Mutations

PCa can be either hereditary or sporadic. A large body of work has indicated that there are multiple complex genomic "hot spots" producing heritable sequence changes which are linked to disease risk [1]. Linkage studies have been used as a

valuable source to identify candidate regions of the genome involved in hereditary PCa. Recently, genome-wide association studies (GWAS) have served as a powerful tool in PCa genomic research [2].

Candidate Genes and Susceptibility Loci Identified by Linkage Analyses

RNASEL: The *RNASEL* gene, within the hereditary prostate cancer 1 (*HPC1*) locus on 1q25, mediates antiviral and proapoptotic activities of the IFN-inducible 2-5A system [3]. A nonsense truncating mutation Glu265X and an initiation codon mutation Met1Ile in the *RNASEL* gene segregate in PCa families that were linked to the *HPC1* locus. Functional studies showed that both mutations were associated with a reduction in *RNASEL* activity [4].

ELAC2: The *ELAC2* gene, on the hereditary prostate cancer 2 (*HPC2*) locus on 17p11, encodes a tRNA 3′ processing endoribonuclease. An association between PCa and two common missense variants, a serine to leucine change (Ser217Leu) and an alanine to threonine change (Ala541Thr), has been reported in families with hereditary PCa [5].

MSR1: The macrophage scavenger receptor 1 (*MSR1*) gene, located at 8p22, has been reported as a strong candidate for PCa susceptibility. Besides the positive linkage findings of this gene in hereditary PCa, the p22 band of chromosome 8 is also frequently deleted in PCa. Mutations in

M.Y. Gabril, M.D.
Department of Pathology and Laboratory Medicine, University Hospital, 339 Windermere Road, London, ON, Canada N6A 5A5
e-mail: manal.gabril@lhsc.on.ca

G.M. Yousef, M.D., Ph.D. (✉)
Department of Laboratory Medicine and Pathobiology, University of Toronto, Medical Sciences Building, 1 King's College Circle, Toronto, ON, Canada M5S 1A8
e-mail: yousefg@smh.ca

G.M. Yousef and S. Jothy (eds.), *Molecular Testing in Cancer*, DOI 10.1007/978-1-4899-8050-2_17, © Springer Science+Business Media New York 2014

MSR1 have been shown to be associated with PCa risk in both hereditary and sporadic cases in European and African-American men [6].

Homeobox B13 (*HOXB13*): The novel rare mutation, homeobox B13 (*HOXB13*) Gly84Glu, was reported to co-segregate with cancer in hereditary PCa families and was associated with a significantly increased risk of hereditary PCa. Several additional rare missense HOXB13 variants (Tyr88Asp, Leu144Pro, Gly216Cys, and Arg229Gly) were also identified. The recurrent nature of the Gly84Glu change and a reported lack of any truncating mutations in HOXB13 in patients with PCa suggest a carcinogenic mechanism that is more consistent with a gain of function (oncogenic) than with a loss of function. Although HOXB13 mutations could be identified in a minority of men with PCa, rare genetic lesions can identify pathways that are found to be abnormal in more common, sporadic cases [7].

CHEK2: The CHEK2 gene (22q) is an upstream regulator of p53 in the DNA damage signaling pathway. CHEK2 mutations have been identified in both sporadic and familial cases of PCa and are associated with a small increased risk of PCa [8].

Low-Penetrance Genes: Mutations in high-penetrance susceptibility genes are relatively uncommon in PCa. On the other hand, polymorphisms in low-penetrance genes increase the risk of developing the disease only modestly but occur at greater frequency:
1. The polymorphic CAG (cytosine–adenosine–guanine) repeat in the *androgen receptor* (*AR*) *gene* has been studied extensively. Studies have shown an inverse relationship between the CAG repeat length and PCa risk. Short CAG length has been also correlated with high-grade, high-stage, metastasis, and fatal outcome. The prevalence of PCa is higher in African Americans with higher prevalence of shorter CAG repeats in the AR gene and lower in Chinese men with a higher prevalence of longer CAG repeats. A recent study showed that this risk factor is less important than previously thought [9, 10].

2. Polymorphisms in the *SRD5A2*, the gene that codes for the enzyme 5α-reductase type II, have been reported to be associated with an increased risk of developing PCa [11]. 5α-reductase is responsible for the conversion of testosterone to its more active metabolite dihydrotestosterone.
3. The *vitamin D receptor* (*VDR*) gene is also a polymorphic steroid hormone receptor implicated in PCa. Whether the *VDR* polymorphisms confer an increased susceptibility to PCa remains a challenge. VDR alleles have been strongly associated with advanced cancers [12].

Other polymorphisms reported to influence the risk of developing PCa include the cytochrome P450 family genes (*CYP3A4* and *CYP17*). *CYP17* encodes cytochrome P450c17α, an enzyme responsible for the biosynthesis of testosterone. A variant *CYP17* allele is associated with both hereditary and sporadic PCas [13]. Others regions detected by linkage analysis are *Predisposing for CAncer of Prostate* (PCAP) at 1q42.2-43 [14]; CABP at 1p36 [15], 16q23 [16], and 19p13 [17]; and HPC20 at 20q13 [18]. Other loci linked to PCa are chromosomal location 3p26, 3q26, 4q35, 7q32-33, 11q14, 17q22, and 22q12-13.

Candidate Genes and Susceptibility Loci Identified by GWAS

Hepatocyte nuclear factor 1B (HNF1B) is encoded by the transcription factor 2 TCF2 gene (17q12). This gene has been reported to be associated with increase PCa risk by 20 %. Interestingly, the HNF1B risk allele (or SNP allele) for PCa was associated with protection against type 2 diabetes, and likewise, the risk allele for type 2 diabetes is associated with decreased risk for PCa. HNF1B/TCF2/MODY5 contains a homeobox domain and is classified as a beta helix-loop-helix transcription factor [19].

Some SNP alleles are not associated with identifiable genes. Studies indicate that there are up to seven distinct loci within the 8q24 region in which SNP alleles correlated with up to a 50 % increased risk of PCa [20]. Recent studies have identified enhancer elements within 8q24 which are conserved in primates and canine species.

The c-Myc proto-oncogene is located 200 kb upstream of 8q24 and has been proposed to be regulated by elements in this region in other cancers. Sotelo et al. linked the enhancers in the region to gene expression in vitro in PCa cells [21]. Another study showed that chromosomal looping leads to a direct interaction between PCa-associated SNP alleles and the c-Myc promoter [22]. Currently, there are conflicting reports on whether or not these SNP alleles change c-Myc expression in vivo. A meta-analysis confirmed that a subset of risk-associated SNPs at 8q24 displays differing patterns of risk association based on race [23].

GWAS have also identified two potential loci on chromosome 10, one of which encompasses a SNP in the proximal promoter of the B-microseminoprotein gene (MSMB). There is a correlation between a reduced level of PSP94 (the protein product of MSMB) and progression after radical prostatectomy [24].

The breast cancer susceptibility genes BRCA1 (17q21) and BRCA2 (13q12.3) confer a relative risk of PCa of 3.0 and 2.6–7.0, respectively. The UK/Canadian/Texan Consortium found up to 30 % of familial clusters may be linked to BRAC1/2, although the confidence intervals were wide and included one. The UK Familial Prostate Cancer Study was unable to find any mutations in the BRAC1 gene but identified two germline mutations in BRCA2. An association between breast and PCa clearly exists; the molecular basis for this association is not yet fully understood [25].

Somatic Molecular Alterations

Chromosomal Aberrations

Most PCas exhibit somatic copy number alterations (SCNAs), with genomic deletions outnumbering amplifications in early stages of disease. Conventional karyotyping identified recurrent chromosomal changes including trisomy 7, loss of Y, deletions of 7q and 10q, and double minutes. Using FISH, gains of chromosomes 1, 7, 8, 8q, 17, X, and Y and loss of chromosomes 1, 7, 8, 8p, 10, 10q, 16q, 17q, 17, and Y have been reported [26]. Recently, comparative genomic hybridization and high-density single-nucleotide

polymorphism arrays have allowed high-resolution genome-wide analysis of SCNAs.

Visakorpi et al. reported loss of 8p and 13q in prostatic intraepithelial neoplasia (PIN) [27]. Also recurrent losses and rearrangements on chromosome 22q between the TMPRSS2 and ERG gene loci are described in PCa, as discussed below in details.

The highest rate of LOH has been detected at the chromosomal regions of 8p, 13q, and 16q [28]. Within 8p, at least two minimal regions of deletions are reported: the first at 8p22, with concurrent gain of 8c (8 centromere), has been associated with adverse disease outcome [29]. The second region at 8p21, the site of a prostate-specific homeobox gene NKX3.1, correlated with tumor progression [30]. LOH at 8p has been also reported in high PIN.

Deletion of 13q21 was also associated with aggressive disease [31]. More than half of PCa cases show LOH at 13p [32, 33]. This region harbors the Rb and BRCA2 genes. Loss of BRCA2 was relatively uncommon in localized PCa, but deletion of Rb was more frequent [33]. Also, allelic loss on chromosome 13q14, q21-22, and q33 occurred frequently in metastatic and aggressive cancers [34].

LOH at 16q (16q22.1-22.3, 16q23.2-24.1, and 16q24.3-ter) is often observed in advanced PCa and is associated with poor prognosis [35]. In 10q, the highest rate of LOH has been reported at region 10q23-q24, harboring the phosphatase and tensin homolog (PTEN) tumor suppressor gene [36]. Another candidate gene, MXII, has been identified which is an antagonist of MYC [37].

Isochromosome 17 was one of the earliest discovered chromosomal abnormalities associated with PCa. Subsequently, a deletion was identified in peak regions of the short arm of chromosome 17. One of these regions harbors a potential metastasis suppressor gene (MKK4/SEK1). p53 (17p13.1) is also mutated in a subset of advanced-stage prostate carcinomas, but does not appear to play a major role in cancer development [38].

Almost 90 % of hormone-refractory and metastatic cancers show 8q gain, compared to 5 % of primary tumors [27, 39–41]. The MYC oncogene located at 8q24 has been associated with aggressive disease [39]. FISH showed MYC overexpression in ~9 % of localized and ~75 % of advanced PCas.

Another gene on chromosome 8q is PSCA, encoding prostate stem cell antigen. Elongin C [42] and EIF3S3 [43] genes are located on chromosome 8q and have also been implicated as potential targets of amplification. Other genes seem to be overexpressed in hormone-refractory prostate carcinomas include TCEB1 (8q21), KIAA0196, and RAD21 (8q23-q24) [44, 45]. Thirty percent of hormone-refractory PCas have shown amplification of region Xq11-13 which encodes androgen receptor and 50 % of cases show gains in regions of 7q/7p [27].

Epigenetic Changes
Hypermethylation

Hypermethylation is a common event in PCa. A list of commonly hypermethylated genes and their functional categories is shown in Box 17.1.

Hormone Signaling: The androgen receptor (AR) is a critical effector in PCa development and progression. Recent studies demonstrated the role of the AR in driving PCa cell growth even in low androgen levels and castrate-resistant PCa [46]. Epigenetic changes including CpG methylation and histone acetylation play important roles in the regulation of AR pathway signaling. Hypermethylation of the AR gene is more frequent in castrate-resistant tumors (29 %) compared with untreated primary tissues (10 %) [47].

DNA Repair Genes: The GSTP1 gene encodes the π-class glutathione S-transferase (GST). The associated loss of its function likely sensitizes prostatic epithelial cells to cell and genome damage. No mutations or deletions have been reported for GSTP1 gene in PCa; however the gene is inactivated and both alleles are commonly methylated [48]. Hypermethylation of CpG island within GSTP1 promoter region is one of the earliest changes in the pathogenesis of PCa. GSTP1 methylation is absent in normal epithelium and present in 70 % of high-grade prostatic intraepithelial neoplasia (HGPIN) and 90 % of PCas [48].

Box 17.1 Commonly Hypermethylated Genes in Prostate Cancer and their Functional Categories

DNA repair genes
  GSTP1
  MGMT
Tumor suppressor genes
  APC
  RARβ
  RASSF1
Hormone receptors
  AR
  ESR1,2
Cell adhesion genes
  CDH1
  CDH13
  CD44
Cell cycle control genes
  CCND2
  CDKN1B
  SFN
Apoptotic genes
  GADD45a
  PYCARD
  RPRM
  GLIPR1

Tumor Suppressor Genes: Promoter methylation in the APC tumor suppressor genes has been identified as markers for PCa prognosis. Patients with APC methylation had higher mortality [49]. Also, inactivation of the tumor suppressor gene RASSF1A has been associated with hypermethylation of its CpG island promoter region. The encoded RASSF1A protein was found to interact with DNA repair protein XPA. It has also been shown to counteract stimulation of cell proliferation by RAS-linked pathways and inhibit the accumulation of cyclin D1 and thus induce cell cycle arrest [50].

Cell Adhesion Genes: E-cadherin (CDH1) is a strong suppressor of invasion. Decreased CDH1 expression has been associated with more extensive metastases and poor overall survival in PCa. The 5′ CpG island of CDH1 is densely methylated in PCa cell lines [51]. CD44 encodes for another membrane protein involved in matrix adhesion and signal transduction. In PCa, CD44 hypermethylation is seen in 78 % of patients compared to only 10 % of normal [52].

Cell Cycle and Proapoptotic Genes: Hypermethylation of the CCND2 promoter is significantly higher in PCas compared to normal prostate tissues (32 % vs. 6 %, respectively) [53]. High CCND2 methylation levels correlate with tumor aggressiveness [54]. A number of genes including GSTP1, APC, PTGS2, MDR1, and RASSF1a are hypermethylated in PCa samples. Importantly, these aberrantly methylated genes positively correlated with disease stage and are unique to PCa. A combined assay for GSTP1 and APC hypermethylation has shown great promise for detecting PCa in clinical samples with up to 100 % certainty [55].

Hypomethylation

Promoter hypomethylation and subsequent upregulation of oncogenes such as WNT5A have been reported in PCa. Among the members of polycomb repressive complex (PRC), the most studied is the polycomb protein enhancer of zeste homologue 2 (EZH2), an essential component of a protein complex that catalyzes methylation of histone H3 at K9 contributing to transcriptional repression of a large number of specific genes. PRC1 complex was also required for trimethylation at H3K27, which is responsible for stable maintenance of gene repression [56]. Increased levels of H3K27me3 in PCa are associated with repression of tumor suppressor genes such as DAB2IP, a member of the Ras GTPase family [57].

Tumor Suppressor Genes

NKX3.1: NKX3.1 is an androgen-regulated tumor suppressor gene on chromosome 8p21.2. It binds to DNA and represses expression of the PSA. In addition to 8p21 LOH, there is evidence that NKX3.1 undergoes epigenetic downregulation through promoter methylation [58].

PTEN: The PTEN gene is mutated in up to 1/3 of hormone-refractory PCas, and homozygous deletions and mutations have been identified in a subset of primary PCas. PTEN loss correlates with high Gleason score and advanced stage [59].

CDKN1B (p27): Reduced concentrations of p27 are common in PCas, particularly in those with poor prognosis. Somatic loss at 12p12–3, encompassing CDKN1B, has been described in 23 % of localized PCas, 30 % of PCa metastases in regional lymph nodes, and 47 % of distant metastases [60].

KLF6: KLF6 comprises a group of transcription factors that appear to be involved in different biological processes including carcinogenesis. Important genetic alterations of KLF6 have been reported, including deletions and loss of expression in a minority of high-grade PCas [61].

Genetic inactivation of the classic tumor suppressor genes *p53*, *RB1*, *p16* is rarely seen in primary cancers but occur at higher frequencies in metastatic and/or hormone-refractory lesions, suggesting that these genes may be involved in PCa progression.

Oncogenes

MYC: Recent studies have suggested a role for MYC overexpression in cancer initiation. Nuclear MYC protein is upregulated in many PIN lesions and the majority of carcinomas in the absence of gene amplification [62]. Several important MYC target genes have been identified which regulate numerous pathways involved in PCa progression and metastasis. FOXP3 is a newly identified X-linked tumor suppressor gene in both prostate and breast cancers. MYC overexpression has been correlated with FOXP3 downregulation, and deletion of FOXP3 resulted in concomitant increase in MYC. FOXP3 binds to the promoter region of MYC and represses its transcription and hence loss of FOXP3 increased MYC expression [63].

Androgen Receptor (AR): Luminal cells in HGPIN and the vast majority of prostatic adenocarcinoma cells express AR at relatively high levels.

Androgen independence eventually develops in advanced cancers. Despite that, AR expression and AR signaling remain intact in most hormone-refractory cancers. In fact, AR expression itself is often increased in hormone-refractory cancers. Somatic mutations of AR have been reported, especially in androgen-independent cancers, and these are often "activating" mutations that can result in altered ligand specificity, thus permitting activation by non-androgens or even antiandro-gens. In addition, AR gene amplification can lead to increasing the sensitivity of the cells to low androgen levels. Androgen-independent PCa cells can also activate AR signaling in the absence of androgens through posttranslational modifica-tions of the AR and/or AR coactivators in response to other growth factor signaling [64–66]. Steroid receptor coactivators (SRCs) have been studied extensively. In addition to interact-ing with nuclear receptors, SRCs coactivate other transcription factors including nuclear factor-κB (NF-κB), STATs, HIF1, and Smads. SRCs have been found to be highly overexpressed or ampli-fied in PCa [67]. Recent studies have also sug-gested that PCa cells may manufacture androgens.

TMPRSS2-ERG Gene Fusion Rearrangement: Gene fusions between the androgen-regulated gene TMPRSS2 and the ETS oncogenic transcription factor family members ERG, ETV1, and ETV4 are the most prevalent gene fusion in PCa and have been reported as a criti-cal event in PCa development. TMPRSS2 is an androgen-regulated gene on chromosome 21q22.2; its upstream regulatory elements and promoter drive the overexpression of ERG upon the formation of gene fusion. Androgen signal-ing has been shown to induce the proximity of TMPRSS2 and ERG locus in androgen respon-sive cells and in combination with agents causing DNA double-strand breaks induces TMPRSS2-ERG gene fusions. PCas are molecularly divided into "fusion-positive" and "fusion-negative" can-cers. Expression of TMPRSS2-ERG fusion tran-script has been found in low-grade PIN and 16–20 % of HGPIN, suggesting it to be an early event in prostate carcinogenesis. It is also present in 65 % of localized PCas. Studies have also

documented increased ERG and ETV1 expression in metastatic PCa, suggesting ETS gene fusions can be maintained in advanced disease [68, 69]. The majority (70 %) of cases demonstrated heterogeneous TMPRSS2 gene rearrangements between different tumor foci, thus supporting multifocal PCa as a heterogeneous group of dis-eases [70].

Activated WNT signaling was recently described to be among the most highly enriched pathways in ERG-overexpressing tumors [71]. In addition, a sig-nificant upregulation of the TGF-β/BMP signal-ing pathways is identified in fusion-positive patients [72]. Clinically, the prognostic importance of ETS gene rearrangement is still controversial, and additional studies are needed to identify and verify different variants of translocations. Furthermore, differential regulatory networks that drives ETS oncogenic rearrangements with respect to androgen signaling need to be elucidated.

Telomere Shortening: Telomeres become markedly shortened during the development of most cancers, most likely to the point where chromosomal insta-bility ensues. In the prostate, somatic telomere shortening occurs in the luminal cells of most of the cases of HGPIN and carcinoma. Telomere shorten-ing may be a nearly universal feature of early PCa and may promote chromosomal instability leading to disease progression [73].

Molecular Pathways of Prostate Cancer

1. Phosphoinositide-3 Kinase/Akt: Phosphoi-nositide-3 kinase (PI3K) is a critical mediator of multiple oncogenic signaling pathways. The most critical negative regulator of PI3K-Akt pathway is PTEN. In PCa, PTEN is fre-quently lost resulting in hyperactive PI3K/Akt pathway promoting cancer progression [74]. Other potential role for AKT in PCa is the phosphorylation of p27Kip1 protein, resulting in cytoplasmic retention of p27Kip1 and lack of p27Kip1 mediated cell cycle arrest. p27Kip1, encoded by the CDKN1b gene, is often downregulated in the nucleus of PCa and high-grade PIN cells [75].

2. Wnt-B Catenin-TCF Signaling and MYC: The Wnt/B catenin pathway is an important player in prostate oncogenesis, particularly tumor cells' invasiveness. In PCa, APC and β-catenin mutations are quite rare (~5 % or less in most studies). Despite this, APC appears to be inactivated in most PCas; APC hypermethylation was reported in 57–85 % of PCas [55, 76] and in 30 % of HGPIN. Interestingly, APC hypermethylation was observed more frequently in cases with high Gleason scores and high serum PSA levels.

3. The IGF Pathway: IGF-I plays an important role in cellular proliferation, differentiation, and apoptosis. Obesity is associated with increased free or bioavailable IGF-I [77], and several epidemiologic studies have reported a positive association between IGF-1 and PCa risk, although data from recent studies are much weaker [78].

4. Obesity and the Inflammatory Pathway: Accumulating data support the hypothesis that chronic inflammation contributes to prostate carcinogenesis. In addition, studies of genetic susceptibility have shown that variants of genes in the inflammation pathway, including MSR1, tumor necrosis factor-α (TNF-α), and IL6, are associated with a higher risk of PCa [79–81].

It is now recognized that adipose tissue is an active organ that secretes a large number of proteins, including cytokines and hormone-like factors, such as leptin and adiponectin [80]. It has been shown that obesity is associated with a state of low-grade chronic inflammation, with infiltrating macrophages within adipose tissue and elevated concentrations of inflammatory cytokines, including TNF-α, interleukin-6, and C-reactive protein [82]. The subclinical inflammatory condition related to obesity promotes the production of proinflammatory factors involved in the pathogenesis of insulin resistance [83]. Furthermore, in obesity, the proinflammatory effects of cytokines involve the NF-κB and c-Jun N-terminal kinase (JNK) systems. Coincidentally, NF-κB is a strong inducer of antiapoptotic gene activity (BCL-XL) and cell cycle genes (cyclin D1) [84]. Nuclear localization of NF-κB is associated with PCa [85].

5. Cholesterol Biosynthesis: Several studies have shown that cholesterol homeostasis gets disturbed in the prostate with advancing age and with the transition from a benign to a malignant state. Elevated cholesterol levels in PCa cells have been shown to be the result of an aberrant regulation of the cholesterol metabolism. Furthermore, the cholesterol metabolism appeared to be involved in PCa recurrence.

Numerous signaling proteins have been identified to associate with plasma membrane lipid rafts, including the EGFR, the AR, heterotrimeric G-protein subunits, the T-cell receptor, as well as the interleukin-6 (IL-6) receptor. The EGFR leads to the activation of the PI3K/Akt pathway and therefore serves as mediator of solid tumor growth [86, 87].

6. Epithelial-to-Mesenchymal Transition: Several recent studies provide evidence that EMT is linked to cancer progression, invasion, and metastasis. EMT is characterized by the repression of E-cadherin expression and increased cell motility. The loss of E-cadherin seems to correlate with dedifferentiation, local invasiveness, and metastasis of PCa cells [88, 89].

Furthermore, EMT coordinates the cooperation between oncogenic Ras and receptor tyrosine kinases to induce downstream Raf/mitogen-activated protein kinase (MAPK) signaling that is strongly associated with tumor progression and poor prognosis [90]. Overexpression of the EGFR family has been associated with disease progression of numerous malignancies including PCa. In PCa, EGFR has been shown to initiate EMT in cooperation with TGF-β and to enhance the invasiveness of cancer cells. In the presence of androgens, endogenous and ectopically expressed AR directly associates with EGFR and alters the activation of downstream PI3K signaling leading to cancer cell growth and survival. EGFR may also sensitize PCa cells to low levels of androgens by enhancing coactivator binding and transcriptional activation of endogenous and ectopically expressed AR. Therefore, the observed cross talk between the AR and EGFR axes leads to the assumption that EGFR-induced EMT, and androgen independence could occur simultaneously in prostatic tumor cells [88].

The link between EMT and tumor progression has been circumstantial, but definitive evidence is emerging. For instance, new data indicate that expression of the fusion protein TMPRSS2-ERG can lead to activation of the beta-catenin pathway and EMT [72]. Additionally, overexpression of the polycomb repressive complex protein EZH2 has been linked to EMT, metastasis, and castration resistance [91]. In PCa model systems, activated stromal signaling from the tumor microenvironment may induce EMT and stemness properties, contributing to castration resistance and metastatic progression through this molecular cross talk, often mediated by cytokines and other paracrine factors [92].

7. MicroRNAs (miRNAs): Several miRNAs have been reported to be deregulated in PCa. Downregulation of let-7b, miR-1, miR-133a, miR-143, miR-145, miR-221, and miR-222 and upregulation of miR-25, miR-93, mir-96, miR-183, miR-182, or miR-301b have been reported in PCa compared with benign prostate hyperplasia and normal prostate. Recent evidence has also shown that miRNAs are involved in PCa pathogenesis and can be potential biomarkers. For instance, overexpression of miR-96 and reduced expression of miR-221 have been associated with increased risk of biochemical recurrence and aggressive PCa. miR-205 is strongly downregulated in PCa and its expression is completely abolished in metastatic tumors. It has been suggested that the tumor-suppressive function of miR-205 takes place through counteracting epithelial-to-mesenchymal transition and reducing cell migration and invasion. miR-183 expression was found to be significantly higher in PCa compared to matched adjacent normal prostate tissues, and higher miR-183 expression was associated with higher PSA at diagnosis, higher pT, and shorter overall survival after radical prostatectomy. Also, different miRNA expression signatures were reported in the high-grade tumors (Gleason score ≥8) compared with tumors Gleason score 6. Upregulation of miR-122, miR-335, miR-184, miR-193, miR-34, miR-138, miR-373, miR-9, miR-198, miR-144, and miR-215 and downregulation of miR-96, miR-222, miR-148, miR-92, miR-27, miR-125, miR-126, and miR-27 were found in the high-grade tumors [93–96].

8. Other Pathways: The *MAPK pathway* also plays a role in PCa pathogenesis, especially advanced and castration-resistant tumors. MAPK pathway activation is associated with higher stage and grade and recurrent disease. In the setting of castration resistance, PI3K and MAPK signaling are often coordinately dysregulated [97].

Another important pathway is the HIV-I NEF pathway. This pathway comprises the tumor necrosis factor (TNF) and FAS receptor signaling pathways and seems to be particularly dysregulated in androgen-independent metastatic cancers [98]. Upregulation of RAS family members *RAF1* and *BRAF*, or downregulation of *SPRY1* or *SPRY2* genes, is enriched in PCa metastases [99]. In some cases, expression of *RAS*, *RAF1*, and *BRAF* is activated by oncogenic fusions with highly expressed promoters. Repression of the RAS-GAP gene *DAB2IP* by EZH2 may activate MAPK signaling and drive progression and metastasis.

Like the Wnt pathway, matrix metalloproteinases (MMPs) are essential in facilitating the invasiveness of PCa. These proteins are important in the degradation of the extracellular matrix, whereby the invasive PCa cells can metastasize to distant sites. Additionally, this protease activity plays a role in facilitating angiogenesis. In bone metastases, prostatic tissue can promote angiogenesis via the MMP9 derived from osteoclasts. As such, metalloproteases are particularly important players later on in PCa, when the cancer is most invasive [100].

Prostate Cancer Initiation and Progression

PCa is thought to develop through a stepwise progression by which the benign prostatic epithelium changes to high-grade PIN, invasive

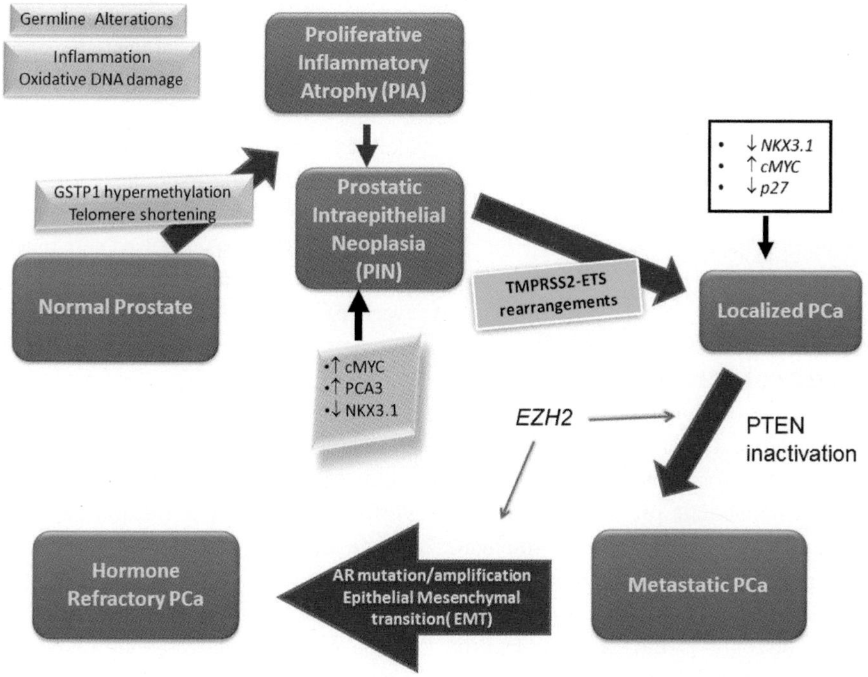

Fig. 17.1 A schematic showing the sequence of molecular events in prostate cancer (PCa) pathogenesis. The earliest somatic molecular alterations that begin to occur just before or at the onset of prostatic intraepithelial neoplasia (PIN)/proliferative inflammatory atrophy (PIA) include silencing of gene expression through epigenetic changes, such as GSTP1 promoter hypermethylation, then telomere shortening, and the activation of the proto-oncogene MYC. Oncogenic ETS family transcription factors are activated by gene fusions at or near the onset of invasive adenocarcinoma in a significant subset of patients. Other common genetic changes found in PCas include deletions of regions harboring putative tumor suppressors on chromosome 8p (NKX3.1), 10q23 (PTEN), 12p13 (CDKN1B-p27), 13q (RB1), and 17q (p53); gains in regions of oncogenes on chromosome 8q24 (MYC) and Xq (AR); and point mutations (e.g., p53 and AR)

adenocarcinoma, distant metastatic disease, and finally androgen refractory metastatic disease. The sequence of the most established molecular events is shown in Fig. 17.1.

Proliferative Inflammatory Atrophy as a Precursor Lesion to Prostate Cancer

Epidemiological studies indicate that prostate inflammation is associated with increased risk of PCa. Recently, a new hypothesis has been proposed for prostate carcinogenesis. It proposes that exposure to environmental factors such as infectious agents, dietary carcinogens, and hormonal imbalances leads to injury of the prostate and to the development of chronic inflammation and regenerative "risk factor" lesions, referred to as proliferative inflammatory atrophy (PIA) [101]. Areas of PIA have epithelial cells that fail to differentiate into columnar cells. Also, it may show morphological transitions in continuity with HGPIN lesions which are putative PCa precursors [101].

Regardless of the cause of PIA (infection, ischemia, or toxin exposure), epithelial cells in these lesions exhibit molecular signs of stress expressing high levels of stress response genes GSTP1, GSTA1, and COX-2. There are increases in chromosome 8 centromere signals, loss of chromosome 8p14, and a gain of chromosome 8q24 in focal atrophy, indicating that chromosomal abnormalities similar to those found in

PIN and carcinoma occur in a subset of these atrophic lesions. Furthermore, these atrophic lesions, which frequently merge with HGPIN, have some of the somatic alterations found in PCa and PIN. Morphological transitions between PIA, PIN, and PCa have been also described. Furthermore, PIA directly merging with cancer was identified in 28 % of the cases [101].

Prostatic Intraepithelial Neoplasia as a Precursor of Carcinoma

PIN is recognized as a continuum between low-grade and high-grade forms, with HGPIN thought to represent the immediate precursor of invasive carcinoma. Several lines of evidence implicate HGPIN as a preneoplastic lesion. First, it is primarily found in the peripheral zone, in proximity to invasive carcinoma [102]. Second, HGPIN lesions generally precede the appearance of carcinoma, consistent with the concept of cancer progression [103]. Third, the chromosomal abnormalities found in PIN resemble those found in early invasive carcinoma, although less prevalent [104]. Fourth, the architectural and cytological features of PIN closely resemble those of invasive carcinoma. Finally, markers of differentiation that are commonly altered in early invasive carcinoma are also altered in HGPIN, including E-cadherin and vimentin [105].

Tumor-Initiating Cells and Cancer Stem Cells

The preferential survival of basal cells following androgen ablation has led to the traditionally held hypothesis that prostate stem cells reside within the basal cell layer of the gland. Substantial evidence indicates that these cells which have a basal phenotype can possess some stem cell behavior like the ability for self-renewal and differentiation into luminal cells [106]. In PCa, however, the majority of cancer cells express luminal, rather than basal, cell markers. For example, PCa and PIN cells express fairly high levels (as compared to basal cells) of AR, PSA,

and NKX3.1. Furthermore, only luminal cells in PIN lesions show the characteristic somatic DNA alteration of telomere shortening. Finally, only luminal cells show the characteristic FISH abnormalities of the ETS family gene rearrangements. This has led to the hypothesis that PCa can be derived from a luminal cell progenitor or mature luminal cell that has acquired self-renewal activity through mutation [107]. Some reports, however, have identified intermediate cells that coexpress both basal and luminal cell markers within PCas [108].

Both cancer stem cells and metastatic cells share traits, such as the migration ability and the ability to differentiate into different cell types. In vitro studies revealed that metastatic PCa cells invade matrigel through an EMT process, are $CD44^+$, and exhibit gene expression profiles consistent with those of $CD44^+CD24^-$ PCa stem cells [109]. While in contrast, noninvasive cells do not express high levels of "stemness" genes. Moreover, purified $CD44^+$, but not $CD44^-$ cells, are invasive. Furthermore, the invasive cell subpopulation was tumorigenic in NOD/SCID mice, whereas the noninvasive cells were only weakly tumorigenic. Thus, these data strongly suggest that the stem cell-like component of cancer cells is responsible for invasion, the first step in metastasis.

Genomic Heterogeneity of Prostate Cancer

PCa is a heterogeneous disease. Independent cancerous foci with distinct morphological features often coexist in a single prostate. The course of disease also varies widely; some cancers remain indolent for decades, while others rapidly progress to lethality. Distinct molecular features appear to underlie these clinical and histological differences. PCa may arise in multiple foci from independent precursor cells that are driven to neoplastic transformation by carcinogenic exposures or genetic predisposition [110]. The presence of genomic lesions can vary between foci, including *TMPRSS2-ERG* fusion, *MYC* amplification, and *TP53* mutation [40, 70, 111]. Multiple distinct clones can be identified in a single biopsy [112], but most metastatic PCas appear to originate from a single clone within a primary tumor [113]. Among other lesions, subclonal *p53* mutations may define cells in the primary tumor with metastatic potential [111]. Intratumoral heterogeneity complicates efforts to define prognostic mutations or expression signatures from primary tumors [114].

Prostate Cancer Biomarkers

There are a number of challenges in PCa management in which molecular markers are expected to provide significant help. These include (1) cancer detection and the determination of who may require an initial prostate biopsy and who may require rebiopsy after an initial negative biopsy; (2) prediction of recurrence after initial treatment to stratify patients into risk groups for emerging adjuvant therapies; (3) detection of recurrence after treatment; and (4) assessing the efficacy of treatments in advanced disease [115].

PSA remains an inexpensive, sensitive biomarker for disease detection and monitoring after curative therapy of localized disease. The pros and cons of PSA testing have been extensively discussed in recent literature [116–118]. Advances in molecular profiling have shifted the biomarker research field to a number of "-omics" approaches, with discoveries based on aberrations in DNA, RNA, or epigenetic DNA methylation states [119–121].

Biomarkers for Screening and Diagnosis of Prostate Cancer

Germline Mutational Screening for Prostate Cancer Risk

To date, more than 50 SNPs have been proposed as putative risk loci for PCa, of which ~30 have been validated in multiple studies. Although each individual SNP is likely to contribute a minor degree to disease risk (generally <1.5-fold), combining multiple SNPs may yield more informative results. In a retrospective study,

Zheng et al. defined a set of five disease-associated SNPs that were then combined with family history to predict risk (up to tenfold) for developing PCa [122]. To date, reported GWAS have evaluated only common inherited variants (minor allele frequency >1–5 % in the population studied) and describe only a minority of the genetic component of risk. Coding variants in the homeobox B13 (HOXB13) gene, an AR gene cofactor, which were recently discovered by targeted exonic sequencing of genes in a region of PCa linkage at chromosome 17q21-22, were found in <0.1 % of controls, but 1.4 % of patients with a very strong family history or early-onset PCa [7].

Serum Diagnostic Markers

PSA: The most common current screening test for PCa is measurement of the serum concentration of PSA. However, there is no single threshold value for PSA that can reliably distinguish patients with PCa from those without, and thus an unfortunate consequence of population-wide PSA screening is the cost of and morbidity from diagnostic biopsies in patients without cancer. The European Randomized Study of Screening for Prostate Cancer trial reported that PSA screening without digital rectal examination was associated with a 20 % relative reduction in the death rate from PCa but was associated with a high risk of overdiagnosis [123]. A GWAS showed an association of certain SNPs with higher probability of a negative biopsy in patients with high PSA, suggesting that PSA thresholds for biopsy could be personalized based on genotype at these loci [124]. It should be also noted that prostate biopsy is still the gold standard test with approximately 80–85 % sensitivity. This reflects the reality that prostate biopsies are typically carried out in a blinded fashion and may miss cancer in up to 15–20 % of patients. Therefore the test performance (sensitivity, specificity, and positive and negative predictive values) of molecular tests is necessarily only relevant to the prediction of a positive prostate needle biopsy and not specifically to the presence or absence of cancer [115].

There has been significant research into improving the performance of PSA, including measuring % free PSA, PSA density, PSA velocity (PSAV), and truncated forms of PSA. PSAV and PSA doubling time (PSADT) have also prognostic value. PSAV is defined as the change in PSA concentration per year, with a high PSAV being strongly associated with PCa and a ninefold elevated risk of cancer-related death after prostatectomy. PSADT is defined as the time necessary for the serum PSA level to double. PSADT is most commonly used to monitor disease progression after curative therapy for organ-confined disease. A more rapid PSADT (<10 months) is associated with reduced survival. Also PSADT may become a useful biomarker to better stratify patients with positive biopsies into risk groups such that more men may safely elect active surveillance as opposed to immediate surgery [125].

Early Prostate Cancer Antigen (*EPCA*): Early PCa antigen is one of the most promising new PCa serum biomarkers. Immunostaining of this antigen could differentiate men with from those without cancer by evaluating histologically normal-appearing tissue adjacent to areas of cancer. EPCA staining occurs only in cancer patients and not in normal controls. EPCA's sensitivity for detecting PCa is 84 %, and its specificity is 85 % [126]. The value of EPCA, however, recently became questionable [127].

Circulating Tumor Cells (*CTCs*): One area of expanding investigation is CTCs. The number of CTCs in blood can be a biomarker for cancer detection, and these cells are a source of molecular information, such as measuring TMPRSS2-ERG, AR, and PTEN copy number status. An increased abundance of CTCs in the blood of castration-resistant PCa patients has predicted worse overall survival. However, detecting CTCs and extracting molecular information are currently labor intensive and expensive, and it is not known if CTC abundance in blood represents aggressive disease undergoing hematogenous spread or simply cells that have dislodged from the tumor bulk. Enumeration of CTCs, measured by the CellSearch® (Veridex LLC, Warren, NJ, USA) is the only assay that is analytically valid and FDA-approved for patient use [128, 129]. Technical aspects of CTCs are provided in the corresponding chapter of this book.

Exosomes: Prostate-derived exosomes (also called prostatosomes) are small vesicles (50–150 nm in diameter) generated from internalized parts of the cellular membrane, which are subsequently secreted into the blood, semen, or urine. PCa patients exhibit increased number of exosomes in their serum compared to men with no disease, and elevated levels of exosomes may also correlate with increasing Gleason score. PCa RNA biomarkers, including PCA3 and TMPRSS2-ERG, can also be detected in urine-derived exosomes from PCa patients [130]. Recent studies also showed that the circulating exosomal miRNAs can serve as cancer biomarkers [131, 132]. Although these efforts remain mainly research oriented at the time being, they provide promising future directions for biomarker discovery.

Urinary Diagnostic Markers
Epigenetic Markers

GSTP1 is a test to quantitate the methylation status of GSTP1 gene in biopsy and radical prostatectomy specimens and from the cells derived from serum, urine, and seminal plasma. GSTP1 has been shown to be sensitive in detecting the presence of PIN and PCa, thereby distinguishing patients with these diseases from those with benign prostatic hyperplasia. It has 75 % sensitivity and 98 % specificity for detecting PCa in urine and 88 % specificity and 91 % sensitivity in biopsy specimens [133]. It can help improving specificity of PSA testing.

DAB2IP is a Ras GTPase-activating protein that is downregulated in PCa due to altered methylation patterns in its promoter region. This methylation leads to transcriptional silencing and also may also contribute to cancer progression [134].

Other putative epigenetic markers include pITX2, sprout 1, PMEPA1, EFEMP1, and PTGS2. Genome-wide methylation analysis has also resulted in the discovery of new epigenetic markers. In contrast to genomic alterations, epigenetic alterations can be reversed. Reactivation of tumor suppressor genes by demethylating agents and histone deacetylase inhibitors could be a potential treatment option for patients with advanced PCa.

A number of studies have tested urine sediment DNA for aberrant methylation. Hoque et al. examined the methylation of nine gene promoters and found that a combination of four genes (p16, ARF [p14], MGMT, and GSTP1) detected 87 % of PCas with a specificity of 100 % [135]. They suggested a four-gene combination (GSTP1, RASSF1a, RARB, and APC) as the best discriminative panel, with 86 % sensitivity and 89 % specificity. On testing a panel of four genes, Payne et al. did not find a combination that significantly improved performance over that of single biomarkers [136]. Of the markers included in these panels, GSTP1 methylation offered the best diagnostic performance. Larger clinical studies including a prospective screening cohort are warranted to validate the clinical utility of this approach.

RNA Markers

PCA3: Prostate cancer antigen 3 (PCA3) is a noncoding RNA with expression confined to the prostate and is highly overexpressed in 95 % of PCa cases compared with normal or benign hyperplastic prostate tissue [137]. Progensa PCA3 (urinary RT-PCR assay for PCA3, Gen-Probe Inc., San Diego, CA) is a commercially available diagnostic test that quantitatively detects PCA3 RNA expression in urine and prostatic fluid after prostatic massage. A quantitative PCA3 score was developed to assess the probability of cancer detection in prostate biopsy. The score is defined as PCA3-RNA/PSA-mRNA ratio. A PCA3 score >35 in the urine correlated with an average sensitivity and specificity of 66 % and 76 %, respectively, for the diagnosis of PCa (compared to a specificity of 47 % for serum PSA at the cut off for 65 % sensitivity). Elevated PCA3 scores have also been demonstrated to increase the probability of a positive repeat biopsy in men with one or two prior negative biopsy results [138]. PCA3 has been incorporated into an FDA-approved test.

α-Methylacyl Coenzyme A Racemase (AMACR): AMACR is a commonly used immunohistochemical marker for PCa which can also be detected in the urine of PCa patients [139]. AMACR, also known as P504S, is involved in β-oxidation of branched-chain fatty acids [140]. It is upregulated at both the mRNA and protein levels in PCa tissue [141]; however, its usefulness as a urine biomarker is controversial. Western blot analysis for AMACR was used on voided urine after TRUS and biopsy, showing a 100 % sensitivity and 58 % specificity for PCa detection in patients with negative biopsy [139].

TMPRSS2-ERG: Detection of the TMPRSS2-ERG fusion in urine has been reported to yield >90 % specificity and 94 % positive predictive value for PCa detection, although a clinical diagnostic test is not yet available. Hessels et al. analyzed TMPRSS2-ETS fusion transcripts in the urinary sediments of 108 PCa cases and found a sensitivity of 37 % and a specificity of 93 %. Negative and positive predictive values were 36 % and 94 %, respectively [142]. No significant correlation was found between the TMPRSS2-ETS fusion transcripts and Gleason score. The sensitivity of a combined PCA3 and TMPRSS2-ETS testing for detecting PCa was 73 % [142]. Additional studies are needed to better determine the association of ETS fusions with prognosis and disease aggressiveness, including the likelihood of extraprostatic disease, Gleason score, and tumor volume.

GOLPH2: GOLPH2 is a gene coding for Golgi phosphoprotein 2, which is a Golgi membrane antigen. It is upregulated in about 90 % of PCa patients. GOLPH2 is a potential diagnostic biomarker that can be assayed in urine. GOLPH2 immunohistochemical staining shows a perinuclear pattern that is more intense in PCa compared to normal glands [143].

Urinary PSA: The presence of urinary PSA after radical prostatectomy was shown to be associated with disease recurrence [144]. Studies by Irani et al. found that the ratio of serum to urinary PSA is clinically useful, especially in the 4–10 ng/mL range of PSA (sensitivity of 42–84 % and specificity of 80–89 %). Other reports confirmed the ability of this ratio to discriminate between BPH and PCa, while others were unable to reproduce these findings.

Telomerase Activity: Botchkina et al. studied urine samples from patients with PCa using a quantitative PCR telomeric repeat amplification protocol assay and reported sensitivity and specificity of 100 % and 88.6 %, respectively, for detection of cancer [145]. mRNA expression of *TERT* in urine has also been analyzed. Sensitivity and specificity were only 36 % and 66 %, respectively [146].

Annexin A3: Annexin A3 level in urine was complementary to serum PSA level. A study showed that it has a potential to avoid unnecessary biopsies in the clinically relevant group of patients with negative digital rectal examination and prostate-specific antigen in the lower range of values. Combined readouts of PSA and urinary annexin A3 were superior to all other combinations [147].

MMPs: Matrix metalloproteinase MMP9 was independent predictors for distinguishing between patients with prostate and bladder cancers. A study found that MMPs were detected significantly more often in urine from PCa compared with healthy controls. The presence of any matrix metalloproteinase showed a specificity of 82 % and a sensitivity of 74 % for PCa [148].

PIM1: Although there is little or no PIM1 expression in the benign prostatic epithelium, there is significant PIM1 expression in advanced PCa, suggesting PIM1 as a potential prognostic marker. It can be also a target for drug development [149].

Hepsin: The gene for hepsin encodes a type II integral membrane protease that has been observed to take part in cell migration and invasion. Hepsin is upregulated in PCa. The lack of detection of hepsin in either urine or serum makes its use as a biomarker difficult [149, 150].

SPINK1: SPINK1 (also referred to as TAT1) is a biomarker for PCa that can be detected in prostatic massage urine. Laxman et al. showed that a multiplexed qPCR assay including SPINK1 on sedimented urine from patients presenting for prostate biopsy or prostatectomy outperformed serum PSA or PCA3 alone [151].

Urinary miRNAs Biomarkers: Five PCa-associated miRNAs (miR-107, miR-141, miR-200b, miR-375, and miR-574-3p) were measured in the urine of PCa patients and healthy controls. All of them were detectable in urine, but only miR-107 and miR-574-3p showed differential expression in cancer [152]. In this cohort, the diagnostic value of these miRNAs exceeded PCA3. miRNAs can also be utilized as prognostic markers. miR-141 and miR-375 were shown to be associated with metastatic disease [152]. Utilizing miRNA signatures rather than a single miRNAs can significantly enhance their performance.

Tissue Diagnostic Markers

The most commonly used basal cell-specific markers in PCa are high-molecular-weight cytokeratin (HMWCK) and p63. HMWCK is expressed in virtually all normal basal cells of the prostate. The use of HMWCK decreased the "atypical" diagnosis rate from 8.3 to 0.4 % [153]. p63 is a nuclear transcription, the expression of which is limited to basal cells of prostate glands. AMACR is strongly positive in PCas with diffuse cytoplasmic staining or circumferential apical granular staining pattern. In contrast, little or no immunoreactivity was observed in benign glands. However, there is a wide variation in the sensitivity and specificity of AMACR immunoreactivity in prostate biopsies. In addition, AMACR expression has been demonstrated in HGPIN [153]. (a partial list of new potential diagnostic markers is summarized in Box 17.2.)

Molecular Predictors of Malignancy in Negative Biopsies

Several attempts were done to determine whether assessment of methylation of GSTP1 and/or other genes (e.g., APC) in DNA isolated from negative biopsy specimens can aid in predicting a positive repeat biopsy, to avoid unnecessary repeat biopsies. Laboratory Corporation of America (Labcorp®) recently announced the availability of a commercial test using this approach. As with all of the other approaches that do not examine the cells directly under the microscope, it is not clear whether the assay is detecting cancer cells, HGPIN cells, or rare methylated atrophic cells that were not originally sampled by microscopic pathology sections, or, whether it is detecting a "field effect," whereby normal-appearing prostate tissues harbor molecular alterations that are predictive of cancer on subsequent biopsies [154].

A study suggested that GSTP1 that is being detected in negative biopsy specimens is likely to be un-sampled carcinoma or PIN cells that remain in the paraffin block after standard histological sections have been obtained [154]. In a preliminary study, APC methylation status appeared to perform better than GSTP1 in predicting the biopsy results of a repeat biopsy in men with risk factors suggestive of cancer (e.g. high serum PSA, previous PIN, or atypical glands on biopsy), suggesting that APC methylation

occurs in nonneoplastic cells and can represent a useful predictor of cancer. The potential of APC methylation to reduce unnecessary repeat biopsies warrants validation in a larger prospective cohort [155].

NKX3.1: Bowen et al. reported that loss of NKX3.1 protein expression correlates with PCa progression. Complete loss of NKX3.1 was found in 20 % of HGPIN, 6 % of stage T1 tumors, 22 % of stage T3/4, 34 % of hormone-refractory cancers, and 78 % of metastatic lesions [30]. By contrast, Korkmaz et al. reported that a vast majority of prostatic adenocarcinomas were positive for NKX3.1 with no correlation with tumor grade or stage [156]. Gelmann et al., reported that NKX3.1 protein was expressed in 66 % of primary untreated tumors, 44 % of untreated metastatic tumors, and 27.3 % of castrate-resistant/hormone-refractory tumors [157]. Chuang et al. found that the sensitivity for NKX3.1 staining in high-grade prostate adenocarcinoma (Gleason score 8–10) ranged from 92 to 95 % [158].

Metabolomics and Imaging Markers

Metabolomics has recently emerged as a novel approach to early and noninvasive PCa detection based on changes in the metabolites including citrate, polyamines, lactate, choline, creatine, sarcosine, and alanine [159–162]. The field of imaging is continuously evolving. FDG-PET imaging, which measures the extent of change in glucose utilization in many cancer types, appears to be associated with increasing Gleason grade, clinical stage, and serum PSA level [163] ImmunoPET imaging for antibody drug conjugates offers exciting potential diagnostic applications [164]. However, these studies are based on relatively small cohorts of patients and the results require further prospective validation.

Radioimmunoscintigraphy (RIS) imaging with Indium-111 capromab pendetide (ProstaScint) is an alternative imaging modality for patients with PCa that is intended to assist in determining the extent and location of disease. For determining whether disease is present in the lymph nodes, RIS has a modest sensitivity

(50–75 %) and specificity is about 80 %. RIS has been proposed to be used for staging prior to curative treatment. For patients with biochemical failure following curative treatment, RIS has been proposed to help differentiate between local and distant recurrence [165].

Multiparametric Approaches to Improve Diagnostic Accuracy

Despite the large number of emerging molecular markers, none has the desired sensitivity and specificity for clinical use. Hessels et al. reported that by combining PCA3 and TMPRSS2-ERG, the sensitivity of PCa detection markedly increased from 63 to 73 % without compromising specificity [142]. Clark et al. observed that diagnostic performance to predict the prostate biopsy outcome might be increased by combining TMPRSS2-ERG with PSA and DRE [166]. Another study used four biomarkers to achieve 66 % specificity and 76 % sensitivity [151]. Similarly, ERG, PCA3, and AMACR created a promising PCa biomarker panel [167]. Other similar models have been also created [151].

Incorporation of molecular markers to nomograms is another interesting application. A study showed that adding PCA3 level in urine helps to improve the accuracy of nomogram that identifies men at risk of harboring PCa and assists in deciding whether further biopsy evaluation is necessary [168]. In a subsequent study Auprich et al. assessed the accuracy of the previously reported PCA3-based nomogram in a large European cohort of men. The nomogram helped identify PCa in 255 of 621 men (41.1 %) [169]. Other groups observed that incorporating PCA3 improved the diagnostic accuracy of the Prostate Cancer Prevention Trial risk calculator.

Prognostic Markers

Distinguishing between indolent and aggressive PCas at the time of diagnosis would be very helpful in formulating the management plan. To date, the Gleason score has been the most commonly used indicator of survival. However, a number of patients with Gleason scores of 6 or 7 who will develop aggressive tumors shortly after diagnosis and have poor survival. A method to detect these patients at diagnosis would be helpful. A number of putative prognostic molecular markers have been identified. There is also significant interest in incorporating molecular markers to current predictive models to more precisely stratify patients to assess the need for therapy, the intensity of therapy, and the extent of surveillance required either before or after initial treatment. However, none are currently employed in clinical practice.

AMACR is reported to have a prognostic value. Decreasing AMACR levels have been linked to increased risk of biochemical recurrence and worse prognosis [170]. *SPINK1* expression in urine is also an independent predictor of biochemical recurrence after resection [171]. *EZH2* is a histone methyltransferase that interacts with DNA methyltransferases. It is overexpressed in hormone-refractory, metastatic PCa. In addition, clinically localized PCas that express higher concentrations of EZH2 show a poorer prognosis [172]. *Cav-1* is an integral membrane protein that is overexpressed in PCa cells. It has been observed to be upregulated in metastatic cancers and is related to disease progression [173].

Overexpression of *HER2 and TOP2A genes*, located on 17q, has been reported in high-grade, androgen-resistant cancers. TOP2A amplification in advanced cancer was associated with androgen resistance and decreased survival by multivariate analysis [174]. There is also evidence that PCa aggressiveness has a heritable component. A germline mutation has been associated with aggressive PCa and cancer-specific mortality is located in the kallikrein-related peptidase 2 and kallikrein-related peptidase 3 (PSA) intergenic region. The PCa-risk SNP rs2735839 (G) was one of the six loci that were associated with higher PSA levels in patients without PCa [124].

Certain genetic alterations have been also correlated with poor prognosis, including amplification of the MYC locus at 8q24 and p53 overexpression. The impact of other known genetic alterations on clinical behavior of tumors remains unclear and somewhat controversial; for example, TMPRSS2-ERG has been implicated as both a negative and positive prognostic marker. While ETS gene fusions seem to drive PCa development, their contribution to progression and the behavior of advanced cancers remain unclear.

Expression signatures have been proposed that delineate histologically aggressive disease or predict outcome independently of clinical variables. However, the overlap between signatures from independent studies is moderate. Some genomic alterations appear to have prognostic value as well. The *TMPRSS2-ERG* fusion, *MYC* amplification, and *PTEN* or *TP53* deletion predict cancer-specific death [175].

Recently, 11 National Cancer Institute-funded prostate SPORE (Specialized Projects of Research Excellence Awards) programs have begun to accrue moderate- to high-risk patients with PCa to a prospective study ($n=700$). This study will hopefully determine whether selected markers applied to prostate needle biopsies may be clinically useful to predict outcome beyond typical clinic-pathological measurements such as Gleason score, serum PSA, and number of positive cores.

Other prognostic markers include loss of the PTEN tumor suppressor or gain of ETS transcription factor gene fusions. PTEN deletion is associated with poor outcome and hormone-refractory disease. Combining multiple biomarkers was also investigated, e.g., PTEN deletion with the TMPRSS2-ERG fusion. Two independent groups found that patients with neither lesion had a favorable prognosis. However, the combination of both lesions did not result in augmented worse prognosis. Inconsistency among studies can be attributed to the different techniques used (for example, genetic deletion of the PTEN locus vs. loss of protein expression) or the different criteria to assess outcome. Other markers tested in combination with PTEN loss include tumor protein p27 gene loss, hemoxygenase-1 overexpression, and HER2/3 overexpression. A four-protein signature, PTEN, SMAD4, cyclin D1, and SPP1, was found to predict biochemical recurrence

significantly better than Gleason score alone. A recent study also identified a miRNA signature that can distinguish between patients with early vs. late biochemical failure based on miRNA expression profile [95].

Molecular Subtyping Based on Gene Expression Profiling

Gene expression profiling is an attractive new tool that allows tumor subclassification based on simultaneous analysis of many genes and thus the biological behavior of the tumor. A number of studies reported gene expression signatures that correlate with poorer prognosis in retrospective analysis. However, the overlap between gene lists generated in these studies was minimal and has yet to be validated for clinical use.

A recent study clustering analysis of gene expression was able to classify PCa into biological subgroups with distinct prognosis [175]. Two hundred and eighty one tumors from the active surveillance cohort were robustly stratified into five molecular subtypes based on their gene expression profiles. The class with the worst survival outcome is characterized by an embryonic stem cell signature together with p53 and PTEN inactivation signatures and strong proliferation and MYC activation signals (ESC | p53– | PTEN–). Although this group is enriched for high Gleason scores (55 %), this molecular signature and Gleason score-based classifications are clearly not identical and not dependent as variables [175].

Given the proven importance of the Gleason score in prediction clinical course, Penney et al. assessed gene expression differences in Gleason ≤6 versus Gleason ≥8 cancers to help predict clinical behavior in patients with Gleason 7 cancer by similarity to more or less aggressive disease [176]. Another study analyzed the miRNA expression profiles and identified a number of miRNAs that are differentially expressed between Gleason grades 3–5 and can serve as prognostic biomarkers (our data, submitted for publication).

Personalized Medicine in Prostate Cancer

Molecular analysis is now being investigated as a tool to identify predictive markers for PCa. The PI3K-PTEN signaling pathway is a noteworthy example [177]. PTEN loss of function has been observed in 40–70 % of advanced PCa, accompanied by frequent alterations in the pathway network such as INPP4B, PHLPP, and PIK3R1 [99]. The fact that PTEN-null prostate tumors respond to inhibition of PI3K has demonstrated the possible role of PTEN loss as a predictive biomarker in clinical trials testing PI3K pathway inhibitors [178]. Like other targeted therapies, resistance eventually occurs, leading to treatment failure. For instance, c-Myc elevation confers resistance to PI3K inhibitors [179] and overrides the mTOR dependence of prostate lesions arising from constitutive AKT activation [180]. More importantly, allelic loss of PTEN and gain of c-Myc coexisted in 3 % human PCa, suggesting innate resistance to PI3K inhibitors in this subtype [181]. Thus, deciphering the genetic makeup of prostate tumors may facilitate patient stratification for PI3K-targeted therapies. Indeed, biomarker-driven drug development has been encouraged by the regulatory authorities as exemplified by the fast-track approval of Trastuzumab for the treatment of Her2-positive breast cancer.

Recently, a feasibility study was published showing the value of a comprehensive sequencing strategy to obtain multimolecular level data that is then integrated to answer the question of the eligibility of metastatic patients with refractory or end-stage disease to certain clinical trials. Thus the assignment of specific patients to their most potentially useful clinical trials can be based on biological signatures rather than anatomical location of the tumor [182].

References

1. Berger MF, Lawrence MS, Demichelis F, et al. The genomic complexity of primary human prostate cancer. Nature. 2011;470(7333):214–20.
2. Bruner DW, Moore D, Parlanti A, Dorgan J, Engstrom P. Relative risk of prostate cancer for men with affected relatives: systematic review and meta-analysis. Int J Cancer. 2003;107(5):797–803.
3. Hassel BA, Zhou A, Sotomayor C, Maran A, Silverman RH. A dominant negative mutant of 2-5A-dependent RNase suppresses antiproliferative and antiviral effects of interferon. EMBO J. 1993;12(8):3297–304.
4. Rokman A, Ikonen T, Seppala EH, et al. Germline alterations of the RNASEL gene, a candidate HPC1 gene at 1q25, in patients and families with prostate cancer. Am J Hum Genet. 2002;70(5):1299–304.
5. Meitz JC, Edwards SM, Easton DF, et al. HPC2/ELAC2 polymorphisms and prostate cancer risk: analysis by age of onset of disease. Br J Cancer. 2002;87(8):905–8.
6. Rennert H, Zeigler-Johnson CM, Addya K, et al. Association of susceptibility alleles in ELAC2/HPC2, RNASEL/HPC1, and MSR1 with prostate cancer severity in European American and African American men. Cancer Epidemiol Biomarkers Prev. 2005;14(4):949–57.
7. Ewing CM, Ray AM, Lange EM, et al. Germline mutations in HOXB13 and prostate-cancer risk. N Engl J Med. 2012;366(2):141–9.
8. Dong X, Wang L, Taniguchi K, et al. Mutations in CHEK2 associated with prostate cancer risk. Am J Hum Genet. 2003;72(2):270–80.
9. Freedman ML, Pearce CL, Penney KL, et al. Systematic evaluation of genetic variation at the androgen receptor locus and risk of prostate cancer in a multiethnic cohort study. Am J Hum Genet. 2005;76(1):82–90.
10. Zeegers MP, Kiemeney LA, Nieder AM, Ostrer H. How strong is the association between CAG and GGN repeat length polymorphisms in the androgen receptor gene and prostate cancer risk? Cancer Epidemiol Biomarkers Prev. 2004;13(11 Pt 1):1765–71.
11. Li Z, Habuchi T, Mitsumori K, et al. Association of V89L SRD5A2 polymorphism with prostate cancer development in a Japanese population. J Urol. 2003;169(6):2378–81.
12. Chen L, Davey Smith G, Evans DM, et al. Genetic variants in the vitamin d receptor are associated with advanced prostate cancer at diagnosis: findings from the prostate testing for cancer and treatment study and a systematic review. Cancer Epidemiol Biomarkers Prev. 2009;18(11):2874–81.
13. Chang B, Zheng SL, Isaacs SD, et al. Linkage and association of CYP17 gene in hereditary and sporadic prostate cancer. Int J Cancer. 2001;95(6):354–9.
14. Berthon P, Valeri A, Cohen-Akenine A, et al. Predisposing gene for early-onset prostate cancer, localized on chromosome 1q42.2-43. Am J Hum Genet. 1998;62(6):1416–24.
15. Gibbs M, Stanford JL, McIndoe RA, et al. Evidence for a rare prostate cancer-susceptibility locus at chromosome 1p36. Am J Hum Genet. 1999;64(3):776–87.

16. Lange EM, Beebe-Dimmer JL, Ray AM, et al. Genome-wide linkage scan for prostate cancer susceptibility from the University of Michigan prostate cancer genetics project: suggestive evidence for linkage at 16q23. Prostate. 2009;69(4):385–91.

17. Wiklund F, Gillanders EM, Albertus JA, et al. Genome-wide scan of Swedish families with hereditary prostate cancer: suggestive evidence of linkage at 5q11.2 and 19p13.3. Prostate. 2003;57(4): 290–7.

18. Bock CH, Cunningham JM, McDonnell SK, et al. Analysis of the prostate cancer-susceptibility locus HPC20 in 172 families affected by prostate cancer. Am J Hum Genet. 2001;68(3):795–801.

19. Kang J, Chen MH, Zhang Y, et al. Type of diabetes mellitus and the odds of gleason score 8 to 10 prostate cancer. Int J Radiat Oncol Biol Phys. 2012;82(3):e463–7.

20. Yeager M, Orr N, Hayes RB, et al. Genome-wide association study of prostate cancer identifies a second risk locus at 8q24. Nat Genet. 2007;39(5): 645–9.

21. Sotelo J, Esposito D, Duhagon MA, et al. Long-range enhancers on 8q24 regulate c-myc. Proc Natl Acad Sci USA. 2010;107(7):3001–5.

22. Ahmadiyeh N, Pomerantz MM, Grisanzio C, et al. 8q24 prostate, breast, and colon cancer risk loci show tissue-specific long-range interaction with MYC. Proc Natl Acad Sci USA. 2010;107(21):9742–6.

23. Troutman SM, Sissung TM, Cropp CD, et al. Racial disparities in the association between variants on 8q24 and prostate cancer: a systematic review and meta-analysis. Oncologist. 2012;17(3):312–20.

24. Reeves JR, Dulude H, Panchal C, Daigneault L, Ramnani DM. Prognostic value of prostate secretory protein of 94 amino acids and its binding protein after radical prostatectomy. Clin Cancer Res. 2006;12(20 Pt 1):6018–22.

25. Eeles RA. Genetic predisposition to prostate cancer. Prostate Cancer Prostatic Dis. 1999;2(1):9–15.

26. Visakorpi T, Hyytinen E, Kallioniemi A, Isola J, Kallioniemi OP. Sensitive detection of chromosome copy number aberrations in prostate cancer by fluorescence in situ hybridization. Am J Pathol. 1994;145(3):624–30.

27. Visakorpi T, Kallioniemi AH, Syvanen AC, et al. Genetic changes in primary and recurrent prostate cancer by comparative genomic hybridization. Cancer Res. 1995;55(2):342–7.

28. Bergerheim US, Kunimi K, Collins VP, Ekman P. Deletion mapping of chromosomes 8, 10, and 16 in human prostatic carcinoma. Genes Chromosomes Cancer. 1991;3(3):215–20.

29. Macoska JA, Trybus TM, Wojno KJ. 8p22 loss concurrent with 8c gain is associated with poor outcome in prostate cancer. Urology. 2000;55(5):776–82.

30. Bowen C, Bubendorf L, Voeller HJ, et al. Loss of NKX3.1 expression in human prostate cancers correlates with tumor progression. Cancer Res. 2000;60(21):6111–5.

31. Dong JT, Chen C, Stultz BG, Isaacs JT, Frierson Jr HF. Deletion at 13q21 is associated with aggressive prostate cancers. Cancer Res. 2000;60(14):3880–3.

32. Cooney KA, Wetzel JC, Merajver SD, Macoska JA, Singleton TP, Wojno KJ. Distinct regions of allelic loss on 13q in prostate cancer. Cancer Res. 1996;56(5):1142–5.

33. Li C, Larsson C, Futreal A, et al. Identification of two distinct deleted regions on chromosome 13 in prostate cancer. Oncogene. 1998;16(4):481–7.

34. Hyytinen ER, Frierson Jr HF, Boyd JC, Chung LW, Dong JT. Three distinct regions of allelic loss at 13q14, 13q21-22, and 13q33 in prostate cancer. Genes Chromosomes Cancer. 1999;25(2):108–14.

35. Miyauchi T, Nagayama T, Maruyama K. Chromosomal abnormalities in carcinoma and hyperplasia of the prostate. Nihon Hinyokika Gakkai Zasshi. 1992;83(1):66–74.

36. Wang SI, Parsons R, Ittmann M. Homozygous deletion of the PTEN tumor suppressor gene in a subset of prostate adenocarcinomas. Clin Cancer Res. 1998;4(3):811–5.

37. Eagle LR, Yin X, Brothman AR, Williams BJ, Atkin NB, Prochownik EV. Mutation of the MXI1 gene in prostate cancer. Nat Genet. 1995;9(3):249–55.

38. Visakorpi T, Kallioniemi OP, Heikkinen A, Koivula T, Isola J. Small subgroup of aggressive, highly proliferative prostatic carcinomas defined by p53 accumulation. J Natl Cancer Inst. 1992;84(11):883–7.

39. Cher ML, Bova GS, Moore DH, et al. Genetic alterations in untreated metastases and androgen-independent prostate cancer detected by comparative genomic hybridization and allelotyping. Cancer Res. 1996;56(13):3091–102.

40. Jenkins RB, Qian J, Lieber MM, Bostwick DG. Detection of c-myc oncogene amplification and chromosomal anomalies in metastatic prostatic carcinoma by fluorescence in situ hybridization. Cancer Res. 1997;57(3):524–31.

41. Sato K, Qian J, Slezak JM, et al. Clinical significance of alterations of chromosome 8 in high-grade, advanced, nonmetastatic prostate carcinoma. J Natl Cancer Inst. 1999;91(18):1574–80.

42. Porkka K, Saramaki O, Tanner M, Visakorpi T. Amplification and overexpression of elongin C gene discovered in prostate cancer by cDNA microarrays. Lab Invest. 2002;82(5):629–37.

43. Saramaki O, Willi N, Bratt O, et al. Amplification of EIF3S3 gene is associated with advanced stage in prostate cancer. Am J Pathol. 2001;159(6):2089–94.

44. Nupponen N, Visakorpi T. Molecular biology of progression of prostate cancer. Eur Urol. 1999;35(5–6):351–4.

45. Porkka KP, Tammela TL, Vessella RL, Visakorpi T. RAD21 and KIAA0196 at 8q24 are amplified and overexpressed in prostate cancer. Genes Chromosomes Cancer. 2004;39(1):1–10.

46. Chen CD, Welsbie DS, Tran C, et al. Molecular determinants of resistance to antiandrogen therapy. Nat Med. 2004;10(1):33–9.

47. Nakayama T, Watanabe M, Suzuki H, et al. Epigenetic regulation of androgen receptor gene expression in human prostate cancers. Lab Invest. 2000;80(12):1789–96.

48. Millar DS, Ow KK, Paul CL, Russell PJ, Molloy PL, Clark SJ. Detailed methylation analysis of the glutathione S-transferase pi (GSTP1) gene in prostate cancer. Oncogene. 1999;18(6):1313–24.

49. Richiardi L, Fiano V, Vizzini L, et al. Promoter methylation in APC, RUNX3, and GSTP1 and mortality in prostate cancer patients. J Clin Oncol. 2009;27(19):3161–8.

50. Dammann R, Schagdarsurengin U, Seidel C, et al. The tumor suppressor RASSF1A in human carcinogenesis: an update. Histol Histopathol. 2005;20(2):645–63.

51. Graff JR, Herman JG, Lapidus RG, et al. E-cadherin expression is silenced by DNA hypermethylation in human breast and prostate carcinomas. Cancer Res. 1995;55(22):5195–9.

52. Woodson K, Hayes R, Wideroff L, Villaruz L, Tangrea J. Hypermethylation of GSTP1, CD44, and E-cadherin genes in prostate cancer among US Blacks and Whites. Prostate. 2003;55(3):199–205.

53. Padar A, Sathyanarayana UG, Suzuki M, et al. Inactivation of cyclin D2 gene in prostate cancers by aberrant promoter methylation. Clin Cancer Res. 2003;9(13):4730–4.

54. Henrique R, Costa VL, Cerveira N, et al. Hypermethylation of cyclin D2 is associated with loss of mRNA expression and tumor development in prostate cancer. J Mol Med (Berl). 2006;84(11):911–8.

55. Yegnasubramanian S, Kowalski J, Gonzalgo ML, et al. Hypermethylation of CpG islands in primary and metastatic human prostate cancer. Cancer Res. 2004;64(6):1975–86.

56. Schulz WA, Hoffmann MJ. Epigenetic mechanisms in the biology of prostate cancer. Semin Cancer Biol. 2009;19(3):172–80.

57. Min J, Zaslavsky A, Fedele G, et al. An oncogene-tumor suppressor cascade drives metastatic prostate cancer by coordinately activating ras and nuclear factor-kappaB. Nat Med. 2010;16(3):286–94.

58. Asatiani E, Huang WX, Wang A, et al. Deletion, methylation, and expression of the NKX3.1 suppressor gene in primary human prostate cancer. Cancer Res. 2005;65(4):1164–73.

59. McMenamin ME, Soung P, Perera S, Kaplan I, Loda M, Sellers WR. Loss of PTEN expression in paraffin-embedded primary prostate cancer correlates with high Gleason score and advanced stage. Cancer Res. 1999;59(17):4291–6.

60. Kibel AS, Faith DA, Bova GS, Isaacs WB. Loss of heterozygosity at 12P12-13 in primary and metastatic prostate adenocarcinoma. J Urol. 2000; 164(1):192–6.

61. Chen C, Hyytinen ER, Sun X, et al. Deletion, mutation, and loss of expression of KLF6 in human prostate cancer. Am J Pathol. 2003;162(4):1349–54.

62. Gurel B, Iwata T, Koh CM, et al. Nuclear MYC protein overexpression is an early alteration in human prostate carcinogenesis. Mod Pathol. 2008;21(9): 1156–67.

63. Wang L, Liu R, Li W, et al. Somatic single hits inactivate the X-linked tumor suppressor FOXP3 in the prostate. Cancer Cell. 2009;16(4):336–46.

64. Xu K, Shimelis H, Linn DE, et al. Regulation of androgen receptor transcriptional activity and specificity by RNF6-induced ubiquitination. Cancer Cell. 2009;15(4):270–82.

65. Kaarbo M, Klokk TI, Saatcioglu F. Androgen signaling and its interactions with other signaling pathways in prostate cancer. Bioessays. 2007;29(12): 1227–38.

66. Chmelar R, Buchanan G, Need EF, Tilley W, Greenberg NM. Androgen receptor coregulators and their involvement in the development and progression of prostate cancer. Int J Cancer. 2007; 120(4):719–33.

67. Xu J, Wu RC, O'Malley BW. Normal and cancer-related functions of the p160 steroid receptor co-activator (SRC) family. Nat Rev Cancer. 2009;9(9):615–30.

68. Dasgupta S, Srinidhi S, Vishwanatha JK. Oncogenic activation in prostate cancer progression and metastasis: molecular insights and future challenges. J Carcinog. 2012;11:4. Epub 2012 Feb 17.

69. Mehra R, Tomlins SA, Yu J, et al. Characterization of TMPRSS2-ETS gene aberrations in androgen-independent metastatic prostate cancer. Cancer Res. 2008;68(10):3584–90.

70. Mehra R, Han B, Tomlins SA, et al. Heterogeneity of TMPRSS2 gene rearrangements in multifocal prostate adenocarcinoma: molecular evidence for an independent group of diseases. Cancer Res. 2007;67(17):7991–5.

71. Iljin K, Wolf M, Edgren H, et al. TMPRSS2 fusions with oncogenic ETS factors in prostate cancer involve unbalanced genomic rearrangements and are associated with HDAC1 and epigenetic reprogramming. Cancer Res. 2006;66(21):10242–6.

72. Xu J, Lamouille S, Derynck R. TGF-beta-induced epithelial to mesenchymal transition. Cell Res. 2009;19(2):156–72.

73. Koeneman KS, Pan CX, Jin JK, et al. Telomerase activity, telomere length, and DNA ploidy in prostatic intraepithelial neoplasia (PIN). J Urol. 1998;160(4):1533–9.

74. Vivanco I, Sawyers CL. The phosphatidylinositol 3-kinase AKT pathway in human cancer. Nat Rev Cancer. 2002;2(7):489–501.

75. Fujita N, Sato S, Katayama K, Tsuruo T. Akt-dependent phosphorylation of p27Kip1 promotes binding to 14-3-3 and cytoplasmic localization. J Biol Chem. 2002;277(32):28706–13.

76. Kang GH, Lee S, Lee HJ, Hwang KS. Aberrant CpG island hypermethylation of multiple genes in prostate cancer and prostatic intraepithelial neoplasia. J Pathol. 2004;202(2):233–40.

77. Nelson WG, De Marzo AM, DeWeese TL, Isaacs WB. The role of inflammation in the pathogenesis of prostate cancer. J Urol. 2004;172(5 Pt 2):S6–11; discussion S11–2.

78. Kaaks R, Lukanova A, Sommersberg B. Plasma androgens, IGF-1, body size, and prostate cancer risk: a synthetic review. Prostate Cancer Prostatic Dis. 2000;3(3):157–72.

79. Lindmark F, Zheng SL, Wiklund F, et al. Interleukin-1 receptor antagonist haplotype associated with prostate cancer risk. Br J Cancer. 2005;93(4):493–7.

80. Sun J, Hsu FC, Turner AR, et al. Meta-analysis of association of rare mutations and common sequence variants in the MSR1 gene and prostate cancer risk. Prostate. 2006;66(7):728–37.

81. Xu J, Lowey J, Wiklund F, et al. The interaction of four genes in the inflammation pathway significantly predicts prostate cancer risk. Cancer Epidemiol Biomarkers Prev. 2005;14(11 Pt 1):2563–8.

82. Greenberg AS, Obin MS. Obesity and the role of adipose tissue in inflammation and metabolism. Am J Clin Nutr. 2006;83(2):461S–5.

83. Shoelson SE, Lee J, Goldfine AB. Inflammation and insulin resistance. J Clin Invest. 2006; 116(7):1793–801.

84. Fradet V, Lessard L, Begin LR, Karakiewicz P, Masson AM, Saad F. Nuclear factor-kappaB nuclear localization is predictive of biochemical recurrence in patients with positive margin prostate cancer. Clin Cancer Res. 2004;10(24):8460–4.

85. Lessard L, Begin LR, Gleave ME, Mes-Masson AM, Saad F. Nuclear localisation of nuclear factor-kappaB transcription factors in prostate cancer: an immunohistochemical study. Br J Cancer. 2005; 93(9):1019–23.

86. Hager MH, Solomon KR, Freeman MR. The role of cholesterol in prostate cancer. Curr Opin Clin Nutr Metab Care. 2006;9(4):379–85.

87. Zhuang L, Kim J, Adam RM, Solomon KR, Freeman MR. Cholesterol targeting alters lipid raft composition and cell survival in prostate cancer cells and xenografts. J Clin Invest. 2005;115(4):959–68.

88. Lawrence MG, Veveris-Lowe TL, Whitbread AK, Nicol DL, Clements JA. Epithelial-mesenchymal transition in prostate cancer and the potential role of kallikrein serine proteases. Cells Tissues Organs. 2007;185(1–3):111–5.

89. Vernon AE, LaBonne C. Tumor metastasis: a new twist on epithelial-mesenchymal transitions. Curr Biol. 2004;14(17):R719–21.

90. Zhu ML, Kyprianou N. Role of androgens and the androgen receptor in epithelial-mesenchymal transition and invasion of prostate cancer cells. FASEB J. 2010;24(3):769–77.

91. Cao Q, Yu J, Dhanasekaran SM, et al. Repression of E-cadherin by the polycomb group protein EZH2 in cancer. Oncogene. 2008;27(58):7274–84.

92. Giannoni E, Bianchini F, Masieri L, et al. Reciprocal activation of prostate cancer cells and cancer-associated fibroblasts stimulates epithelial-mesenchymal transition and cancer stemness. Cancer Res. 2010;70(17):6945–56.

93. Martens-Uzunova ES, Jalava SE, Dits NF, et al. Diagnostic and prognostic signatures from the small non-coding RNA transcriptome in prostate cancer. Oncogene. 2012;31(8):978–91.

94. White NM, Fatoohi E, Metias M, Jung K, Stephan C, Yousef GM. Metastamirs: a stepping stone towards improved cancer management. Nat Rev Clin Oncol. 2011;8(2):75–84.

95. Fendler A, Jung M, Stephan C, et al. miRNAs can predict prostate cancer biochemical relapse and are involved in tumor progression. Int J Oncol. 2011;39(5):1183–92.

96. Fendler A, Stephan C, Yousef GM, Jung K. MicroRNAs as regulators of signal transduction in urological tumors. Clin Chem. 2011;57(7):954–68.

97. Oka H, Chatani Y, Kohno M, Kawakita M, Ogawa O. Constitutive activation of the 41- and 43-kDa mitogen-activated protein (MAP) kinases in the progression of prostate cancer to an androgen-independent state. Int J Urol. 2005;12(10):899–905.

98. Setlur SR, Royce TE, Sboner A, et al. Integrative microarray analysis of pathways dysregulated in metastatic prostate cancer. Cancer Res. 2007;67(21):10296–303.

99. Taylor BS, Schultz N, Hieronymus H, et al. Integrative genomic profiling of human prostate cancer. Cancer Cell. 2010;18(1):11–22.

100. Pulukuri SM, Rao JS. Matrix metalloproteinase-1 promotes prostate tumor growth and metastasis. Int J Oncol. 2008;32(4):757–65.

101. De Marzo AM, Platz EA, Sutcliffe S, et al. Inflammation in prostate carcinogenesis. Nat Rev Cancer. 2007;7(4):256–69.

102. Bostwick DG, Brawer MK. Prostatic intra-epithelial neoplasia and early invasion in prostate cancer. Cancer. 1987;59(4):788–94.

103. Sakr WA, Haas GP, Cassin BF, Pontes JE, Crissman JD. The frequency of carcinoma and intraepithelial neoplasia of the prostate in young male patients. J Urol. 1993;150(2 Pt 1):379–85.

104. Qian J, Bostwick DG, Takahashi S, et al. Chromosomal anomalies in prostatic intraepithelial neoplasia and carcinoma detected by fluorescence in situ hybridization. Cancer Res. 1995;55(22):5408–14.

105. Haggman MJ, Macoska JA, Wojno KJ, Oesterling JE. The relationship between prostatic intraepithelial neoplasia and prostate cancer: critical issues. J Urol. 1997;158(1):12–22.

106. Xin L, Lawson DA, Witte ON. The sca-1 cell surface marker enriches for a prostate-regenerating cell subpopulation that can initiate prostate tumorigenesis. Proc Natl Acad Sci USA. 2005;102(19):6942–7.

107. Lawson DA, Witte ON. Stem cells in prostate cancer initiation and progression. J Clin Invest. 2007;117(8):2044–50.

108. Verhagen AP, Ramaekers FC, Aalders TW, Schaafsma HE, Debruyne FM, Schalken JA.

Colocalization of basal and luminal cell-type cytokeratins in human prostate cancer. Cancer Res. 1992;52(22):6182–7.

109. Hurt EM, Kawasaki BT, Klarmann GJ, Thomas SB, Farrar WL. CD44+ CD24(−) prostate cells are early cancer progenitor/stem cells that provide a model for patients with poor prognosis. Br J Cancer. 2008;98(4):756–65.

110. Andreoiu M, Cheng L. Multifocal prostate cancer: biologic, prognostic, and therapeutic implications. Hum Pathol. 2010;41(6):781–93.

111. Mirchandani D, Zheng J, Miller GJ, et al. Heterogeneity in intratumor distribution of p53 mutations in human prostate cancer. Am J Pathol. 1995;147(1):92–101.

112. Ruiz C, Lenkiewicz E, Evers L, et al. Advancing a clinically relevant perspective of the clonal nature of cancer. Proc Natl Acad Sci USA. 2011;108(29): 12054–9.

113. Liu W, Laitinen S, Khan S, et al. Copy number analysis indicates monoclonal origin of lethal metastatic prostate cancer. Nat Med. 2009;15(5):559–65.

114. Sboner A, Demichelis F, Calza S, et al. Molecular sampling of prostate cancer: a dilemma for predicting disease progression. BMC Med Genomics. 2010;3:8.

115. Gurel B, Iwata T, Koh CM, Yegnasubramanian S, Nelson WG, De Marzo AM. Molecular alterations in prostate cancer as diagnostic, prognostic, and therapeutic targets. Adv Anat Pathol. 2008;15(6): 319–31.

116. Vickers AJ, Roobol MJ, Lilja H. Screening for prostate cancer: early detection or overdetection? Annu Rev Med. 2012;63:161–70.

117. Stephan C, Jung K, Lein M, Diamandis EP. PSA and other tissue kallikreins for prostate cancer detection. Eur J Cancer. 2007;43(13):1918–26.

118. Shariat SF, Semjonow A, Lilja H, Savage C, Vickers AJ, Bjartell A. Tumor markers in prostate cancer I: blood-based markers. Acta Oncol. 2011;50 Suppl 1:61–75.

119. Diamandis M, White NM, Yousef GM. Personalized medicine: marking a new epoch in cancer patient management. Mol Cancer Res. 2010;8(9):1175–87.

120. Pasic MD, Samaan S, Yousef GM. Genomic medicine: new frontiers and new challenges. Clin Chem. 2013;59(1):158–67.

121. Prensner JR, Chinnaiyan AM, Srivastava S. Systematic, evidence-based discovery of biomarkers at the NCI. Clin Exp Metastasis. 2012;29(7): 645–52.

122. Zheng SL, Sun J, Wiklund F, et al. Cumulative association of five genetic variants with prostate cancer. N Engl J Med. 2008;358(9):910–9.

123. Schroder FH, Hugosson J, Roobol MJ, et al. Screening and prostate-cancer mortality in a randomized European study. N Engl J Med. 2009; 360(13):1320–8.

124. Gudmundsson J, Besenbacher S, Sulem P, et al. Genetic correction of PSA values using sequence variants associated with PSA levels. Sci Transl Med. 2010;2(62):62ra92.

125. Cooperberg MR, Cowan JE, Hilton JF, et al. Outcomes of active surveillance for men with intermediate-risk prostate cancer. J Clin Oncol. 2011;29(2):228–34.

126. Dhir R, Vietmeier B, Arlotti J, et al. Early identification of individuals with prostate cancer in negative biopsies. J Urol. 2004;171(4):1419–23.

127. Diamandis EP. Early prostate cancer antigen-2: a controversial prostate cancer biomarker? Clin Chem. 2010;56(4):542–4.

128. Danila DC, Pantel K, Fleisher M, Scher HI. Circulating tumors cells as biomarkers: progress toward biomarker qualification. Cancer J. 2011;17(6):438–50.

129. Allard WJ, Matera J, Miller MC, et al. Tumor cells circulate in the peripheral blood of all major carcinomas but not in healthy subjects or patients with nonmalignant diseases. Clin Cancer Res. 2004;10(20):6897–904.

130. Tomlins SA, Rhodes DR, Perner S, et al. Recurrent fusion of TMPRSS2 and ETS transcription factor genes in prostate cancer. Science. 2005; 310(5748):644–8.

131. Taylor DD, Gercel-Taylor C. MicroRNA signatures of tumor-derived exosomes as diagnostic biomarkers of ovarian cancer. Gynecol Oncol. 2008;110(1): 13–21.

132. Mo MH, Chen L, Fu Y, Wang W, Fu SW. Cell-free circulating miRNA biomarkers in cancer. J Cancer. 2012;3:432–48.

133. Woodson K, O'Reilly KJ, Hanson JC, Nelson D, Walk EL, Tangrea JA. The usefulness of the detection of GSTP1 methylation in urine as a biomarker in the diagnosis of prostate cancer. J Urol. 2008;179(2):508–11; discussion 511–2.

134. Tomlins SA, Laxman B, Varambally S, et al. Role of the TMPRSS2-ERG gene fusion in prostate cancer. Neoplasia. 2008;10(2):177–88.

135. Hoque MO, Topaloglu O, Begum S, et al. Quantitative methylation-specific polymerase chain reaction gene patterns in urine sediment distinguish prostate cancer patients from control subjects. J Clin Oncol. 2005;23(27):6569–75.

136. Payne SR, Serth J, Schostak M, et al. DNA methylation biomarkers of prostate cancer: confirmation of candidates and evidence urine is the most sensitive body fluid for non-invasive detection. Prostate. 2009;69(12):1257–69.

137. Bussemakers MJ, van Bokhoven A, Verhaegh GW, et al. DD3: a new prostate-specific gene, highly overexpressed in prostate cancer. Cancer Res. 1999;59(23):5975–9.

138. Marks LS, Fradet Y, Deras IL, et al. PCA3 molecular urine assay for prostate cancer in men undergoing repeat biopsy. Urology. 2007;69(3):532–5.

139. Rogers CG, Yan G, Zha S, et al. Prostate cancer detection on urinalysis for alpha methylacyl coenzyme a racemase protein. J Urol. 2004;172(4 Pt 1): 1501–3.

140. Luo J, Zha S, Gage WR, et al. Alpha-methylacyl-CoA racemase: a new molecular marker for prostate cancer. Cancer Res. 2002;62(8):2220–6.

141. Jamaspishvili T, Kral M, Khomeriki I, Student V, Kolar Z, Bouchal J. Urine markers in monitoring for prostate cancer. Prostate Cancer Prostatic Dis. 2010;13(1):12–9.

142. Hessels D, Smit FP, Verhaegh GW, Witjes JA, Cornel EB, Schalken JA. Detection of TMPRSS2-ERG fusion transcripts and prostate cancer antigen 3 in urinary sediments may improve diagnosis of prostate cancer. Clin Cancer Res. 2007;13(17):5103–8.

143. Kristiansen G. Immunohistochemical algorithms in prostate diagnostics: what's new? Pathologe. 2009;30 Suppl 2:146–53.

144. Patel A, Dorey F, Franklin J, deKernion JB. Recurrence patterns after radical retropubic prostatectomy: clinical usefulness of prostate specific antigen doubling times and log slope prostate specific antigen. J Urol. 1997;158(4):1441–5.

145. Botchkina GI, Kim RH, Botchkina IL, Kirshenbaum A, Frischer Z, Adler HL. Noninvasive detection of prostate cancer by quantitative analysis of telomerase activity. Clin Cancer Res. 2005;11(9):3243–9.

146. Crocitto LE, Korns D, Kretzner L, et al. Prostate cancer molecular markers GSTP1 and hTERT in expressed prostatic secretions as predictors of biopsy results. Urology. 2004;64(4):821–5.

147. Schostak M, Schwall GP, Poznanovic S, et al. Annexin A3 in urine: a highly specific noninvasive marker for prostate cancer early detection. J Urol. 2009;181(1):343–53.

148. Roy R, Louis G, Loughlin KR, et al. Tumor-specific urinary matrix metalloproteinase fingerprinting: identification of high molecular weight urinary matrix metalloproteinase species. Clin Cancer Res. 2008;14(20):6610–7.

149. Dhanasekaran SM, Barrette TR, Ghosh D, et al. Delineation of prognostic biomarkers in prostate cancer. Nature. 2001;412(6849):822–6.

150. Holt SK, Kwon EM, Lin DW, Ostrander EA, Stanford JL. Association of hepsin gene variants with prostate cancer risk and prognosis. Prostate. 2010;70(9):1012–9.

151. Laxman B, Morris DS, Yu J, et al. A first-generation multiplex biomarker analysis of urine for the early detection of prostate cancer. Cancer Res. 2008;68(3):645–9.

152. Bryant RJ, Pawlowski T, Catto JW, et al. Changes in circulating microRNA levels associated with prostate cancer. Br J Cancer. 2012;106(4):768–74.

153. Varma M, Jasani B. Diagnostic utility of immunohistochemistry in morphologically difficult prostate cancer: review of current literature. Histopathology. 2005;47(1):1–16.

154. Nakayama M, Bennett CJ, Hicks JL, et al. Hypermethylation of the human glutathione S-transferase-pi gene (GSTP1) CpG island is present in a subset of proliferative inflammatory atro-

phy lesions but not in normal or hyperplastic epithelium of the prostate: a detailed study using laser-capture microdissection. Am J Pathol. 2003;163(3):923–33.

155. Trock BJ, Brotzman MJ, Mangold LA, et al. Evaluation of GSTP1 and APC methylation as indicators for repeat biopsy in a high-risk cohort of men with negative initial prostate biopsies. BJU Int. 2012;110(1):56–62.

156. Korkmaz CG, Korkmaz KS, Manola J, et al. Analysis of androgen regulated homeobox gene NKX3.1 during prostate carcinogenesis. J Urol. 2004; 172(3):1134–9.

157. Gelmann EP, Bowen C, Bubendorf L. Expression of NKX3.1 in normal and malignant tissues. Prostate. 2003;55(2):111–7.

158. Chuang AY, DeMarzo AM, Veltri RW, Sharma RB, Bieberich CJ, Epstein JI. Immunohistochemical differentiation of high-grade prostate carcinoma from urothelial carcinoma. Am J Surg Pathol. 2007; 31(8):1246–55.

159. Roberts MJ, Schirra HJ, Lavin MF, Gardiner RA. Metabolomics: a novel approach to early and noninvasive prostate cancer detection. Korean J Urol. 2011;52(2):79–89.

160. Spratlin JL, Serkova NJ, Eckhardt SG. Clinical applications of metabolomics in oncology: a review. Clin Cancer Res. 2009;15(2):431–40.

161. Sreekumar A, Poisson LM, Rajendiran TM, et al. Metabolomic profiles delineate potential role for sarcosine in prostate cancer progression. Nature. 2009;457(7231):910–4.

162. Tessem MB, Swanson MG, Keshari KR, et al. Evaluation of lactate and alanine as metabolic biomarkers of prostate cancer using 1H HR-MAS spectroscopy of biopsy tissues. Magn Reson Med. 2008;60(3):510–6.

163. Jadvar H. FDG PET, in prostate cancer. PET Clin. 2009;4(2):155–61.

164. Nakajima T, Mitsunaga M, Bander NH, Heston WD, Choyke PL, Kobayashi H. Targeted, activatable, in vivo fluorescence imaging of prostate-specific membrane antigen (PSMA) positive tumors using the quenched humanized J591 antibody-indocyanine green (ICG) conjugate. Bioconjug Chem. 2011;22(8):1700–5.

165. Wilkinson S, Chodak G. The role of 111indium-capromab pendetide imaging for assessing biochemical failure after radical prostatectomy. J Urol. 2004;172(1):133–6.

166. Clark JP, Munson KW, Gu JW, et al. Performance of a single assay for both type III and type VI TMPRSS2:ERG fusions in noninvasive prediction of prostate biopsy outcome. Clin Chem. 2008;54(12):2007–17.

167. Petrovics G, Liu A, Shaheduzzaman S, et al. Frequent overexpression of ETS-related gene-1 (ERG1) in prostate cancer transcriptome. Oncogene. 2005;24(23):3847–52.

168. Chun FK, de la Taille A, van Poppel H, et al. Prostate cancer gene 3 (PCA3): development and internal validation of a novel biopsy nomogram. Eur Urol. 2009;56(4):659–67.

169. Auprich M, Haese A, Walz J, et al. External validation of urinary PCA3-based nomograms to individually predict prostate biopsy outcome. Eur Urol. 2010;58(5):727–32.

170. Rubin MA, Bismar TA, Andren O, et al. Decreased alpha-methylacyl CoA racemase expression in localized prostate cancer is associated with an increased rate of biochemical recurrence and cancer-specific death. Cancer Epidemiol Biomarkers Prev. 2005;14(6):1424–32.

171. Tomlins SA, Rhodes DR, Yu J, et al. The role of SPINK1 in ETS rearrangement-negative prostate cancers. Cancer Cell. 2008;13(6):519–28.

172. Varambally S, Dhanasekaran SM, Zhou M, et al. The polycomb group protein EZH2 is involved in progression of prostate cancer. Nature. 2002;419(6907):624–9.

173. Tahir SA, Yang G, Ebara S, et al. Secreted caveolin-1 stimulates cell survival/clonal growth and contributes to metastasis in androgen-insensitive prostate cancer. Cancer Res. 2001;61(10):3882–5.

174. Murphy AJ, Hughes CA, Barrett C, et al. Low-level TOP2A amplification in prostate cancer is associated with HER2 duplication, androgen resistance, and decreased survival. Cancer Res. 2007;67(6): 2893–8.

175. Markert EK, Mizuno H, Vazquez A, Levine AJ. Molecular classification of prostate cancer using curated expression signatures. Proc Natl Acad Sci USA. 2011;108(52):21276–81.

176. Penney KL, Sinnott JA, Fall K, et al. mRNA expression signature of gleason grade predicts lethal prostate cancer. J Clin Oncol. 2011;29(17):2391–6.

177. Jia S, Liu Z, Zhang S, et al. Essential roles of PI(3) K-p110beta in cell growth, metabolism and tumorigenesis. Nature. 2008;454(7205):776–9.

178. Ilic N, Utermark T, Widlund HR, Roberts TM. PI3K-targeted therapy can be evaded by gene amplification along the MYC-eukaryotic translation initiation factor 4E (eIF4E) axis. Proc Natl Acad Sci USA. 2011;108(37):E699–708.

179. Liu P, Cheng H, Santiago S, et al. Oncogenic PIK3CA-driven mammary tumors frequently recur via PI3K pathway-dependent and PI3K pathway-independent mechanisms. Nat Med. 2011;17(9):1116–20.

180. Clegg NJ, Couto SS, Wongvipat J, et al. MYC cooperates with AKT in prostate tumorigenesis and alters sensitivity to mTOR inhibitors. PLoS One. 2011;6(3):e17449.

181. Zafarana G, Ishkanian AS, Malloff CA, et al. Copy number alterations of c-MYC and PTEN are prognostic factors for relapse after prostate cancer radiotherapy. Cancer. 2012;118(16):4053–62.

182. Roychowdhury S, Iyer MK, Robinson DR, Lonigro RJ, Wu YM, Cao X, Kalyana-Sundaram S, Sam L, Balbin OA, Quist MJ, Barrette T, Everett J, Siddiqui J, Kunju LP, Navone N, Araujo JC, Troncoso P, Logothetis CJ, Innis JW, Smith DC, Lao CD, Kim SY, Roberts JS, Gruber SB, Pienta KJ, Talpaz M, Chinnaiyan AM. Personalized oncology through integrative high-throughput sequencing: a pilot study. Sci Transl Med. 2011 Nov 30;3(111).

Manal Y. Gabril and George M. Yousef

Genomics of Urinary Bladder Cancer

Chromosomal Aberrations

Loss of heterozygosity (LOH) and deletions of chromosome 9 are the most frequently described genetic alteration in more than 50 % of UC. LOH of 9q and 9p are reported more in low-grade noninvasive papillary tumors and urothelial hyperplasia than carcinoma in situ and invasive cancers. Even the adjacent normal-appearing urothelium harbors these chromosomal abnormalities. Other studies, however, detected chromosome 9 deletions in both low-grade urothelium and CIS lesions, indicating that this abnormality cannot distinguish between noninvasive and high-grade invasive types [1]. Therefore, chromosome 9 deletions may set the stage for tumorigenesis and contribute to both pathways of urothelial carcinogenesis by predisposing urothelial cells to a cascade of

M.Y. Gabril, M.D.
Department of Pathology and Laboratory Medicine,
University Hospital, 339 Windermere Road,
London, ON, Canada N6A 5A5
e-mail: manal.gabril@lhsc.on.ca

G.M. Yousef, M.D., Ph.D. (✉)
Department of Laboratory Medicine and Pathobiology,
University of Toronto, Medical Sciences Building,
1 King's College Circle, Toronto, ON, Canada M5S 1A8
e-mail: yousefg@smh.ca

genetic alterations. Chromosome 9 contains critical regions that harbor tumor suppressor genes on both 9p and 9q regions. For instance, p16 (cyclin-dependent kinase inhibitor 2A, *CDKN2A*) resides on 9p21.3 and encodes two alternatively spliced products, INK4A and ARF, which induce cell cycle arrest through the retinoblastoma protein and p53 signaling pathways. Other candidate genes include *PTCH* (9q22), *DBC1* (9q32-33), and *TSC1* (9q34) [2, 3].

The importance of trisomy 7 as a tumor-associated aberration remains controversial, since it has been also found repeatedly in some unquestionably nonneoplastic lesions. Trisomy 7 can lead to increased number of alleles of the epidermal growth factor (EGF) receptor gene [4].

Deletion of the p arm and gain of the q arm of chromosome 8 are reported in UC. LOH of 8p is associated with more aggressive tumors. The 8p21-22 locus contains several candidate genes, including DBC2, LZTS1, and TRAIL-R2 [5, 6]. A commonly gained region in 8q24 involves the c-myc proto-oncogene. Higher c-myc copy number was associated with advanced tumor stage and grade [7].

Chromosome 11 polysomy and amplifications of 11q13 have been reported in 70 % of bladder tumors. The 11q13 locus contains several candidate genes including cyclin D1, EMS1, FGF3, and FGF4 [8]. Polysomy 17, gene amplification, and HER2/neu protein overexpression are associated with poor prognosis. Bolenz et al. found that HER2-positive muscle-invasive urothelial carcinoma was at twice increased risk for recurrence and cancer-specific mortality in multivariate analyses [9]. Mechanisms other than gene amplification may be also responsible for HER2/neu protein overexpression.

In muscle-invasive tumors, there is association between metastasis and 10q loss (a region that harbors *PTEN*). In preclinical models, LOH within PTEN locus on chromosome 10 appears to be much more common in muscle invasive compared to superficial tumors, and a genetic signature of PTEN loss predicts poor clinical prognosis with metastasis [10]. Alteration 5p13 region, which results in downregulation of a candidate tumor suppressor gene DOC-2/DAB2, has also been reported in bladder cancer.

Epigenetic Alterations

DNA Methylation

Widespread instability of DNA promoter methylation was reported in 86 % of UC and occurs frequently in upper genitourinary tract tumors (94 %) than in bladder tumor (76 %). Hypermethylation of CpG islands is associated with transcriptional repression of tumor suppressor genes and was commonly found in invasive tumors. A number of tumor suppressor genes, including *p16*, *CDH1*, *CDH13*, *INK4A* (*CDKN2A*), *RASSF1A*, *APC*, *ARF*, *MLH1*, and *DAPK*, have been reported to be frequently hypermethylated. Hypermethylation of *CDH1*, *CDK2AP2*, or *RASSF1A* in urine sediment DNA was detected in 85 % of superficial low-grade bladder tumors, 79 % of high-grade tumors, and 75 % of invasive bladder cancer [11].

Many of the hypomethylated loci are non-CpG island promoters of tissue-specific genes and may lead to increased potential for gene activity or chromosomal instability and are found in noninvasive tumors. In addition to global hypomethylation of repetitive elements, such as long interspersed nuclear elements (LINE-1) [12], a study has demonstrated that a specific LINE-1 located within the mesenchymal-epithelial transition factor (MET) oncogene

(L1-MET) is hypomethylated and transcriptionally active in UC, accompanied by the presence of a nucleosome-depleted region (NDR) just upstream of the transcription start site (TSS), active histone marks, and the histone variant H2A.Z [13].

miRNAs and Urothelial Carcinoma

Dysregulated miRNAs have been reported in bladder cancer and may confer a "tumor signature" that can be exploited for diagnostic purposes [14]. Several recent reports have shown that miRNAs are associated with tumor stage, grade, as well as prognosis, although investigating the utility of miRNA as diagnostic tools are limited. Hanke et al. reported that miR-126: miR-152 ratio enabled the detection of bladder cancer in urine samples with 82 % specificity and 72% sensitivity [15].

Molecular Pathways of Urothelial Carcinoma

Recent evidence supports the presence of two distinct pathways of UC (Fig. 18.1). The majority of tumors (70 %) are superficial noninvasive low-grade tumors which are often multifocal with high recurrence rate. These tumors infrequently progress to muscle invasion (10–15 %). Muscle-invasive disease (Stages pT2–pT4), on the other hand, represents 20 % of tumors with approximately 50 % chance of developing metastases. Most invasive tumors arise through sequences of events starting from normal to dysplasia, to carcinoma in situ, and then to invasion. Stage pT1 tumors have lamina propria invasion and represent 10–20 % of cases. A significant number of these pT1 tumors recur with muscle-invasive disease and require radical treatment. The molecular changes in T1 high-grade tumors are challenging and complex. They have overlapping molecular features between the above two groups.

As summarized in Box 18.1, a number of critical molecules/pathways were reported to be associated with noninvasive superficial urothelial carcinoma including FGFR3, phosphatidylinositol-3 kinase

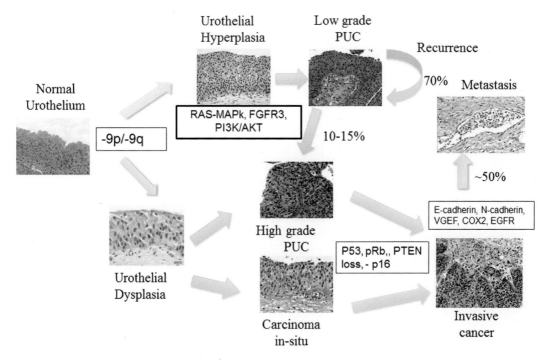

Fig. 18.1 Recent evidence suggests that there are two biologically distinct pathways of urothelial tumor pathogenesis. The majority of the tumors follow the superficial noninvasive pathway of tumorigenesis, where as ~20 % show unique alterations of the high-grade, muscle-invasive pathway. High-grade T1 tumors exhibit alterations that are overlapping between these two pathways

---

Box 18.1: Summary of the Most Common Molecular Abnormalities in Low-Grade and High-Grade Urothelial Tumors

– Low-grade tumors:

  The most frequent activating mutations detected in low-grade tumors constitutively upregulate the activity of receptor-tyrosine kinase- RAS pathway.

  Overexpression of FGFR-3 in up to 70 % of tumors, HRAS in 30–40 % and PIK3CA in 10 %.

  Chromosome 9 loss is seen in both low-grade and high-grade tumors.

– High-grade tumors:

  The deletion and mutation of tumor suppressor genes *p53* and *pRB* are the most frequent abnormalities in high-grade tumors and contribute to tumor progression.

  High-grade lesions may have *PTEN* and *p16* loss as well.

  Changes in the microenvironment promote invasion and progression though aberrant N- and E-cadherin expression and production of vascular endothelial growth factor.

(continued)

(PI3K)/AKT pathway, and RAS/mitogen-activated protein kinase (MAPK) pathway. In invasive UC, changes are related to cell cycle and a number of tumor suppressor genes, including p53, p16, and RB.

FGFR3 Pathway

Seventy to 80 % of low-grade noninvasive papillary urothelial carcinomas exhibit activating fibroblast growth factor receptor 3 (FGFR3) mutations compared to 10–20 % of invasive tumors. Mutations between the IgII and IgIII domains (exon 7) are by far the most common, accounting for 50–80 % of all mutations of FGFR3. Mutations affecting the transmembrane domain (exon 10) account for 15–40 %, and those affecting tyrosine kinase 2 domain (exon 15) account for 5–10 %. FGFR3 activation triggers several downstream kinase pathways [16].

High-grade tumors with FGFR3 mutation have unique histologic features characterized by a bulky, exophytic component with branching papillary architecture as well as irregular nuclei with a koilocytotic appearance which can facilitate the identification of this subset of tumors [17]. Tomlinson et al. reported that 42 % of tumors with no detectable mutation showed overexpression of the wild-type receptor, including many muscle-invasive tumors [18]. Activated FGFR3 can also trigger the *STAT* pathway and interact with proline-rich tyrosine kinase 2 (*PYK2*), leading to further STAT pathway activation [19].

RAS

Mutations in *HRAS* constitutively activate the *HRAS* protein and enable propagation of the growth factor signal. Earlier studies showed that *HRAS* mutations dominate over *KRAS* mutations in bladder cancers. A recent study, however, showed that *KRAS* and *HRAS* mutations occurred with equal frequency [20]. *NRAS* mutations are not frequent in bladder cancer. Mutations in HRAS are primarily associated with non-muscle-invasive disease.

PI3K/AKT Pathway

The PI3K/AKT pathway regulates a number of biological activities, including cellular growth, survival, and proliferation [21]. Activated FGFR3 triggers the downstream PI3K pathway. PI3KCA

hot spot mutations in codons 542, 545, and 1047 have been found in approximately 20 % of superficial bladder tumors in contrast to a very low incidence in invasive cancers. *PIK3CA* mutations tend to occur in a subset of cases harboring *FGFR3* mutations. The lower prevalence of *PIK3CA* mutations in muscle-invasive tumors further strengthens the notion that papillary non-invasive and muscle-invasive tumors are two different molecular entities [22].

TSC1, TSC2, and the mTOR Pathway

The tumor suppressor gene TSC1 has been reported to be mutated in 16 % of UC [23]. TSC1 is a negative regulator of them TOR pathway, which is important for cell proliferation and is frequently activated in tumors including UC. Notably, TSC1 is regulated by AKT1 and is therefore a potential downstream target of the FGFR3 signaling pathway. Additional proteins in this pathway include PIK3R1, PTEN, and TSC2. PIK3R1 is a negative regulator of PIK3CA while PTEN is a negative regulator of AKT1. TSC2 forms a complex with TSC1 that functions as a negative regulator of the mTOR pathway. So far no mutation data on *PIK3R1* or *TSC2* in UC is available. Sjödahl et al. reported *APC/CTNNB1* mutations in both *FGFR3* and *p53* wild-type and mutated cases, indicating that activation of the APC/CTNNB1 signaling pathway occur independent of *FGFR3* and *TP53* mutations. All detected *APC* mutations were missense mutations [23].

p53 Pathway

p53 mutations induce a series of downstream effects, including decreased expression or loss of p21, leading to cell cycle arrest. This important downstream target of p53 is downregulated in the majority of urothelial carcinomas with p53 mutations. Multiple codons seemed to be preferentially mutated, including codons 280 and 285. These two mutations are rare in other epithelial tumors, suggesting that they are urothelial specific. Accumulation of p53 within the nucleus and p53 gene mutations is very common in high-grade invasive urothelial carcinoma (>50 %) and flat CIS. In addition, p53 has been implicated as an important predictor of recurrence, progression, and survival of patients with high-grade recurrent superficial papillary UC, independent of tumor grade and stage [24].

In addition to mutational inactivation, p53 can be functionally inactivated by MDM2. UC overexpresses this oncoprotein which is more frequent with high-grade than low-grade tumor [25]. The molecular changes in T1 high-grade tumors are challenging. In one study, these tumors had *FGFR3* mutations in only 16.8 % of cases, whereas inactivating p53 mutations occur in 58 %, supporting the notion that these tumors resemble invasive bladder cancers at the molecular level [26].

RB Gene and Cell Cycle

The Rb protein is a key player in regulating the G1-S phase of cell cycle. LOH of Rb gene locus is associated with a higher grade and stage tumors. Moreover, there is generally either a lack of Rb expression or overexpression of a hyperphosphorylated version of the protein. In both situations, Rb is dysfunctional, leading to an increase in cell proliferation [25]. Also, CDK activity is reduced through interaction with several small inhibitor proteins as p15/INK4b, p16/INK4a, p21, p27, and p57 in bladder cancer.

Epidermal Growth Factor Receptor and the RAS-MAPK Pathway

Cancer progression is associated with dysregulation of signaling pathways of various growth factors and pro-inflammatory cytokines such as EGF, transforming growth factor-β (TGFβ) and interleukin-6 (IL-6). EGFR activation leads to downstream signaling that influences cell proliferation, angiogenesis, invasion, and metastasis.

Several pathways participate in EGFR signaling such as PI3K, extracellular signal-regulated kinase (ERK), and MAPK [27].

In normal urothelium EGFR is expressed only by the basal cells, and EGF is physiologically excreted in the urine, but a layer of EGFR-negative cells prevents its binding to EGFR. The disruption of this barrier allows ligand-receptor binding, which may play a role in tumorigenesis. In invasive UC, there is continuous activation of the RAS-MAPK pathway, typically through the activation of EGFR. MAPK regulates cell proliferation and survival. Binding of EGF causes activation of already overexpressed EGFR. The activated receptor then recruits proteins that activate RAS which can transmit a mitogenic signal via the RAS-MAPK pathway. The function of activated RAS protein can be inhibited by a tumor suppressor gene, RASSFIA which is usually methylated in bladder cancer [28].

EGFR expression level correlates with higher tumor grade and stage, disease progression, and worse prognosis in UC. Many studies showed that EGFR overexpression is an independent predictor of survival and disease-specific mortality [27]. Black and Dinney concluded that EGFR and HER2 expressions appear to indicate poor prognosis, while HER4 and FGFR3 are favorable prognostic indicators [29]. Another study revealed that high EGFR or low HER4 expression was associated with non-papillary, high-grade, and invasive tumors, as well as with significantly lower recurrence-free and overall survival. HER2 and HER3 were not associated with overall or recurrence-free survival [30].

Molecular Aspects of Multifocality and Heterogeneity

Cancer Stem Cells

Cancer stem cells (CSCs) are a subpopulation of tumor cells with tumor-initiating potential, self-renewal properties, and the ability to generate cellular tumor heterogeneity via differentiation. CSCs do not necessarily arise from embryonic stem cells; they can be also derived from differentiated progenies that have acquired tumorigenic properties via genetic or epigenetic alteration. Evidence suggests that CSCs in bladder urothelial carcinomas can give rise to biological heterogeneity within a tumor by differentiating into different downstream differentiated tumor cells.

Advances relating to molecular and functional characterization of CSCs in UC have revealed insights into understanding a two-pathway model of carcinogenesis. Ho et al. demonstrated that CK14+ cells constitute a subpopulation of CK5+ basal cells and could represent a stem cell population. UC with a higher frequency of CK14+ CSCs have been associated with poor survival. It was also shown that activation of the STAT3 signaling pathway directed urothelial cells towards the CIS-invasive urothelial carcinoma pathway. STAT3-driven invasive urothelial carcinomas are heavily populated with primitive CK14+ stem cells. Additionally, retrospective studies have demonstrated the potential of several CSC markers particularly CK14, ALDH1A1, and p63 as prognostic markers for stratifying high-risk bladder UC. It seems probable that low-grade noninvasive urothelial carcinomas arise from a more differentiated cell of origin, whereas invasive carcinomas arise from more primitive cells [31].

A study has shown that the tumorigenic potential of CD44+ cells is higher than CD44− cells from the same tumor [32]. Ho et al. identified a panel of 477 genes upregulated in CD44+ CSCs (referred to as a bladder CSC gene signature) [31], which can be highly reliable for predicting clinical outcomes. Additionally, CSC gene signatures can be used to identify subgroups of patients with noninvasive bladder cancers who are at risk of shorter progression-free survival. Another study showed that high-grade poorly differentiated UC have an enriched embryonic stem cell gene signature, although this signature did not effectively segregate noninvasive from invasive carcinomas [33]. These findings suggest that genes that are upregulated in CSCs could have a key role in bladder cancer cell invasion, whereas genes enriched in embryonic stem cells are associated with poorly differentiated tumors.

Multifocality, Heterogeneity, and Recurrence

One of the important features of UC is the high frequency of synchronous and metachronous multifocal occurrence. It is common for UC to be associated with surrounding abnormal urothelium that ranges from dysplasia to CIS. There are two hypotheses to explain multifocality; the first is the "field cancerization effect" where the entire bladder urothelium is exposed to carcinogens causing independent transforming genetic alterations at different sites of the urothelial lining leading to multiple genetically unrelated tumors [34]. The second hypothesis is a monoclonal theory suggesting that multiple tumors arise from a single transformed progenitor cell that proliferates and spreads throughout the urothelium either by intraluminal implantation or by intraepithelial migration. Multiple tumors might be characterized by early genetic instability and loss of cell adhesion, leading to the migration of neoplastic cells through wide areas of the urothelium [35]. Many studies investigating multifocal urothelial lesions have demonstrated a monoclonal origin. Other studies have shown that field cancerization contributes to urothelial carcinogenesis as well, leading to "oligoclonal" tumors. The term "oligoclonality" should be preferred over polyclonality because the number of unrelated clones detected in a single tumor is usually low [36].

Also, it has been suggested that expansion of tumor cells could be a late event in pathogenesis, following acquisition of complex genetic alterations, but still can occur before clinical manifestation of the disease. After initial carcinogenesis, clonally related tumor cells can accumulate additional genetic alterations, resulting either in intratumoral genetic heterogeneity or the development of topologically distinct subclones with different genetic alterations [36].

With the discovery of CSCs, the field cancerization concept has been modified. It is now suggested that clonal expansions of different CSCs result in multifocality and recurrent tumors. Current data suggest that UC recurrence may arise from CSCs remaining in an affected field after gross tumor ablation. Most current therapies eliminate differentiated cells, which are more sensitive to therapy than CSCs. Clonal expansion of fugitive CSCs results in the recurrent neoplasm wherever the surviving cells find a favorable niche [37].

The remaining urothelium in bladder with cancer is no longer normal, but instead it has undergone widespread epigenetic alterations mainly consisting of aberrant hypermethylation, which can be responsible for such high recurrence rate in some cases. Altered methylation of a significant number of loci was observed not only in tumors but also in normal-appearing urothelium taken at least 5 cm away from the corresponding primary tumor, with the majority of the loci, such as ZO2, MYOD1, and CDH13, being aberrantly hypermethylated [38]. In one study, 145 loci displayed a trend of increasing methylation in invasive tumors and 41 loci were methylated in noninvasive tumors [13].

Molecular Mechanisms of Aggressive Behavior

Superficial urothelial tumors almost invariably display an "epithelial" phenotype, whereas muscle-invasive tumors are heterogeneous. The sarcomatoid phenotype is relatively rare and occurs in less than 10 % of high-grade invasive bladder cancers. Such tumors are characterized by complex chromosomal abnormalities, pronounced aneuploidy, and clinical aggressiveness. These tumors exhibit epithelial to mesenchymal transition (EMT) associated with partial or complete loss of epithelial phenotype and the development of mesenchymal features. The hallmark feature of EMT is loss of E-cadherin, which is the canonical marker of an "epithelial" phenotype. EMT can be induced by a variety of developmental signals, but TGFβ is the best-studied stimulus [39].

Many tumor microenvironmental changes are considered features of invasive urothelial tumor pathways. These include decreased cell-cell adhesions. Loss or reduced expression of E-cadherin is seen in 78 % of high-grade invasive UC. Hypermethylation of CpG in the promoter which encodes E-cadherin occurs in 84 % of UC.

In vitro studies showed that forced expression of N-cadherin in E-cadherin-expressing urothelial carcinoma cell lines increased their invasiveness; therefore, a competing effect can be expected, and the net effect will depend on the qualitative ratio and functional status of both molecules. Also, matrix metalloproteinases (MMPs) particularly MMP99 and MMP2 are increased in urine and serum of patients with invasive tumors. Other mechanisms include increased angiogenesis and overexpression of cyclooxygenase 2 [16].

Divergent Differentiation in Urothelial Carcinoma

Urothelial carcinoma can demonstrate divergent differentiation to glandular, squamous, or other elements. The relationship between urothelial carcinoma and its various divergent elements has been investigated recently. Molecular genetic evidence has emerged supporting a close relationship between urothelial carcinoma and various divergent elements [40]. Two principal theories have been proposed. One is that divergent elements develop initially as monoclonal proliferations derived from a single multipotent CSC, subsequently diverging into morphologically distinct components. The second theory proposes that these components are similar to the main tumor only in their location and synchrony, and both develop independently from two separate CSCs of different histologic types.

Molecular Profiling and Biological Classification of Urothelial Tumors

High-throughput analysis of various levels of molecular changes in urothelial tumors showed the potential of developing new classification based on gene and chromosomal aberrations rather than morphology. Earlier studies showed the existence of two distinct groups of UC based on chromosomal alterations [16]. Recently Hurst et al. [40] showed presence of distinct genomic changes between low-grade pTa tumors (with low complexity of chromosomal changes, frequent FGFR3 mutation, and infrequent p53 mutations) and muscle-invasive cancers (with more complex chromosomal changes, infrequent FGFR3 mutations, and frequent p53 mutations).

Furthermore, hierarchical clustering analysis of high-grade stage T1 tumors showed that they can be separated into three major subgroups that differ with respect to copy-number alterations, FGFR3, and p53 mutation status. The first cluster had frequent FGFR3 mutations (70 %), with few chromosomal alterations. Tumors of the third cluster were FGFR3 wild-type and mostly p53 mutant (71 %), with more complex chromosomal changes but strikingly low frequency of chromosome 9 loss. The second cluster had fewer alterations than the third cluster but showed the highest rate of stage progression/metastasis [40].

Integrated genomic analysis also showed that FGFR3 mutant tumors are more chromosomally stable than their wild-type counterparts, and a mutually exclusive relationship between FGFR3 mutation and overrepresentation of 8q was observed in non-muscle-invasive tumors. In muscle-invasive tumors, metastasis was positively associated with losses of regions on 10q (including PTEN), 16q, and 22q and gains on 10p, 11q, 12p, 19p, and 19q. Concomitant copy-number alterations positively associated with p53 mutation in muscle-invasive tumors [40].

Microarray gene expression analysis showed the presence of distinct, clinically relevant subgroups. In a study by Blaveri et al., unsupervised hierarchical clustering successfully classified tumors into two subgroups containing superficial (pTa and pT1) versus muscle-invasive (pT2–pT4) tumors. Also, supervised classification had a 91 % success rate separating superficial from muscle-invasive tumors based on expression of a gene panel. Tumors could also be classified into transitional versus squamous subtypes (89 % success rate) and good versus bad prognosis (78 % success rate) [41].

Molecular Markers for Screening, Early Diagnosis, and Surveillance

The standard practice in the follow-up of patients with UC requires cystoscopy at regular intervals. Cytology is the most widely used noninvasive test. Cytology is very specific but limited by its low sensitivity (28–100 %). In recent years, a number of urinary markers are investigated for their potential utility in early tumor detection or follow-up of bladder cancer. The scope of applications of molecular markers in bladder cancer is summarized in Fig. 18.2. They can be divided into two categories based on whether urine

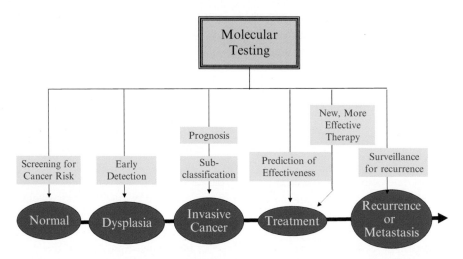

Fig. 18.2 The scope of applications of molecular testing in urothelial tumors is broad. Molecular markers either alone or combined with clinical parameters can signifi-cantly improve treatment decision and patient outcome at multiple steps of the disease process

(soluble urine markers) or exfoliated cells (cell-associated markers) are used for the assay. To date, six urine markers have been approved for clinical use in the detection of bladder cancer. ImmunoCyt/uCyt™ and UroVysion™ are currently the most common commercial markers used in the clinical setting.

Soluble Urine Markers

1. *Nuclear matrix proteins*: NMP-22 is an FDA-approved quantitative sandwich ELISA test. The sensitivity is 50–70 % and specificity is 60–90 %. It has lower sensitivity to detect low-grade tumors (30–50 %). False-positive cases are seen in inflammatory conditions [42]. *BLCA-4 and BLCA-1* are promising markers for bladder cancer, with a high sensitivity and specificity. BLCA-4 is measured in urine using ELISA. Sensitivity ranges between 89 and 96 %, with 100 % specificity [43, 44].
2. *Bladder tumor-associated antigen* (*BTA*): The *BTA test* (BardéBion Diagnostics) is an agglutination assay that qualitatively detects the presence of complexes of disrupted basement membrane in patient's urine. Advantages include high sensitivity for invasive tumors. Disadvantages are the high rate of false-positive results due to inflammatory conditions and a low overall sensitivity for lower-grade tumors. *BTA-Stat* is a point-of-care immunoassay using two monoclonal antibodies to detect human complement factor H-related protein that is frequently released into urine by urothelial neoplasms. It has 36–89 % sensitivity and 90 % specificity. *BTA-TRAK* is a quantitative ELISA assay [45, 46].
3. *HA-HAse* is an ELISA-like test that combines the analysis of hyaluronic acid and hyaluronidase. HA-HAse is expressed by tumors and is involved in angiogenesis, tumor growth, and invasion. The test has a high sensitivity to detect low- and high-grade and stage tumors. In one study, HA-HAse was reported to have

83 % sensitivity, 78 % specificity, 64 % positive predictive value, and 90 % negative predictive value [47].
4. *Survivin* is an antiapoptotic endogenous protein which is a promising marker for the diagnosis and follow-up of bladder cancer. The sensitivity and specificity for detecting recurrence were 100 % and 78 %, respectively [48]. Urinary assays detecting Survivin mRNA by RT-PCR have shown sensitivities ranging from 53 to 94 % and specificities from 88 to 100 %. This protein also correlates with unfavorable prognosis. It is associated with higher-stage, lymphovascular invasion, lymph node metastasis, and recurrence in patients treated with radical cystectomy [49].
5. *Mutations in the FGFR3* occur in 50 % of primary bladder tumors and is associated with good prognosis. FGFR3 mutations are especially prevalent in low-grade/stage tumors, with pTa tumors harboring mutations in 85 % of cases. van Oers et al. [50] described a simple assay for the simultaneous detection of nine different FGFR3 mutations in bladder cancer and voided urine with 62 % sensitivity. Zuiverloon et al. evaluated the ability of FGFR3 mutation in voided urine to detect recurrences during surveillance in patients with low-grade non-muscle-invasive tumors. The assay sensitivity (58 %) was higher than urinary cytology only but still far from perfect [51].

Cell-Based Markers

Molecular and Protein Assays

1. Microsatellite DNA analysis: Microsatellites are short tandem DNA repeats (2–4 bp) found throughout the human genome. Microsatellite DNA loci are useful markers for the detection of LOH and microsatellite instability (MSI). In UC, LOH is often found in chromosome 4p, 8p, 9q, 9p, 11p, 13p, 16q, and 17p. The test is carried out by PCR. This test offers interesting sensitivities (72–97 %) and specificities

(80–100 %) but requires expensive equipment and trained personnel. Studies reported that deletions in 9q21 correlated with invasive tumor growth. LOH at 18q21.1 and 9p21-22 correlated with poor prognosis and higher death rate. Microsatellite analysis of urine samples has been used for surveillance after treatment. The 2-year risk of developing recurrence reached 83 % if microsatellite results were persistently positive and declined to 22 % when result of microsatellite analysis was persistently negative.

Studies showed that MSI was observed in 73 % of tumors at BAT-26, BAT-40, D2S123, D9S283, D9S1851, and D18S58 loci. Good association of MSI was seen with stage and grade. MSI-high (instability at >30 % of loci) was frequently observed in high-stage (41 %) and high-grade (59 %) tumors. MSI is a good prognostic marker that correlates with risk of recurrence in superficial (Ta-T1) tumors irrespective of the grade [52].

2. Telomerase activity assessment: Urine telomerase activity is a good marker for early detection and follow-up of bladder tumors. The expression of the telomerase subunits such as human telomerase reverse transcriptase (hTERT) and human telomerase RNA component (hTR) may be associated with tumor development and progression. The hTERT/GAPDH ratio and hTERT mRNA/total RNA were significantly lower in superficial compared to invasive bladder tumors. The hTR/GAPDH mRNA ratio and hTR mRNA/total RNA were significantly lower in superficial compared to invasive tumors. The hTERT, but not hTR mRNA expression, significantly correlated with tumor grade [53]. The telomeric repeat amplification protocol assay for telomerase in exfoliated cells has 70–86 % sensitivity and 60–90 % specificity [54].

3. Cytokeratins: Major tests include the UBC test (a sandwich ELISA targeting cytokeratins 8 and 18), the cytokeratin 20 test (RT-PCR analysis) and CYFRA 21-1 (an immunoradiometric and electrochemiluminescent assay targeting cytokeratin 19). Their use is, however, limited by their high false-positive rates [54]. Studies have shown that CK20 has 78–87 % sensitivity for detecting bladder cancer in urine. The specificity of CK20 ranges from 56 to 98 % [55]. Mckenney et al. suggested the use of CK20 along with p53 markers for distinguishing CIS from reactive atypia which show sensitivity of 82–87 % in detecting UC [56].

Cytology-Based Tests

1. *The UroVysion™* is a multitarget multicolor fluorescent in situ hybridization (FISH) assay that is developed for the determination of chromosome specific anomalies in cells obtained from urine specimens. Two types of probes are used: *centromeric numeration probes* to detect urinary cells that have chromosomal numerical abnormalities consistent with a diagnosis of bladder cancer (chromosomes 3, 7, and 17) and *locus-specific probes* to detect specific mutations in known tumor suppressor genes, like 9p21 which harbors p16. Studies have shown that UroVysion is more sensitive than urine cytology for the detection of all stages and grades of bladder cancer. It is FDA approved for the detection of new or recurrent bladder cancer in voided urine specimens. Recent studies also suggest that UroVysion may be useful for assessing superficial bladder cancer patients' response to BCG therapy and in detecting upper tract urothelial carcinoma. Moonen et al. showed that sensitivity and specificity were 39 % and 90 %, respectively, for UroVysion™, 41 and 90 % for cytology, and 42 and 68 % for quantitative cytology. When the UroVysion™ test and cytology were combined, sensitivity increased to 53 %, but specificity decreased to 80 %. Detection of Ta tumors was equal for cytology and UroVysion™ (27 %); detection of T1 and T2–T4 by UroVysion™ was 60 % and 50 %, respectively. Detection of grade 1, 2, and 3 tumors by UroVysion™ was 21 %, 37 %, and 67 %, respectively [57]. The test was also particularly useful at predicting tumor recurrence. In patients with a history of UC and negative cystoscopy, UroVysion™ predicted recurrence in 39 % of patients with a positive cytology test and in 21 % of patients with a negative test [58]. In another study, 27 % of patients under UC surveillance without

evidence of tumor recurrence had a positive UroVysion™, and 65 % of these patients had recurrent carcinoma within 29 months [59].

2. *ImmunoCyt/uCyt™* is a very promising FDA-approved fluorescence test that combines three monoclonal antibodies against mucin-like antigens (M344, LDQ10, and 19A211) [60]. A major advantage of this test is its sensitivity to detect both low-grade and high-grade tumors. ImmunoCyt/uCyt™ sensitivity reached 79 % for grade 1, 84 % for grade 2, and 92 % for grade 3 tumors [61]. Limitations of this test are that it is operator dependent, time-consuming, and requires at least 500 cells to call a case negative. Test sensitivity is 53–100 % and specificity is 64–95 %. Whereas up to 50 % of patients were either negative or suspicious by cytology, all CIS are detected by combining cytology and ImmunoCyt/uCyt™ [62]. The test is less sensitive in the follow-up of patients under BCG therapy; however, the combination with cytology leads to sensitivity of 100 % for recurrences. ImmunoCyt/uCyt™ may also help to predict UC recurrence. With a history of urothelial tumor and negative cystoscopy, 18 % of patients with positive test developed a recurrence 2–6 months after the negative cystoscopy; compared to 7 % only in those with negative test. Forty-seven percent of test positive developed a recurrence at 1 year, as opposed to 12 % of those who are negative [63].

3. *DNA flow cytometry and digital imaging analysis (DIA)*: DNA ploidy studies demonstrate that the majority of low-grade papillary urothelial carcinomas are diploid or near-diploid while most of the high-grade and invasive UC are aneuploid. Aneuploid cells can be detected by DNA flow cytometry or DIA. The sensitivity of flow cytometry is limited by the fact it will fail to detect UC cells if small proportion of aneuploid cells are represented in urine. In DIA, cells are stained, followed by image analysis to assess aneuploid cells. Cajulis et al. showed that sensitivity of DIA and flow cytometry are 91 and 72 %, compared to 61 % for cytology, and specificities are 83 and 80 %, compared to 100 % for cytology [64].

Emerging Urine Biomarkers

1. DNA methylation: The first study demonstrating the feasibility of diagnosing bladder cancer through methylation analysis using DNA from voided urine came from Chan et al. [65]. A panel of markers (DAPK, RARβ, E-cadherin, and p16) was analyzed by methylation-sensitive PCR and showed 91 % sensitivity and 76 % specificity. Subsequently, studies have reported methylation markers with an increased sensitivity but a lower specificity compared to cytology. In another study, a panel of markers (DAPK, BCL2, and TERT) achieved a sensitivity of 78 % and a specificity of 100 % [66, 67].

   The advantages of DNA methylation include stability and sensitive detection by real-time PCR. In a study by Reinert et al., a four-marker panel (ZNF154, HOXA9, POU4F2, and EOMES) achieved a sensitivity of 84 % and a specificity of 96 % [68]. Another study identified a subset of genes specifically methylated in non-muscle-invasive UC recurrences. A four-gene panel (APC_a, TERT_a, TERT_b, and EDNRB) achieved an area under the receiver operating characteristic curve (AUC) of 0.82 in the test set and 0.69 in the validation set [69].

2. miRNAs: miRNAs represent ideal bladder cancer biomarkers since they are secreted in urine, require little handling care, and are more stable against nuclease degradation due to their small size. Recently, urinary miRNA expression was reported, and the upregulation of miRs-126, 182, and 199a was found to distinguish bladder cancer patients from disease-free controls. The combination of miR-126 and -182 identified up to 77 % of bladder cancer cases. Larger-scale validations are necessary to further define these markers [67, 70].

   To summarize, DNA methylation markers have the highest sensitivity (94 %) followed by ImmunoCyt (81 %), NMP22 (69 %), UroVysion (64 %), and cytology (38 %). Cytology has the highest specificity (94 %) followed by NMP22 (81 %), ImmunoCyt (75 %), UroVysion (73 %), and DNA methylation markers (66 %).

3. Circulating tumor cells: Due to imprecise clinical staging, the finding of extravesical and node-positive disease at the time of radical cystectomy for patients with clinically localized bladder cancer is not uncommon. Circulating tumor cells (CTCs) have been shown to be present in the peripheral blood of patients with metastatic urothelial carcinoma. Guzzo et al. detected CTCs in low numbers in 21 % of patients prior to radical cystectomy. CTC status was not a robust predictor of extravesical or node-positive disease in this cohort, with sensitivity, specificity, and PPV of 27 %, 88 %, and 78 %, respectively [71]. Several bladder cancer cell markers such as Uroplakin II (UPII), CK20, EGFR, and MUC-7 have been analyzed for use as candidate detection molecules found in CTCs. The sensitivity of these techniques is high, but their specificity for diagnostic purposes remains debatable [72].

Molecular Predictors of Outcome of Bladder Cancer

Lymph node metastasis is an important determinant of survival in patients with muscle-invasive UC. Histologically undetected micrometastasis may be present in regional lymph nodes. A study evaluated the expression of UPII, an urothelial-specific gene, in perivesical and lymph node samples at radical surgery as a predictor of clinical recurrence [73]. Pathologically node-negative cases had a UPII perivesical positivity of 27 % and a lymph node positivity of 33 %. UPII node positivity was a significant predictor of tumor recurrence in multivariate analysis. Marin-Aguilera et al. identified a number of genes which could indicate dissemination to lymph nodes [74]. The combination of FXYD3 and KRT20 yielded a 100 % sensitivity and specificity differentiating lymph nodes with urothelial cancer dissemination from controls. The combined expression of both genes allowed the identification of urothelial cells in lymph nodes in 21 % of patients with histologically negative lymph nodes [74].

Plastiras et al. reported that both p53 and PCNA were significant predictors of disease-related mortality in superficial tumors compared to tumor grade, size, and multiplicity. They were not, however, of prognostic significance in invasive tumors [75]. p21 status is an independent predictor of recurrence and survival after RC. Moreover, patients with p53-altered/p21-negative tumors have a higher rate of recurrence and worse survival than those with p53-altered/p21-positive tumors [76].

p27 is the second most powerful cell cycle regulator after p53 for prediction of recurrence and survival in patients with muscle-invasive bladder cancer treated with radical cystectomy. However, it has limited predictive value in non-muscle-invasive disease. Furthermore, the status of individual cell cycle regulators did not add significantly to predictions of outcome in patients with advanced disease (node positive and T4). Studies found that Ki-67 proliferation index is an independent predictor of recurrence-free survival among pTa and pT1 tumors [77]. In muscle-invasive disease, Ki-67 overexpression was significantly associated with advanced stage, higher tumor grade, lymphovascular invasion, lymph node metastasis, as well as both disease recurrence and cancer-specific mortality. Higher expression of Ki-67 appears to correlate with decreased expression of p27/kip1 and lower cyclin E. These features are observed in poorly differentiated tumors, muscle invasion, lymph node metastasis, and poor survival. Also Ki-67 expression correlated with the recurrence in superficial tumors [78]. Studies have shown that more accurate prediction of outcome can be achieved by combinations of markers as p53, Rb, and CDKs like p16 and p21. Alterations of two or more of these molecules cause a significant increase in recurrence and shorter survival.

A summary of the tissue-based prognostic markers is shown in Table 18.1. Studies have shown that any single molecular biomarker will not provide reliable prognostic stratification, and there is a strong trend towards simultaneous assessment of multiple biomarkers and incorporating both clinical and molecular parameters to improve prediction of bladder cancer outcome.

Table 18.1 Tissue-based prognostic markers in bladder tumors

Molecular mechanisms	Markers
Cell cycle	p53, pRb, Ki-67, p21, p27, cyclins
Apoptosis	Fas (CD95), caspase-3, Bcl-, survivin
Angiogenesis	MVD, thrombospondin-1, VEGF, bFGF
Signaling proteins	EGFR, FGFR3
Hormone receptors	HER2, AR, ER

A nomogram incorporating urinary NMP22, cytology, age, and gender was able to predict with high accuracy the probability of disease recurrence and progression in patients with non-muscle-invasive bladder cancer (www.nomogram.org). Assessment of a panel of p53, Rb, p21, p27, and cyclin E1 in radical cystectomy specimens improved the prediction of recurrence and survival in patients with pTa-3N0M0 disease [79]. Addition of a number of biomarkers increased the predictive accuracy of nomograms based on the TNM staging system for disease recurrence and cancer-specific mortality by 11 % [79].

Individual mutations in FGFR3 or PIK3CA and the different mutated combinations FGFR3-PIK3CA/AKT1 and PIK3CA-RAS can activate the AKT. Combinations of mutated genes in the RAS-MAPK and PI3K-AKT signaling pathways represent mutually exclusive events. FGFR3 mutations and the FGFR3-PIK3CA combined mutation, but not single PIK3CA mutation, characterize low-grade bladder tumors, and mutations in PIK3CA-KRAS and AKT1 are present exclusively in high-grade tumors [17].

Bcl-2, caspase-3, p53, and survivin have a cooperative effect on progression of bladder cancer [80]. Higher VEGF expression was associated with increasing tumor stage, grade, progression, and recurrence in patients treated with transurethral resection [81]. Recently, it has also been showed that VEGF is overexpressed in a large number of patients treated with radical cystectomy.

Thrombospondin-1 (TSP-1) is a potent inhibitor of angiogenesis that is independently associated with disease recurrence and all-cause mortality after cystectomy. Grossfeld et al. reported that p53 alterations are associated with low TSP-1 expression, and these patients are more likely to demonstrate high microvessel density [82]. Microvascular density is a surrogate marker for angiogenesis and has also been shown to be a prognostic marker associated with highest risk of recurrence and cancer-specific mortality in muscle-invasive cancer. Also, vascular density was associated with p53 alterations [82].

Targeted Therapy

Results of clinical trials of targeted agents for urothelial cancers thus far have generally been disappointing, and to date, no biologic agents have been approved either as monotherapy or in combination with cytotoxic chemotherapy for advanced UC, despite the identification of genetic alterations thought to drive high-grade, muscle-invasive disease. Classes of agents in recent and ongoing clinical trials include antiangiogenic antibodies;,multitargeted tyrosine kinase inhibitors against VEGFR2 and PDGFR, EGFR and HER2 inhibitors, and other inhibitors targeting mTOR, FGFR3, IGFR1, and Src. Novel vaccine strategies are also being tested.

Multiple agents are available that target angiogenesis and the VEGF pathway. Agents such as bevacizumab, which targets VEGF, and sunitinib and sorafenib, which target the VEGF receptor, are being tested in advanced urothelial cancer. To enhance the success of targeted antiangiogenic therapy, new strategies include the combination of multiple inhibitors against different targets or the use of single inhibitors directed against multiple targets [83].

Clinical trials evaluating EGFR targeting therapy are limited. Inhibitory monoclonal antibodies raised against the extracellular domains of EGFR, Erb-B-1, and Her-2/neu have been tried, but the results were not very promising. Similarly, results of a phase II evaluation of cisplatin, gemcitabine, and gefitinib as first-line treatment for advanced urothelial carcinoma showed no improvement in response rates or survival [84].

FGFR-3 and IGF1R are known to be overexpressed in urothelial carcinoma and may represent clinically useful therapeutic targets. TKI12458 is currently being studied in a phase II trial as second- and third-line therapy for patients with FGFR-3 mutated and wild-type urothelial carcinoma [85].

Molecular-based testing can be also used for predicting treatment efficiency. A prospective trial incorporating p53 status in the selection of adjuvant chemotherapy for patients with muscle-invasive, node-negative urothelial carcinoma following radical cystectomy failed to demonstrate prognostic or predictive value of p53. In contrast, a recent report of over 3,000 patients demonstrated that p53 had predictive value in advanced bladder cancer but not in superficial (Ta) disease. As a mechanism to overcome platinum resistance, overexpression of p53 through adenoviral gene transfer has been successful in human bladder cancer cell lines and demonstrated synergy with cisplatin. Adenoviral p53 gene transfer has also been combined with the use of antisense oligodeoxynucleotide targeting of the antiapoptotic gene clustering in a bladder cancer model in nude mice where it resulted in eradication of tumors and lymph node metastases following treatment with cisplatin, suggesting that this strategy may have clinical efficacy [83].

A vaccine against survivin, an inhibitor of apoptosis protein (IAP) that targets caspases, was recently tested in a phase I trial and was shown to be safe without adverse events reported. While this trial was not designed to assess clinical efficacy, one patient experienced a slight reduction in tumor burden, and five patients had a significant increase in the peptide-specific CTL frequency [86].

References

1. Hartmann A, Schlake G, Zaak D, et al. Occurrence of chromosome 9 and p53 alterations in multifocal dysplasia and carcinoma in situ of human urinary bladder. Cancer Res. 2002;62(3):809–18.
2. Schulze A, Zerfass K, Spitkovsky D, Henglein B, Jansen-Durr P. Activation of the E2F transcription factor by cyclin D1 is blocked by p16INK4, the product of the putative tumor suppressor gene MTS1. Oncogene. 1994;9(12):3475–82.
3. Keen AJ, Knowles MA. Definition of two regions of deletion on chromosome 9 in carcinoma of the bladder. Oncogene. 1994;9(7):2083–8.
4. Johansson B, Heim S, Mandahl N, Mertens F, Mitelman F. Trisomy 7 in nonneoplastic cells. Genes Chromosomes Cancer. 1993;6(4):199–205.
5. Adams J, Cuthbert-Heavens D, Bass S, Knowles MA. Infrequent mutation of TRAIL receptor 2 (TRAIL-R2/DR5) in transitional cell carcinoma of the bladder with 8p21 loss of heterozygosity. Cancer Lett. 2005;220(2):137–44.
6. Knowles MA, Aveyard JS, Taylor CF, Harnden P, Bass S. Mutation analysis of the 8p candidate tumour suppressor genes DBC2 (RHOBTB2) and LZTS1 in bladder cancer. Cancer Lett. 2005;225(1):121–30.
7. Mahdy E, Pan Y, Wang N, Malmstrom PU, Ekman P, Bergerheim U. Chromosome 8 numerical aberration and C-MYC copy number gain in bladder cancer are linked to stage and grade. Anticancer Res. 2001;21(5):3167–73.
8. Watters AD, Latif Z, Forsyth A, et al. Genetic aberrations of c-myc and CCND1 in the development of invasive bladder cancer. Br J Cancer. 2002;87(6):654–8.
9. Bolenz C, Shariat SF, Karakiewicz PI, et al. Human epidermal growth factor receptor 2 expression status provides independent prognostic information in patients with urothelial carcinoma of the urinary bladder. BJU Int. 2010;106(8):1216–22.
10. McConkey DJ, Lee S, Choi W, et al. Molecular genetics of bladder cancer: emerging mechanisms of tumor initiation and progression. Urol Oncol. 2010;28(4):429–40.
11. Lin HH, Ke HL, Huang SP, Wu WJ, Chen YK, Chang LL. Increase sensitivity in detecting superficial, low grade bladder cancer by combination analysis of hypermethylation of E-cadherin, p16, p14, RASSF1A genes in urine. Urol Oncol. 2010;28(6):597–602.
12. Wilhelm CS, Kelsey KT, Butler R, et al. Implications of LINE1 methylation for bladder cancer risk in women. Clin Cancer Res. 2010;16(5):1682–9.
13. Wolff EM, Byun HM, Han HF, et al. Hypomethylation of a LINE-1 promoter activates an alternate transcript of the MET oncogene in bladders with cancer. PLoS Genet. 2010;6(4):e1000917.
14. Fendler A, Stephan C, Yousef GM, Jung K. MicroRNAs as regulators of signal transduction in urological tumors. Clin Chem. 2011;57(7):954–68.
15. Hanke M, Hoefig K, Merz H, et al. A robust methodology to study urine microRNA as tumor marker: microRNA-126 and microRNA-182 are related to urinary bladder cancer. Urol Oncol. 2010;28(6):655–61.
16. Wu XR. Urothelial tumorigenesis: a tale of divergent pathways. Nat Rev Cancer. 2005;5(9):713–25.
17. Al-Ahmadie HA, Iyer G, Janakiraman M, et al. Somatic mutation of fibroblast growth factor receptor-3 (FGFR3) defines a distinct morphological subtype of high-grade urothelial carcinoma. J Pathol. 2011;224(2):270–9.
18. Tomlinson DC, Baldo O, Harnden P, Knowles MA. FGFR3 protein expression and its relationship to mutation status and prognostic variables in bladder cancer. J Pathol. 2007;213(1):91–8.

19. Hart KC, Robertson SC, Kanemitsu MY, Meyer AN, Tynan JA, Donoghue DJ. Transformation and stat activation by derivatives of FGFR1, FGFR3, and FGFR4. Oncogene. 2000;19(29):3309–20.

20. Kompier LC, Lurkin I, van der Aa MN, van Rhijn BW, van der Kwast TH, Zwarthoff EC. FGFR3, HRAS, KRAS, NRAS and PIK3CA mutations in bladder cancer and their potential as biomarkers for surveillance and therapy. PLoS One. 2010;5(11):e13821.

21. Park S, Chapuis N, Tamburini J, et al. Role of the PI3K/AKT and mTOR signaling pathways in acute myeloid leukemia. Haematologica. 2010;95(5):819–28.

22. Lopez-Knowles E, Hernandez S, Malats N, et al. PIK3CA mutations are an early genetic alteration associated with FGFR3 mutations in superficial papillary bladder tumors. Cancer Res. 2006;66(15):7401–4.

23. Sjödahl G, Lauss M, Gudjonsson S, et al. A systematic study of gene mutations in urothelial carcinoma; inactivating mutations in TSC2 and PIK3R1. PLoS One. 2011;6(4):e18583.

24. van Rhijn BW, van der Kwast TH, Vis AN, et al. FGFR3 and P53 characterize alternative genetic pathways in the pathogenesis of urothelial cell carcinoma. Cancer Res. 2004;64(6):1911–4.

25. Williams SG, Stein JP. Molecular pathways in bladder cancer. Urol Res. 2004;32(6):373–85.

26. Hernandez S, Lopez-Knowles E, Lloreta J, et al. FGFR3 and Tp53 mutations in T1G3 transitional bladder carcinomas: independent distribution and lack of association with prognosis. Clin Cancer Res. 2005;11(15):5444 50.

27. Grivas PD, Day M, Hussain M. Urothelial carcinomas: a focus on human epidermal receptors signaling. Am J Transl Res. 2011;3(4):362–73.

28. Mitra AP, Datar RH, Cote RJ. Molecular pathways in invasive bladder cancer: new insights into mechanisms, progression, and target identification. J Clin Oncol. 2006;24(35):5552–64.

29. Black PC, Dinney CP. Growth factors and receptors as prognostic markers in urothelial carcinoma. Curr Urol Rep. 2008;9(1):55–61.

30. Kassouf W, Black PC, Tuziak T, et al. Distinctive expression pattern of ErbB family receptors signifies an aggressive variant of bladder cancer. J Urol. 2008;179(1):353–8.

31. Ho PL, Kurtova A, Chan KS. Normal and neoplastic urothelial stem cells: getting to the root of the problem. Nat Rev Urol. 2012;9(10):583–94.

32. Chan KS, Espinosa I, Chao M, et al. Identification, molecular characterization, clinical prognosis, and therapeutic targeting of human bladder tumor-initiating cells. Proc Natl Acad Sci USA. 2009; 106(33):14016–21.

33. Ben-Porath I, Thomson MW, Carey VJ, et al. An embryonic stem cell-like gene expression signature in poorly differentiated aggressive human tumors. Nat Genet. 2008;40(5):499–507.

34. Steiner G, Schoenberg MP, Linn JF, Mao L, Sidransky D. Detection of bladder cancer recurrence by microsatellite analysis of urine. Nat Med. 1997;3(6):621–4.

35. Simon R, Eltze E, Schafer KL, et al. Cytogenetic analysis of multifocal bladder cancer supports a monoclonal origin and intraepithelial spread of tumor cells. Cancer Res. 2001;61(1):355–62.

36. Hafner C, Knuechel R, Stoehr R, Hartmann A. Clonality of multifocal urothelial carcinomas: 10 years of molecular genetic studies. Int J Cancer. 2002;101(1):1–6.

37. Cheng L, Zhang S, Davidson DD, et al. Molecular determinants of tumor recurrence in the urinary bladder. Future Oncol. 2009;5(6):843–57.

38. Wolff EM, Chihara Y, Pan F, et al. Unique DNA methylation patterns distinguish noninvasive and invasive urothelial cancers and establish an epigenetic field defect in premalignant tissue. Cancer Res. 2010;70(20):8169–78.

39. Singh A, Settleman J. EMT, cancer stem cells and drug resistance: an emerging axis of evil in the war on cancer. Oncogene. 2010;29(34):4741–51.

40. Hurst CD, Platt FM, Taylor CF, Knowles MA. Novel tumor subgroups of urothelial carcinoma of the bladder defined by integrated genomic analysis. Clin Cancer Res. 2012;18(21):5865–77.

41. Blaveri E, Simko JP, Korkola JE, et al. Bladder cancer outcome and subtype classification by gene expression. Clin Cancer Res. 2005;11(11):4044–55.

42. Shariat SF, Marberger MJ, Lotan Y, et al. Variability in the performance of nuclear matrix protein 22 for the detection of bladder cancer. J Urol. 2006;176(3): 919–26; discussion 926.

43. Van Le TS, Miller R, Barder T, Babjuk M, Potter DM, Getzenberg RH. Highly specific urine-based marker of bladder cancer. Urology. 2005;66(6):1256–60.

44. Guo B, Che T, Shi B, et al. Screening and identification of specific markers for bladder transitional cell carcinoma from urine urothelial cells with suppressive subtractive hybridization and cDNA microarray. Can Urol Assoc J. 2011;5(6): E129–37.

45. Konety BR, Getzenberg RH. Urine based markers of urological malignancy. J Urol. 2001;165(2):600–11.

46. Lokeshwar VB, Soloway MS. Current bladder tumor tests: does their projected utility fulfill clinical necessity? J Urol. 2001;165(4):1067–77.

47. Hautmann S, Toma M, Lorenzo Gomez MF, et al. Immunocyt and the HA-HAase urine tests for the detection of bladder cancer: a side-by-side comparison. Eur Urol. 2004;46(4):466–71.

48. Hausladen DA, Wheeler MA, Altieri DC, Colberg JW, Weiss RM. Effect of intravesical treatment of transitional cell carcinoma with bacillus Calmette-Guerin and mitomycin C on urinary survivin levels and outcome. J Urol. 2003;170(1):230–4.

49. Moussa O, Abol-Enein H, Bissada NK, Keane T, Ghoneim MA, Watson DK. Evaluation of survivin reverse transcriptase-polymerase chain reaction for noninvasive detection of bladder cancer. J Urol. 2006;175(6):2312–6.

50. van Oers JM, Zwarthoff EC, Rehman I, et al. FGFR3 mutations indicate better survival in invasive upper

urinary tract and bladder tumours. Eur Urol. 2009;55(3):650–7.

51. Zuiverloon TC, van der Aa MN, van der Kwast TH, et al. Fibroblast growth factor receptor 3 mutation analysis on voided urine for surveillance of patients with low-grade non-muscle-invasive bladder cancer. Clin Cancer Res. 2010;16(11):3011–8.

52. Vaish M, Mandhani A, Mittal RD, Mittal B. Microsatellite instability as prognostic marker in bladder tumors: a clinical significance. BMC Urol. 2005;5:2.

53. Takihana Y, Tsuchida T, Fukasawa M, Araki I, Tanabe N, Takeda M. Real-time quantitative analysis for human telomerase reverse transcriptase mRNA and human telomerase RNA component mRNA expressions as markers for clinicopathologic parameters in urinary bladder cancer. Int J Urol. 2006;13(4):401–8.

54. Lokeshwar VB, Habuchi T, Grossman HB, et al. Bladder tumor markers beyond cytology: international consensus panel on bladder tumor markers. Urology. 2005;66(6 Suppl 1):35–63.

55. Retz M, Lehmann J, Amann E, Wullich B, Roder C, Stockle M. Mucin 7 and cytokeratin 20 as new diagnostic urinary markers for bladder tumor. J Urol. 2003;169(1):86–9.

56. McKenney JK, Desai S, Cohen C, Amin MB. Discriminatory immunohistochemical staining of urothelial carcinoma in situ and non-neoplastic urothelium: an analysis of cytokeratin 20, p53, and CD44 antigens. Am J Surg Pathol. 2001;25(8):1074–8.

57. Moonen PM, Merkx GF, Peelen P, Karthaus HF, Smeets DF, Witjes JA. UroVysion compared with cytology and quantitative cytology in the surveillance of non-muscle-invasive bladder cancer. Eur Urol. 2007;51(5):1275–80; discussion 1280.

58. Zellweger T, Benz G, Cathomas G, et al. Multi-target fluorescence in situ hybridization in bladder washings for prediction of recurrent bladder cancer. Int J Cancer. 2006;119(7):1660–5.

59. Yoder BJ, Skacel M, Hedgepeth R, et al. Reflex UroVysion testing of bladder cancer surveillance patients with equivocal or negative urine cytology: a prospective study with focus on the natural history of anticipatory positive findings. Am J Clin Pathol. 2007;127(2):295–301.

60. Allard P, Fradet Y, Tetu B, Bernard P. Tumor-associated antigens as prognostic factors for recurrence in 382 patients with primary transitional cell carcinoma of the bladder. Clin Cancer Res. 1995;1(10):1195–202.

61. Mian C, Maier K, Comploj E, et al. uCyt+/ImmunoCyt in the detection of recurrent urothelial carcinoma: an update on 1991 analyses. Cancer. 2006;108(1):60–5.

62. Mian C, Lodde M, Comploj E, et al. The value of the ImmunoCyt/uCyt+ test in the detection and follow-up of carcinoma in situ of the urinary bladder. Anticancer Res. 2005;25(5):3641–4.

63. Piaton E, Daniel L, Verriele V, et al. Improved detection of urothelial carcinomas with fluorescence immunocytochemistry (uCyt+ assay) and urinary cytology:

results of a French prospective multicenter study. Lab Invest. 2003;83(6):845–52.

64. Cajulis RS, Haines GK III, Frias-Hidvegi D, McVary K, Bacus JW. Cytology, flow cytometry, image analysis, and interphase cytogenetics by fluorescence in situ hybridization in the diagnosis of transitional cell carcinoma in bladder washes: a comparative study. Diagn Cytopathol. 1995;13(3): 214–23; discussion 224.

65. Chan MW, Chan LW, Tang NL, et al. Hypermethylation of multiple genes in tumor tissues and voided urine in urinary bladder cancer patients. Clin Cancer Res. 2002;8(2):464–70.

66. Reinert T. Methylation markers for urine-based detection of bladder cancer: the next generation of urinary markers for diagnosis and surveillance of bladder cancer. Adv Urol. 2012;2012:503271.

67. Friedrich MG, Weisenberger DJ, Cheng JC, et al. Detection of methylated apoptosis-associated genes in urine sediments of bladder cancer patients. Clin Cancer Res. 2004;10(22):7457–65.

68. Reinert T, Modin C, Castano FM, et al. Comprehensive genome methylation analysis in bladder cancer: identification and validation of novel methylated genes and application of these as urinary tumor markers. Clin Cancer Res. 2011;17(17):5582–92.

69. Zuiverloon TC, Beukers W, van der Keur KA, et al. A methylation assay for the detection of non-muscle-invasive bladder cancer (NMIBC) recurrences in voided urine. BJU Int. 2012;109(6):941–8.

70. Schaefer A, Stephan C, Busch J, Yousef GM, Jung K. Diagnostic, prognostic and therapeutic implications of microRNAs in urologic tumors. Nat Rev Urol. 2010;7(5):286–97.

71. Guzzo TJ, McNeil BK, Bivalacqua TJ, Elliott DJ, Sokoll LJ, Schoenberg MP. The presence of circulating tumor cells does not predict extravesical disease in bladder cancer patients prior to radical cystectomy. Urol Oncol. 2012;30(1):44–8.

72. Cheng L, Zhang S, MacLennan GT, Williamson SR, Lopez-Beltran A, Montironi R. Bladder cancer: translating molecular genetic insights into clinical practice. Hum Pathol. 2011;42(4):455–81.

73. Copp HL, Chin JL, Conaway M, Theodorescu D. Prospective evaluation of the prognostic relevance of molecular staging for urothelial carcinoma. Cancer. 2006;107(1):60–6.

74. Marin-Aguilera M, Mengual L, Burset M, et al. Molecular lymph node staging in bladder urothelial carcinoma: impact on survival. Eur Urol. 2008; 54(6):1363–72.

75. Plastiras D, Moutzouris G, Barbatis C, Presvelos V, Petrakos M, Theodorou C. Can p53 nuclear overexpression, bcl-2 accumulation and PCNA status be of prognostic significance in high-risk superficial and invasive bladder tumours? Eur J Surg Oncol. 1999;25(1):61–5.

76. Stein JP, Ginsberg DA, Grossfeld GD, et al. Effect of p21WAF1/CIP1 expression on tumor progression in bladder cancer. J Natl Cancer Inst. 1998;90(14):1072–9.

77. Youssef RF, Lotan Y. Predictors of outcome of non-muscle-invasive and muscle-invasive bladder cancer. ScientificWorldJournal. 2011;11:369–81.

78. van Rhijn BW, Vis AN, van der Kwast TH, et al. Molecular grading of urothelial cell carcinoma with fibroblast growth factor receptor 3 and MIB-1 is superior to pathologic grade for the prediction of clinical outcome. J Clin Oncol. 2003;21(10):1912–21.

79. Shariat SF, Karakiewicz PI, Ashfaq R, et al. Multiple biomarkers improve prediction of bladder cancer recurrence and mortality in patients undergoing cystectomy. Cancer. 2008;112(2):315–25.

80. Karam JA, Lotan Y, Karakiewicz PI, et al. Use of combined apoptosis biomarkers for prediction of bladder cancer recurrence and mortality after radical cystectomy. Lancet Oncol. 2007;8(2):128–36.

81. Chen JX, Deng N, Chen X, et al. A novel molecular grading model: combination of Ki67 and VEGF in predicting tumor recurrence and progression in non-invasive urothelial bladder cancer. Asian Pac J Cancer Prev. 2012;13(5):2229–34.

82. Grossfeld GD, Ginsberg DA, Stein JP, et al. Thrombospondin-1 expression in bladder cancer: association with p53 alterations, tumor angiogenesis, and tumor progression. J Natl Cancer Inst. 1997;89(3):219–27.

83. Guancial EA, Chowdhury D, Rosenberg JE. Personalized therapy for urothelial cancer: review of the clinical evidence. Clin Investig (Lond). 2011;1(4):546–55.

84. Petrylak DP, Tangen CM, Van Veldhuizen Jr PJ, et al. Results of the southwest oncology group phase II evaluation (study S0031) of ZD1839 for advanced transitional cell carcinoma of the urothelium. BJU Int. 2010;105(3):317–21.

85. Rochester MA, Patel N, Turney BW, et al. The type 1 insulin-like growth factor receptor is over-expressed in bladder cancer. BJU Int. 2007;100(6):1396–401.

86. Honma I, Kitamura H, Torigoe T, et al. Phase I clinical study of anti-apoptosis protein survivin-derived peptide vaccination for patients with advanced or recurrent urothelial cancer. Cancer Immunol Immunother. 2009;58(11):1801–7.

Molecular Testing in Thyroid Cancer

Matthew T. Olson, Jason D. Prescott, and Martha A. Zeiger

Introduction

Several differentiated tumor subtypes can arise from the thyroid gland, including papillary thyroid carcinoma (PTC), follicular thyroid carcinoma (FTC), and medullary thyroid carcinoma (MTC). Each of these tumors demonstrates both unique clinical and pathological features and genetic mutations, as shown in Table 19.1. Well-studied molecular models of tumor progression from normal thyroid follicular cells to well-differentiated thyroid malignancies include the mitogen-activated protein kinase (MAPK) [1] and the phosphatidylinositol-3 kinase (PI3K) signaling pathways [2]. The MAPK pathway includes well-known oncogenes and tumor suppressor genes, including the rearranged during transfection (RET) tyrosine kinase [3]; Rat Sarcoma (RAS) isotypes H, N, and K [4]; and serine/threonine-protein kinase B-Raf (BRAF) [5], all of which have been linked to the development of PTC. The PI3K pathway also includes RET, RAS, in addition to p110a (PI3KCA) [6], inhibitory phosphatase and tensin homolog (PTEN) [7], and protein kinase B (AKT) [8]; the latter pathway is

thought to be a significant driver in FTC. MTC is primarily a RET oncogene-driven disease and is often a hereditary disease. Besides MAPK and PI3K, other signaling transduction pathways are also under investigation (primarily the mammalian target of rapamycin (mTOR) pathway) [9] for their potential involvement in the development of poorly differentiated and anaplastic thyroid carcinomas (ATC). Depending on the type of cancer within the thyroid gland, molecular diagnostics can have several roles in the diagnosis and management. Given the broad range of molecular aberrations, different technologies have recently been proposed in the workup of thyroid cancer. As such, each role of molecular diagnostics is described separately from diagnosis through prognosis and management. The newest application of molecular markers—preoperative diagnosis of thyroid nodules—is described last because it builds on knowledge developed in the specific tumor subtypes.

Papillary Thyroid Carcinoma

Diagnostics

Approximately 45 % of PTC tumors harbor the *BRAF* point mutation V600E (c.1799T>A), approximately 20 % harbor clonal RET/PTC translocations, and approximately 10 % harbor *RAS* mutations [10, 11]. *BRAF* is the strongest known activator of the MAPK signaling pathway [12]. The associated high frequency and the specificity of the V600E mutation in PTC are thought

M.T. Olson, M.D.
Departments of Pathology, Johns Hopkins University School of Medicine, Baltimore, MD, USA

J.D. Prescott, M.D., Ph.D. (✉) • M.A. Zeiger, M.D.
Department of Surgery, John Hopkins University School of Medicine, 600 North Wolfe Street, Baltimore, MD 21287, USA
e-mail: jpresco5@jhmi.edu

G.M. Yousef and S. Jothy (eds.), *Molecular Testing in Cancer*,
DOI 10.1007/978-1-4899-8050-2_19, © Springer Science+Business Media New York 2014

Table 19.1 Most common mutations for the most common histological types of thyroid cancer

Histological type	Most common mutations
Papillary thyroid carcinoma	*BRAF*
	RAS (isotypes H, N, and K)
	RET/PTC translocation
Follicular thyroid carcinoma	*RAS* (isotypes H, N, and K)
	PAX8/PPARγ translocation
	PIK3CA
Medullary thyroid carcinoma	*RET*
Anaplastic thyroid carcinoma	*RAS* (isotypes H, N, and K)
	BRAF
	PIK3CA
	p53
	β-catenin

to be useful in the diagnosis of this malignancy. Additionally, there is some evidence that the incidence of *BRAF* mutations in PTC is increasing [13] and that such mutations could be related to environmental exposures, including iodide excess [14, 15] and volcanic ash [16]. In contrast, *RET/PTC* translocations are known to be associated with ionizing radiation [17, 18] and are thus relatively uncommon in PTC cases unassociated with radiation exposure. These translocations involve fusion of the *RET* oncogene with an active promoter, which leads to the overproduction of a functionally intact *RET* tyrosine kinase [19]. The two most common *RET/PTC* translocations—*RET/PTC1* and *RET/PTC3*—are paracentric intrachromosomal inversions in the long arm of chromosome 10 [20]. Numerous other *RET/PTC* translocations have also been described [21–25], all of which result from translocation of an activating promoter from a chromosome other than chromosome 10.

BRAF

BRAF mutational analysis is rapidly becoming routine in thyroid surgical pathology specimens. While Sanger sequencing [26] is the traditional gold-standard method for mutational analysis, this method has largely been replaced by pyrosequencing [27], since the latter is faster, more sensitive, and more quantitative [28]. Pyrosequencing involves a "sequencing by synthesis" approach that follows a preset program of

deoxynucleotide triphosphate injections (called a dispensation sequence) into a reaction vessel containing the template DNA and DNA polymerase; when a synthesis occurs, the DNA is extended by one nucleotide, and the liberated pyrophosphate is converted to light through sulfurylase, luciferin, and luciferase [29]. When used with a well-designed dispensation sequence coupled with data interpretation software, pyrosequencing can identify most mutants without the need for any additional testing [30].

As the demand for *BRAF* testing grows, direct and indirect cost considerations become important. Direct costs such as polymerase chain reaction (PCR) amplification and assay-specific reagents will likely decrease as more protocols become available and are streamlined. However, the pre-analytical, indirect costs, such as specialized PCR-compatible microtomy and PCR-clean workspaces, involve substantial labor and infrastructure expenditures that will likely not decrease over time. Thus, low-cost alternatives to sequencing are highly desirable. In a recent small trial, a monoclonal antibody specific for the mutant *BRAF* V600E protein performed better than Sanger sequencing [31] for mutation identification. While cost-effective, the monoclonal antibody specificity is limited to the V600E epitope and so can miss some clinically relevant but less common *BRAF* mutations [32]. Additionally, the associated immunohistochemical interpretation is a visual and possibly subjective process for which standardization and guidelines do not exist. Regardless of these drawbacks, the monoclonal antibody carries a theoretical advantage in that the genetic mutation can be seen directly in the tumor cells and absent in cells that do not harbor the mutation.

RET/PTC Translocation

RET/PTC translocations can be detected with karyotyping, southern blotting, interphase fluorescence in situ hybridization, reverse transcription PCR (RT-PCR), in situ hybridization, or immunohistochemistry. An excellent review compares and contrasts these techniques in greater detail [25]. Data about the incidence of *RET/PTC* translocations is confounded by the availability and use of numerous analytical methods and the fact that sensitive techniques such as RT-PCR detect these translocations in a small percentage of non-clonal tumors. *RET/PTC* translocations have also been detected in benign thyroid tissue, which limits the diagnostic usefulness of this marker [33]. Accurate detection of the *RET/PTC* translocations is also confounded by the possibility of numerous distinct breakpoints, many of which may not be detected by standard assays: currently, the presence of *RET/PTC* translocations is most commonly assayed using RT-PCR, with primers that flank only the most well-characterized fusion points in the *RET* oncogene [34].

Prognosis and Management

Among the various mutations associated with PTC, only *BRAF* mutational status has been associated with tumor behavior. Aggressive tumor characteristics, including local tumor invasion, advanced disease stage at diagnosis, and the presence of distant metastases, have been correlated with the *BRAF* V600E mutation [35, 36]. Similarly, *BRAF* V600E mutation frequency has been linked to aggressive histological PTC subtype: in one study, 83 % of tumors demonstrating tall cell histology, an aggressive PTC variant, harbored the *BRAF* V600E mutation, while this mutation was found to be much less frequent in the more indolent follicular variant [37]. Postoperative radioiodine therapy, which has been shown to increase survival in advanced stage PTC, appears to be less efficacious in the context of *BRAF* mutation. This is presumably the result of decreased tumor cell iodine avidity and may be mediated by *BRAF*-directed repression of the sodium-iodine symporter gene [38, 39]. In keeping with these findings, *BRAF* mutation has been associated with disease-specific mortality: a recent multi-institutional study found that 80 % of PTC-related mortalities in their series were associated with the *BRAF* V600E mutation [40].

Despite these findings, controversy remains regarding the relationship between *BRAF* mutational status and aggressive PTC behavior. A recent multivariant analysis did not reveal a relationship between *BRAF* V600E mutational status and the presence of central neck lymph node metastases [46]. Moreover, interpretation of studies in which the *BRAF* V600E mutation has been linked to aggressive PTC clinicopathologic

features is limited in most cases by retrospective design, by inconsistent and unstandardized central neck dissection use, and by failure to subcategorize according to histological subtype [47]. Further, positive correlations between *BRAF* mutation and PTC behavior are almost always based on univariate analysis and should thus be interpreted with caution.

Surgical resection that remains the standard treatment for PTC and total thyroidectomy, with or without postoperative radioiodine therapy, is indicated in all cases (regardless of mutational status). Compartment-oriented lymph node dissection at the time of thyroidectomy should be performed whenever cervical lymph node metastasis is discovered preoperatively, usually by neck ultrasound or physical exam [41]. Prophylactic lymph node dissection of the central neck (level 6), the most probable initial site of PTC metastasis at the time of thyroidectomy, has been advocated as a means of decreasing PTC recurrence and improving disease-specific survival [42]. Some experts hypothesize that *BRAF* V600E mutation may be associated with an increased risk of central neck nodal metastasis [36, 43]. However, other studies refute this association [44, 45]. Similarly, studies examining the need for postoperative radioiodine therapy on the basis of *BRAF* mutational status have yet to be reported. Taken together, the preponderance of data does not yet support specific alterations in the surgical or postsurgical management of PTC based on genetic abnormalities, and additional studies defining this relationship are needed.

Follicular Thyroid Carcinoma

Diagnostics
PAX8/PPARγ
Approximately 50 % of FTC cases harbor a *RAS* mutation and 30 %, a translocation of the paired homeobox protein 8 gene and peroxisome proliferator-activated receptor subtype-γ *PAX8/PPARγ*, t(2;3)(q13;p25) [11, 46]. *RAS* mutations are part of the paradigm of MAPK and PI3K signaling pathways and function as drivers of thyroid cancer while the oncogenic significance of *PAX8/PPARγ* is less clear. There is some evidence

that the PPARγ moiety is more oncogenic than is the PAX8 component. This hypothesis is based on the finding of another translocation [CREB3L2/PPARγ t(3;7)(p25;q34)] [47] in FTC that involves the same breakpoint in the *PPARγ* gene, the fact that several PAX8 breakpoints have been described in the *PAX8/PPARγ* translocation and the breakpoint within the PPARγ gene is uniformly conserved [46]. If PPARγ is responsible for mediating oncogenesis, it is unclear whether malignancy results from PPARγ over- or underactivity [48] and thus how therapeutics might be designed for PPARγ-associated FTC [49]. Regardless, this translocation appears to correlate well with FTC morphology and is also seen in the follicular variant of PTC [50], a subtype that demonstrates both FTC and PTC histopathological features and behaves clinically like FTC. There is little evidence showing a therapeutic or prognostic usefulness in detecting either mutations or translocations in FTC, including the *PAX8/PPARγ* rearrangement. In addition, *PAX8/PPARγ* translocations are known to occur in some follicular adenomas [51], benign neoplasms that overlap cytomorphologically with FTC.

Prognosis and Management

While the presence of the PAX8/PPARγ translocation in a follicular adenoma may provide some clues about an associated progression to carcinoma, the clinical relevance of this translocation remains unclear. Even if PAX8/PPARγ has a role in the evolution of follicular adenomas to FTC, the latency and probability of such a progression has yet to be investigated. For these reasons, consideration of mutational status has not yet been shown to be useful in directing the clinical management of patients with FTC, and total thyroidectomy, with or without radioiodine therapy, is indicated in all cases.

Medullary Thyroid Carcinoma

Diagnostics
RET
In contrast to the diverse mutation profiles associated with PTC and FTC, MTC appears to be purely a *RET* oncogene-associated tumor.

MTC has a special place in the history of cancer genetics, as assays identifying germline *RET* oncogene mutations were some of the first clinically applicable genetic tests to be developed for the diagnosis of multiple endocrine neoplasia type 2 (MEN2) and, more recently, familial MTC [52, 53]. Assessment of *RET* gene mutations can be used to estimate the risk of MTC development among relatives of patients diagnosed with MTC and thus may guide serum calcitonin surveillance (serum calcitonin levels are frequently elevated in MTC patients) and/or the need for prophylactic thyroidectomy [54, 55]. Although *RET* oncogene mutations are also found in approximately one half of sporadic MTC tumors, verifying the absence of a *RET* mutation in a patient with sporadic MTC obviates the need for family screening. Finally, in the postoperative setting, *RET* mutations are becoming increasingly useful in directing additional clinical management; several different tyrosine kinase inhibitors show promise in the treatment of disseminated disease [56]. The *RET* oncogene has numerous gain-of-function germline mutations, including mutations in exons 10, 11, 13, 14, 15, and 16, and all of these are associated with MTC [52, 57, 58]. Thus, assays detecting *RET* mutations must be sufficiently multiplexed in order to capture all mutations. The majority of *RET* polymorphism assays are designed to identify germline mutations where analytical sensitivity is less of a concern than for tissue and fine needle aspiration (FNA) analysis. Sanger sequencing [59], pyrosequencing [60], and denaturing high-performance liquid chromatography [61] methods have all been described and each is used routinely.

Prognosis and Management

As is the case for PTC and FTC, surgical resection is the treatment standard for MTC. All sporadic MTC cases should be managed with total thyroidectomy and prophylactic central neck (Level VI) dissection, with more extensive lateral neck dissection reserved for cases in which nodal metastases are detected laterally [62]. Cases in which hereditary transmission of *RET* mutations is suspected require identification of the specific mutations involved. Because the penetrance of hereditary MTC can approach 100 %, the goal of surgery in these cases is to prevent disease development through prophylactic thyroidectomy. Further, because correlations between specific hereditary *RET* gene mutations and disease course have been well defined, the surgeon can optimize timing of prophylactic surgery to minimize the probability of disease development and spread. Aggressive mutations, such as those involving codons 883, 918, and 922, for example, merit prophylactic thyroidectomy with central neck dissection within the first month of life, while surgery may be deferred up to the age of 5 years when the causative mutation is limited to codons 611, 618, 620, 634, or 891 [63, 64].

Poorly Differentiated and Anaplastic Thyroid Carcinoma

Diagnostics

The molecular genetics of poorly differentiated thyroid cancer and ATC are not well understood. This is due to the relative rarity of these diseases and to difficulty standardizing inclusion criteria for studying these tumors (in light of their significant morphological heterogeneity) [65]. Thus, much of the research to date has focused on models of progression whereby well-differentiated thyroid cancers may evolve into ATC and current evidence suggests that progression to ATC from well-differentiated disease occurs more frequently than does de novo development of anaplastic tumors.

Prognosis and Management

Evidence regarding the prognostic significance of molecular changes in these very aggressive tumors is lacking, so routine genetic analysis is not the standard of care and does not guide clinical management. One study has shown that *RAS* mutations portend a poor prognosis in ATC, although only 53 patients were evaluated [66]. Other mutations overlapping between ATC and well-differentiated tumors include *BRAF* [67] and *PIK3CA* [68], although the prognostic and therapeutic significance of these mutations in ATC remains unknown. Additional mutations classically associated with poorly differentiated and anaplastic thyroid carcinoma are *p53* and

β-catenin [69], and β-catenin mutations have also been described in the rare cribriform-morular variant of PTC [70, 71].

Molecular Tests for Preoperative Testing for Cytologically Indeterminate or Suspicious Thyroid Nodules

Diagnostics

The previous sections have focused on molecular alterations associated with the different tumor subtypes, with emphasis on underlying pathophysiology and potential treatment schemes. There is yet another burgeoning application for molecular diagnostics in thyroid cancer: preoperative assessment of malignancy risk for cytologically indeterminate or suspicious thyroid nodules. Thyroid FNA is widely accepted as the standard of care for the evaluation of thyroid nodules, since it is rapid, safe, cost-effective, and accurate when definitive [41, 72–74]. When the cytomorphological diagnosis is benign, thyroid FNA has a negative predictive value that exceeds 95 %, and when the cytomorphological diagnosis is malignant, thyroid FNA positive predictive value exceeds 99 % [73, 75–78]. Nonetheless, approximately 20 % of all thyroid aspirates yield an indeterminate or suspicious only result, with associated malignancy rates that range from 5 to 85 % [73, 75, 76]. While there is clearly a place for morphological risk stratification in the indeterminate or suspicious categories, as outlined by the Bethesda System for Reporting Thyroid Cytopathology [73], disagreement and uncertainty often persist, even after expert review [79]. Indeterminate diagnoses result from three failures inherent to cytopathology: first, cytopathologic material represents a very limited sampling of a heterogeneous lesion; second, the limited sampling present in FNA material is not uniformly distributed, so interobserver bias can be expected, and this nonuniform distribution has the potential to limit more objective ancillary testing, such as molecular markers; and finally, the diagnosis of follicular and Hürthle cell malignancy requires histological evidence of vascular or capsular invasion, which cannot be assessed in cytological material.

Somatic Mutation Panel

Somatic mutation panel (SMP) testing has recently been introduced as an adjunct to thyroid cytological diagnosis [34, 80]. The most commonly used SMP currently includes *BRAF*, *HRAS*, *NRAS*, and *KRAS* point mutation testing as well as testing for *RET/PTC* and *PAX8/PPARγ* translocations [34]. In a single institutional trial, the SMP was shown to have a positive predictive value ranging from 87 to 95 % and a negative predictive value ranging from 72 to 94 %, depending on the associated indeterminate or suspicious FNA category [81]. In this study, the best positive predictive value (95 %) and the worst negative predictive value (72 %) were seen in the suspicious for malignancy (SFM) category. This is not surprising, given that the SFM category is overwhelmingly comprised of cases that are suspicious for well-differentiated PTC, a tumor that is commonly *BRAF* positive [67, 81–83]. As others have shown, *BRAF* mutations correlate well with morphological findings (nuclear grooves, inclusions, and elongation) that are already classically associated with a high malignancy risk [73, 84]. Consequently, the true added value of SMP testing in the categories that are suspicious for PTC remains unclear because morphology alone may have similar predictive values in these diagnostic categories [73, 84, 85]. The worst positive predictive value for SMP (87 %) was seen in the SFN category, a finding that underlies the difficulties in clearly showing distinct genetic drivers in follicular malignancy, as well as the molecular and morphological continuum between benign, follicular adenomas, follicular variant of PTC, and follicular carcinomas [86, 87]. Consequently, the true value of SMP testing in follicular neoplasms remains unclear because the predictive values are low. Performance of the SMP in the atypia of undetermined significance (AUS) category is not well characterized. In a single institutional trial, the SMP demonstrated only slightly worse performance for AUS than in the SFM category. However, this study included a high rate of *BRAF* mutation, the number of AUS nodules was small,

and the subcategories of AUS were not described. As such, it is also not clear if the management for AUS would be altered based on SMP testing alone.

Gene Expression Classifier

In addition to SMP testing, a gene expression classifier (GEC) has been developed [88, 89], validated [90], and tested in a multicenter clinical trial [91]. The GEC differs from the SMP in several ways. First, the GEC is based on patterns of quantitative mRNA expression. Second, data about specific transcript expression is incorporated into a proprietary model that yields a binomial answer ("benign" or "suspicious"); no data about individual transcripts are available. Third, while SMP is based on readily available assays that any laboratory can develop or send out to any reference laboratory at the request of the patient's pathologist and/or clinician, the GEC is proprietary, is only performed at one laboratory, and can only be performed at the discretion of a single group of cytopathologists after centralized morphological review. Finally, in contrast to SMP, which has a high positive predictive value, the GEC has a high negative predictive value and is thus most useful when negative in allowing patients with solitary asymptomatic cytomorphologically indeterminate nodules to avoid surgery safely. In a multicenter clinical trial [91], GEC was shown to have an overall negative predictive value of 95 % for AUS and 94 % for SFN. While a 5 % risk of malignancy may seem high given that TBSRTC envisions AUS as a diagnosis that confers a 5–15 % risk of malignancy, the true risk of malignancy in nodules diagnosed as AUS is higher—in the randomized multicenter trial, it was 32 %. Thus, the high negative predictive value could represent a significant stratification of some patients into low risk. The high negative predictive value of GEC is attributable to high sensitivity and low specificity; it is only 52 % specific for malignancy overall. The nonspecificity of the GEC is critical in any clinical practice setting because it means that approximately one third of cytomorphologically benign nodules will be positive by the GEC [91]. Thus, the GEC should not be performed in cytomorphologically benign nodules. Even in the setting of the cytomorphologically indeterminate categories, AUS and SFN, the usefulness of a positive result remains questionable. Furthermore, the nonspecificity of GEC renders it unnecessary in the context of the SFM category, which is known to have a substantially higher positive predictive value, on the basis of cytology alone, than does the GEC [92].

Limitations of Molecular Testing

A summary of the SMP and GEC tests is shown in Table 19.2. Beyond individual performance characteristics for each test, genetic testing of thyroid FNA material currently has several critical technological limitations that need to be considered before any test is performed and interpreted. The most significant limitation for both GEC and SMP is how specimen adequacy is determined. This limitation manifests differently in each assay. In the SMP, the main concern is allele dropout [93], a false-negative result due to preferential amplification of the wild-type allele. Given its multiplex design, SMP has the potential for allele dropout, as FNA specimens are scant, and multiplexing requires separation of the few cells harvested into multiple wells. The potential for allele dropout is the rationale for specimen adequacy control done in the pretesting phase, a real-time PCR assay that shows the difference in amplification between *KRT7* and *GADPH* [81]. In contrast to the SMP, the GEC lacks a stringent adequacy control (it uses only total mRNA content assessed by the RNA integrity number [94]); this is a possible explanation for why false-negative specimens obtained from GEC appear to correlate with scant specimens [91]. Beyond adequacy, vis-à-vis the number of follicular cells or total mRNA content, there is no direct way to correlate molecular results with associated cytological morphology, since the material used for molecular analysis cannot be used to assess morphology and vice versa. This limitation is most marked for the GEC, since it is primarily used as

Table 19.2 Summary of advantages and disadvantages of molecular tests for cytologically indeterminate thyroid nodules

	SMP	GEC
Analyte	DNA	mRNA
Type of result	List of mutations	Binomial ("benign" or "suspicious")
Compatible with existing pathology workflow	Yes, any pathologist or clinician can submit	No, centralized pathology only
Laboratory performing assay	Numerous	Single laboratory
Theoretical basis	Published mutations	Proprietary algorithm
Direct correlation of morphology with molecular results	No	No
Quality control	Thyroid origin of cells verified by difference in amplification between *KRT7* and *GADPH*	Quantity of mRNA, no verification of thyroid origin
Most useful result	Positive predictive value	Negative predictive value

a negative predictor, and one cannot yet determine if morphologically atypical or benign follicular cells were sampled. Although recent developments may enable concurrent SMP testing and cytological review of the same cells [95], this is unlikely with GEC since it requires immediate fixation in RNA preservative.

Prognosis and Management

Both GEC and SMP add significant incremental cost. While these costs have been justified for both GEC and SMP in cost-effectiveness models [96, 97], their true value in clinical practice remains to be shown. As discussed above, both tests require awareness of the technological shortcomings and performance characteristics of the test as well as the sophistication to correlate the results with the cytomorphology and the constellation of clinical findings. The incorporation of the results from these tests into a clinical or surgical algorithm is further encumbered by the paucity of good evidence and guidelines on how this should be done [98, 99]. In summary, molecular tests for cytomorphologically indeterminate thyroid are promising, but their true impact on clinical management remains to be determined.

References

1. Pearson G. Mitogen-activated protein (MAP) kinase pathways: regulation and physiological functions. Endocr Rev. 2001;22(2):153–83.
2. Whitman M, Kaplan DR, Schaffhausen B, Cantley L, Roberts TM. Association of phosphatidylinositol kinase activity with polyoma middle-T competent for transformation. Nature. 1985;315(6016):239–42.
3. Takahashi M, Ritz J, Cooper GM. Activation of a novel human transforming gene, ret, by DNA rearrangement. Cell. 1985;42(2):581–8.
4. Chang EH, Gonda MA, Ellis RW, Scolnick EM, Lowy DR. Human genome contains four genes homologous to transforming genes of Harvey and Kirsten murine sarcoma viruses. Proc Natl Acad Sci U S A. 1982;79(16):4848–52.
5. Sithanandam G, Kolch W, Duh FM, Rapp UR. Complete coding sequence of a human B-raf cDNA and detection of B-raf protein kinase with isozyme specific antibodies. Oncogene. 1990;5(12):1775–80.
6. Hiles ID, Otsu M, Volinia S, Fry MJ, Gout I, Dhand R, et al. Phosphatidylinositol 3-kinase: structure and expression of the 110 kd catalytic subunit. Cell. 1992; 70(3):419–29.
7. Steck PA, Pershouse MA, Jasser SA, Yung WKA, Lin H, Ligon AH, et al. Identification of a candidate tumour suppressor gene, MMAC1, at chromosome 10q23.3 that is mutated in multiple advanced cancers. Nat Genet. 1997;15(4):356–62.
8. Staal SP. Molecular cloning of the akt oncogene and its human homologues AKT1 and AKT2: amplification of AKT1 in a primary human gastric adenocarcinoma. Proc Natl Acad Sci U S A. 1987;84(14):5034–7.
9. Brown EJ, Albers MW, Bum Shin T, Ichikawa K, Keith CT, Lane WS, et al. A mammalian protein targeted by G1-arresting rapamycin–receptor complex. Nature. 1994;369(6483):756–8.
10. Adeniran AJ, Zhu Z, Gandhi M, Steward DL, Fidler JP, Giordano TJ, et al. Correlation between genetic alterations and microscopic features, clinical manifestations, and prognostic characteristics of thyroid papillary carcinomas. Am J Surg Pathol. 2006;30(2): 216–22.
11. Nikiforov YE, Nikiforova MN. Molecular genetics and diagnosis of thyroid cancer. Nat Rev Endocrinol. 2011;7(10):569–80.
12. Sithanandam G, Druck T, Cannizzaro LA, Leuzzi G, Huebner K, Rapp UR. B-raf and a B-raf pseudogene are located on 7q in man. Oncogene. 1992;7(4): 795–9.
13. Mathur A, Moses W, Rahbari R, Khanafshar E, Duh Q-Y, Clark O, et al. Higher rate of BRAF mutation in papillary thyroid cancer over time: a single-institution study. Cancer. 2011;117(19):4390–5.
14. Guan H, Ji M, Bao R, Yu H, Wang Y, Hou P, et al. Association of high iodine intake with the T1799A BRAF mutation in papillary thyroid cancer. J Clin Endocrinol Metab. 2009;94(5):1612–7.
15. Lind P, Langsteger W, Molnar M, Gallowitsch HJ, Mikosch P, Gomez I. Epidemiology of thyroid diseases in iodine sufficiency. Thyroid. 1998;8(12): 1179–83.
16. Pellegriti G, De Vathaire F, Scollo C, Attard M, Giordano C, Arena S, et al. Papillary thyroid cancer incidence in the volcanic area of Sicily. J Natl Cancer Inst. 2009;101(22):1575–83.
17. Thomas GA, Bunnell H, Cook HA, Williams ED, Nerovnya A, Cherstvoy ED, et al. High prevalence of RET/PTC rearrangements in Ukrainian and Belarussian post-Chernobyl thyroid papillary carcinomas: a strong correlation between RET/PTC3 and the solid-follicular variant. J Clin Endocrinol Metab. 1999;84(11):4232–8.
18. Rabes HM, Demidchik EP, Sidorow JD, Lengfelder E, Beimfohr C, Hoelzel D, et al. Pattern of radiation-induced RET and NTRK1 rearrangements in 191 post-chernobyl papillary thyroid carcinomas: biological, phenotypic, and clinical implications. Clin Cancer Res. 2000;6(3):1093–103.
19. Santoro M, Carlomagno F, Hay ID, Herrmann MA, Grieco M, Melillo R, et al. Ret oncogene activation in human thyroid neoplasms is restricted to the papillary cancer subtype. J Clin Invest. 1992;89(5):1517–22.
20. Minoletti F, Butti MG, Coronelli S, Miozzo M, Sozzi G, Pilotti S, et al. The two genes generating RET/PTC3 are localized in chromosomal band 10q11.2. Genes Chromosomes Cancer. 1994;11(1):51–7.
21. Bongarzone I, Monzini N, Borrello MG, Carcano C, Ferraresi G, Arighi E, et al. Molecular characterization of a thyroid tumor-specific transforming sequence formed by the fusion of ret tyrosine kinase and the regulatory subunit RI alpha of cyclic AMP-dependent protein kinase A. Mol Cell Biol. 1993;13(1):358–66.
22. Klugbauer S, Demidchik EP, Lengfelder E, Rabes HM. Detection of a novel type of RET rearrangement (PTC5) in thyroid carcinomas after Chernobyl and analysis of the involved RET-fused gene RFG5. Cancer Res. 1998;58(2):198–203.
23. Klugbauer S, Rabes HM. The transcription coactivator HTIF1 and a related protein are fused to the RET receptor tyrosine kinase in childhood papillary thyroid carcinomas. Oncogene. 1999;18(30):4388–93.
24. Klugbauer S, Jauch A, Lengfelder E, Demidchik E, Rabes HM. A novel type of RET rearrangement (PTC8) in childhood papillary thyroid carcinomas

and characterization of the involved gene (RFG8). Cancer Res. 2000;60(24):7028–32.

25. Nikiforov YE. RET/PTC rearrangement in thyroid tumors. Endocr Pathol. 2002;13(1):3–16.

26. Sanger F, Nicklen S, Coulson AR. DNA sequencing with chain-terminating inhibitors. Proc Natl Acad Sci U S A. 1977;74(12):5463–7.

27. Tan YH, Liu Y, Eu KW, Ang PW, Li WQ, Salto-Tellez M, et al. Detection of BRAF V600E mutation by pyrosequencing. Pathology. 2008;40(3):295–8.

28. Tsiatis AC, Norris-Kirby A, Rich RG, Hafez MJ, Gocke CD, Eshleman JR, et al. Comparison of sanger sequencing, pyrosequencing, and melting curve analysis for the detection of KRAS mutations. J Mol Diagn. 2010;12(4):425–32.

29. Harrington CT, Lin EI, Olson MT, Eshleman JR. Fundamentals of pyrosequencing. Arch Pathol Lab Med. 2013;137(9):1296–303.

30. Chen G, Olson MT, O'Neill A, Norris A, Beierl K, Harada S, et al. A virtual pyrogram generator to resolve complex pyrosequencing results. J Mol Diagn. 2012;14(2):149–59.

31. Bullock M, O'Neill C, Chou A, Clarkson A, Dodds T, Toon C, et al. Utilization of a MAB for BRAF(V600E) detection in papillary thyroid carcinoma. Endocr Relat Cancer. 2012;19(6):779–84.

32. Amanuel B, Grieu F, Kular J, Millward M, Iacopetta B. Incidence of BRAF p.Val600Glu and p.Val600Lys mutations in a consecutive series of 183 metastatic melanoma patients from a high incidence region. Pathology. 2012;44(4):357–9.

33. Ishizaka Y, Kobayashi S, Ushijima T, Hirohashi S, Sugimura T, Nagao M. Detection of retTPC/PTC transcripts in thyroid adenomas and adenomatous goiter by an RT-PCR method. Oncogene. 1991;6(9):1667–72.

34. Nikiforov YE, Steward DL, Robinson-Smith TM, Haugen BR, Klopper JP, Zhu Z, et al. Molecular testing for mutations in improving the fine-needle aspiration diagnosis of thyroid nodules. J Clin Endocrinol Metab. 2009;94(6):2092–8.

35. Kim K-M, Park J-B, Bae K-S, Kang S-J. Analysis of prognostic factors in patients with multiple recurrences of papillary thyroid carcinoma. Surg Oncol. 2012;21(3):185–90.

36. Xing M, Westra WH, Tufano RP, Cohen Y, Rosenbaum E, Rhoden KJ, et al. BRAF mutation predicts a poorer clinical prognosis for papillary thyroid cancer. J Clin Endocrinol Metab. 2005;90(12):6373–9.

37. Lupi C, Giannini R, Ugolini C, Proietti A, Berti P, Minuto M, et al. Association of BRAF V600E mutation with poor clinicopathological outcomes in 500 consecutive cases of papillary thyroid carcinoma. J Clin Endocrinol Metab. 2007;92(11):4085–90.

38. Chakravarty D, Santos E, Ryder M, Knauf JA, Liao X-H, West BL, et al. Small-molecule MAPK inhibitors restore radioiodine incorporation in mouse thyroid cancers with conditional BRAF activation. J Clin Invest. 2011;121(12):4700–11.

39. Ho AL, Grewal RK, Leboeuf R, Sherman EJ, Pfister DG, Deandreis D, et al. Selumetinib-enhanced radioiodine uptake in advanced thyroid cancer. N Engl J Med. 2013;368(7):623–32.

40. Xing M, Alzahrani AS, Carson KA, Viola D, Elisei R, Bendlova B, et al. Association between BRAF V600E mutation and mortality in patients with papillary thyroid cancer. JAMA. 2013;309(14):1493–501.

41. Cooper DS, Doherty GM, Haugen BR, Hauger BR, Kloos RT, Lee SL, et al. Revised American Thyroid Association management guidelines for patients with thyroid nodules and differentiated thyroid cancer. Thyroid. 2009;19(11):1167–214.

42. Tisell LE, Nilsson B, Mölne J, Hansson G, Fjälling M, Jansson S, et al. Improved survival of patients with papillary thyroid cancer after surgical microdissection. World J Surg. 1996;20(7):854–9.

43. O'Neill CJ, Bullock M, Chou A, Sidhu SB, Delbridge LW, Robinson BG, et al. BRAF(V600E) mutation is associated with an increased risk of nodal recurrence requiring reoperative surgery in patients with papillary thyroid cancer. Surgery. 2010;148(6):1139–45. discussion 1145–6.

44. Hughes DT, Doherty GM. Central neck dissection for papillary thyroid cancer. Cancer Control. 2011;18(2): 83–8.

45. Lee KC, Li C, Schneider EB, Wang Y, Somervell H, Krafft M, et al. Is BRAF mutation associated with lymph node metastasis in patients with papillary thyroid cancer? Surgery. 2012;152(6):977–83.

46. Kroll TG, Sarraf P, Pecciarini L, Chen CJ, Mueller E, Spiegelman BM, et al. PAX8-PPARgamma1 fusion oncogene in human thyroid carcinoma [corrected]. Science. 2000;289(5483):1357–60.

47. Lui W-O, Zeng L, Rehrmann V, Deshpande S, Tretiakova M, Kaplan EL, et al. CREB3L2-PPARgamma fusion mutation identifies a thyroid signaling pathway regulated by intramembrane proteolysis. Cancer Res. 2008;68(17):7156–64.

48. Eberhardt NL, Grebe SKG, McIver B, Reddi HV. The role of the PAX8/PPARgamma fusion oncogene in the pathogenesis of follicular thyroid cancer. Mol Cell Endocrinol. 2010;321(1):50–6.

49. Shen WT, Chung W-Y. Treatment of thyroid cancer with histone deacetylase inhibitors and peroxisome proliferator-activated receptor-gamma agonists. Thyroid. 2005; 15(6):594–9.

50. Caria P, Vanni R. Cytogenetic and molecular events in adenoma and well-differentiated thyroid follicular-cell neoplasia. Cancer Genet Cytogenet. 2010;203(1): 21–9.

51. Nikiforova MN, Lynch RA, Biddinger PW, Alexander EK, Dorn GW, Tallini G, et al. RAS point mutations and PAX8-PPAR gamma rearrangement in thyroid tumors: evidence for distinct molecular pathways in thyroid follicular carcinoma. J Clin Endocrinol Metab. 2003;88(5):2318–26.

52. Mulligan LM, Kwok JB, Healey CS, Elsdon MJ, Eng C, Gardner E, et al. Germ-line mutations of the RET

proto-oncogene in multiple endocrine neoplasia type 2A. Nature. 1993;363(6428):458–60.

53. Hu MI, Cote GJ. Medullary thyroid carcinoma: who's on first? Thyroid. 2012;22(5):451–3.

54. Elisei R, Romei C, Renzini G, Bottici V, Cosci B, Molinaro E, et al. The timing of total thyroidectomy in RET gene mutation carriers could be personalized and safely planned on the basis of serum calcitonin: 18 years experience at one single center. J Clin Endocrinol Metab. 2012;97(2):426–35.

55. Skinner MA, Moley JA, Dilley WG, Owzar K, DeBenedetti MK, Wells J, Samuel A. Prophylactic thyroidectomy in multiple endocrine neoplasia type 2A. N Engl J Med. 2005;353(11):1105–13.

56. Wells SA, Robinson BG, Gagel RF, Dralle H, Fagin JA, Santoro M, et al. Vandetanib in patients with locally advanced or metastatic medullary thyroid cancer: a randomized, double-blind phase III trial. J Clin Oncol. 2012;30(2):134–41.

57. Eng C. RET proto-oncogene in the development of human cancer. J Clin Oncol. 1999;17(1):380–93.

58. Donis-Keller H, Dou S, Chi D, Carlson KM, Toshima K, Lairmore TC, et al. Mutations in the RET proto-oncogene are associated with MEN 2A and FMTC. Hum Mol Genet. 1993;2(7):851–6.

59. Vierhapper H, Bieglmayer C, Heinze G, Baumgartner-Parzer S. Frequency of RET proto-oncogene mutations in patients with normal and with moderately elevated pentagastrin-stimulated serum concentrations of calcitonin. Thyroid. 2004;14(8):580–3.

60. Kruckeberg KE, Thibodeau SN. Pyrosequencing technology as a method for the diagnosis of multiple endocrine neoplasia type 2. Clin Chem. 2004;50(3): 522–9.

61. Pazaitou-panayiotou K, Kaprara A, Sarika L, Zovoilis T, Belogianni I, Vainas I, et al. Efficient testing of the RET gene by DHPLC analysis for MEN 2 syndrome in a cohort of patients. Anticancer Res. 2005;25(3B): 2091–5.

62. Machens A, Dralle H. Biomarker-based risk stratification for previously untreated medullary thyroid cancer. J Clin Endocrinol Metab. 2010;95(6):2655–63.

63. Zenaty D, Aigrain Y, Peuchmaur M, Philippe-Chomette P, Baumann C, Cornelis F, et al. Medullary thyroid carcinoma identified within the first year of life in children with hereditary multiple endocrine neoplasia type 2A (codon 634) and 2B. Eur J Endocrinol. 2009;160(5):807–13.

64. Roman S, Mehta P, Sosa JA. Medullary thyroid cancer: early detection and novel treatments. Curr Opin Oncol. 2009;21(1):5–10.

65. Garcia-Rostan G, Sobrinho-Simões M. Poorly differentiated thyroid carcinoma: an evolving entity. Diagn Histopathol. 2011;17(3):114–23.

66. Volante M, Rapa I, Gandhi M, Bussolati G, Giachino D, Papotti M, et al. RAS mutations are the predominant molecular alteration in poorly differentiated thyroid carcinomas and bear prognostic impact. J Clin Endocrinol Metab. 2009;94(12):4735–41.

67. Nikiforova MN, Kimura ET, Gandhi M, Biddinger PW, Knauf JA, Basolo F, et al. BRAF mutations in thyroid tumors are restricted to papillary carcinomas and anaplastic or poorly differentiated carcinomas arising from papillary carcinomas. J Clin Endocrinol Metab. 2003;88(11):5399–404.

68. Wu G, Mambo E, Guo Z, Hu S, Huang X, Gollin SM, et al. Uncommon mutation, but common amplifications, of the PIK3CA gene in thyroid tumors. J Clin Endocrinol Metab. 2005;90(8):4688–93.

69. Nikiforov YE. Genetic alterations involved in the transition from well-differentiated to poorly differentiated and anaplastic thyroid carcinomas. Endocr Pathol. 2004;15(4):319–28.

70. Boonyaarunnate T, Olson MT, Bishop JA, Yang GCH, Ali SZ. Cribriform morular variant of papillary thyroid carcinoma: clinical and cytomorphological features on fine-needle aspiration. Acta Cytol. 2013; 57(2):127–33.

71. Sastre-Perona A, Santisteban P. Role of the wnt pathway in thyroid cancer. Front Endocrinol (Lausanne). 2012;3:31.

72. Hamberger B, Gharib H, Melton LJ, Goellner JR, Zinsmeister AR. Fine-needle aspiration biopsy of thyroid nodules. Impact on thyroid practice and cost of care. Am J Med. 1982;73(3):381–4.

73. Olson MT, Clark DP, Erozan YS, Ali SZ. Spectrum of risk of malignancy in subcategories of 'atypia of undetermined significance'. Acta Cytol. 2011;55(6): 518–25.

74. Cibas ES, Bibbo M. Thyroid FNA: challenges and opportunities. Acta Cytol. 2011;55(6):489–91.

75. Jo VY, Stelow EB, Dustin SM, Hanley KZ. Malignancy risk for fine-needle aspiration of thyroid lesions according to the Bethesda system for reporting thyroid cytopathology. Am J Clin Pathol. 2010;134(3): 450–6.

76. Theoharis CGA, Schofield KM, Hammers L, Udelsman R, Chhieng DC. The Bethesda thyroid fine-needle aspiration classification system: year 1 at an academic institution. Thyroid. 2009;19(11): 1215–23.

77. Baloch ZW, Cibas ES, Clark DP, Layfield LJ, Ljung B-M, Pitman MB, et al. The National Cancer Institute thyroid fine needle aspiration state of the science conference: a summation. Cytojournal. 2008;5:6.

78. Yassa L, Cibas ES, Benson CB, Frates MC, Doubilet PM, Gawande AA, et al. Long-term assessment of a multidisciplinary approach to thyroid nodule diagnostic evaluation. Cancer. 2007;111(6):508–16.

79. Olson MT, Boonyaarunnate T, Aragon Han P, Umbricht CB, Ali SZ, Zeiger MA. A tertiary center's experience with second review of 3885 thyroid cytopathology specimens. J Clin Endocrinol Metab. 2013; 98(4):1450–7.

80. Ohori NP, Nikiforova MN, Schoedel KE, LeBeau SO, Hodak SP, Seethala RR, et al. Contribution of molecular testing to thyroid fine-needle aspiration cytology of "follicular lesion of undetermined significance/atypia

of undetermined significance". Cancer Cytopathol. 2010;118(1):17–23.

81. Nikiforov YE, Ohori NP, Hodak SP, Carty SE, LeBeau SO, Ferris RL, et al. Impact of mutational testing on the diagnosis and management of patients with cytologically indeterminate thyroid nodules: a prospective analysis of 1056 FNA samples. J Clin Endocrinol Metab. 2011;96(11):3390–7.

82. Davies H, Bignell GR, Cox C, Stephens P, Edkins S, Clegg S, et al. Mutations of the BRAF gene in human cancer. Nature. 2002;417(6892):949–54.

83. Puxeddu E. BRAFV599E mutation is the leading genetic event in adult sporadic papillary thyroid carcinomas. J Clin Endocrinol Metab. 2004;89(5): 2414–20.

84. Kleiman DA, Sporn MJ, Beninato T, Crowley MJ, Nguyen A, Uccelli A, et al. Preoperative BRAF (V600E) mutation screening is unlikely to alter initial surgical treatment of patients with indeterminate thyroid nodules: a prospective case series of 960 patients. Cancer. 2013;119(8):1495–502.

85. Kloos RT, Reynolds JD, Walsh PS, Wilde JI, Tom EY, Pagan M, et al. Does addition of BRAF V600E mutation testing modify sensitivity or specificity of the Afirma gene expression classifier in cytologically indeterminate thyroid nodules? J Clin Endocrinol Metab. 2013;98(4):E761–8.

86. Zhu Z, Gandhi M, Nikiforova MN, Fischer AH, Nikiforov YE. Molecular profile and clinical-pathologic features of the follicular variant of papillary thyroid carcinoma. An unusually high prevalence of ras mutations. Am J Clin Pathol. 2003;120(1):71–7.

87. Burns JS, Blaydes JP, Wright PA, Lemoine L, Bond JA, Dillwyn Williams E, et al. Stepwise transformation of primary thyroid epithelial cells by a mutant Ha-ras oncogene: an in vitro model of tumor progression. Mol Carcinog. 1992;6(2):129–39.

88. Barden CB, Shister KW, Zhu B, Guiter G, Greenblatt DY, Zeiger MA, et al. Classification of follicular thyroid tumors by molecular signature: results of gene profiling. Clin Cancer Res. 2003;9(5):1792–800.

89. Finley DJ, Zhu B, Fahey I, Thomas J. Molecular analysis of Hurthle cell neoplasms by gene profiling. Surgery. 2004;136(6):1160–8.

90. Chudova D, Wilde JI, Wang ET, Wang H, Rabbee N, Egidio CM, et al. Molecular classification of thyroid nodules using high-dimensionality genomic data. J Clin Endocrinol Metab. 2010;95(12):5296–304.

91. Alexander EK, Kennedy GC, Baloch ZW, Cibas ES, Chudova D, Diggans J, et al. Preoperative diagnosis of benign thyroid nodules with indeterminate cytology. N Engl J Med. 2012;367(8):705–15.

92. Jameson JL. Minimizing unnecessary surgery for thyroid nodules. N Engl J Med. 2012;367(8):765–7.

93. Findlay I, Ray P, Quirke P, Rutherford A, Lilford R. Allelic drop-out and preferential amplification in single cells and human blastomeres: implications for preimplantation diagnosis of sex and cystic fibrosis. Hum Reprod. 1995;10(6):1609–18.

94. Schroeder A, Mueller O, Stocker S, Salowsky R, Leiber M, Gassmann M, et al. BMC molecular biology | full text | the RIN: an RNA integrity number for assigning integrity values to RNA measurements. BMC Mol Biol. 2006;7(1):3.

95. Ferraz C, Rehfeld C, Krogdahl A, Precht Jensen EM, Bösenberg E, Narz F, et al. Detection of PAX8/PPARG and RET/PTC rearrangements is feasible in routine air-dried fine needle aspiration smears. Thyroid. 2012; 22(10):1025–30.

96. Yip L, Farris C, Kabaker AS, Hodak SP, Nikiforova MN, McCoy KL, et al. Cost impact of molecular testing for indeterminate thyroid nodule fine-needle aspiration biopsies. J Clin Endocrinol Metab. 2012; 97(6):1905–12.

97. Li H, Robinson KA, Anton B, Saldanha IJ, Ladenson PW. Cost-effectiveness of a novel molecular test for cytologically indeterminate thyroid nodules. J Clin Endocrinol Metab. 2011;96(11):E1719–26.

98. Hodak SP, Rosenthal DS, The American Thyroid Association Clinical Affairs Committee. Information for clinicians: commercially available molecular diagnosis testing in the evaluation of thyroid nodule fine-needle aspiration specimens. Thyroid. 2013; 23(2):131–4.

99. Duick DS. Overview of molecular biomarkers for enhancing the management of cytologically indeterminate thyroid nodules and thyroid cancer. Endocr Pract. 2012;18(4):611–5.

Molecular Testing of Head and Neck Tumors

20

Diana Bell and Ehab Y. Hanna

Introduction

Per cubic centimeter, the head and neck region gives rise to a greater diversity of neoplasms than any other site in the human body does. The diversity is due partly to the anatomic complexity of and highly varied tissues in this compact area. Two unique areas of study within the head and neck region are squamous mucosal lesions and salivary gland tumors. Results of morphologic, histologic, and immunohistochemical analyses are the mainstay of diagnosis, but recent advances in molecular pathology are being used to identify potential targets, and for pathologists as aid for the diagnostic approach. This chapter provides contemporary information on the molecular characterization and testing of head and neck squamous epithelial lesions and salivary gland tumors for clinical management.

Squamous Mucosal Lesions

The most common neoplastic process in the head and neck region involves the squamous epithelium. Tumorigenesis of head and neck squamous cell cancer (HNSCC) is the sixth most common neoplasm worldwide [2, 26, 30, 64]. Risk factors play an important role in the susceptibility to and the development of squamous carcinoma. Tobacco and alcohol abuse are epidemiologically linked to HNSCC.

Traditional pathologic classification and diagnosis of HNSCC are based on evaluation with a light microscope and, rarely, selective use of immunohistochemical markers. The traditional clinicopathologic factors used to guide the management of the disease are limited. New tools are needed to improve the early detection of HNSCC, treatment stratification, and patient outcome [2, 64].

Conventional (Non-viral) Squamous Carcinomas

Although no definitive molecular events or pathways have been firmly established for HCNS tumorigenesis, significant progress has been made in identifying critical chromosomal genomic alterations [2, 22, 35]. Squamous tumorigenesis is a multistage process: an accumulation of successive genomic alterations precede or coincide with the development of epithelial alterations (i.e., dysplasia) [2, 22, 35]. The type, order, and composition of these events

D. Bell, M.D. (✉)
Department of Pathology, The University
of Texas MD Anderson Cancer Center,
1515 Holcombe Boulevard, Houston,
TX 77030, USA
e-mail: diana.bell@mdanderson.org

E.Y. Hanna, M.D.
Department of Head and Neck Surgery,
The University of Texas MD Anderson Cancer
Center, Houston, TX, USA

G.M. Yousef and S. Jothy (eds.), *Molecular Testing in Cancer*,
DOI 10.1007/978-1-4899-8050-2_20, © Springer Science+Business Media New York 2014

are unknown, although temporal accumulation of certain genetic and epigenetic events has been associated with the progressive development of premalignant lesions and invasive carcinoma. Efforts to identify the genetic and phenotypic alterations associated with the biological progression of these lesions have led to the characterization of several markers associated with the development of this cancer.

Cellular Related Molecular Markers
Loss of Heterozygosity

Comparative analysis of DNA extracted from histologically normal mucosa or lymphocytes to tumor has identified loss of heterozygosity at chromosomes 3p, 9p, or 17p in more than 30 % of HNSCC tumors [22, 35]. These chromosomal regions house the p16 and p53 tumor suppressor genes, respectively, and the loss of these loci suggests early involvement of these genes in HNSCC and tumor progression. Loss of heterozygosity at loci 4p, 8p, 11q, 13q, or 18q has been found predominantly in a subset of advanced HNSC cases [22, 35]. Patterns of chromosomal aberrations in loci 3q24, 8p23.1, and 8q12.2k and gain of chromosome 20 distinguish between two major HNSCC subgroups with different biological progression and metastatic features [22, 35].

Tumor Suppressor Genes
p53 Gene

Mutations at certain exons of the p53 gene, which is located on chromosome 17p13, appear in about half of HSNCCs [18]. These hotspot mutations have been identified in exons 5–9 of the p53 gene [22, 76]. Alterations of p53 have been detected in premalignant squamous lesions, suggesting that this gene is involved in the early development of this carcinoma. The p53 mutation alterations have been correlated with poor survival at a different site [22, 76].

p16 Gene

The p16 gene is located in the chromosome 9p21 region and plays a central role in the regulation of cell cycle. Loss of this gene is most commonly due to methylation of its promoter. The first exons have been frequently found in HNSC [40, 48, 51, 74–76].

Oncogenes
Cyclin D1 Gene

Located on chromosome 11p, the Cyclin D1 gene is critical to the cell cycle [47, 49, 79]. Cyclin D1 amplification and overexpression have been reported for approximately a third of HNSCs and are associated with advanced and more aggressive tumors [79].

p63 Gene

The p63 gene is a putative oncogene located in the chromosome 3q27 region [21, 57, 58]. Two main isotopes created with alternative promoters and six with alternative splicing at the carboxyl end have been identified. The P36ΔN isotype was highly expressed in progressive premalignant lesions and aggressive HNSC [21, 57, 58].

c-Met Gene

c-Met is an oncogene that mediates angiogenesis, cell motility, invasion, and metastasis. Overexpression of c-Met has been reported for 80 % of HNSCCs but its amplification in only 13 % [19, 22, 25, 28, 29, 39, 42, 52, 59]. Because c-Met intersects with the epidermal growth factor receptor (EGFR) and phosphoinositol 3-kinase (PI3K) pathways in HNSC, it may be a viable target for combined therapy [25].

Epigenetic Alterations

Epigenetic modifications, such as methylation of 5-cystosine at CpG islands, chromatin modeling, and histone acetylation, play a major role in tumorigenesis [40]. Several genes have been identified to be hypermethylated in HNSCC, including CDKN1, p16, DAP-K, E-cadherin, cyclin-A1, and MGMT [40, 48, 51]. A profile of these genes was recently tested with DNA extracted from saliva and mouthwash. Methylation was associated with an increased risk of squamous carcinoma and was predictive of tumor recurrence [20, 40, 62].

EGFR

EGFR contains an extracellular ligand-binding transmembrane, a nuclear localizing signal, and cytoplasmic tyrosine kinase domains. Activation of these elements is tightly associated with the binding of EGFR to epidermal growth factor

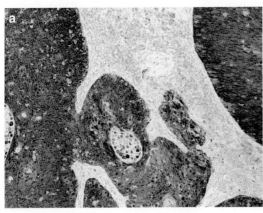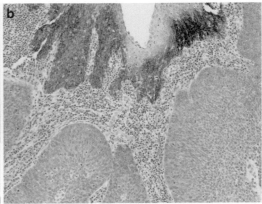

Fig. 20.1 EGFR heterogeneity in head and neck squamous carcinoma as illustrated with immunohistochemistry. (**a**) Strong diffuse homogeneous pattern. (**b**) Scattered weak/intermediate staining of a few cell nests/or negative

family members such as transforming growth factor α, amphiregulin, B-cellulin, heparin-binding epidermal growth factor, and epiregulin [31].

Dysregulation of the EGFR pathway by overexpression or constitutive activation can induce angiogenesis, invasion, and metastasis. Overexpression of EGFR has been associated with tumor cell invasiveness and metastasis via the stimulation of metalloproteinases [44]. EGFR overexpression has also been positively correlated with nodal metastasis, high tumor stage, and poor outcome [5]. Therefore, inhibition or blockade of EGFR by monoclonal antibodies or small-molecule tyrosine kinase inhibitors could be used to inhibit these processes and treat certain patients with head and neck carcinoma [44].

EGFR is a candidate marker for HNSC. Assessing for EGFR on clinical materials is performed with immunohistochemical analysis (for expression) or in situ hybridization (for amplification). Although more practical and economical than in situ hybridization, immunohistochemical evaluation of EGFR suffers from a lack of performance guidelines and acceptable interpretive criteria. Nonetheless, immunohistochemical evaluation of EGFR is being performed for clinical trials to determine its extent and localization in tumor cells. The scoring can be done by eye or by imaging. The results can be broadly categorized as strong, uniform, and membranous and cytoplasmic staining; intermediate, patchy, and

variable membranous and cytoplasmic staining; and weak/negative with scattered weak/intermediate staining of a few cell nests/or negative [53] (Fig. 20.1). An alternative or complementary method of amplifying the EGFR gene is chromogenic in situ hybridization. Gene amplification of EGFR with this method was reported for 10–60 % of HNSCs and has been associated with response to tyrosine kinase inhibitors [70, 71].

Signaling Pathways
PI3K/AKT/mTOR Pathway

The PI3K/AKT/mTOR pathway has been shown to be activated in the majority of HNSCs (>70 %) [24, 27]. Loss of the PTEN gene, a negative regulator of PI3K that lies on chromosome 10q, results in the upregulation of AKT and mTOR and is associated with poor behavior of these tumors [27, 63]. Development of a tyrosine kinase inhibitor that targets multiple components of diverse pathways or a combination of agents is a likely strategy for successfully managing these tumors [24, 41].

Virus-Associated Squamous Carcinomas

Carcinomas arising at lymphoid-rich stromal sites are phenotypically, etiologically, and epidemiology distinct from conventional (non-viral) squamous carcinomas.

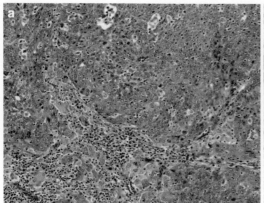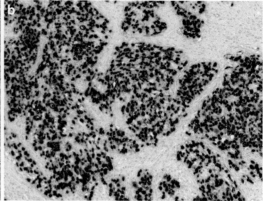

Fig. 20.2 Histologic features of nasopharyngeal undifferentiated carcinoma. (**a**) Hematoxylin and eosin staining showing syncytial pattern. (**b**) Epstein–Barr virus-associated nasopharyngeal carcinoma (in situ hybridization, nuclear blue signal)

Nasopharyngeal Carcinoma

Nasopharyngeal carcinoma is characterized by a unique geographic and ethnic distribution worldwide and is closely associated with Epstein–Barr virus infection, especially in endemic location [9]. Genetic susceptibility, dietary factor, and environmental factors may also play a major role in the development of this entity.

Histopathologically, nasopharyngeal carcinoma is graded according to the World Health Organization's classification system as grade I (differentiated squamous carcinoma) or grades II and III (undifferentiated carcinoma) [9]. Epstein–Barr virus-encoded RNA and keratin, which are tested for in situ, are important diagnostic markers (Fig. 20.2). These tumors are radiosensitive and are rarely surgically removed in the Western countries.

Oropharyngeal Carcinoma

A rise in the incidence of poorly differentiated carcinoma of Waldeyer's ring has been reported [34]. The mucosa is lymphoid based, and these tumors have a different histologic appearance than most tumors of the oral cavity in that human papilloma virus (HPV)-associated squamous cell carcinomas are more likely to appear nonkeratinizing or basaloid and to have limited or absent keratinization. A subset of tumors of the tonsil or base of tongue that resemble undifferentiated nasopharyngeal carcinoma, with morphologic features of lymphoepithelial carcinoma, are HPV positive.

The detection of HPV-16 by in situ hybridization, polymerase chain reaction (PCR), or p16 overexpression in tumor cells is important to the diagnosis of oropharyngeal carcinoma [23, 35]. The majority of patients are young adults, are well educated, and do not have the typical risk factors of patients with HNSCC. For these patients, sexual practice may be associated with this disease.

Pathogenesis of HPV-Associated Squamous Cell Carcinoma

Activation of HPV-16 involves the integration of the circular double-stranded DNA virus into the host DNA genome [8], which results in the loss of the regulatory exon 2 of the virus genome and thus unregulated expression of E6 and E7 viral oncogenes [37, 43, 54]. These viral genes bind and degrade the host's tumor suppressor proteins p53 and Rb, respectively. Loss of the cell regulatory functions of these genes underlies the pathogenesis of oropharyngeal carcinoma. Presumably the degradation of the Rb protein, as well as the release of the E2F transcription factor, upregulates p16 protein [8].

HPV infection has been detected in more than 70 % of oropharyngeal carcinomas. These cancers tend to have high-grade morphologic features, although patients with HPV-positive tumors have

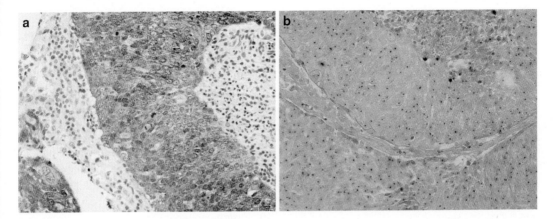

Fig. 20.3 HPV-associated head and neck squamous carcinoma. (**a**) In situ hybridization for high-risk HPV (nuclear blue signal). (**b**) Immunohistochemical analysis for p16 (homogeneous diffuse nuclear and cytoplasmic brown staining)

a better prognosis than patients with HPV-negative tumors do [6, 33, 56]. Clinical manifestations are heterogeneous due to variability in the viral load or the activated viral oncogenes [6].

HPV-Associated Genomic Alterations

A few genomic studies of oropharyngeal carcinoma have been conducted. Compared with HPV-negative tumors, HPV-positive tumors were found to have a significantly lower number of copy number alterations [35] or common chromosomal alterations at regions 3p, 11q, and 16q [66]. Generally, findings have supported the idea that the association between HPV in a population with no risk factors and better outcome [6, 33, 36]. A recent study of genome-wide methylation and gene expression of these tumors revealed hypermethylation in HPV-positive tumors compared with HPV-negative tumors and a correlation between methylation status and gene expression [55, 60]. Differential gene expression studies have also shown distinct patterns of DNA replication and cell cycle regulation genes, viral resistance, and immune response between HPV-positive and HPV-negative tumors. Dysregulation of the DNA replication and cell cycle regulation genes and those related to immune regulation, including those of natural killer cells, Toll-like receptor, and JAK-STAT, may be relevant to the pathogenesis of HPV in oropharyngeal cancer patients.

The lack of alterations to the p53 gene in HPV-associated tumors may render tumor cells susceptible to chemotherapy and radiotherapy as compared with HPV-negative tumors with p53 mutations [32]. The E6 viral oncogene was reported to sensitize tumor cells to radiation-induced apoptosis independent of p53 status [78]. An inverse correlation between p53 alterations and HPV status has been reported in several studies [3, 77, 78].

Biomarkers in HPV-Associated Cancer

The results from molecular and immunohistochemical analyses are critical to a diagnosis of virus-associated oropharyngeal carcinoma. Currently three procedures are used by most pathology laboratories to detect viral DNA and RNA: quantitative or qualitative PCR, in situ hybridization, and p16 protein expression. PCR-based techniques are highly sensitive but may result in a relatively high number of false-positive cases. In situ hybridization is less sensitive, but it allows for the localization of the virus in tumor nuclei and a qualitative view of the viral load [23, 35]. Upregulated p16 protein is currently considered a reliable surrogate marker for HPV-positive oropharyngeal cancer [23]. Immunohistochemical analysis for p16 is emerging as a supportive or practical substitute for viral detection. Strong and homogenous p16 staining in both the nucleus and cytoplasm is consistent with HPV positivity [23]. Heterogeneous, patchy, and strictly nuclear staining require additional HPV testing with PCR or in situ hybridization (Fig. 20.3).

In addition to identifying viral DNA or RNA, biomarkers are critical for guiding and improving tumor therapy. Patients with oropharyngeal cancer that does not respond to chemotherapy and radiotherapy or both may undergo salvage surgery or receive palliative therapy. To more accurately stratify patients for treatment and improve tumor response to therapy, the biological predictors need to be determined [68].

Salivary Gland Lesions

The salivary glands are the site of origin for a wide variety of neoplasms. The histopathology of these tumors may be the most complex and diverse of any organ in the body. Salivary gland neoplasms are uncommon, with an estimated annual incidence in the United States of 2.2–2.5 cases per 100,000 people; they constitute approximately 5 % of all head and neck neoplasms [1, 67]. Nearly 80 % of these tumors occur in the parotid glands, 15 % in the submandibular glands, and the remaining 5 % in the sublingual and minor salivary glands. Benign neoplasms make up about 80 %, 50 %, and less than 40 % of these tumor types [67].

The primary management of salivary gland lesions is surgical resection. Postoperative radiotherapy may be performed for patients with close margins or perineural invasion. The treatment options for patients presenting with locally advanced, recurrent, or distant metastatic disease are limited and generally palliative [1, 4]. Attempts to understand the genetics and biology of salivary gland tumors in order to identify molecular targets have been limited due to the rarity of these tumors and the inconsistency of findings to date.

Tumor-Specific Translocations and Fusion Oncogenes in Salivary Carcinomas

Chromosomal aberrations are a characteristic feature of neoplasia. Recurrent, nonrandom chromosomal translocations and the creation of novel chimeric fusion oncogenes are well recognized and causally implicated in carcinogenesis. Tumor-specific chromosomal rearrangements often produce potent fusion oncogenes, which induce tumorigenesis by deregulating the cell cycle, resulting in overexpression of a gene in one of the breakpoints, or by fusion of two genes, one in each breakpoint, resulting in a hybrid, chimeric gene [16]. Almost 400 critical gene fusions have been identified in human cancers, such as those of the prostate, thyroid, kidney, breast, bronchus, lung, and salivary glands. These oncogenes account for 20 % of human cancer morbidity. Fusion oncogenes are often derived from, and encode for, transcription factors, transcription regulators, and receptor tyrosine kinases, all of which are frequently involved in oncogenesis [16]. In solid tumors, most fusion oncogenes encode aberrant transcription factors, while other fusion oncogenes express chimeric proteins that deregulate growth factor signaling. Both types represent important diagnostic and prognostic biomarkers as well as potential therapeutic targets. As sequencing technology advances, it is anticipated that the number of known fusion oncogenes identified will rise exponentially.

Highly specific chromosomal translocations resulting in pathognomonic fusion oncogenes have been reported for salivary gland tumors, namely, mucoepidermoid carcinoma (MEC), adenoid cystic carcinoma (AdCC), hyalinizing clear cell carcinoma (HCCC), and mammary analogue secretory carcinoma (MASC) [Table 20.1]. These translocations target transcription factors involved in growth factor signaling and cell cycle regulation, transcriptional coactivators, or tyrosine kinase receptors [16].

Mucoepidermoid Carcinoma

The most common salivary gland malignancy, MEC arises in the upper aerodigestive tract and tracheobronchial tree [11]. The patient's age and conventional clinicopathologic parameters, such as tumor stage and grade, influence management. Low-grade, low-stage tumors require surgical resection alone, whereas high-grade, high-stage tumors necessitate adjuvant radiation and neck dissection. MECs are graded based on histologic

Table 20.1 Tumor-specific fusion oncogenes in salivary carcinomas

	Mucoepidermoid carcinoma (MEC)	Adenoid cystic carcinoma (AdCC)	Hyalinizing clear cell carcinoma (HCCC)	Mammary analogue secretory carcinoma (MASC)
Cell of origin	Precursor cells of exocrine glands in the head and neck	Epithelial and myoepithelial cells of the salivary glands	Epithelial (squamous) cells of the salivary glands	Epithelial cells of the salivary glands
Site of tumor	Exocrine glands in the upper aerodigestive tract and tracheobronchial tree	Salivary glands	Salivary glands oral cavity	Salivary glands
Pathognomonic translocation	t(11;19)(q21;p13)	t(6;9)(q22-23;p23-24)	t(12;22) (q13;q12)	t(12;15) (p13;q25)
Proto-oncogene	Mucoepidermoid carcinoma translocated-1 (MECT1)—also known as CRTC1, TORC1, WAMTP1	MYB	EWSR	ETV6
Promoter gene	MAML2	NFIB	ATF1	NTRK3
Fusion oncogene	MECT1–MAML2	MYB–NFIB	EWSR–ATF1	ETV6–NTRK3
Diagnostic modality	RT-PCR, FISH	RT-PCR, FISH, immunohistochemistry	RT-PCR, FISH	RT-PCR, FISH
Prognosis	t(11;19) associated with improved survival	Histologic grade influences prognosis	Low-grade salivary carcinoma	Intermediate-grade salivary carcinoma (resembles secretory carcinoma of breast)

features. Adverse histologic parameters include perineural invasion, angiolymphatic invasion, coagulative necrosis, high mitotic rate, cystic component <20 %, anaplasia, and infiltrative growth pattern [11]. The great variability in and poor reproducibility of histologic grading schemes are reflected by suboptimal treatment planning and prognostication [11].

t(11;19) MECT1–MAML2 Fusion Transcript in MEC

First described by Nordkvist et al. in 1994 [46] and characterized by Tonon et al. in 2003 [73], the recurrent t(11;19)(q12;p13) translocation involving the MECT1 and MAML2 genes has been identified as the underlying pathogenetic event in the majority of MECs. Both genes participate in cell cycle regulation: MECT1 (mucoepidermoid carcinoma translocated-1, also known as CRTC1, TORC1, and WAMTP1) is a

75-kDa protein that activates cAMP response element-binding (CREB)-mediated transcription, and MAML2 (mastermind-like 2) is a 125-kDa protein involved in Notch signaling pathways. The MECT1–MAML2 fusion protein is comprised of the N-terminal CREB protein-binding domain (exon 1) of MECT1 at 19p13 and the C-terminal transcriptional activation domain (exons 2–5) of the Notch coactivator MAML2 at 11q21 [73]. The MECT1–MAML2 fusion protein may activate both cAMP-CERB targets and Notch signaling targets, disrupting both cell cycle and differentiation functions [73]. Because CREB regulates cell proliferation and differentiation and MECT1 deletion abolishes transforming activity, it is likely that CREB dysregulation mediates tumorigenesis [73].

Several studies have found a greater than 55 % detection rate for MECT1–MAML2 fusion in MECs [10, 61, 72]. Fusion-positive cases have demonstrated significantly longer patient survival than fusion-negative cases do, suggesting that MECT1–MAML2 represents a specific prognostic molecular marker in MEC. Behboudi et al. reported median survival times of 10 and 1.6 years in fusion-positive and fusion-negative patients, respectively, as well as a significantly lower risk of local recurrence, metastases, and tumor-related death in fusion-positive patients [10]. Seethala et al. found that while translocation-positive patients had a better disease-specific survival rate than translocation-negative patients did, the disease-free survival rate was not significantly affected by translocation status [61].

Clinical and Diagnostic Significance of Fusion Transcript MECT1–MAML2 in MEC

Detection of the MECT1–MAML2 fusion transcript in a significant number of MECs may affect the diagnosis, prognosis, and treatment of this disease [11]. Results from fine-needle aspiration cytology analysis are increasingly being used as part of a diagnostic triage for putative salivary gland tumors, although the diagnostic role of this assessment is controversial. For MECs, such results may be diagnostically accurate for high- or intermediate-grade tumors but unsatisfactory for low-grade tumors. The application of molecular techniques to cytological material to detect the MECT1–MAML2 fusion transcript or protein may be helpful when the diagnosis is uncertain, although clinical studies will be required to validate this approach.

The fact that high-grade MEC can express the MECT1–MAML2 fusion transcript suggests that detection of this transcript may help in distinguishing this tumor type from poorly differentiated adenocarcinoma or clear cell carcinomas when conventional histological distinction is difficult. High-grade MEC is prone to diagnostic confusion with adenosquamous carcinoma, adenoid (acantholytic) squamous carcinoma, and sometimes adenocarcinoma not otherwise specified or salivary duct carcinoma [38]. In the initial series, the fusion transcript was observed for only low- and intermediate-grade MEC, but in our experience and as recently confirmed by other researchers, the translocation can occur in high-grade MEC, although at a lower rate. Histologically low-grade MEC may behave aggressively [38]. However, the most challenging category of MEC in terms of prognosis and management is the intermediate grade. Histologic grading criteria are most useful for morphologic classification, and the inclusion of molecular findings provides submicroscopic information and, hence, more accurate assessment. Integrating molecular findings allows for biological stratification within individual grades [11]. The translocation can be regarded as a biomarker of favorable prognosis, which could influence the decision for neck dissection or radiotherapy. Although retrospective data support the usefulness of identifying this translocation, its prognostic value remains to be verified prospectively [11].

In clinical practice, assessment for the MECT1–MAML2 fusion transcript is an ancillary test that is performed using reverse transcriptase-PCR or fluorescent in situ hybridization (FISH) with paraffin-embedded tissue. The translocation status can support a diagnosis of high-grade MEC or MEC with variant morphologies.

Adenoid Cystic Carcinoma

AdCC is a biphasic salivary gland malignancy that is characterized by cellular, morphologic, and clinical heterogeneity [67]. Despite the relative infrequency of these tumors, AdCCs are the second most common salivary gland malignancy, are the most common malignancy of minor salivary glands, and comprise 15–25 % of all salivary carcinomas. Histologic architecture alone determines the grade of AdCC: tubular and cribriform growth patterns are associated with a longer survival time than solid forms are. Despite locally aggressive growth with frequent perineural invasion, AdCCs demonstrate slow biologic progression and lymph node metastasis is rare [67].

Numerous cytogenetic studies have explored the molecular events in the development and progression of AdCC with the aim of identifying management targets (reviewed in [13]). Deletions or translocations of the terminal regions of the long arm of chromosome 6 are consistently found in salivary AdCC [13]. A subset of AdCCs shows reciprocal translocations or loss of chromosome 6q terminal loci; chromosome 9p is the most frequent translocation partner in these tumors. The t(6;9) translocation is the sole genetic alteration in this subset of AdCCs, suggesting involvement of the 6q region during the early development of AdCCs (reviewed in [13]).

t(6;9) MYB–NFIB Fusion Transcript in AdCC

A reciprocal t(6;9)(q22-23;p23-24) translocation resulting in formation of the MYB–NFIB fusion oncogene was recently described [50]. MYB is a leucine zipper transcription factor at 6q22-24 that participates in the regulation of cell proliferation, apoptosis, and differentiation [50]. MYB–NFIB fusion results in the loss of the MYB 3′-untranslated region (exon 15), which normally contains highly conserved target sequences for certain microRNAs; these target sites negatively regulate MYB expression. Loss of MYB repression results in overexpression of the fusion transcripts and protein, thereby inducing transcriptional activation of MYB target genes [50]. These target genes are associated with cell cycle control (CCNB1, CDC2, MAD1L1), apoptosis (API5, BCL2, BIRC3, HSPA8, SET), and cell growth and angiogenesis (MYC, KIT, VEGFA, FGF2, CD53). MYB–NFIB transcriptional downstream targets represent potential diagnostic biomarkers and therapeutic targets in AdCC [50].

Persson et al. reported a 100 % incidence of MYB–NFIB in a study of 11 AdCCs. However, Mitani et al. could demonstrate the presence of MYB–NFIB fusion transcripts in only 33 % of primary and metastatic AdCCs, although this work confirmed the role of the fusion transcript in the development of a subset of AdCCs [45, 50]. In the study by Mitani et al., a total of 14 fusion transcripts that involved different exons of MYB and NFIB were found in fusion-positive AdCCs. For the MYB gene, the most frequent fusion variants involved exons 13, 8b, 11, 15, 9b, 8a, 14, and 16. For the NFIB gene, most variants involved exons 12 and 11. The presence of multiple fusion variants can be explained by the presence of multiple break points within the MYB gene and alternative splicing in the last exons of the NFIB gene. The ability of MYB–NFIB fusion to cause a dramatic rise in MYB expression can be attributed to the loss of the MYB sequences containing the regulatory microRNA binding sites in MYB–NFIB transcripts (Mitani et al.). Several studies have reported increased expression of MYB RNA in fusion-positive AdCCs (reviewed in [13]).

A monoclonal antibody against the NH2-terminal domain of human MYB was shown to demonstrate strong nuclear MYB staining in 85 % and 61 % of MYB–NFIB fusion-positive and fusion-negative AdCCs, respectively [14]. In tubular and cribriform AdCCs composed of both epithelial and myoepithelial cell populations, MYB expression was limited to the myoepithelial cells [14].

Identification of the MYB–NFIB Fusion Transcript and Therapeutic Applications

RT-PCR or FISH can be used to detect MYB–NFIB fusions. FISH complemented by immunohistochemical analysis using anti-MYB or anti-MYB–NFIB proteins may provide ancillary diagnostic information. Few therapeutic options are available to directly target MYB, but preliminary reports of DNA vaccines and antisense MYB oligodeoxynucleotides suggest a potential role for them in the treatment of AdCCs. Therapy directed against MYB–NFIB transcriptional downstream targets may prove to be more feasible. Various antibodies and inhibitors, such as those directed against BCL2, FGF2, MYC, and COX-2, have emerged as potential chemotherapeutic agents, but their efficacy in AdCC requires further investigation.

Other Genetic Mutations in AdCC

Most AdCCs overexpress both c-Kit and EGFR [12, 13, 15]. In AdCCs, c-Kit expression is mostly limited to inner epithelial cells, while EGFR expression typically occurs in myoepithelial cells [15]. The mechanism of c-Kit expression in AdCCs may involve multiple genetic, epigenetic, and biologic events as well as gene copy numbers. EGFR, which facilitates carcinogenesis in humans by blocking apoptosis and promoting angiogenesis, can be modified by anti-EGFR therapies such as cetuximab and erlotinib. Histogenetic differences between the two cell populations may influence biologic heterogeneity

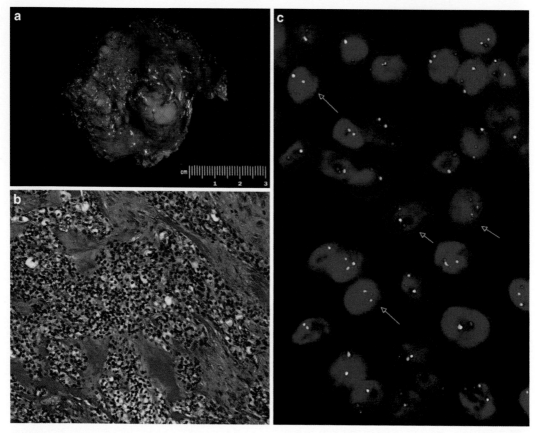

Fig. 20.4 HCCC. (**a**) Submucosal, rubbery, firm tumor of the base of the tongue. (**b**) Histological analysis reveals nests, trabeculae, and islands of clear cells embedded in a hyalinized, fibrotic stroma. (**c**) Consistent EWSR rearrangement by FISH as the result of EWSR–ATF1 fusion oncogene (FISH with break-apart probe for EWSR)

as well as response to treatment. Better clinical outcomes with EGFR expression and with concomitant EGFR and c-Kit positivity have been reported in AdCCs with myoepithelial cells, whereas epithelial c-Kit expression confers a worse prognosis regardless of the histologic features of the tumors [15]. Specific therapies targeting c-Kit or EGFR may require individualization in patients with AdCC, depending on biomarker stratification and tumor cell composition [15].

Hyalinizing Clear Cell Carcinoma

HCCC is a rare salivary tumor that consists of clear cells and hyalinized stroma. It is recognized as a separate entity than clear cell variants of epithelial–myoepithelial carcinoma, myoepithelial carcinoma, and MEC. Other clear cell tumor variants are clear cell-containing tumors of the salivary glands, odontogenic tumors, and metastatic renal cell carcinoma. HCCC cells are immunoreactive for keratins and do not express myoepithelial markers. Although morphologic and immunohistochemical studies can distinguish HCCC from other clear cell variants, establishing a correct diagnosis can be challenging in difficult cases or with small biopsy specimens [7, 69].

Several studies using FISH have indicated that HCCC has a consistent EWSR rearrangement as the result of an EWSR–ATF1 fusion oncogene. The fact that this finding has been consistent for HCCC can be used to distinguish this tumor from its potential mimics, as most other clear cell tumors do not exhibit EWSR or ATF1 rearrangement according to FISH analysis [7, 69] (Fig. 20.4).

Mammary Analogue Secretory Carcinoma of the Salivary Gland

MASC is a recently described salivary gland neoplasm that is characterized by its striking morphologic and molecular similarities to secretory carcinoma of the breast [65]. Retrospective studies have found that MASC has been most often diagnosed as acinic cell carcinoma (ACC), MEC, or adenocarcinoma/cystadenocarcinoma not otherwise specified. The resemblance of MASC to ACC is particularly striking: both tumors show overlapping architectural features (microcystic, follicular, and papillary-cystic), and MASC cells can resemble many of the cell types seen in ACC (intercalated duct-like, vacuolated, clear cells) [17, 65]. Additional studies are needed to clarify whether the clinical behavior of MASC matches the tumor's low-grade histologic appearance.

MASC characteristically harbors a balanced translocation, t(12,15)(p13;q25), which results in the formation of the ETV–NTRK3 fusion gene that encodes a chimeric oncoprotein tyrosine kinase [17, 65]. The same translocation is encountered in secretory breast carcinoma, infantile fibrosarcoma, congenital mesoblastic nephroma, and sometimes myelogenous leukemia [17]. This chromosomal alteration may be detected by ETV6 break-apart FISH, or the ETV6–NTRK3 fusion transcript can be detected by RT-PCR [17, 65].

Conclusion

Expanding understanding of the pathogenesis and molecular alterations in different head and neck tumor types will allow new targets to be proposed for diagnostic, prognostic, and therapeutic applications. The multidisciplinary healthcare team needs to be familiar with molecular alterations that could be successfully integrated into diagnostic algorithms with good clinical applications.

References

1. Adelstein DJ, Koyfman SA, El-Naggar AK, Hanna EY. Biology and management of salivary gland cancers. Semin Radiat Oncol. 2012;22:245–53.
2. Adelstein DJ, Ridge JA, Gillison ML, Chaturvedi AK, D'Souza G, Gravitt PE, Westra W, Psyrri A, Kast WM, Koutsky LA, et al. Head and neck squamous cell cancer and the human papillomavirus: summary of a National Cancer Institute State of the Science Meeting, November 9-10, 2008, Washington, DC. Head Neck. 2009;31:1393–422.
3. Agrawal Y, Koch WM, Xiao W, Westra WH, Trivett AL, Symer DE, Gillison ML. Oral human papillomavirus infection before and after treatment for human papillomavirus 16-positive and human papillomavirus 16-negative head and neck squamous cell carcinoma. Clin Cancer Res. 2008;14:7143–50.
4. Andry G, Hamoir M, Locati LD, Licitra L, Langendijk JA. Management of salivary gland tumors. Expert Rev Anticancer Ther. 2012;12:1161–8.
5. Ang KK, Berkey BA, Tu X, Zhang HZ, Katz R, Hammond EH, Fu KK, Milas L. Impact of epidermal growth factor receptor expression on survival and pattern of relapse in patients with advanced head and neck carcinoma. Cancer Res. 2002;62:7350–6.
6. Ang KK, Harris J, Wheeler R, Weber R, Rosenthal DI, Nguyen-Tan PF, Westra WH, Chung CH, Jordan RC, Lu C, et al. Human papillomavirus and survival of patients with oropharyngeal cancer. N Engl J Med. 2010;363:24–35.
7. Antonescu CR, Katabi N, Zhang L, Sung YS, Seethala RR, Jordan RC, Perez-Ordonez B, Have C, Asa SL, Leong IT, et al. EWSR1-ATF1 fusion is a novel and consistent finding in hyalinizing clear-cell carcinoma of salivary gland. Genes Chromosomes Cancer. 2011;50:559–70.
8. Barbosa MS, Vass WC, Lowy DR, Schiller JT. In vitro biological activities of the E6 and E7 genes vary among human papillomaviruses of different oncogenic potential. J Virol. 1991;65:292–8.
9. Barnes L, Eveson JW, Reichart P, et al., editors. Head and neck tumours. Lyon: IARC; 2005.
10. Behboudi A, Enlund F, Winnes M, Andren Y, Nordkvist A, Leivo I, Flaberg E, Szekely L, Makitie A, Grenman R, et al. Molecular classification of mucoepidermoid carcinomas—prognostic significance of the MECT1-MAML2 fusion oncogene. Genes Chromosomes Cancer. 2006;45:470–81.
11. Bell D, El-Naggar AK. Molecular heterogeneity in mucoepidermoid carcinoma: conceptual and practical implications. Head Neck Pathol. 2013;7:23–7.
12. Bell D, Hanna EY. Salivary gland cancers: biology and molecular targets for therapy. Curr Oncol Rep. 2012;14:166–74.

13. Bell D, Hanna EY. Head and neck adenoid cystic carcinoma: what is new in biological markers and treatment? Curr Opin Otolaryngol Head Neck Surg. 2013;21:124–9.

14. Bell D, Roberts D, Karpowicz M, Hanna EY, Weber RS, El-Naggar AK. Clinical significance of Myb protein and downstream target genes in salivary adenoid cystic carcinoma. Cancer Biol Ther. 2011;12:569–73.

15. Bell D, Roberts D, Kies M, Rao P, Weber RS, El-Naggar AK. Cell type-dependent biomarker expression in adenoid cystic carcinoma: biologic and therapeutic implications. Cancer. 2010;116:5749–56.

16. Bhaijee F, Pepper DJ, Pitman KT, Bell D. New developments in the molecular pathogenesis of head and neck tumors: a review of tumor-specific fusion oncogenes in mucoepidermoid carcinoma, adenoid cystic carcinoma, and NUT midline carcinoma. Ann Diagn Pathol. 2011;15:69–77.

17. Bishop JA. Unmasking MASC: bringing to light the unique morphologic, immunohistochemical and genetic features of the newly recognized mammary analogue secretory carcinoma of salivary glands. Head Neck Pathol. 2013;7:35–9.

18. Brennan JA, Mao L, Hruban RH, Boyle JO, Eby YJ, Koch WM, Goodman SN, Sidransky D. Molecular assessment of histopathological staging in squamous-cell carcinoma of the head and neck. N Engl J Med. 1995;332:429–35.

19. Chen X, Kong W, Cai G, Zhang S, Zhang D. The expressions of K-ras in human laryngeal squamous cell carcinoma cell lines (Hep-2) and its significance. Lin Chuang Er Bi Yan Hou Ke Za Zhi. 2005; 19:417–9.

20. Coombes MM, Briggs KL, Bone JR, Clayman GL, El-Naggar AK, Dent SY. Resetting the histone code at CDKN2A in HNSCC by inhibition of DNA methylation. Oncogene. 2003;22:8902–11.

21. DeYoung MP, Johannessen CM, Leong CO, Faquin W, Rocco JW, Ellisen LW. Tumor-specific p73 up-regulation mediates p63 dependence in squamous cell carcinoma. Cancer Res. 2006;66:9362–8.

22. El-Naggar AK. Pathobiology of head and neck squamous tumorigenesis. Curr Cancer Drug Targets. 2007;7:606–12.

23. El-Naggar AK, Westra WH. p16 Expression as a surrogate marker for HPV-related oropharyngeal carcinoma: a guide for interpretative relevance and consistency. Head Neck. 2012;34:459–61.

24. Emerling BM, Akcakanat A. Targeting PI3K/mTOR signaling in cancer. Cancer Res. 2011;71:7351–9.

25. Engelman JA, Zejnullahu K, Mitsudomi T, Song Y, Hyland C, Park JO, Lindeman N, Gale CM, Zhao X, Christensen J, et al. MET amplification leads to gefitinib resistance in lung cancer by activating ERBB3 signaling. Science. 2007;316:1039–43.

26. Forastiere A, Koch W, Trotti A, Sidransky D. Head and neck cancer. N Engl J Med. 2001;345:1890–900.

27. Gan YH, Zhang S. PTEN/AKT pathway involved in histone deacetylases inhibitor induced cell growth inhibition and apoptosis of oral squamous cell carcinoma cells. Oral Oncol. 2009;45:e150–4.

28. Hirano T, Steele PE, Gluckman JL. Low incidence of point mutation at codon 12 of K-ras proto-oncogene in squamous cell carcinoma of the upper aerodigestive tract. Ann Otol Rhinol Laryngol. 1991; 100:597–9.

29. Hoa M, Davis SL, Ames SJ, Spanjaard RA. Amplification of wild-type K-ras promotes growth of head and neck squamous cell carcinoma. Cancer Res. 2002;62:7154–6.

30. Jemal A, Siegel R, Xu J, Ward E. Cancer statistics, 2010. CA Cancer J Clin. 2010;60:277–300.

31. Kalyankrishna S, Grandis JR. Epidermal growth factor receptor biology in head and neck cancer. J Clin Oncol. 2006;24:2666–72.

32. Kessis TD, Slebos RJ, Nelson WG, Kastan MB, Plunkett BS, Han SM, Lorincz AT, Hedrick L, Cho KR. Human papillomavirus 16 E6 expression disrupts the p53-mediated cellular response to DNA damage. Proc Natl Acad Sci USA. 1993;90:3988–92.

33. Kostareli E, Holzinger D, Hess J. New concepts for translational head and neck oncology: lessons from HPV-related oropharyngeal squamous cell carcinomas. Front Oncol. 2012;2:36.

34. Kreimer AR, Clifford GM, Boyle P, Franceschi S. Human papillomavirus types in head and neck squamous cell carcinomas worldwide: a systematic review. Cancer Epidemiol Biomarkers Prev. 2005;14: 467–75.

35. Leemans CR, Braakhuis BJ, Brakenhoff RH. The molecular biology of head and neck cancer. Nat Rev Cancer. 2011;11:9–22.

36. Licitra L, Perrone F, Bossi P, Suardi S, Mariani L, Artusi R, Oggionni M, Rossini C, Cantu G, Squadrelli M, et al. High-risk human papillomavirus affects prognosis in patients with surgically treated oropharyngeal squamous cell carcinoma. J Clin Oncol. 2006;24:5630–6.

37. Lindquist D, Romanitan M, Hammarstedt L, Nasman A, Dahlstrand H, Lindholm J, Onelov L, Ramqvist T, Ye W, Munck-Wikland E, et al. Human papillomavirus is a favourable prognostic factor in tonsillar cancer and its oncogenic role is supported by the expression of E6 and E7. Mol Oncol. 2007;1:350–5.

38. Luna MA. Salivary mucoepidermoid carcinoma: revisited. Adv Anat Pathol. 2006;13:293–307.

39. Lyronis ID, Baritaki S, Bizakis I, Krambovitis E, Spandidos DA. K-ras mutation, HPV infection and smoking or alcohol abuse positively correlate with esophageal squamous carcinoma. Pathol Oncol Res. 2008;14:267–73.

40. Maruya S, Issa JP, Weber RS, Rosenthal DI, Haviland JC, Lotan R, El-Naggar AK. Differential methylation status of tumor-associated genes in head and neck squamous carcinoma: incidence and potential implications. Clin Cancer Res. 2004;10:3825–30.

41. Matta A, Ralhan R. Overview of current and future biologically based targeted therapies in head and neck

squamous cell carcinoma. Head Neck Oncol. 2009;1:6.

42. McDonald JS, Jones H, Pavelic ZP, Pavelic LJ, Stambrook PJ, Gluckman JL. Immunohistochemical detection of the H-ras, K-ras, and N-ras oncogenes in squamous cell carcinoma of the head and neck. J Oral Pathol Med. 1994;23:342–6.

43. McLaughlin-Drubin ME, Munger K. Oncogenic activities of human papillomaviruses. Virus Res. 2009;143:195–208.

44. Mendelsohn J. Epidermal growth factor receptor inhibition by a monoclonal antibody as anticancer therapy. Clin Cancer Res. 1997;3:2703–7.

45. Mitani Y, Li J, Rao PH, Zhao YJ, Bell D, Lippman SM, Weber RS, Caulin C, El-Naggar AK. Comprehensive analysis of the MYB-NFIB gene fusion in salivary adenoid cystic carcinoma: incidence, variability, and clinicopathologic significance. Clin Cancer Res. 2010;16:4722–31.

46. Nordkvist A, Gustafsson H, Juberg-Ode M, Stenman G. Recurrent rearrangements of 11q14-22 in mucoepidermoid carcinoma. Cancer Genet Cytogenet. 1994;74:77–83.

47. Opitz OG, Suliman Y, Hahn WC, Harada H, Blum HE, Rustgi AK. Cyclin D1 overexpression and p53 inactivation immortalize primary oral keratinocytes by a telomerase-independent mechanism. J Clin Invest. 2001;108:725–32.

48. Pai SI, Westra WH. Molecular pathology of head and neck cancer: implications for diagnosis, prognosis, and treatment. Annu Rev Pathol. 2009;4:49–70.

49. Papadimitrakopoulou VA, Izzo J, Mao L, Keck J, Hamilton D, Shin DM, El-Naggar A, den Hollander P, Liu D, Hittelman WN, et al. Cyclin D1 and p16 alterations in advanced premalignant lesions of the upper aerodigestive tract: role in response to chemoprevention and cancer development. Clin Cancer Res. 2001;7:3127–34.

50. Persson M, Andren Y, Mark J, Horlings HM, Persson F, Stenman G. Recurrent fusion of MYB and NFIB transcription factor genes in carcinomas of the breast and head and neck. Proc Natl Acad Sci USA. 2009;106:18740–4.

51. Poage GM, Houseman EA, Christensen BC, Butler RA, Avissar-Whiting M, McClean MD, Waterboer T, Pawlita M, Marsit CJ, Kelsey KT. Global hypomethylation identifies loci targeted for hypermethylation in head and neck cancer. Clin Cancer Res. 2011; 17:3579–89.

52. Pochylski T, Kwasniewska A. Absence of point mutation in codons 12 and 13 of K-RAS oncogene in HPV-associated high grade dysplasia and squamous cell cervical carcinoma. Eur J Obstet Gynecol Reprod Biol. 2003;111:68–73.

53. Psyrri A, Yu Z, Weinberger PM, Sasaki C, Haffty B, Camp R, Rimm D, Burtness BA. Quantitative determination of nuclear and cytoplasmic epidermal growth factor receptor expression in oropharyngeal squamous cell cancer by using automated quantitative analysis. Clin Cancer Res. 2005;11:5856–62.

54. Rampias T, Sasaki C, Weinberger P, Psyrri A. E6 and E7 gene silencing and transformed phenotype of human papillomavirus 16-positive oropharyngeal cancer cells. J Natl Cancer Inst. 2009;101:412–23.

55. Richards KL, Zhang B, Baggerly KA, Colella S, Lang JC, Schuller DE, Krahe R. Genome-wide hypomethylation in head and neck cancer is more pronounced in HPV-negative tumors and is associated with genomic instability. PLoS One. 2009;4:e4941.

56. Richards L. Human papillomavirus—a powerful predictor of survival in patients with oropharyngeal cancer. Nat Rev Clin Oncol. 2010;7:481.

57. Rocco JW, Ellisen LW. p63 and p73: life and death in squamous cell carcinoma. Cell Cycle. 2006;5: 936–40.

58. Rocco JW, Leong CO, Kuperwasser N, DeYoung MP, Ellisen LW. p63 Mediates survival in squamous cell carcinoma by suppression of p73-dependent apoptosis. Cancer Cell. 2006;9:45–56.

59. Ruiz-Godoy RL, Garcia-Cuellar CM, Herrera Gonzalez NE, Suchil BL, Perez-Cardenas E, Sacnchez-Perez Y, Suarez-Roa ML, Meneses A. Mutational analysis of K-ras and Ras protein expression in larynx squamous cell carcinoma. J Exp Clin Cancer Res. 2006;25:73–8.

60. Sartor MA, Dolinoy DC, Jones TR, Colacino JA, Prince ME, Carey TE, Rozek LS. Genome-wide methylation and expression differences in HPV(+) and HPV(−) squamous cell carcinoma cell lines are consistent with divergent mechanisms of carcinogenesis. Epigenetics. 2011;6:777–87.

61. Seethala RR, Dacic S, Cieply K, Kelly LM, Nikiforova MN. A reappraisal of the MECT1/MAML2 translocation in salivary mucoepidermoid carcinomas. Am J Surg Pathol. 2010;34:1106–21.

62. Sethi S, Benninger MS, Lu M, Havard S, Worsham MJ. Noninvasive molecular detection of head and neck squamous cell carcinoma: an exploratory analysis. Diagn Mol Pathol. 2009;18:81–7.

63. Shao X, Tandon R, Samara G, Kanki H, Yano H, Close LG, Parsons R, Sato T. Mutational analysis of the PTEN gene in head and neck squamous cell carcinoma. Int J Cancer. 1998;77:684–8.

64. Shibuya K, Mathers CD, Boschi-Pinto C, Lopez AD, Murray CJ. Global and regional estimates of cancer mortality and incidence by site: II. Results for the global burden of disease 2000. BMC Cancer. 2002;2:37.

65. Skalova A, Vanecek T, Sima R, Laco J, Weinreb I, Perez-Ordonez B, Starek I, Geierova M, Simpson RH, Passador-Santos F, et al. Mammary analogue secretory carcinoma of salivary glands, containing the ETV6-NTRK3 fusion gene: a hitherto undescribed salivary gland tumor entity. Am J Surg Pathol. 2010;34:599–608.

66. Smeets SJ, Braakhuis BJ, Abbas S, Snijders PJ, Ylstra B, van de Wiel MA, Meijer GA, Leemans CR,

Brakenhoff RH. Genome-wide DNA copy number alterations in head and neck squamous cell carcinomas with or without oncogene-expressing human papillomavirus. Oncogene. 2006;25:2558–64.

67. Speight PM, Barrett AW. Salivary gland tumours. Oral Dis. 2002;8:229–40.

68. Takes RP, Rinaldo A, Rodrigo JP, Devaney KO, Fagan JJ, Ferlito A. Can biomarkers play a role in the decision about treatment of the clinically negative neck in patients with head and neck cancer? Head Neck. 2008;30:525–38.

69. Tanguay J, Weinreb I. What the EWSR1-ATF1 fusion has taught us about hyalinizing clear cell carcinoma. Head Neck Pathol. 2013;7:28–34.

70. Temam S, Kawaguchi H, El-Naggar AK, Jelinek J, Tang H, Liu DD, Lang W, Issa JP, Lee JJ, Mao L. Epidermal growth factor receptor copy number alterations correlate with poor clinical outcome in patients with head and neck squamous cancer. J Clin Oncol. 2007;25:2164–70.

71. Tinhofer I, Klinghammer K, Weichert W, Knodler M, Stenzinger A, Gauler T, Budach V, Keilholz U. Expression of amphiregulin and EGFRvIII affect outcome of patients with squamous cell carcinoma of the head and neck receiving cetuximab-docetaxel treatment. Clin Cancer Res. 2011;17:5197–204.

72. Tirado Y, Williams MD, Hanna EY, Kaye FJ, Batsakis JG, El-Naggar AK. CRTC1/MAML2 fusion transcript in high grade mucoepidermoid carcinomas of salivary and thyroid glands and Warthin's tumors: implications for histogenesis and biologic behavior. Genes Chromosomes Cancer. 2007;46:708–15.

73. Tonon G, Modi S, Wu L, Kubo A, Coxon AB, Komiya T, O'Neil K, Stover K, El-Naggar A, Griffin JD, et al. t(11;19)(q21;p13) translocation in mucoepidermoid carcinoma creates a novel fusion product that disrupts a notch signaling pathway. Nat Genet. 2003;33:208–13.

74. Wang D, Grecula JC, Gahbauer RA, Schuller DE, Jatana KR, Biancamano JD, Lang JC. p16 Gene alterations in locally advanced squamous cell carcinoma of the head and neck. Oncol Rep. 2006;15:661–5.

75. Weber A, Bellmann U, Bootz F, Wittekind C, Tannapfel A. Expression of p53 and its homologues in primary and recurrent squamous cell carcinomas of the head and neck. Int J Cancer. 2002;99:22–8.

76. Weber F, Xu Y, Zhang L, Patocs A, Shen L, Platzer P, Eng C. Microenvironmental genomic alterations and clinicopathological behavior in head and neck squamous cell carcinoma. JAMA. 2007;297:187–95.

77. Westra WH. The changing face of head and neck cancer in the 21st century: the impact of HPV on the epidemiology and pathology of oral cancer. Head Neck Pathol. 2009;3:78–81.

78. Westra WH, Taube JM, Poeta ML, Begum S, Sidransky D, Koch WM. Inverse relationship between human papillomavirus-16 infection and disruptive p53 gene mutations in squamous cell carcinoma of the head and neck. Clin Cancer Res. 2008;14:366–9.

79. Yu Z, Weinberger PM, Haffty BG, Sasaki C, Zerillo C, Joe J, Kowalski D, Dziura J, Camp RL, Rimm DL, et al. Cyclin d1 is a valuable prognostic marker in oropharyngeal squamous cell carcinoma. Clin Cancer Res. 2005;11:1160–6.

Molecular Testing in Bone and Soft Tissue Tumors

21

Brendan C. Dickson, Gino R. Somers,
and Rita A. Kandel

Introduction

Tumours of bone and soft tissue represent a
heterogenous population of relatively uncommon
neoplasms. Accurate classification is imperative
for ensuring proper treatment; this can be complicated by their rarity, frequent overlap with
other entities and limitations imposed by certain
methods of tissue sampling (e.g. needle core
biopsy). In recent decades our understanding of
the molecular pathophysiology of these entities
has rapidly expanded. Paralleling this advance, the
importance of molecular diagnostics in the diagnosis of soft tissue tumours is ostensibly greater
than any other specialty in pathology [1]. On the
precipice of a revolution in molecular diagnostics—
typified by next generation sequencing and expression array analysis—that will soon be ushered into
routine clinical use, the purpose of this chapter is
to summarize the *current* state of clinically

relevant molecular diagnostics in bone and soft
tissue pathology.

Mesenchymal tissues are not restricted to the
musculoskeletal system. Indeed, they support
every organ of the body. Discussion of organ-
based soft tissue tumours can be found within
their respective organ chapters. This chapter is
restricted to representation of those typically
found in the musculoskeletal system.

It is convenient to broadly classify bone and
soft tissue tumours based on the nature of their
underlying molecular abnormality: tumours with
specific recurrent translocations, tumours with
oncogenic mutations and tumours with nonspecific genetic findings and complex unbalanced
karyotypes [2]. In evaluating a case, it is necessary to have a unifying approach that includes
integration of the clinical, radiologic and histopathologic attributes of the tumour. The latter is
largely influenced by tumour morphology and
supported by ancillary studies such as immunohistochemistry, molecular and cytogenetic analysis, as well as other techniques (e.g. electron
microscopy and special stains). This chapter
offers a diagnostic approach to tumours of bone
and soft tissue; following the classification
scheme of the World Health Organization [3], in
which tumours are organized based on their putative cell of origin. This space does not permit an
in-depth coverage of all of the characterized
molecular alterations in bone and soft tissue
tumours so this review is predominantly focused
on molecular diagnostic tests used currently.

B.C. Dickson, M.D. (✉) • R.A. Kandel, M.D.
Department of Pathology and Laboratory Medicine
and Pathobiology, Mount Sinai Hospital, University
of Toronto, Toronto, ON, Canada M5G 1X5
e-mail: bdickson@mtsinai.on.ca;
rkandel@mtsinai.on.ca

G.R. Somers, M.D., Ph.D.
Department of Paediatric Laboratory Medicine and
Pathobiology, Hospital for Sick Children,
University of Toronto, Toronto, ON,
Canada M5G 1X8
e-mail: gino.somers@sickkids.ca

Adipocytic Tumours

Atypical Lipomatous Tumour, Well-Differentiated and Dedifferentiated Liposarcoma

Liposarcoma is the most common type of soft tissue sarcoma. It typically occurs in middle-aged adults and affects males and females equally [4, 5]. Atypical lipomatous tumour (ALT) and well-differentiated liposarcoma (WD-LPS) are synonymous, with the former term employed for extremity-based lesions [6]. Histologically, tumours are composed of sheets of adipocytes of variable size and shape. Scattered lipoblasts and enlarged hyperchromatic nuclei are typical of the 'lipoma-like variant' but can be less conspicuous in the 'sclerosing' and 'inflammatory' subtypes. Dedifferentiation (DD-LPS) more frequently occurs in the retroperitoneum and mediastinum. Histologically this is typified by spindle cells with a storiform pattern and a greater degree of pleomorphism, mitotic activity and necrosis. This heralds a more aggressive tumour with the potential for metastatic spread. The diagnosis of ALT/WD-LPS is largely based on morphology; the presence of staining for p16 by immunohisto-

chemistry is a potentially helpful adjunct [7]. The diagnosis of DD-LPS is facilitated by a history, or radiology or histologic evidence of a well-differentiated component. The immunohistochemical profile tends to be nonspecific, with variable expressions of S100, CD34 and smooth muscle actin and desmin.

The cytogenetic findings in WD-LPS and DD-LPS are similar (reviewed in [4]). One or two 'marker chromosomes' with a supernumerary ring or giant rod, containing regions of chromosome 12, may be observed [8]. Dedifferentiation may include added numbers of marker chromosomes, in addition to a greater degree of cytogenetic complexity [4]. Fluorescence in situ hybridization (FISH) and comparative genomic hybridization (CGH) consistently show amplification in the q14–15 region (Fig. 21.1). Amplification of this region results in increased cell proliferation and decreased apoptosis [4]. *MDM2* falls within this region and is almost invariably amplified [9], while other genes in this area are less consistently amplified, such as *HMGA2* and *CDK4* [4]. Immunohistochemistry is available for each of these products, but it is less sensitive and specific than FISH. FISH for

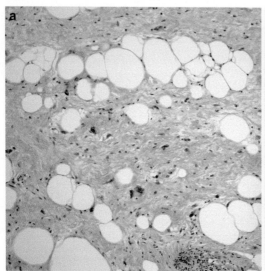
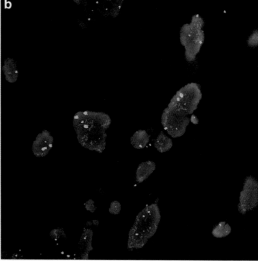

Fig. 21.1 (**a**) Haematoxylin and eosin stained section demonstrating a well-differentiated liposarcoma. (**b**) Interphase fluorescence in situ hybridization for *MDM2* showing amplification of MDM2. The spectrum orange signal is amplified *MDM2* (12q15) relative to the spectrum green cen(12) signal (Probe: LSI MDM2 CEP12, Vysis, Abbott; image courtesy Ms. M. Wood)

MDM2 amplification is now routinely used to facilitate the diagnosis of WD-LPS/DD-LPS as over 90 % of these tumours will show this alteration [10, 11]. Polymerase chain reaction (PCR)-based techniques have also been shown to be diagnostically useful [10, 12].

Myxoid/Round Cell Liposarcoma

Less common than the conventional subtype of liposarcoma, myxoid/round cell liposarcoma represents approximately 15–20 % of liposarcomas [3]. It tends to occur at a younger age, with a median of 45 years, and possible male predominance [13]. The most common location is the deep soft tissues of the extremities, with 90 % arising in the lower limb [13]. Tumours are composed of hypocellular sheets of spindle-polygonal cells with pale eosinophilic cytoplasm. The nuclei are round-ovoid and small with minimal atypia and rare mitotic activity. Scattered mono- and multi-vacuolated lipoblasts are generally readily identified. The background typically contains a 'chicken wire-like' vasculature and pools of myxoid stroma. Round cell liposarcoma is characterized by cellular areas with a high nuclear cytoplasmic ratio and lacking intervening stroma [3]. If this is greater or equal to 5 %, this feature is correlated with poorer outcome [14]. Immunohistochemistry is of limited value in confirming the diagnosis; however, over-expression of p53 is an independent predictor of poor outcome in localized disease [14].

Over 90 % of cases contain a recurrent t(12;16) (q13;p11) translocation involving *DDIT3* (formerly *CHOP*) and *TLS* (formerly *FUS*) [15]. Less commonly, cytogenetics reveal a t(12;22) (q13;q12) translocation, whereby *DDIT3* is partnered with *EWSR1*. Other structural rearrangements have also been described [16]. Diagnosis of myxoid/round cell is readily confirmed by FISH for *TLS* (and *EWS* when presented with a negative TLS result and classic histomorphology); alternatively, a *DDIT3* break-apart probe can be used to cover both forms of rearrangements [17]. *TLS* has several common variable breakpoints fusing exons 5, 7 and 8, with exon 2 of *DDIT3*; this leads to three basic transcript types: type I (7-2), type 2 (5-2) and type 3 (8-2), which do not appear to have prognostic significance [14]. Other fusion transcripts have been reported for both *FUS-DDIT3* and *EWSRI-DDIT3* [14, 18], thereby complicating use of PCR as a diagnostic method (Fig. 21.2) [17]. Of interest, this fusion product, when transfected into cells in culture, induces a myxoid liposarcoma phenotype [19, 20]. It is possible that this is accomplished via dysregulation of the nuclear factor-kappaB (NFKB) pathway through interactions with the FUS-DDIT3 product [21, 22].

Fibroblastic/Myofibroblastic Tumours

Nodular Fasciitis

Nodular fasciitis is a common and benign soft tissue tumour which can occur at any age, affecting children to the elderly, but is most common in young adults. It typically forms in the subcutis, but may present anywhere on the body, predominately in the upper limbs and head and neck region [23]. Histologically it is composed of spindle cell lesion arranged in short fascicles, in a storiform or with a patternless distribution. The cytoplasm is pale and wispy with bland ovoid nuclei showing conspicuous mitotic activity; atypical mitotic figures and pleomorphism are not a feature of nodular fasciitis. Interspersed between the cells is stroma that is variably myxoid-collagenous, scattered lymphocytes, osteoclast-like giant cells as well as extravasated erythrocytes. Immunohistochemistry generally confirms a myofibroblast-type phenotype, with expression of smooth muscle actin.

Historically, nodular fasciitis was thought to be a reactive lesion, perhaps instigated by trauma. Recently, it was found that most cases are characterized by rearrangement of *USP6* (ubiquitin-specific peptidase 6). In approximately 90 % of cases there is fusion with *MYH9* (myosin heavy chain 9, non-muscle) [23–25]. Both FISH-and PCR-based assays have proved useful as diagnostic markers for nodular fasciitis [23–25]. The translocation leads to over-expression of *USP6*, a protein shown to be involved in proliferation, inflammation and cell signalling [23].

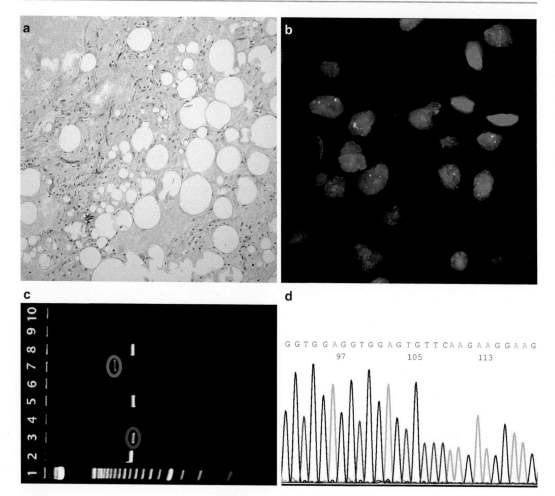

Fig. 21.2 (**a**) Haematoxylin and eosin stained section demonstrating a myxoid liposarcoma. (**b**) Interphase fluorescence in situ hybridization showing *FUS* rearrangement with a dual colour break-apart probe. Many of the cells contain both a fusion signal, where the probes are closely approximated, and a break-apart signal, where the spectrum orange and spectrum green signals are widely separated within the nucleus (Probe: LSI FUS, Vysis, Abbott; image courtesy Ms. M. Wood). (**c**) Composite image of gel electrophoresis showing representative bands positive and negative for two forms of *TLS-DDIT3* fusion transcripts: Lane 1: 25 bp ladder. Lanes 2–4: *Case 1*, *PGK* (247 bp), type II positive (245 bp), type I negative. Lanes 5–7: *Case 2*, *PGK* (247 bp), type II negative, type I positive (338 bp). Lanes 8–10: *Case 3*, *PGK* (247 bp), type I and type II negative. D. Sequencing confirming presence of type II fusion transcript: *TLS* exon 5 GGTGGAGGTGGAG//TGTTCAAGAAGGAAG*DDIT3* exon 2 (C & D courtesy Mr. D. Swanson)

Low-Grade Fibromyxoid Sarcoma

Low-grade fibromyxoid sarcoma (LGFMS) and hyalinizing spindle cell tumour with giant rosettes fall on a histologic continuum. These malignant fibroblastic tumours are rare and frequently characterized by a long clinical history prior to presentation and late metastases. They predominate in young adults (range from 2 to 70 years) [26] without an obvious sex predilection [27]. Tumours maybe deep or superficial; they are frequently located in the trunk and extremities, but can occasionally be intra-abdominal [27]. The morphology is deceptively bland, with monomorphic spindle cells showing a streaming or whorled pattern, frequently condensed along a delicate curvilinear vasculature. The nuclei are ovoid and mitotic activity is typically rare. The stroma is largely fibrous, but myxoid areas are typically present. Unusual findings, including collagen rosettes, sheets of spindle cells, pleomorphism, ossification and multinucleation are less common [27]. Tumours frequently show focal immunoreactivity for actin and epithelial membrane antigen; more recently, MUC4 has been described as specific and sensitive marker [28].

The majority of cases of LGFMS are characterized by a t(7;16)(q32–34;p11) translocation derived from fusion of *FUS* and *CREB3L2*, with a minority exhibiting a t(11;16)(p11;p11) translocation that results in the pairing of *FUS* and *CREB3L1*. Recently two cases exhibiting fusion of *EWSR1*and *CREB3L1* were described [29]. Both FISH and RT-PCR are useful diagnostic techniques for identifying this translocation. Given the possibility of multiple different fusion products, the use of commercially available EWSR1 and FUS break-apart probes represents a convenient means of diagnostic confirmation. The different fusion products do not appear to be associated with morphologic or immunohistochemical differences; at present there is insufficient information to know if the fusion product is associated with differences in clinical behaviour [29]. CREB3L2 is similar in structure and function to CREB3L1 [30]; the role of these chimaeric proteins remains unclear, but is likely related to altering transcriptional activation [31].

Inflammatory Myofibroblastic Tumour

Inflammatory myofibroblastic tumour (IMT) is a neoplasm showing (myo)fibroblastic differentiation. This tumour spans a broad demographic, ranging from prenatal to the elderly, but is most common in children with a similar frequency amongst both sexes. Tumours are not restricted by anatomic location, but most frequently involve the abdominal and chest cavities, followed by the viscera, head and neck and soft tissues. Roughly 10–30 % cases are associated with a fever and weight loss along with a number of haematologic findings [32]. Histologically, tumours generally fall into one of three basic histologic subtypes. The first resembles granulation tissue or nodular fasciitis; it contains loosely organized spindle cells set within a myxoid stroma with small vessels and a mixed inflammatory infiltrate. The second pattern is more cellular and contains fascicles of spindle cells in a variably myxoid and collagenous background. There is a diffuse inflammatory infiltrate that largely includes plasma cells and lymphocytes. Finally, the third pattern contains prominent collagen deposition resembling scar or fibromatosis, with scattered lymphocytes, plasma cells and eosinophils [3, 32]. Immunohistochemistry frequently demonstrates expression of smooth muscle actin, desmin and keratin [32]. Roughly half of the cases are positive for ALK by immunohistochemistry [32].

Approximately half of inflammatory myofibroblastic tumours contain rearrangement of the 2p23 region corresponding to the *ALK* gene [33]. Molecular diagnostic confirmation is becoming imperative given the emergence of targeted therapies based on inhibition of ALK tyrosine kinase [34]. Numerous fusion partners have been reported, including *TPM3* and *TPM4* [35], *CLTC* [14], *RANBP2* [36], *ATIC* [37], *CARS* [38], *SEC31L1* [39] and *PPFIBP* [40], with new fusion partners continually being identified. The mechanism of tumorigenesis in cases without ALK rearrangement, remains to be explained. Given the large percentage of ALK negative cases, it should be emphasized that the diagnosis frequently rests on morphologic and immunohistochemical criteria. Some fusion products have been reported to be associated with a worse prognosis, such as *RANBP2-ALK* [41]. Interestingly, at least some of these cases are associated with an epithelioid morphology; in addition, rather than showing the typical cytoplasmic pattern of ALK expression, they may be a perinuclear or nuclear membrane decoration [41]. Other molecular changes have been described in inflammatory myofibroblastic tumour, including p53 mutations and MDM2 amplification [42]. The various fusion partners are reported to share an N-terminal oligomerization motif that leads to ALK kinase catalytic activation [36].

Smooth Muscle Tumours

Currently there is no diagnostic molecular marker routinely available for smooth muscle neoplasms. It has, however, recently been demonstrated that about 70 % of uterine leiomyomas contain mutations in the mediator complex sub-unit 12 (*MED12*) gene [43]. Subsequent reports found that mutations also occurred in 7–20 % of uterine leiomyosarcoma [44, 45], implying that this test cannot be used to differentiate benign from malignant uterine smooth muscle tumours. The presence, albeit rare, of mutations in extra-uterine leiomyomas [46, 47] further suggests this cannot be used to differentiate the site of origin of smooth muscle tumours.

Skeletal Muscle Tumours

Alveolar Rhabdomyosarcoma

Alveolar rhabdomyosarcoma (ARMS) is a sar-coma that occurs predominantly in older chil-dren (median age at diagnosis 9 years) [48]. It usually presents as a mass in the extremities, although the head and neck, trunk and retroperi-toneum can also be affected [48]. The diagnosis rests upon a combination of light microscopy, immunohistochemistry and molecular diagnos-tics. The morphology has been extensively reviewed elsewhere [49, 50]; in short, ARMS comprises nests of round cells with central discohesion, peripheral palisading and a fine col-lagenous stroma. The original description emphasized the alveolar architecture and nested, discohesive pattern of the tumour cells [51]. Cells are usually round to oval hyperchromatic nuclei and scant to moderate amounts of dense eosinophilic cytoplasm. Multinucleation is com-monly seen, and solid variants of ARMS are described [49]. Immunohistochemistry shows positivity for MyoD1, myogenin (nuclear, major-ity of cells) and desmin [52, 53]. Further, certain immunohistochemical markers can be used to aid in subclassification of rhabdomyosarcoma. Diffuse myogenin, p-cadherin and AP2 beta pos-itivity are associated with ARMS, whereas EGFR, fibrillin-2 and IGF-2 expression are asso-ciated with embryonal rhabdomyosarcoma (ERMS) [54, 55].

Molecular diagnostics demonstrates a rear-rangement involving the *FOXO1* gene with a member of the *PAX* family of genes [49]. Approximately 50 % harbour a t(2;13)(q35;q14) rearrangement with the formation of a

FOXO1/PAX3 fusion gene, whereas approxi-mately 25 % will harbour a t(1;13)(p36;q14) rearrangement and a *FOXO1/PAX7* fusion gene [56]. The remaining tumours do not harbour diagnostic rearrangements and are termed 'translocation-negative' ARMSs [57, 58]. Translocation-negative ARMS has a better out-come than translocation-positive ARMS [59, 60], and some suggest that such tumours are clinically indistinguishable from ERMS [59]. Recently it has been shown that PAX3/FOXO1-positive non-metastatic patients had a significantly worse out-come than those whose tumours were either translocation negative or PAX7/FOXO1 positive. Interestingly, a 'clinicomolecular risk score' incorporating fusion gene status, TNM stage and age was a better predictor of outcome compared to the current risk-stratification scheme [60, 61]. The *PAX3/FOXO1* transcript is thought to con-tribute to tumorigenesis via pleiotropic mecha-nisms, including stimulation of cell proliferation, promotion of cell survival, suppression of differ-entiation and, perhaps, increased angiogenesis (reviewed in [62]). A recent study using gene ontology analysis of microarray data and other studies showed that the presence of the PAX3/FOXO1 translocation resulted in changes in apoptosis, cell death, development and signal transduction genes which may contribute to the worse prognosis [63, 64].

Tumours of Nerve Sheath Origin

Malignant Peripheral Nerve Sheath Tumours (MPNST)

MPNST is a malignancy that occurs predomi-nantly in adults, with 10–20 % being diagnosed in the first 2 decades of life [65]. It accounts for between 5 and 17 % of all paediatric soft tissue sarcomas [65]. Typically, MPNST occurs as a mass in the subcutaneous or deep soft tissues [65, 66], and if the patient has neurofibromatosis (NF1), it may arise in association with a pre-existing neurofibroma [66]. Risk factors for the development of MPNST include a diagnosis of NF1 and prior irradiation, and patients with NF1 generally develop MPNST 10 years earlier than non-NF1 patients [67].

The diagnosis of MPNST relies upon one or more of the following clinicopathological criteria being present: (1) the tumour arises within a peripheral nerve; (2) the tumour arises from a pre-existing benign or malignant peripheral nerve tumour; (3) the tumour arises in a patient with NF1 or (4) the tumour arises in a patient without NF1, but has the same histologic features of MPNST, and shows evidence of Schwannian or perineurial cell differentiation by immunohistochemistry or ultrastructural analysis [66]. Histologically, MPNSTs are tumours composed of spindle cells with a sheet-like architecture [66, 67]. The cells are tightly packed and nuclei are oval, tapered or wavy. Many different architectures have been noted in MPNST, and MPNST is a great mimic of other spindle cell neoplasms including fibrosarcoma and synovial sarcoma [66, 67]. Numerous morphologic subtypes of MPNST are recognized, including epithelioid, mesenchymal, perineurial, rhabdomyosarcomatous and glandular [67, 68]. Immunohistochemistry shows focal neural differentiation (S100 protein, CD57) in up to 70 % of cases, and EMA and CD34 staining may also be seen (reviewed in [65, 67]).

Molecular genetic analysis of MPNSTs has failed to show diagnostic recurrent rearrangements. However, MPNSTs are characterized by markedly complex karyotypes, encompassing multiple chromosomal losses, gains and rearrangements. Losses involving the short arms of chromosomes 1, 3, 9, 10, 11, 15, 17 and 22 have been reported, as well as loss of material on the long arms of chromosomes 11, 13, 16, 17 and 22 (reviewed in [67]). Rearrangements have been reported, most commonly involving 1p, 7p22, 11q13–23, 20q13 and 22q11–13 (reviewed in [67]). By CGH analysis, gains of 17q23–25 and 7p15–21 have been associated with a poorer prognosis [69].

The role of NF1 is intriguing. NF1 is a canonical tumour suppressor, and loss of function leads to activation of the Ras pathway [70]. This activity promotes the development of multiple peripheral nerve sheath tumours, as seen in patients with NF1 [68, 70]. Loss of the second copy of NF1 may contribute to the development of MPNST in these tumours, but additional genetic alterations are required for malignant transformation (e.g. *TP53*, *RB* and *CDCKC*) [71, 72]. Certainly, expression array studies have found a marked dysregulation of several genes when comparing MPNST to Schwann cells, with downregulation of differentiation-associated genes and upregulation of neural crest-associated proteins such as TWIST and SOX9 [73].

Tumours of Vascular Origin

Haemangioma of Bone

Haemangiomas represent an eclectic population of benign vascular neoplasms occurring throughout the body, spanning virtually the entire life cycle and without obvious sex predilection. Diagnosis is typically made on clinical-radiologic grounds and can readily be confirmed on biopsy. Occasionally, on needle core samples, the presence of obscuring adipose and fibrous tissue can complicate interpretation.

Despite their high prevalence, not much is known about their pathophysiology. Recently a t(18;22)(q23;q12) translocation bridging the *EWSR1-NFATC1* genes was identified in a case of haemangioma of bone [74]. The prevalence of this translocation in other vascular lesions remains to be determined. *NFATC1* is a member of the NFAT transcription factor family which has pleiotropic effect on cells; *EWSR1-NFATC1* chimaeras have rarely been reported in Ewing Family of Tumours [74].

Recently, through whole genome sequencing, so-called port wine stains arising within and without a background of Sturge-Weber syndrome have been linked to somatic activating mutation in *GNAQ* [75].

Epithelioid Haemangioendothelioma

Epithelioid haemangioendothelioma is a malignant vascular neoplasm that can occur at essentially any age, but which predominates in the second decade. There is no obvious sex predisposition and tumours can ostensibly arise anywhere in the body. Histologically, lesions frequently contain a prominent myxohyaline background and can arise within, or in association with a vessel.

a

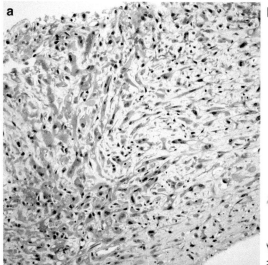

b

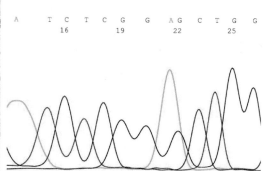

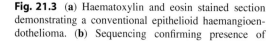

Fig. 21.3 (**a**) Haematoxylin and eosin stained section demonstrating a conventional epithelioid haemangioendothelioma. (**b**) Sequencing confirming presence of fusion transcript: *WWTR1* exon 4 ATCTCG//GAGCTGG *CAMTA1* exon 9 (courtesy Mr. D. Swanson)

The tumour is composed of individual and cords of epithelioid cells with abundant eosinophilic cytoplasm, some of which contain clear cytoplasmic vacuoles with erythrocytes. The nucleus is ovoid with mild pleomorphism and prominent nucleoli; mitotic activity is frequently conspicuous. A subset of cases may show greater atypia, well-formed vascular lumens lined by plump epithelioid cells, and nested and/or solid growth. Tumours typically express CD31, CD34, Factor VIII, ERG and FLI-1 immunoreactivity.

A recurrent t(1;3)(p36.3;q25) translocation was identified in epithelioid haemangioendothelioma [76] which results in a *WWTR1-CAMTA1* gene fusion [77, 78]. This involves fusion of exon 3 or 4 of *WWTR1* with exon 8 or 9 of *CAMTA1* [77–79]. Both break-apart FISH and RT-PCR are effective diagnostic tools for detecting the fusion (Fig. 21.3). Interestingly, recently a subset of epithelioid haemangioma showing an atypical morphology was discovered to contain a *YAP-TFE3* fusion partner [80]. Parenthetically, these tumours are readily identified using immunohistochemistry for TFE3, which is diffusely and strongly positive [80]. At present, given the limited number of cases, it is unclear whether this will translate into a difference in clinical presentation or prognosis.

Cytogenetic studies have raised the possibility of other potential fusion products, but this remains to be characterized [76, 81–83].

Angiosarcoma

Malignant vascular tumours show a wide range in morphologic findings, but are frequently characterized by vascular channels with multilayering of cells, nuclear pleomorphism, nuclear hyperchromasia and mitotic activity. Tumours can arise at any age but predominate in the elderly. Excluding discussion of Kaposi's sarcoma, which is associated with HHV8 infection, angiosarcomas may arise de novo or be associated with radiation exposure, lymphoedema or exposure to certain chemicals. Tumours are typically positive for CD31, CD34, ERG and FLI-1.

No comprehensive molecular studies have been undertaken for angiosarcoma to date [84]; hence little is known regarding the pathogenesis of tumours arising de novo in the deep soft tissues. In the head and neck region, a single case with a t(12;22) translocation involving *EWSR1-ATF1* has been reported [85]. In bone, there is a single report of a t(1;14)(p21;q24) translocation [86]. In the setting of radiation-induced angiosarcoma, MYC amplification has been detected by FISH [87].

Tumours of Cartilage

With some exceptions, tumours of cartilage show a continuum in clinical and histologic findings. The conventional spectrum includes the benign enchondroma which is a cartilaginous tumour that affects individuals at all ages and most commonly occurs in the short and long tubular bones. At the malignant end of the spectrum is chondrosarcoma, which is most common in late adulthood. It can arise secondary to enchondroma particularly in the setting of Ollier's disease, but most are primary tumours. The most common locations include the pelvis and long tubular bones. Histologically, enchondroma is hypocellular and composed of bland chondrocytes with pale eosinophilic cytoplasm and bland nuclei lacking mitotic activity. The background is avascular and composed of hyaline cartilage. The tumour does not permeate between existing bone trabeculae, and if this feature is present, the findings warrant consideration of a diagnosis of low-grade chondrosarcoma. The diagnosis of chondrosarcoma is dependent on the presence of nuclear pleomorphism, bi- or multinucleated cells and mitotic activity, the severity of which dictates the histologic grade of these tumours.

Despite their frequency, only recently are the genetic mechanisms underlying these tumours being elucidated. Mutations in the isocitrate dehydrogenase genes *IDH1* or *IDH2* have been described in roughly half of enchondromas and chondrosarcomas [88, 89]. This mutation does not occur in potential mimics, thus, when present, may permit a means of differentiation from chordoma [90] and chondroblastic osteosarcoma [91]. Whole exome sequencing has confirmed this observation, and it has further revealed mutations in *COL2A1* in 37 % of cases; in addition, mutations were confirmed in *TP53* and the RB1 and Hedgehog pathways [92]. Subtypes of chondrosarcoma have been associated with different molecular findings. For example, mesenchymal chondrosarcoma has been reported to frequently show *HEY1-NCOA2* fusion products [93, 94].

Tumours of Bone

Aneurysmal Bone Cyst

Aneurysmal bone cyst may arise de novo, or secondary to another underlying lesion such as giant cell tumour of bone. It is most common in the first 2 decades and most frequently involves the metaphysis of long bones and the spine. The name of this tumour is somewhat misleading as soft tissue variants have also been encountered; in addition, there are solid variants. Histologically, it generally consists of fibrous septae containing bland spindle cells, osteoclast-type multinucleated giant cells and osteoblasts rimming delicate woven bone surrounding cavities containing pools of blood. The diagnosis is not difficult when diagnostic imaging and adequate sampling are obtained; however, limited sampling and unusual variants can occasionally pose a diagnostic challenge.

Recurrent clonal karyotypic abnormalities have been reported in primary aneurysmal bone cyst, including a t(16;17)(q22;p13) translocation [95, 96], which involves production of a *CDH11-USP6* fusion product [97]; other reported translocations include t(1;17)(p34.1–34.3;p13), t(3;17) (q21;p13), t(5;17)(q33;p13), t(9;17)(q22;p11–12), t(11;16)(q13;q22–23) and t(17;17)(q12;p13) and t(6;13)(q15;q34) translocations [86, 87, 98–100]. Based on the fact that most translocations involve *USP6*, and a varied number of fusion partners, break-apart FISH for *USP6* would be the most diagnostically helpful.

Osteosarcoma

Osteosarcoma represents a malignant bone forming neoplasm for which numerous subtypes exist. The molecular biology of conventional subtypes is generally characterized by complex and unbalanced chromosomal abnormalities, and to date, few findings have translated into diagnostic markers. Specific subtypes have, however, limited diagnostic molecular applications. For example, parosteal osteosarcoma is associated with ring chromosomes and the majority have amplification of *MDM2* and *CDK4* [86, 87, 101, 102], which can readily be confirmed by FISH and/or immunohistochemistry. Interestingly, there is a single report of small cell osteosarcoma harbouring an *EWSR1-CREB3L1* fusion product [103].

Tumour of Uncertain Origin

Synovial Sarcoma

Synovial sarcoma occurs in older children, adolescents and young adults [104], with its incidence peaking in the third to fourth decade [105]. It usually occurs as a mass in the soft tissues of the extremities, particularly around the knee and ankle, although the upper extremity, trunk and head and neck can also be affected [105, 106]. It is not a tumour of synovium, and the name remains as a historical anachronism [107]. Microscopically, it is a sarcoma that in its classical form is biphasic, with both epithelial and mesenchymal components [105, 106]. The epithelioid portion comprises nests or glands of cuboidal or columnar cells; occasionally, such cells form a network of whorls or strands throughout the tumour [105]. Ultrastructurally, the epithelioid component has features of true epithelial differentiation, including desmosomes, microvilli and tight junctions [108]. The mesenchymal component comprises spindle cells forming sheets with scant collagen [96, 97]. Monophasic forms exist, usually composed of spindle mesenchymal cells without an epithelial component, and can mimic fibrosarcoma or malignant peripheral nerve sheath tumour [106]. SS can occur as a monophasic epithelial tumour, in which case it would be indistinguishable from adenocarcinoma without cytogenetics [106]. Other morphologic variants include myxoid, calcifying and poorly differentiated [106, 109]. The poorly differentiated form is particularly difficult to diagnose, and without coexisting foci of classical SS, requires the use of ancillary investigations for correct diagnosis. Immunohistochemistry is helpful and demonstrates focal and variable positivity for epithelial markers, including cytokeratins and EMA. Bcl-2 is usually diffusely positive, but this finding is less specific. More recently, TLE1 has been touted as a very specific marker for SS [110], with some authors suggesting positive nuclear staining may avoid the need for molecular confirmation of the presence of the fusion transcript [111]. However, others have not found a significant association between TLE1 positivity and SS [112], so the diagnostic utility of using TLE1 immunostaining rather than molecular analysis requires further study.

Molecular genetic analysis of synovial sarcoma demonstrates recurrent rearrangements involving the *SYT* gene on 18q11.2 and the SSX family of genes on Xp11.2. The latter includes *SSX1*, *SSX2* and rarely *SSX4* [104]. The biologic function of the fusion genes is not clear, although SYT has been suggested to have a role in chromatin remodelling [104, 113] and expression of various transcription factors. The SSX genes, of which there are nine recognized members, function as transcriptional repressors [114, 115]. Various studies describing gene expression profiles in synovial sarcoma have demonstrated upregulation of proteins involved in several oncologically important pathways, including *IGF*, *ERBB2* and beta-catenin (reviewed in [104]), as well as possible involvement of *NMYC* [116]. Further, constitutive expression of the chimaeric protein promotes phenotypic transformation in rat fibroblasts in culture, with a histologic appearance similar to SS [117]. The translocation type influences the histology, with SYT/SSX1 transcripts more frequently associated with the biphasic subtype and the SYT/SSX2 transcript with the monophasic subtype [118]. Prognostically, the fusion transcript subtype does not influence outcome as shown in several studies [114, 119].

Alveolar Soft Part Sarcoma

This is a very rare neoplasm that occurs across a broad age range, but predominantly affects young adults. Despite being relatively indolent, this tumour has a high rate of metastases, particularly late. Tumours are characterized histologically by small groups of cells with a nested or pseudoalveolar pattern; these are separated by thin fibrovascular septae. The cells are typically polygonal with pale cytoplasm, and the nuclei are round with macronucleoli. Periodic acid Schiff stain with diastase highlights the cytoplasmic crystals. Immunohistochemistry for desmin and S100 are occasionally positive, and there is almost always strong nuclear expression of TFE3 [120].

Tumours are defined by the presence of a typically, but not invariably, unbalanced der(17) t(X;17)(p11;q25) translocation [94, 95], resulting in a *ASPL-TFE3* fusion product [121]. This translocation is readily identified using a TFE3 breakapart probe, or via RT-PCR [122].

Clear Cell Sarcoma

Clear cell sarcoma is a malignant neoplasm with melanocytic differentiation. Tumours generally occur in young adults, without significant sex predilection, and are typically found in the deep tissues of the extremities [123]; however, unusual locations such as the trachea, skin, gastrointestinal tract and kidney occur. Histologically, tumours generally have a nested pattern of growth of spindle-epithelioid cells with hyalinized collagen interspersed between groups of tumour. The cytoplasm is often amphophilic and the nuclei monomorphic with macronucleoli. Scattered multinucleated giant cells are a frequent finding. Immunohistochemistry is almost invariably positive for S100, HMB45, MART-1 and MiTF, making molecular analysis critical for differentiation from melanoma.

Tumours are characterized by reciprocal t(12;22)(q13;q13) translocations [94, 95, 124]. This leads to the formation of a *EWSR1-ATF1* fusion product [125–127]. Exons 8, 7 and 10 of *EWSR1* have been reported to fuse with exon 4 or 5 of *ATF1* (the pubmed ID is stated in the text) 18300804. More recently, *EWSR1-CREB1* fusion products have been described for clear cell in clear cell sarcomas arising in both the soft tissues and gastrointestinal locations [123, 128, 129]. RT-PCR remains an excellent means of diagnosing this tumour [129, 130]. Given the presence of multiple fusion partners, fluorescence in situ hybridization with a break-apart EWSR1 probe is convenient. The fusion type does not appear to be associated with outcome [123, 130]. Expression of the *EWS/ATF1* fusion product in a murine model has been shown to generate tumours similar to those arising spontaneously in humans [131].

Extraskeletal Myxoid Chondrosarcoma

Despite its name, extraskeletal myxoid chondrosarcoma is not of chondrocytic derivation [132]. Indeed, recent cases have been described as arising from bone [133], rather than the more typical deep soft tissues; less commonly it has been reported as arising in the joint space and intracranially. Patients are typically adults without a consistent sex predisposition [134, 135]. Tumours are aggressive, with a high rate of metastasis on presentation and follow-up, in addition to frequent local recurrence [135]. Tumours may show a range of morphologies. The most common is cells arranged in chains, nests or filigree-like, with a lobular pattern; however, cellular lesions have been reported. The cells are usually small and round-spindle shaped. They are set within a chondromyxoid stroma, but lack actual hyaline cartilage. A consistent immunophenotype is not present, but S100, epithelial membrane antigen, synaptophysin and chromogranin are often positive [136]. Of note, in cases with a rhabdoid morphology, INI-1 expression may be lost [137].

Cytogenetic analysis has revealed a t(9;22) (q22;q12) in a majority of cases [138]. This involves rearrangement of *NR4A3* with *EWSR1*. As a result, FISH, using commercially available EWSR1 break-apart probe, is a useful diagnostic marker [139], in addition to RT-PCR. There are, however, additional fusion products that do not involve EWS. For example, t(9;17)(q22;q11) [140] and t(9;15)(q22;q21) [141] translocations were subsequently described. Secondary structural abnormalities are a common feature on cytogenetic analysis [142]. The latter tumours respectively partner *NR4A3* [143] with *TAF15* and *TCF12* [141]. There are commercially available *NR4A3* break-apart probes which help broaden the sensitivity of FISH for this diagnosis. An unusual case of a sarcoma with dual morphologic and molecular features of synovial sarcoma and extraskeletal myxoid chondrosarcoma has been described [144].

Conclusion

Molecular diagnostics—particularly molecular cytogenetics [1] and reverse transcriptase PCR [145]—is now an essential adjunct in the routine characterization of bone and soft tissue tumours. Both techniques can be applied to both fresh frozen and formalin-fixed paraffin-embedded tissues and generally show similar, although not identical, sensitivity and specificity. Fluorescence in situ hybridization break-apart probes have the advantage of allowing detection of tumours possessing multiple possible breakpoints, but the disadvantage of not being able to identify the partner. For example, FISH using an EWSR1 break-apart probe would not be able to differentiate a case of Ewing Family of tumours from extraskeletal myxoid chondrosarcoma, myxoid liposarcoma and/or desmoplastic small round cell tumour harbouring an EWSR1 fusion partner. RT-PCR permits confirmation of the fusion partner, which is arguably of greater diagnostic value. However, one limitation is that the partner must be known, so this method cannot be used in gene discovery. Again, however, there may be cases where the fusion partner is identical in two distinct tumours, thereby precluding differentiation (e.g. clear cell sarcoma and angiomatoid fibrous histiocytoma). For this reason histology, to date, remains the 'gold standard', and molecular diagnostics supplements the morphologic and immunohistochemical attributes of bone and soft tissue tumours [145].

Sanger sequencing is another approach to detecting molecular alterations and is used clinically in the characterization of certain tumour types such as gastrointestinal stromal tumours (covered in Chap. 22), which most commonly are part of companion testing for therapeutic agents. Advances in sequencing methods and the need for less expensive techniques have driven the development of the next generation of sequencing methods (NGS, 'next gen sequencing') [146]. NGS platforms perform massively parallel sequencing during which millions of fragments of DNA, for example, are sequenced at once. This facilitates high throughput sequencing as well as automation, both of which have led to the development of rapid, low cost sequencing that has moved this methodology into clinical diagnostics. The Human Genome Project cost about $3 billion; currently we can sequence a human genome for about $1000 and the price is dropping. NGS approaches include sequencing the whole genome and whole exome, and with the use of RNA-seq also provide microRNA or gene

expression profiling [147]. These methods will allow detection of nucleotide substitutions (point mutations), small insertions and deletions, copy-number alterations and chromosomal translocations and may obviate the use of other methods such as array CGH, SNP arrays and microarrays. Importantly NGS likely is better than Sanger sequencing as it has the potential to provide a deeper characterization of the molecular landscape. A recent study by Marchetti et al. [148] showed that using NGS to re-evaluate lung cancer samples analyzed previously by Sanger sequencing could identify a more complex pattern of EGFR deletions than the current gold standard sequencing method. We are just beginning to appreciate the power of these methods. Recently Beck et al. used expression profiling and aCGH to identify three subtypes of leiomyosarcoma that had distinct genomic changes that allowed for the identification of prognostic biomarkers [149]. Another study from Coindre's group identified two subtypes of leiomyosarcomas and was able to show that molecular profiling using the gene expression signature they developed based on genomic complexity (CINSARC) was prognostic [150, 151]. As the methods are developed to extract DNA and RNA from paraffin-embedded tissues suitable for use in these advanced molecular methods, the translation of advancing sequencing methods into routine diagnostics is inevitable. As NGS can be applied to cytology specimens, it is possible to see how the practice of sarcoma pathology will change [152]. Sequencing, either as targeted panels or more extensively, will allow the application of individualized medicine to those afflicted with soft tissue or bone tumours, and the pathologist will play an important role in the delivery of this care.

References

1. Tanas MR, Rubin BP, Tubbs RR, Billings SD, Downs-Kelly E, Goldblum JR. Utilization of fluorescence in situ hybridization in the diagnosis of 230 mesenchymal neoplasms: an institutional experience. Arch Pathol Lab Med. 2010;134(12):1797–803.
2. Antonescu CR. The role of genetic testing in soft tissue sarcoma. Histopathology. 2006;48(1):13–21.

3. Fletcher CDM, World Health Organization, International Agency for Research on Cancer. WHO classification of tumours of soft tissue and bone. 4th ed. Lyon: IARC Press; 2013.

4. Coindre JM, Pedeutour F, Aurias A. Well-differentiated and dedifferentiated liposarcomas. Virchows Arch. 2010;456(2):167–79.

5. Dalal KM, Antonescu CR, Singer S. Diagnosis and management of lipomatous tumors. J Surg Oncol. 2008;97(4):298–313.

6. Evans HL, Soule EH, Winkelmann RK. Atypical lipoma, atypical intramuscular lipoma, and well-differentiated retroperitoneal liposarcoma: a reappraisal of 30 cases formerly classified as well differentiated liposarcoma. Cancer. 1979;43(2):574–84.

7. He M, Aisner S, Benevenia J, Patterson F, Aviv H, Hameed M. p16 immunohistochemistry as an alternative marker to distinguish atypical lipomatous tumor from deep-seated lipoma. Appl Immunohistochem Mol Morphol. 2009;17(1):51–6.

8. Pedeutour F, Suijkerbuijk RF, Forus A, Van Gaal J, Van de Klundert W, Coindre JM, et al. Complex composition and co-amplification of SAS and MDM2 in ring and giant rod marker chromosomes in well-differentiated liposarcoma. Genes Chromosom Cancer. 1994;10(2):85–94.

9. Oliner JD, Kinzler KW, Meltzer PS, George DL, Vogelstein B. Amplification of a gene encoding a p53-associated protein in human sarcomas. Nature. 1992;358(6381):80–3.

10. Sirvent N, Coindre JM, Maire G, Hostein I, Keslair F, Guillou L, et al. Detection of MDM2-CDK4 amplification by fluorescence in situ hybridization in 200 paraffin-embedded tumor samples: utility in diagnosing adipocytic lesions and comparison with immunohistochemistry and real-time PCR. Am J Surg Pathol. 2007;31(10):1476–89.

11. Weaver J, Rao P, Goldblum JR, Joyce MJ, Turner SL, Lazar AJ, et al. Can MDM2 analytical tests performed on core needle biopsy be relied upon to diagnose well-differentiated liposarcoma? Mod Pathol. 2010;23(10):1301–6.

12. Shimada S, Ishizawa T, Ishizawa K, Matsumura T, Hasegawa T, Hirose T. The value of MDM2 and CDK4 amplification levels using real-time polymerase chain reaction for the differential diagnosis of liposarcomas and their histologic mimickers. Hum Pathol. 2006;37(9):1123–9.

13. Moreau LC, Turcotte R, Ferguson P, Wunder J, Clarkson P, Masri B, et al. Myxoid\round cell liposarcoma (MRCLS) revisited: an analysis of 418 primarily managed cases. Ann Surg Oncol. 2012;19(4):1081–8.

14. Bridge JA, Kanamori M, Ma Z, Pickering D, Hill DA, Lydiatt W, et al. Fusion of the ALK gene to the clathrin heavy chain gene, CLTC, in inflammatory myofibroblastic tumor. Am J Pathol. 2001;159(2):411–5.

15. Lopez-Gines C, Navarro S, Peydro-Olaya A, Pellin A, Llombart-Bosch A. Malignant myxoid liposarcoma: an immunohistochemical, electron-microscopical and cytogenetical analysis. Appl Pathol. 1989;7(5):285–93.

16. Mrozek K, Szumigala J, Brooks JS, Crossland DM, Karakousis CP, Bloomfield CD. Round cell liposarcoma with the insertion (12;16)(q13;p11.2p13). Am J Clin Pathol. 1997;108(1):35–9.

17. Narendra S, Valente A, Tull J, Zhang S. DDIT3 gene break-apart as a molecular marker for diagnosis of myxoid liposarcoma—assay validation and clinical experience. Diagn Mol Pathol. 2011;20(4):218–24.

18. Powers MP, Wang WL, Hernandez VS, Patel KS, Lev DC, Lazar AJ, et al. Detection of myxoid liposarcoma-associated FUS-DDIT3 rearrangement variants including a newly identified breakpoint using an optimized RT-PCR assay. Mod Pathol. 2010;23(10):1307–15.

19. Riggi N, Cironi L, Provero P, Suva ML, Stehle JC, Baumer K, et al. Expression of the FUS-CHOP fusion protein in primary mesenchymal progenitor cells gives rise to a model of myxoid liposarcoma. Cancer Res. 2006;66(14):7016–23.

20. Engstrom K, Willen H, Kabjorn-Gustafsson C, Andersson C, Olsson M, Goransson M, et al. The myxoid/round cell liposarcoma fusion oncogene FUS-DDIT3 and the normal DDIT3 induce a liposarcoma phenotype in transfected human fibrosarcoma cells. Am J Pathol. 2006;168(5):1642–53.

21. Goransson M, Andersson MK, Forni C, Stahlberg A, Andersson C, Olofsson A, et al. The myxoid liposarcoma FUS-DDIT3 fusion oncoprotein deregulates NF-kappaB target genes by interaction with NFKBIZ. Oncogene. 2009;28(2):270–8.

22. Willems SM, Schrage YM, Bruijn IH, Szuhai K, Hogendoorn PC, Bovee JV. Kinome profiling of myxoid liposarcoma reveals NF-kappaB-pathway kinase activity and casein kinase II inhibition as a potential treatment option. Mol Cancer. 2010;9:257.

23. Erickson-Johnson MR, Chou MM, Evers BR, Roth CW, Seys AR, Jin L, et al. Nodular fasciitis: a novel model of transient neoplasia induced by MYH9-USP6 gene fusion. Lab Invest. 2011;91(10):1427–33.

24. Swanson DB, Cohen E, Ramyar L, Kandel RA, Dickson BC. MYH9-USP6 fusion transcript in nodular fasciitis: an institutional review. Mod Pathol. 2012;25(S2):20A.

25. Amary MF, Ye H, Berisha F, Tirabosco R, Presneau N, Flanagan AM. Detection of USP6 gene rearrangement in nodular fasciitis: an important diagnostic tool. Virchows Arch. 2013;463(1):97–8.

26. Billings SD, Giblen G, Fanburg-Smith JC. Superficial low-grade fibromyxoid sarcoma (Evans tumor): a clinicopathologic analysis of 19 cases with a unique observation in the pediatric population. Am J Surg Pathol. 2005;29(2):204–10.

27. Evans HL. Low-grade fibromyxoid sarcoma: a clinicopathologic study of 33 cases with long-term follow-up. Am J Surg Pathol. 2011;35(10):1450–62.

28. Doyle LA, Moller E, Dal Cin P, Fletcher CD, Mertens F, Hornick JL. MUC4 is a highly sensitive

and specific marker for low-grade fibromyxoid sarcoma. Am J Surg Pathol. 2011;35(5):733–41.

29. Lau PP, Lui PC, Lau GT, Yau DT, Cheung ET, Chan JK. EWSR1-CREB3L1 gene fusion: a novel alternative molecular aberration of low-grade fibromyxoid sarcoma. Am J Surg Pathol. 2013;37(5):734–8.

30. Mertens F, Fletcher CD, Antonescu CR, Coindre JM, Colecchia M, Domanski HA, et al. Clinicopathologic and molecular genetic characterization of low-grade fibromyxoid sarcoma, and cloning of a novel FUS/CREB3L1 fusion gene. Lab Invest. 2005;85(3):408–15.

31. Storlazzi CT, Mertens F, Nascimento A, Isaksson M, Wejde J, Brosjo O, et al. Fusion of the FUS and BBF2H7 genes in low grade fibromyxoid sarcoma. Hum Mol Genet. 2003;12(18):2349–58.

32. Coffin CM, Watterson J, Priest JR, Dehner LP. Extrapulmonary inflammatory myofibroblastic tumor (inflammatory pseudotumor). A clinicopathologic and immunohistochemical study of 84 cases. Am J Surg Pathol. 1995;19(8):859–72.

33. Griffin CA, Hawkins AL, Dvorak C, Henkle C, Ellingham T, Perlman EJ. Recurrent involvement of 2p23 in inflammatory myofibroblastic tumors. Cancer Res. 1999;59(12):2776–80.

34. Butrynski JE, D'Adamo DR, Hornick JL, Dal Cin P, Antonescu CR, Jhanwar SC, et al. Crizotinib in ALK-rearranged inflammatory myofibroblastic tumor. N Engl J Med. 2010;363(18):1727–33.

35. Lawrence B, Perez-Atayde A, Hibbard MK, Rubin BP, Dal Cin P, Pinkus JL, et al. TPM3-ALK and TPM4-ALK oncogenes in inflammatory myofibroblastic tumors. Am J Pathol. 2000;157(2):377–84.

36. Ma Z, Hill DA, Collins MH, Morris SW, Sumegi J, Zhou M, et al. Fusion of ALK to the Ran-binding protein 2 (RANBP2) gene in inflammatory myofibroblastic tumor. Genes Chromosom Cancer. 2003;37(1):98–105.

37. Debiec-Rychter M, Marynen P, Hagemeijer A, Pauwels P. ALK-ATIC fusion in urinary bladder inflammatory myofibroblastic tumor. Genes Chromosom Cancer. 2003;38(2):187–90.

38. Debelenko LV, Arthur DC, Pack SD, Helman LJ, Schrump DS, Tsokos M. Identification of CARS-ALK fusion in primary and metastatic lesions of an inflammatory myofibroblastic tumor. Lab Invest. 2003;83(9):1255–65.

39. Panagopoulos I, Nilsson T, Domanski HA, Isaksson M, Lindblom P, Mertens F, et al. Fusion of the SEC31L1 and ALK genes in an inflammatory myofibroblastic tumor. Int J Cancer. 2006;118(5):1181–6.

40. Takeuchi K, Soda M, Togashi Y, Sugawara E, Hatano S, Asaka R, et al. Pulmonary inflammatory myofibroblastic tumor expressing a novel fusion, PPFIBP1-ALK: reappraisal of anti-ALK immunohistochemistry as a tool for novel ALK fusion identification. Clin Cancer Res. 2011;17(10):3341–8.

41. Marino-Enriquez A, Wang WL, Roy A, Lopez-Terrada D, Lazar AJ, Fletcher CD, et al. Epithelioid inflammatory myofibroblastic sarcoma: an aggressive intra-abdominal variant of inflammatory myofibroblastic tumor with nuclear membrane or perinuclear ALK. Am J Surg Pathol. 2011;35(1):135–44.

42. Yamamoto H, Oda Y, Saito T, Sakamoto A, Miyajima K, Tamiya S, et al. p53 mutation and MDM2 amplification in inflammatory myofibroblastic tumours. Histopathology. 2003;42(5):431–9.

43. Makinen N, Mehine M, Tolvanen J, Kaasinen E, Li Y, Lehtonen HJ, et al. MED12, the mediator complex subunit 12 gene, is mutated at high frequency in uterine leiomyomas. Science. 2011;334(6053):252–5.

44. Perot G, Croce S, Ribeiro A, Lagarde P, Velasco V, Neuville A, et al. MED12 alterations in both human benign and malignant uterine soft tissue tumors. PLoS One. 2012;7(6):e40015.

45. Kampjarvi K, Makinen N, Kilpivaara O, Arola J, Heinonen HR, Bohm J, et al. Somatic MED12 mutations in uterine leiomyosarcoma and colorectal cancer. Br J Cancer. 2012;107(10):1761–5.

46. Ravegnini G, Marino-Enriquez A, Slater J, Eilers G, Wang Y, Zhu M, et al. MED12 mutations in leiomyosarcoma and extrauterine leiomyoma. Mod Pathol. 2013;26(5):743–9.

47. Markowski DN, Huhle S, Nimzyk R, Stenman G, Loning T, Bullerdiek J. MED12 mutations occurring in benign and malignant mammalian smooth muscle tumors. Genes Chromosom Cancer. 2013;52(3):297–304.

48. Newton Jr WA, Soule EH, Hamoudi AB, Reiman HM, Shimada H, Beltangady M, et al. Histopathology of childhood sarcomas, Intergroup Rhabdomyosarcoma Studies I and II: clinicopathologic correlation. J Clin Oncol. 1988;6(1):67–75.

49. Parham DM, Barr FG. Alveolar rhabdomyosarcoma. In: Fletcher CD, Unni KK, Mertens F, editors. World Health Organization classification of tumours: tumours of soft tissue and bone. Lyon: IARC Press; 2002. p. 150–2.

50. Kempson RL, Fletcher CDM, Evans HL, Hendrickson MR, Sibley RK. Tumors of the soft tissues. 3rd edn. In: Rosai J, Sobin LH, editors. Washington, DC: Armed Forces Institute of Pathology; 2001. ISBN 1881041603.

51. Raney RB, Oberlin O, Parham DM. An English Translation of Joseph Luc Riopelle, MD, (Hotel-Dieu of Montreal), and Jean Paul Theriault (Hopital General of Verdun, Quebec, Canada): Sur une forme meconnue de sarcome des parties molles: le rhabdomyosarcome alveolaire (concerning an unrecognized form of sarcoma of the soft tissues: alveolar rhabdomyosarcoma). annales d'anatomie pathologique 1956;1:88–111. Pediatr Dev Pathol. 2012;15(5):407–16.

52. Heerema-McKenney A, Wijnaendts LC, Pulliam JF, Lopez-Terrada D, McKenney JK, Zhu S, et al. Diffuse myogenin expression by immunohistochemistry is an independent marker of poor survival in pediatric rhabdomyosarcoma: a tissue microarray study of 71 primary tumors including correlation with molecular phenotype. Am J Surg Pathol. 2008;32(10):1513–22.

53. Cessna MH, Zhou H, Perkins SL, Tripp SR, Layfield L, Daines C, et al. Are myogenin and myoD1 expression specific for rhabdomyosarcoma? A study of 150 cases, with emphasis on spindle cell mimics. Am J Surg Pathol. 2001;25(9):1150–7.

54. Wachtel M, Runge T, Leuschner I, Stegmaier S, Koscielniak E, Treuner J, et al. Subtype and prognostic classification of rhabdomyosarcoma by immunohistochemistry. J Clin Oncol. 2006;24(5):816–22.

55. Morotti RA, Nicol KK, Parham DM, Teot LA, Moore J, Hayes J, et al. An immunohistochemical algorithm to facilitate diagnosis and subtyping of rhabdomyosarcoma: the Children's Oncology Group experience. Am J Surg Pathol. 2006;30(8):962–8.

56. Parham DM, Alaggio R, Coffin CM. Myogenic tumors in children and adolescents. Pediatr Dev Pathol. 2012;15(1 Suppl):211–38.

57. Sorensen PH, Lynch JC, Qualman SJ, Tirabosco R, Lim JF, Maurer HM, et al. PAX3-FKHR and PAX7-FKHR gene fusions are prognostic indicators in alveolar rhabdomyosarcoma: a report from the children's oncology group. J Clin Oncol. 2002;20(11):2672–9.

58. Barr FG, Qualman SJ, Macris MH, Melnyk N, Lawlor ER, Strzelecki DM, et al. Genetic heterogeneity in the alveolar rhabdomyosarcoma subset without typical gene fusions. Cancer Res. 2002;62(16):4704–10.

59. Williamson D, Missiaglia E, de Reynies A, Pierron G, Thuille B, Palenzuela G, et al. Fusion gene-negative alveolar rhabdomyosarcoma is clinically and molecularly indistinguishable from embryonal rhabdomyosarcoma. J Clin Oncol. 2010;28(13):2151–8.

60. Stegmaier S, Poremba C, Schaefer KL, Leuschner I, Kazanowska B, Bekassy AN, et al. Prognostic value of PAX-FKHR fusion status in alveolar rhabdomyosarcoma: a report from the cooperative soft tissue sarcoma study group (CWS). Pediatr Blood Cancer. 2011;57(3):406–14.

61. Missiaglia E, Williamson D, Chisholm J, Wirapati P, Pierron G, Petel F, et al. PAX3/FOXO1 fusion gene status is the key prognostic molecular marker in rhabdomyosarcoma and significantly improves current risk stratification. J Clin Oncol. 2012;30(14):1670–7.

62. Linardic CM. PAX3-FOXO1 fusion gene in rhabdomyosarcoma. Cancer Lett. 2008;270(1):10–8.

63. Lae M, Ahn EH, Mercado GE, Chuai S, Edgar M, Pawel BR, et al. Global gene expression profiling of PAX-FKHR fusion-positive alveolar and PAX-FKHR fusion-negative embryonal rhabdomyosarcomas. J Pathol. 2007;212(2):143–51.

64. Ahn EH, Mercado GE, Lae M, Ladanyi M. Identification of target genes of PAX3-FOXO1 in alveolar rhabdomyosarcoma. Oncol Rep. 2013; 30(2):968–78.

65. Cates JM, Coffin CM. Neurogenic tumors of soft tissue. Pediatr Dev Pathol. 2012;15(1 Suppl):62–107.

66. Scheithauer BW, Woodruff J, Erlandson RA. Tumors of the peripheral nervous system. Washington, DC: Armed Forces Institute of Pathology; 1999.

67. Guillou L, Aurias A. Soft tissue sarcomas with complex genomic profiles. Virchows Arch. 2010;456(2):201–17.

68. Grobmyer SR, Reith JD, Shahlaee A, Bush CH, Hochwald SN. Malignant Peripheral Nerve Sheath Tumor: molecular pathogenesis and current management considerations. J Surg Oncol. 2008;97(4):340–9.

69. Schmidt H, Wurl P, Taubert H, Meye A, Bache M, Holzhausen HJ, et al. Genomic imbalances of 7p and 17q in malignant peripheral nerve sheath tumors are clinically relevant. Genes Chromosomes Cancer. 1999;25(3):205–11.

70. Theos A, Korf BR. Pathophysiology of neurofibromatosis type 1. Ann Intern Med. 2006;144(11):842–9.

71. Kourea HP, Cordon-Cardo C, Dudas M, Leung D, Woodruff JM. Expression of p27(kip) and other cell cycle regulators in malignant peripheral nerve sheath tumors and neurofibromas: the emerging role of p27(kip) in malignant transformation of neurofibromas. Am J Pathol. 1999;155(6):1885–91.

72. Nielsen GP, Stemmer-Rachamimov AO, Ino Y, Moller MB, Rosenberg AE, Louis DN. Malignant transformation of neurofibromas in neurofibromatosis 1 is associated with CDKN2A/p16 inactivation. Am J Pathol. 1999;155(6):1879–84.

73. Miller SJ, Rangwala F, Williams J, Ackerman P, Kong S, Jegga AG, et al. Large-scale molecular comparison of human schwann cells to malignant peripheral nerve sheath tumor cell lines and tissues. Cancer Res. 2006;66(5):2584–91.

74. Arbajian E, Magnusson L, Brosjo O, Wejde J, Folpe AL, Nord KH, et al. A benign vascular tumor with a new fusion gene: EWSR1-NFATC1 in hemangioma of the bone. Am J Surg Pathol. 2013;37(4):613–6.

75. Shirley MD, Tang H, Gallione CJ, Baugher JD, Frelin LP, Cohen B, et al. Sturge-Weber syndrome and port-wine stains caused by somatic mutation in GNAQ. N Engl J Med. 2013;368(21):1971–9.

76. Mendlick MR, Nelson M, Pickering D, Johansson SL, Seemayer TA, Neff JR, et al. Translocation t(1;3)(p36.3;q25) is a nonrandom aberration in epithelioid hemangioendothelioma. Am J Surg Pathol. 2001;25(5):684–7.

77. Errani C, Zhang L, Sung YS, Hajdu M, Singer S, Maki RG, et al. A novel WWTR1-CAMTA1 gene fusion is a consistent abnormality in epithelioid hemangioendothelioma of different anatomic sites. Genes Chromosom Cancer. 2011;50(8):644–53.

78. Tanas MR, Sboner A, Oliveira AM, Erickson-Johnson MR, Hespelt J, Hanwright PJ, et al. Identification of a disease-defining gene fusion in epithelioid hemangioendothelioma. Sci Transl Med. 2011;3(98):98ra82.

79. Errani C, Sung YS, Zhang L, Healey JH, Antonescu CR. Monoclonality of multifocal epithelioid hemangioendothelioma of the liver by analysis of WWTR1-CAMTA1 breakpoints. Cancer Genet. 2012;205(1–2): 12–7.

80. Antonescu CR, Le Loarer F, Mosquera JM, Sboner A, Zhang L, Chen CL, et al. Novel YAP1-TFE3 fusion defines a distinct subset of epithelioid hemangioendothelioma. Genes Chromosom Cancer. 2013; 52(8):775–84.

81. Boudousquie AC, Lawce HJ, Sherman R, Olson S, Magenis RE, Corless CL. Complex translocation [7;22] identified in an epithelioid hemangioendothelioma. Cancer Genet Cytogenet. 1996;92(2):116–21.

82. Rogatto SR, Rainho CA, Zhang ZM, Figueiredo F, Barbieri-Neto J, Georgetto SM, et al. Hemangioendothelioma of bone in a patient with a constitutional supernumerary marker. Cancer Genet Cytogenet. 1999;110(1):23–7.

83. He M, Das K, Blacksin M, Benevenia J, Hameed M. A translocation involving the placental growth factor gene is identified in an epithelioid hemangioendothelioma. Cancer Genet Cytogenet. 2006;168(2):150–4.

84. Young RJ, Brown NJ, Reed MW, Hughes D, Woll PJ. Angiosarcoma. Lancet Oncol. 2010;11(10):983–91.

85. Gru AA, Becker N, Pfeifer JD. Angiosarcoma of the parotid gland with a t(12;22) translocation creating a EWSR1-ATF1 fusion: a diagnostic dilemma. J Clin Pathol. 2013;66(5):452–4.

86. Dunlap JB, Magenis RE, Davis C, Himoe E, Mansoor A. Cytogenetic analysis of a primary bone angiosarcoma. Cancer Genet Cytogenet. 2009;194(1):1–3.

87. Mentzel T, Schildhaus HU, Palmedo G, Buttner R, Kutzner H. Postradiation cutaneous angiosarcoma after treatment of breast carcinoma is characterized by MYC amplification in contrast to atypical vascular lesions after radiotherapy and control cases: clinicopathological, immunohistochemical and molecular analysis of 66 cases. Mod Pathol. 2012;25(1):75–85.

88. Amary MF, Bacsi K, Maggiani F, Damato S, Halai D, Berisha F, et al. IDH1 and IDH2 mutations are frequent events in central chondrosarcoma and central and periosteal chondromas but not in other mesenchymal tumours. J Pathol. 2011;224(3):334–43.

89. Pansuriya TC, van Eijk R, d'Adamo P, van Ruler MA, Kuijjer ML, Oosting J, et al. Somatic mosaic IDH1 and IDH2 mutations are associated with enchondroma and spindle cell hemangioma in Ollier disease and Maffucci syndrome. Nat Genet. 2011;43(12):1256–61.

90. Arai M, Nobusawa S, Ikota H, Takemura S, Nakazato Y. Frequent IDH1/2 mutations in intracranial chondrosarcoma: a possible diagnostic clue for its differentiation from chordoma. Brain Tumor Pathol. 2012;29(4):201–6.

91. Kerr DA, Lopez HU, Deshpande V, Hornicek FJ, Duan Z, Zhang Y, et al. Molecular distinction of chondrosarcoma from chondroblastic osteosarcoma through IDH1/2 mutations. Am J Surg Pathol. 2013; 37(6):787–95.

92. Tarpey PS, Behjati S, Cooke SL, Van Loo P, Wedge DC, Pillay N, et al. Frequent mutation of the major cartilage collagen gene COL2A1 in chondrosarcoma. Nat Genet. 2013;45(8):923–6. PubMed PMID: 23770606.

93. Wang L, Motoi T, Khanin R, Olshen A, Mertens F, Bridge J, et al. Identification of a novel, recurrent HEY1-NCOA2 fusion in mesenchymal chondrosarcoma based on a genome-wide screen of exon-level expression data. Genes Chromosom Cancer. 2012; 51(2):127–39.

94. Nyquist KB, Panagopoulos I, Thorsen J, Haugom L, Gorunova L, Bjerkehagen B, et al. Whole-transcriptome sequencing identifies novel IRF2BP2-CDX1 fusion gene brought about by translocation t(1;5)(q42;q32) in mesenchymal chondrosarcoma. PLoS One. 2012;7(11):e49705.

95. Panoutsakopoulos G, Pandis N, Kyriazoglou I, Gustafson P, Mertens F, Mandahl N. Recurrent t(16;17)(q22;p13) in aneurysmal bone cysts. Genes Chromosom Cancer. 1999;26(3):265–6.

96. Sciot R, Dorfman H, Brys P, Dal Cin P, De Wever I, Fletcher CD, et al. Cytogenetic-morphologic correlations in aneurysmal bone cyst, giant cell tumor of bone and combined lesions. A report from the CHAMP study group. Mod Pathol. 2000;13(11):1206–10.

97. Oliveira AM, Hsi BL, Weremowicz S, Rosenberg AE, Dal Cin P, Joseph N, et al. USP6 (Tre2) fusion oncogenes in aneurysmal bone cyst. Cancer Res. 2004;64(6):1920–3.

98. Dal Cin P, Kozakewich HP, Goumnerova L, Mankin HJ, Rosenberg AE, Fletcher JA. Variant translocations involving 16q22 and 17p13 in solid variant and extraosseous forms of aneurysmal bone cyst. Genes Chromosom Cancer. 2000;28(2):233–4.

99. Nielsen GP, Fletcher CD, Smith MA, Rybak L, Rosenberg AE. Soft tissue aneurysmal bone cyst: a clinicopathologic study of five cases. Am J Surg Pathol. 2002;26(1):64–9.

100. Oliveira AM, Perez-Atayde AR, Dal Cin P, Gebhardt MC, Chen CJ, Neff JR, et al. Aneurysmal bone cyst variant translocations upregulate USP6 transcription by promoter swapping with the ZNF9, COL1A1, TRAP150, and OMD genes. Oncogene. 2005; 24(21):3419–26.

101. Yoshida A, Ushiku T, Motoi T, Shibata T, Beppu Y, Fukayama M, et al. Immunohistochemical analysis of MDM2 and CDK4 distinguishes low-grade osteosarcoma from benign mimics. Mod Pathol. 2010; 23(9):1279–88.

102. Dujardin F, Binh MB, Bouvier C, Gomez-Brouchet A, Larousserie F, Muret A, et al. MDM2 and CDK4 immunohistochemistry is a valuable tool in the differential diagnosis of low-grade osteosarcomas and other primary fibro-osseous lesions of the bone. Mod Pathol. 2011;24(5):624–37.

103. Debelenko LV, McGregor LM, Shivakumar BR, Dorfman HD, Raimondi SC. A novel EWSR1-CREB3L1 fusion transcript in a case of small cell osteosarcoma. Genes Chromosom Cancer. 2011; 50(12):1054–62.

104. Haldar M, Randall RL, Capecchi MR. Synovial sarcoma: from genetics to genetic-based animal modeling. Clin Orthop Relat Res. 2008;466(9):2156–67.

105. Alaggio R, Coffin CM, Vargas SO. Soft tissue tumors of uncertain origin. Pediatr Dev Pathol. 2012;15(1 Suppl):267–305.

106. Kempson RL, Fletcher CDM, Evans HL, Hendrickson MR, Sibley RK. Tumors of the soft tissues. 3rd ed. Washington, DC: Armed Forces Institute of Pathology; 2001.

107. Fisher C. Synovial sarcoma. Ann Diagn Pathol. 1998;2(6):401–21.
108. Fisher C. Synovial sarcoma: ultrastructural and immunohistochemical features of epithelial differentiation in monophasic and biphasic tumors. Hum Pathol. 1986;17(10):996–1008.
109. Fisher C. Soft tissue sarcomas with non-EWS translocations: molecular genetic features and pathologic and clinical correlations. Virchows Arch. 2010;456(2):153–66.
110. Foo WC, Cruise MW, Wick MR, Hornick JL. Immunohistochemical staining for TLE1 distinguishes synovial sarcoma from histologic mimics. Am J Clin Pathol. 2011;135(6):839–44.
111. Jagdis A, Rubin BP, Tubbs RR, Pacheco M, Nielsen TO. Prospective evaluation of TLE1 as a diagnostic immunohistochemical marker in synovial sarcoma. Am J Surg Pathol. 2009;33(12):1743–51.
112. Kosemehmetoglu K, Vrana JA, Folpe AL. TLE1 expression is not specific for synovial sarcoma: a whole section study of 163 soft tissue and bone neoplasms. Mod Pathol. 2009;22(7):872–8.
113. Ishida M, Tanaka S, Ohki M, Ohta T. Transcriptional co-activator activity of SYT is negatively regulated by BRM and Brg1. Genes Cells. 2004;9(5):419–28.
114. Gure AO, Wei IJ, Old LJ, Chen YT. The SSX gene family: characterization of 9 complete genes. Int J Cancer. 2002;101(5):448–53.
115. Smith HA, McNeel DG. The SSX family of cancer-testis antigens as target proteins for tumor therapy. Clin Dev Immunol. 2010;2010:150591.
116. Somers GR, Zielenska M, Abdullah S, Sherman C, Chan S, Thorner PS. Expression of MYCN in pediatric synovial sarcoma. Mod Pathol. 2007;20(7):734–41.
117. Nagai M, Tanaka S, Tsuda M, Endo S, Kato H, Sonobe H, et al. Analysis of transforming activity of human synovial sarcoma-associated chimeric protein SYT-SSX1 bound to chromatin remodeling factor hBRM/hSNF2 alpha. Proc Natl Acad Sci U S A. 2001;98(7):3843–8.
118. Antonescu CR, Kawai A, Leung DH, Lonardo F, Woodruff JM, Healey JH, et al. Strong association of SYT-SSX fusion type and morphologic epithelial differentiation in synovial sarcoma. Diagn Mol Pathol. 2000;9(1):1–8.
119. Guillou L, Benhattar J, Bonichon F, Gallagher G, Terrier P, Stauffer E, et al. Histologic grade, but not SYT-SSX fusion type, is an important prognostic factor in patients with synovial sarcoma: a multicenter, retrospective analysis. J Clin Oncol. 2004;22(20):4040–50.
120. Tsuji K, Ishikawa Y, Imamura T. Technique for differentiating alveolar soft part sarcoma from other tumors in paraffin-embedded tissue: comparison of immunohistochemistry for TFE3 and CD147 and of reverse transcription polymerase chain reaction for ASPSCR1-TFE3 fusion transcript. Hum Pathol. 2012;43(3):356–63.
121. Ladanyi M, Lui MY, Antonescu CR, Krause-Boehm A, Meindl A, Argani P, et al. The der(17)t(X;17)(p11;q25) of human alveolar soft part sarcoma fuses the TFE3 transcription factor gene to ASPL, a novel gene at 17q25. Oncogene. 2001;20(1):48–57.
122. Williams A, Bartle G, Sumathi VP, Meis JM, Mangham DC, Grimer RJ, et al. Detection of ASPL/TFE3 fusion transcripts and the TFE3 antigen in formalin-fixed, paraffin-embedded tissue in a series of 18 cases of alveolar soft part sarcoma: useful diagnostic tools in cases with unusual histological features. Virchows Arch. 2011;458(3):291–300.
123. Hisaoka M, Ishida T, Kuo TT, Matsuyama A, Imamura T, Nishida K, et al. Clear cell sarcoma of soft tissue: a clinicopathologic, immunohistochemical, and molecular analysis of 33 cases. Am J Surg Pathol. 2008;32(3):452–60.
124. Reeves BR, Fletcher CD, Gusterson BA. Translocation t(12;22)(q13;q13) is a nonrandom rearrangement in clear cell sarcoma. Cancer Genet Cytogenet. 1992;64(2):101–3.
125. Zucman J, Delattre O, Desmaze C, Epstein AL, Stenman G, Speleman F, et al. EWS and ATF-1 gene fusion induced by t(12;22) translocation in malignant melanoma of soft parts. Nat Genet. 1993;4(4):341–5.
126. Speleman F, Delattre O, Peter M, Hauben E, Van Roy N, Van Marck E. Malignant melanoma of the soft parts (clear-cell sarcoma): confirmation of EWS and ATF-1 gene fusion caused by a t(12;22) translocation. Mod Pathol. 1997;10(5):496–9.
127. Hiraga H, Nojima T, Abe S, Yamashiro K, Yamawaki S, Kaneda K, et al. Establishment of a new continuous clear cell sarcoma cell line. Morphological and cytogenetic characterization and detection of chimaeric EWS/ATF-1 transcripts. Virchows Arch. 1997;431(1):45–51.
128. Antonescu CR, Nafa K, Segal NH, Dal Cin P, Ladanyi M. EWS-CREB1: a recurrent variant fusion in clear cell sarcoma—association with gastrointestinal location and absence of melanocytic differentiation. Clin Cancer Res. 2006;12(18):5356–62.
129. Wang WL, Mayordomo E, Zhang W, Hernandez VS, Tuvin D, Garcia L, et al. Detection and characterization of EWSR1/ATF1 and EWSR1/CREB1 chimeric transcripts in clear cell sarcoma (melanoma of soft parts). Mod Pathol. 2009;22(9):1201–9.
130. Coindre JM, Hostein I, Terrier P, Bouvier-Labit C, Collin F, Michels JJ, et al. Diagnosis of clear cell sarcoma by real-time reverse transcriptase-polymerase chain reaction analysis of paraffin embedded tissues: clinicopathologic and molecular analysis of 44 patients from the French sarcoma group. Cancer. 2006;107(5):1055–64.
131. Yamada K, Ohno T, Aoki H, Semi K, Watanabe A, Moritake H, et al. EWS/ATF1 expression induces sarcomas from neural crest-derived cells in mice. J Clin Invest. 2013;123(2):600–10.
132. Aigner T, Oliveira AM, Nascimento AG. Extraskeletal myxoid chondrosarcomas do not show a chondrocytic phenotype. Mod Pathol. 2004;17(2):214–21.

133. Demicco EG, Wang WL, Madewell JE, Huang D, Bui MM, Bridge JA, et al. Osseous myxochondroid sarcoma: a detailed study of 5 cases of extraskeletal myxoid chondrosarcoma of the bone. Am J Surg Pathol. 2013;37(5):752–62.

134. Kawaguchi S, Wada T, Nagoya S, Ikeda T, Isu K, Yamashiro K, et al. Extraskeletal myxoid chondrosarcoma: a Multi-Institutional Study of 42 Cases in Japan. Cancer. 2003;97(5):1285–92.

135. Drilon AD, Popat S, Bhuchar G, D'Adamo DR, Keohan ML, Fisher C, et al. Extraskeletal myxoid chondrosarcoma: a retrospective review from 2 referral centers emphasizing long-term outcomes with surgery and chemotherapy. Cancer. 2008;113(12):3364–71.

136. Goh YW, Spagnolo DV, Platten M, Caterina P, Fisher C, Oliveira AM, et al. Extraskeletal myxoid chondrosarcoma: a light microscopic, immunohisto-chemical, ultrastructural and immuno-ultrastructural study indicating neuroendocrine differentiation. Histopathology. 2001;39(5):514–24.

137. Kohashi K, Oda Y, Yamamoto H, Tamiya S, Oshiro Y, Izumi T, et al. SMARCB1/INI1 protein expression in round cell soft tissue sarcomas associated with chromosomal translocations involving EWS: a special reference to SMARCB1/INI1 negative variant extraskeletal myxoid chondrosarcoma. Am J Surg Pathol. 2008;32(8):1168–74.

138. Turc-Carel C, Dal Cin P, Rao U, Karakousis C, Sandberg AA. Recurrent breakpoints at 9q31 and 22q12.2 in extraskeletal myxoid chondrosarcoma. Cancer Genet Cytogenet. 1988;30(1):145–50.

139. Wang WL, Mayordomo E, Czerniak BA, Abruzzo LV, Dal Cin P, Araujo DM, et al. Fluorescence in situ hybridization is a useful ancillary diagnostic tool for extraskeletal myxoid chondrosarcoma. Mod Pathol. 2008;21(11):1303–10.

140. Bjerkehagen B, Dietrich C, Reed W, Micci F, Saeter G, Berner A, et al. Extraskeletal myxoid chondrosarcoma: multimodal diagnosis and identification of a new cytogenetic subgroup characterized by t(9;17)(q22;q11). Virchows Arch. 1999;435(5):524–30.

141. Sjogren H, Wedell B, Meis-Kindblom JM, Kindblom LG, Stenman G. Fusion of the NH2-terminal domain of the basic helix-loop-helix protein TCF12 to TEC in extraskeletal myxoid chondrosarcoma with translocation t(9;15)(q22;q21). Cancer Res. 2000;60(24):6832–5.

142. Sjogren H, Meis-Kindblom JM, Orndal C, Bergh P, Ptaszynski K, Aman P, et al. Studies on the molecular pathogenesis of extraskeletal myxoid chondrosarcoma-cytogenetic, molecular genetic, and cDNA microarray analyses. Am J Pathol. 2003;162(3):781–92.

143. Panagopoulos I, Mertens F, Isaksson M, Domanski HA, Brosjo O, Heim S, et al. Molecular genetic characterization of the EWS/CHN and RBP56/CHN fusion genes in extraskeletal myxoid chondrosarcoma. Genes Chromosom Cancer. 2002;35(4):340–52.

144. Vergara-Lluri ME, Stohr BA, Puligandla B, Brenholz P, Horvai AE. A novel sarcoma with dual differentiation: clinicopathologic and molecular characterization of a combined synovial sarcoma and extraskeletal myxoid chondrosarcoma. Am J Surg Pathol. 2012;36(7):1093–8.

145. Neuville A, Ranchere-Vince D, Dei Tos AP, Cristina Montesco M, Hostein I, Toffolatti L, et al. Impact of molecular analysis on the final sarcoma diagnosis: a study on 763 cases collected during a European Epidemiological Study. Am J Surg Pathol. 2013;37(8):1259–68.

146. Sweeney RT, Zhang B, Zhu SX, Varma S, Smith KS, Montgomery SB, et al. Desktop transcriptome sequencing from archival tissue to identify clinically relevant translocations. Am J Surg Pathol. 2013;37(6):796–803.

147. Dylla L, Jedlicka P. Growth-promoting role of the miR-106a 363 cluster in Ewing sarcoma. PLoS One. 2013;8(4):e63032.

148. Marchetti A, Del Grammastro M, Filice G, Felicioni L, Rossi G, Graziano P, et al. Complex mutations & subpopulations of deletions at exon 19 of EGFR in NSCLC revealed by next generation sequencing: potential clinical implications. PLoS One. 2012;7(7):e42164.

149. Beck AH, Lee CH, Witten DM, Gleason BC, Edris B, Espinosa I, et al. Discovery of molecular subtypes in leiomyosarcoma through integrative molecular profiling. Oncogene. 2010;29(6):845–54.

150. Italiano A, Lagarde P, Brulard C, Terrier P, Lae M, Marques B, et al. Genetic profiling identifies two classes of soft-tissue leiomyosarcomas with distinct clinical characteristics. Clin Cancer Res. 2013;19(5):1190–6.

151. Chibon F, Lagarde P, Salas S, Perot G, Brouste V, Tirode F, et al. Validated prediction of clinical outcome in sarcomas and multiple types of cancer on the basis of a gene expression signature related to genome complexity. Nat Med. 2010;16(7):781–7.

152. Buttitta F, Felicioni L, Del Grammastro M, Filice G, Di Lorito A, Malatesta S, et al. Effective assessment of egfr mutation status in bronchoalveolar lavage and pleural fluids by next-generation sequencing. Clin Cancer Res. 2013;19(3):691–8.

Molecular testing in Cutaneous Melanoma

Margaret Redpath, Leon van Kempen, Caroline Robert, and Alan Spatz

Introduction

Melanoma is one of the solid tumors with the best characterized clinical and histopathological prognostic features. Primary lesion thickness, mitotic rate, and ulceration are all strong, independent prognostic variables [1, 2]. Other robust and easily assessed prognostic factors of melanoma include gender, age at diagnosis, the site of the lesion, mitotic rate, and presence of positive lymph nodes [1–4]. The staging system developed by the American Joint Committee on Cancer, Melanoma Task Force, can be used to effectively categorize patients into risk groups of disease progression. However, the molecular mechanisms driving these prognostic factors are poorly understood. Melanoma is also a paradigm in personalized medicine, illustrating how the discovery and further clinical validation of driving mutations can represent a breakthrough in cancer therapy. In this chapter, we will address the molecular mechanisms that may drive the strongest prognostic features of cutaneous melanoma, describe part of the current knowledge of phenotype–genotype correlations, and summarize the current standards in molecular pathology testing.

Correlations Phenotype–Biology

Tumor Thickness

In 1970, Alexander Breslow reported that thickness, cross-sectional areas, and depth of invasion were prognostic of cutaneous melanoma recurrence or metastasis rate at 5 years [5]. It is notable that although this report identified the most robust and reliable prognostic feature among all histological prognostic features ever described in cancer, this article is based on an error. Breslow considered maximal thickness as an indicator of tumor burden and cross-sectional area as the other important prognostic feature. We now know that the prognostic significance of Breslow's index is actually not related to tumor burden and that cross-sectional area does not predict clinical outcome. In 2009, the AJCC confirmed the prognostic significance of Breslow's thickness; the 10-year survival is 92 % among the patients with

M. Redpath, M.D.
Department of Pathology, McGill University, Duff Medical Building, 3775 University Street, Montreal, QC, Canada, H3A 2B4

L. van Kempen, Ph.D.
Department of Pathology, McGill University and Lady Davis Institute, Jewish General Hospital, 3755 Cote Ste Catherine, Montreal, QC, Canada, H3T 1E2

C. Robert, M.D.
Dermatology Unit, Gustave Roussy Institute, Rue Camille Desmoulins, 94805 Villejuif, France

A. Spatz, M.D. (✉)
Departments of Pathology and Oncology, McGill University and Lady Davis Institute, Jewish General Hospital, 3755 Cote Ste Catherine, Montreal, QC, Canada, H3T 1E2
e-mail: alan.spatz@mcgill.ca

G.M. Yousef and S. Jothy (eds.), *Molecular Testing in Cancer*,
DOI 10.1007/978-1-4899-8050-2_22, © Springer Science+Business Media New York 2014

T1 melanomas (0.1–1.0 mm) and is 50 % in patients with T4 melanomas (≥4.1 mm) [2]. Several studies have attempted to identify an expression signature associated with Breslow's thickness [6–15]. These studies identified only a few genes whose expression changes with increasing thickness and include E- and N-cadherin [8, 13], cadherin-19 [8, 16–20], bcl2a1 [21–25], as well as protocadherin 7 (pcdh7) [26–32], the regulator of G-protein signaling 20 (rgs20) [33], and activated leukocyte cell adhesion molecule (ALCAM/CD166) [34–40]. There is no data to support the view that melanoma thickness and Clark's level of invasion directly promote melanoma metastasis by, for instance, increasing the likelihood for the melanoma cells to encounter vessels. Breslow's thickness is likely an important phenotypic indicator of the biology of the melanoma cells at the leading edge of the tumor. Proteins whose expression correlates with tumor thickness are commonly involved in cell survival and invasion. E-cadherin is a keratinocyte–melanoma adhesion molecule whose loss is required for the acquisition of an invasive phenotype [18, 41–44]. Interestingly, this loss is mediated by the transcription factor Tbx3 that is also involved in suppressing melanocytes senescence through repressing the cyclin-dependent kinase inhibitors p19 (ARF) and p21 (WAF1/CIP1/SDII) [45, 46]. The cadherin switch, especially the decreased expression of E-cadherin and the increased expression of N-cadherin, is an early phenomenon during melanoma progression, which is associated with increased motility and invasiveness of the tumor and altered signaling, leading to decreased apoptosis and evasion of senescence [16, 27, 30, 41, 47–56]. Loss of E-cadherin expression in melanoma can be caused by gene loss, promoter methylation, or inhibition of transcription. Promoter methylation and expression of proteins and micro-RNAs that regulated E-cadherin expression, such as Snail, miRNA-200, and Gli2, are likewise associated with thickness and invasion [9, 13, 57]. Importantly, loss of E-cadherin expression affects β-catenin activity [26, 58–62]. β-Catenin anchors the actin cytoskeleton to E-cadherin, and loss of the latter causes β-catenin to move toward the nucleus where it acts as a transcription factor that drives the expression of a wide variety of genes that promote invasion, such as urokinase-like plasminogen activator (uPA) [63]. However, in contrast to carcinoma cells, the presence of melanocyte-specific MITF can attenuate β-catenin's pro-invasive properties that are otherwise active in nonpigmented tumor cells [64]. In line with this, loss of β-catenin expression is part of a seven-marker signature predicting high risk of disease recurrence [65]. Therefore, one may regard Breslow's index as a quantitative surrogate of the multifactorial biological machinery that drives melanoma progression and invasion.

Melanoma Ulceration

Tumor ulceration is associated with a poor prognosis in melanoma patients [1, 66]. Thick melanomas have a higher incidence of ulceration than thin melanomas [67]. However the prognostic strength of ulceration is independent of thickness [2]. Survival of patients with an ulcerated melanoma is significantly poorer than those of patients with a non-ulcerated melanoma of equivalent T category. Interestingly, this adverse prognostic effect of ulceration remains robust even when the patient has metastatic disease in 2 or 3 lymph nodes. This suggests that ulceration is a phenotypic surrogate of an important biological event rather than directly promoting metastatic evolution.

Several hypotheses have been proposed to explain the molecular changes underlying the adverse prognosis of ulceration. Factors related to the cellular biology of the tumor and the immuno-modulation of the melanoma cells have been identified. Changes in ALCAM-mediated adhesion contribute to melanoma invasion by triggering the expression of genes associated with the innate immune response [68]. Loss of E-cadherin expression induces an imbalance in inflammatory mediators and impairs keratinocyte control of melanocyte proliferation [42, 69, 70]. The N-cadherin-mediated interaction between fibroblasts and melanoma cells creates an imbalance of growth factor production, especially β-FGF, in a microenvironment that is already rich in melanoma-derived TGF-β [71]. The synergy between both growth factors can result in the recruitment of peripheral blood and bone marrow mesenchymal stem cells [72] and may drive the inflammatory response resulting in ulceration. Furthermore, loss of E-cadherin may result in increased β-catenin-regulated gene expression [19, 73–77]. β-catenin is highly expressed in ulcerated melanomas [78], but whether this phenomenon is a cause or effect remains to be determined.

Venous leg ulcers display a persistent stimulation of the innate immune response and a strong Th1-like inflammatory response [79]; however, this is not thought to occur in ulcerating melanomas. On the contrary, a retrospective analysis of 537 consecutive micrometastatic sentinel lymph nodes with melanoma demonstrated that ulceration in the primary melanoma is associated with a lower density of mature dendritic cells in the sentinel node as compared with sentinel nodes from non-ulcerated melanomas [80]. Whether this defect is due to constitutional host characteristics that also favor melanoma ulceration needs further investigations. Post hoc and meta-analyses of several adjuvant interferon (IFN) therapy trials strongly indicate that patients with an ulcerated primary melanoma are far more sensitive to IFN than patients with non-ulcerated primaries [42, 81–84]. This suggests that melanoma ulceration is associated with a defect in Th1 response, rather than a strong, persistent activation thereof. The efficacy of adjuvant IFN in mounting an antitumor Th1 immune response in ulcerated melanomas is currently being studied in a clinical trial. The interaction between inflammation-inducing mediators released by melanoma cells and the lack of activation of a Th1 response indicates complex and poorly understood reciprocal interactions between melanoma and inflammatory cells.

Mitotic Activity

Proliferation of the primary melanomas, defined by the mitotic rate, is a powerful and independent predictor of survival [1, 3, 85]. As a result, primary tumor mitotic rate is now a required element for the 2009 edition of the melanoma staging system. Data from the AJCC melanoma staging database demonstrate a highly significant correlation between increasing mitotic rate and declining survival rates ($p < 10^{-3}$). In a multifactorial analysis of 10,233 patients with clinically localized melanoma, mitotic rate was the second most powerful predictor of survival, after tumor thickness. Two large, validated gene expression profiling studies in melanoma that predict for the risk of metastasis or death reveal a strong representation of genes associated with replication or DNA repair [15, 86]. The expression of proteins involved in initiation of DNA replication, such as DNA unwinding protein complex subunits mini chromosome maintenance helicases MCM4 and MCM6, has a strong prognostic value for progression and metastasis-free melanoma survival [15]. Firing of the origins of DNA replication is tightly regulated to duplicate DNA only once during the S phase and prevent aneuploidy (reviewed in [87]). In human cells, cell division cycle 6 homolog (Cdc6) accumulates in the nucleus during G1 and binds to chromatin via the origin recognition complexes (ORC) that occupy the origins of replication throughout the genome. Subsequent binding of the Cdt1–MCM2-7 complex and phosphorylation by cyclin A/cyclin-dependent kinase 2 (CDK2) results in the release of phosphorylated Cdt1 and phosphorylated Cdc6 from this complex and marks the start of DNA replication [88, 89]. Expression of the kinase that phosphorylates Cdc6, i.e., CDK2, is of high prognostic value [90].

Highly proliferative cells such as aggressive melanoma require an effective DNA repair machinery to correct deleterious errors that compromise genomic integrity. Overexpression of DNA repair genes is associated with metastases or death [91, 92]. Increase in post-replicative DNA repair capacity associated with topoisomerase II alpha could explain spontaneous resistance of most melanomas toward radiotherapy and alkylating agents.

Gender

The gender effect on survival is another unresolved mystery in the melanoma field. The male gender is associated with an adverse outcome that persists even after adjustment for other prognostic variables [2, 93–97]. After adjustment the relative excess risk to die from melanoma is 1.85 (95 % CI=1.65–2.10) in males [93]. This gender impact on mortality risk is observed at all stages, even in patients with visceral metastases. No biological explanation has been identified so far. In particular, it is difficult to evoke a hormonal influence as the adjusted risk estimates are similar among patients below 45 or above 60 years of age. As most of the cancer–testis antigens (CTAs) genes are located on the X chromosome, one possibility would be that CTA expression differs between females and males, but in fact no difference has been observed. Moreover, data regarding the prognostic impact of CTAs expression are conflicting. A possible confounding factor would have been differences in behavior toward UV exposure. But the gender effect is unchanged when body site is introduced in the model strongly suggesting that survival difference among sexes is not due to behavioral differences [96]. A possible explanation may be found in X-linked gene expression. Although one of the two X chromosomes in female cells is inactivated, this inactivation is incomplete and can result in a possible dosage effect of X-inactivation escaping genes in females compared to the expression of the same gene from the one X in males [98]. These escaping genes may be melanoma suppressor genes such as UTX gene, coding for a H3-K27 demethylase, and WTX involved in a subset of Wilms tumor [99, 100]. Whether this would be sufficient to explain the gender difference is still unclear and requires further study.

Solar Elastosis and Location of Melanoma

An important phenotypic variable in melanoma is the presence of histopathological features of chronic sun exposure damage, such as grade 2 or 3 solar elastosis. It has been clearly demonstrated that presence or absence of solar elastosis correlates with the rate and the type of *BRAF* mutations [101–105]. Incidence of mutations is also impacted by the location of a melanoma. Acral

melanomas, aka melanomas of glabrous skin, are associated with more frequent KIT mutations and a lower rate of BRAF mutations [104].

Molecular Biology of Melanoma

Constitutional Defects

Several constitutional susceptibility loci have been associated with an inherited melanoma risk (Fig. 22.1, reviewed in [106]). These include P14 and P16 that are tumor-suppressor proteins encoded by the *CDKN2A* locus [107, 108]. P14 interacts with P53 and P16 with Rb. P14 binds to MDM2 and has an antiapoptotic effect through P53 destabilization, decreasing apoptosis [109]. P16 prevents CDK4 and CDK6 from phosphorylating Rb, which promotes G1–S transition [110, 111]. *CDK4* mutations interfere with Rb pathway and promote cell proliferation [112–114]. *Rb1* mutations predispose to familial melanoma as well as bilateral retinoblastoma [115, 116]. *MC1R* codes for a G-protein-coupled receptor-activating adenyl cyclase after binding of a melanocyte-stimulating hormone, resulting in an upregulation of MITF through the cAMP response element-binding protein [117, 118]. MITF controls the transcription of many genes, including pigmentation genes and HIF1A, and predisposes to melanoma [119, 120].

Somatic Alterations

Receptor tyrosine kinase and downstream kinase pathways are involved in most of the melanomas (reviewed in [121]). The mitogen-activated protein kinase pathway and the PI3K pathway are often activated [121]. There is an association between distinct melanoma subtypes and molecular somatic events that are involved. Mucosal, acral, and, to a lesser extent, the so-called lentigo maligna melanomas can have increased copies of CDK4 and CCND1 downstream of the MAPK pathway, as well as mutations in KIT receptor [122–127]. *NRAS* is mutated in about 18 % of

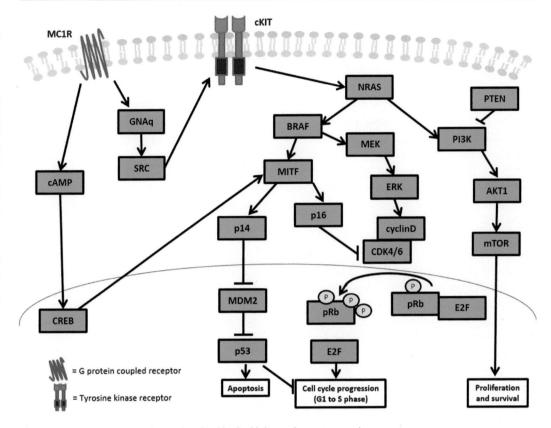

Fig. 22.1 Main molecular pathways involved in the biology of cutaneous melanoma

melanomas and seems to be more frequently activated in melanomas due to chronic sun damage [124, 128, 129]. BRAF is in a family with two other enzymes, ARAF and RAF1, and the gene is located downstream of RAS proteins and upstream of MEK and ERK proteins. *BRAF* has a recurrent gain-of-function mutation V600E in about 7 % of all cancers and 43–50 % of melanomas [121]. This mutational event is frequently reported in benign pigmented nevi, so is not fully sufficient to induce a malignant transformation [130]. *BRAF*-mutated melanomas are usually without nodular elastolysis and associated with a pagetoid appearance rather than lentiginous [105]. MEK1 and MEK2 are downstream from RAS and RAF, on the same MAPK pathway [121]. MEK1 is encoded by *MAP2K1* and MEK2 by *MAP2K2*. Activating mutations of MEK1 and MEK2 are found in 8 % of melanomas [131]. The

PI3K pathway is activated through a PTEN loss-of-function abnormality (most often deletion) in 20–40 % of melanomas [122, 132, 133]. Activating mutations or amplifications of PI3K or of AKT1 can also be found in some melanomas, although inhibitors of this pathway have not yet shown significant efficacy in any melanoma subtype.

Molecular Testing in Melanoma

The identification of a mutation in exon 15 of *BRAF* in 43–50 % of melanomas was an important push toward molecular classification [134, 135]. Although several additional somatic mutations, including driver mutations, have been identified, few have had therapeutic effect [136]. An algorithm for molecular testing should be based on the present therapeutic situation. Without the existence of an active adjuvant targeted treatment, to test a patient without metastases for targetable mutations in routine clinical practice is arguable. Tissue from primary tumors is often scarce and needs to be preserved for testing when necessary. Therefore, if one decide to test a primary melanoma, for instance, associated with a high metastatic risk, it is preferable to use multiplex tests, looking at several gene changes at once. *BRAF* mutations are present in 43–50 % of melanomas, and these are mostly in younger individuals and are on non-chronically sun-damaged skin [103, 121, 137]. Melanomas associated with chronic sun exposure are less often associated with *BRAF* mutations. The effect of chronic sun exposure is histologically signed by the presence of grade 2 or 3 elastolysis. However, this has no effect on clinical practice because all patients with stage IV disease should be screened for *BRAF* mutations. BRAF mutations carry a weak adverse prognostic value [138]. The frequency of BRAF mutations in primary cutaneous melanomas is not significantly different than in metastatic lesions. Few cases of discrepancies between the primary tumor and subsequent metastases or between metastases have been reported, but this appears to be a rare situation [137, 139, 140]. In clinical practice, it is more logical to test the metastasis but the primary tumor can be tested as well. About 90 % of BRAF mutations occur in exon 15 at the Val600, and most of these *BRAF* Val600 mutations lead to an exchange to glutamate BRAF Val600E, whereas 15–30 % of the mutations result in a substituted lysine (BRAF V600K) [141, 142]. The incidence rate for BRAF V600K varies by region, and a higher amount of cumulative sun-induced damage is associated with BRAF V600K, but not with BRAF V600E melanomas [141]. The real-time PCR Cobas 4800 assay has little cross-reactivity for non-V600E profiles [143]. Therefore, when this method is used, tumors with negative results should also be screened for V600K mutations with another technique. Similarly, the V600 mutation-specific VE1 antibody has a high sensitivity (97 %) and specificity (98 %) for detection of the V600E mutation, but

not for V600K [144–149]. Vemurafenib is the first selective BRAF inhibitor developed in the clinical setting. The drug was recently approved for first-line treatment of advanced V600E *BRAF*-mutated melanoma after a clinical trial comparing vemurafenib with dacarbazine showed a significant survival benefit and a median progression-free survival of 5.3 months versus 1.6 months (HR 0.26, $p<0.001$) [150]. Responses are frequent (48 % of patients) and fast. Dabrafenib, another BRAF inhibitor, is associated with a similar increase in progression-free survival [151]. The efficacy of BRAF inhibition for melanomas with non-V600E mutations on exon 15 of *BRAF* is a crucial question since these mutations can account for up to 30 % of the *BRAF* V600 cancer mutants [142]. The major concern for treatment with BRAF inhibitors is of a short median length of response, about 6 months [151]. Nearly all patients relapse, and the overall survival benefit is modest. This is why all efforts focus on combinations of targeted treatments, or targeted therapy and immunotherapy. Combinations of treatments targeting BRAF and MEK have showed a synergistic effect on clinical endpoints [152]. Mutations in *KIT* are noted in less than 1 % of melanomas overall; occurrence is more frequent in acral and mucosal sites [153, 154]. Activating mutations in and gene amplification of *KIT* have been initially reported in 39 % of mucosal site, 36 % of acral site, and 28 % of melanomas from patients with chronically sun-damaged skin, with mutation rates between 11 and 21 %. However, further studies found much lower proportions, of about 15 % in acral sites and below 5 % in mucosal sites [155, 156]. It is likely that these variations reflect both an overestimation of the frequency of KIT mutations in acral melanomas in the initial reports and sensitivity differences in the detection technique. KIT inhibitors can have substantial effects in patients with melanomas that contain *KIT* mutations. Therefore, investigators should systematically screen for *KIT* mutations in metastatic acral lentiginous melanoma and mucosal melanoma. Mutations in exons 11 and 13 make up 85 % of *KIT* mutations reported in melanomas and are associated with sensitivity to imatinib [157, 158].

Other mutations are reported in exon 17. Major differences seen in gastrointestinal stromal tumors are that melanomas have more point mutations than deletions or insertions, have more frequent mutations in exons 13 and 17, and have more amplified wild-type *KIT*. These amplifications seem to be predictive of no response to anti-KIT therapies [159]. Mutations that activate the mitogen-activated protein (MAP) kinase pathways are reported in 20 % of cutaneous melanomas in *NRAS* and in 83 % of uveal melanomas in *GNAQ* or *GNA11* [160, 161]. Treatments that target mutated *NRAS* and *GNAQ* are under investigation.

Conclusion: Multidimensionality of Melanoma Prognostic Biomarkers

There is a strong need to refine prognostication in melanoma. The main reason is that we need to replace outcome clustering, based on artificial biomarker breakpoints, by a continuous multidimensional prognostic model. The pace of new biomarker development will quickly make it impossible to update the list of prognostic variables to assess each time a new biomarker is identified. Major improvement will come from shared computerized tools which will help us in generating continuous likelihood scores for diagnosis, prognosis, and response to treatment predictions ([162] as an example). This will lead to the development of platforms which can be used by scientists from different fields to integrate and share high-quality data in the precompetitive setting and generate new probabilistic causal models.

References

1. Balch CM et al. Multivariate analysis of prognostic factors among 2,313 patients with stage III melanoma: comparison of nodal micrometastases versus macrometastases. J Clin Oncol. 2010;28(14):2452–9.
2. Balch CM et al. Final version of 2009 AJCC melanoma staging and classification. J Clin Oncol. 2009;27(36):6199–206.
3. Balch CM et al. Update on the melanoma staging system: the importance of sentinel node staging and primary tumor mitotic rate. J Surg Oncol. 2011;104(4):379–85.
4. Balch CM, et al. Age as a prognostic factor in patients with localized melanoma and regional metastases. Ann Surg Oncol. 2013;20(12):3961–8.
5. Breslow A. Thickness, cross-sectional areas and depth of invasion in the prognosis of cutaneous melanoma. Ann Surg. 1970;172(5):902–8.
6. Brunner G et al. Increased expression of the tumor suppressor PLZF is a continuous predictor of long-term survival in malignant melanoma patients. Cancer Biother Radiopharm. 2008;23(4):451–9.
7. Hanna JA et al. In situ measurement of miR-205 in malignant melanoma tissue supports its role as a tumor suppressor microRNA. Lab Invest. 2012;92(10):1390–7.
8. Jaeger J et al. Gene expression signatures for tumor progression, tumor subtype, and tumor thickness in laser-microdissected melanoma tissues. Clin Cancer Res. 2007;13(3):806–15.
9. Journe F et al. TYRP1 mRNA expression in melanoma metastases correlates with clinical outcome. Br J Cancer. 2011;105(11):1726–32.
10. Kannengiesser C et al. Gene expression signature associated with BRAF mutations in human primary cutaneous melanomas. Mol Oncol. 2008;1(4):425–30.
11. Lugassy C et al. Gene expression profiling of human angiotropic primary melanoma: selection of 15 differentially expressed genes potentially involved in extravascular migratory metastasis. Eur J Cancer. 2011;47(8):1267–75.
12. Van den Oord JJ et al. Expression profiling of melanoma cell lines: in search of a progression-related molecular signature. Future Oncol. 2007;3(6):609–11.
13. van Kempen LC et al. Loss of microRNA-200a and c, and microRNA-203 expression at the invasive front of primary cutaneous melanoma is associated with increased thickness and disease progression. Virchows Arch. 2012;461(4):441–8.
14. Winnepenninckx V et al. Expression and possible role of hPTTG1/securin in cutaneous malignant melanoma. Mod Pathol. 2006;19(9):1170–80.
15. Winnepenninckx V et al. Gene expression profiling of primary cutaneous melanoma and clinical outcome. J Natl Cancer Inst. 2006;98(7):472–82.
16. Ciolczyk-Wierzbicka D, Gil D, Laidler P. The inhibition of cell proliferation using silencing of N-cadherin gene by siRNA process in human melanoma cell lines. Curr Med Chem. 2012;19(1):145–51.
17. Kumar S et al. A pathway for the control of anoikis sensitivity by E-cadherin and epithelial-to-mesenchymal transition. Mol Cell Biol. 2011;31(19):4036–51.
18. Rodriguez M et al. Tbx3 represses E-cadherin expression and enhances melanoma invasiveness. Cancer Res. 2008;68(19):7872–81.

19. Kreizenbeck GM et al. Prognostic significance of cadherin-based adhesion molecules in cutaneous malignant melanoma. Cancer Epidemiol Biomarkers Prev. 2008;17(4):949–58.

20. Billion K et al. Increased soluble E-cadherin in melanoma patients. Skin Pharmacol Physiol. 2006;19(2): 65–70.

21. Haq R, Fisher DE. Improving apoptotic responses to targeted therapy. Oncotarget. 2013;4(9):1331.

22. Haq R et al. BCL2A1 is a lineage-specific antiapoptotic melanoma oncogene that confers resistance to BRAF inhibition. Proc Natl Acad Sci U S A. 2013; 110(11):4321–6.

23. Cruz-Munoz W et al. Roles for endothelin receptor B and BCL2A1 in spontaneous CNS metastasis of melanoma. Cancer Res. 2012;72(19):4909–19.

24. Timar J, Gyorffy B, Raso E. Gene signature of the metastatic potential of cutaneous melanoma: too much for too little? Clin Exp Metastasis. 2010;27(6): 371–87.

25. Torikai H et al. Aberrant expression of BCL2A1-restricted minor histocompatibility antigens in melanoma cells: application for allogeneic transplantation. Int J Hematol. 2008;87(5):467–73.

26. Lee DJ et al. Peroxiredoxin-2 represses melanoma metastasis by increasing E-cadherin/beta-catenin complexes in adherens junctions. Cancer Res. 2013;73(15):4744–57.

27. Lade-Keller J, et al. E- to N-cadherin switch in melanoma is associated with decreased expression of PTEN and cancer progression. Br J Dermatol. 2013;169(3):618–28.

28. Bosserhoff AK, et al. Loss of T-cadherin (CDH-13) regulates AKT signaling and desensitizes cells to apoptosis in melanoma. Mol Carcinog. 2014 (In Press).

29. Lobos-Gonzalez L et al. E-cadherin determines Caveolin-1 tumor suppression or metastasis enhancing function in melanoma cells. Pigment Cell Melanoma Res. 2013;26(4):555–70.

30. Monaghan-Benson E, Burridge K. Mutant B-RAF regulates a Rac-dependent cadherin switch in melanoma. Oncogene. 2012;32(40):4836–44.

31. Boyd SC et al. Oncogenic B-RAF(V600E) signaling induces the T-Box3 transcriptional repressor to repress E-cadherin and enhance melanoma cell invasion. J Invest Dermatol. 2013;133(5):1269–77.

32. Seleit IA et al. Impact of E-cadherin expression pattern in melanocytic nevi and cutaneous malignant melanoma. Anal Quant Cytol Histol. 2012;34(4): 204–13.

33. Riker AI et al. The gene expression profiles of primary and metastatic melanoma yields a transition point of tumor progression and metastasis. BMC Med Genomics. 2008;1:13.

34. Magnoni C, et al. Stem cell properties in cell cultures from different stage of melanoma progression. Appl Immunohistochem Mol Morphol. 2014 (In Press).

35. Shanesmith RP, Smart C, Cassarino DS. Tissue microarray analysis of ezrin, KBA.62, CD166, nestin, and p-Akt in melanoma versus banal and

atypical nevi, and nonmelanocytic lesions. Am J Dermatopathol. 2011;33(7):663–8.

36. Weidle UH et al. ALCAM/CD166: cancer-related issues. Cancer Genomics Proteomics. 2010;7(5): 231–43.

37. van Kilsdonk JW et al. Attenuation of melanoma invasion by a secreted variant of activated leukocyte cell adhesion molecule. Cancer Res. 2008;68(10): 3671–9.

38. Lunter PC et al. Activated leukocyte cell adhesion molecule (ALCAM/CD166/MEMD), a novel actor in invasive growth, controls matrix metalloproteinase activity. Cancer Res. 2005;65(19):8801–8.

39. van Kempen LC et al. Truncation of activated leukocyte cell adhesion molecule: a gateway to melanoma metastasis. J Invest Dermatol. 2004;122(5):1293–301.

40. van Kempen LC et al. Activated leukocyte cell adhesion molecule/CD166, a marker of tumor progression in primary malignant melanoma of the skin. Am J Pathol. 2000;156(3):769–74.

41. Kim JE et al. Heterogeneity of expression of epithelial-mesenchymal transition markers in melanocytes and melanoma cell lines. Front Genet. 2013;4:97.

42. Spatz A, Batist G, Eggermont AM. The biology behind prognostic factors of cutaneous melanoma. Curr Opin Oncol. 2010;22(3):163–8.

43. Robert G et al. SPARC represses E-cadherin and induces mesenchymal transition during melanoma development. Cancer Res. 2006;66(15):7516–23.

44. Smalley KS et al. Up-regulated expression of zonula occludens protein-1 in human melanoma associates with N-cadherin and contributes to invasion and adhesion. Am J Pathol. 2005;166(5):1541–54.

45. Abrahams A et al. UV-mediated regulation of the anti-senescence factor Tbx2. J Biol Chem. 2008; 283(4):2223–30.

46. Demay F et al. T-box factors: targeting to chromatin and interaction with the histone H3 N-terminal tail. Pigment Cell Res. 2007;20(4):279–87.

47. Perrot CY, et al. GLI2 cooperates with ZEB1 for transcriptional repression of CDH1 expression in human melanoma cells. Pigment Cell Melanoma Res. 2013;26(6):861–73.

48. Hao L et al. Cadherin switch from E- to N-cadherin in melanoma progression is regulated by the PI3K/PTEN pathway through Twist and Snail. Br J Dermatol. 2012;166(6):1184–97.

49. Mougiakakos D et al. High expression of GCLC is associated with malignant melanoma of low oxidative phenotype and predicts a better prognosis. J Mol Med (Berl). 2012;90(8):935–44.

50. Koefinger P et al. The cadherin switch in melanoma instigated by HGF is mediated through epithelial-mesenchymal transition regulators. Pigment Cell Melanoma Res. 2011;24(2):382–5.

51. Fukunaga-Kalabis M, Santiago-Walker A, Herlyn M. Matricellular proteins produced by melanocytes and melanomas: in search for functions. Cancer Microenviron. 2008;1(1):93–102.

52. Augustine CK et al. Targeting N-cadherin enhances antitumor activity of cytoxic therapies in melanoma treatment. Cancer Res. 2008;68(10):3777–84.

53. Kuphal S, Bosserhoff AK. Influence of the cytoplasmic domain of E-cadherin on endogenous N-cadherin expression in malignant melanoma. Oncogene. 2006;25(2):248–59.

54. Haass NK, Smalley KS, Herlyn M. The role of altered cell-cell communication in melanoma progression. J Mol Histol. 2004;35(3):309–18.

55. Hendrix MJ et al. Expression and functional significance of VE-cadherin in aggressive human melanoma cells: role in vasculogenic mimicry. Proc Natl Acad Sci U S A. 2001;98(14):8018–23.

56. Hsu M et al. Cadherin repertoire determines partner-specific gap junctional communication during melanoma progression. J Cell Sci. 2000;113(Pt 9): 1535–42.

57. Alexaki VI et al. GLI2-mediated melanoma invasion and metastasis. J Natl Cancer Inst. 2010;102(15): 1148–59.

58. Grossmann AH et al. The small GTPase ARF6 stimulates beta-catenin transcriptional activity during WNT5A-mediated melanoma invasion and metastasis. Sci Signal. 2013;6(265):ra14.

59. Kuphal S, Bosserhoff AK. Phosphorylation of beta-catenin results in lack of beta-catenin signaling in melanoma. Int J Oncol. 2011;39(1):235–43.

60. Takahashi Y et al. Gene silencing of beta-catenin in melanoma cells retards their growth but promotes the formation of pulmonary metastasis in mice. Int J Cancer. 2008;123(10):2315–20.

61. Torres VA et al. E-cadherin is required for caveolin-1-mediated down-regulation of the inhibitor of apoptosis protein survivin via reduced beta-catenin-Tcf/Lef-dependent transcription. Mol Cell Biol. 2007;27(21):7703–17.

62. Bachmann IM et al. Importance of P-cadherin, beta-catenin, and Wnt5a/frizzled for progression of melanocytic tumors and prognosis in cutaneous melanoma. Clin Cancer Res. 2005;11(24 Pt 1):8606–14.

63. Hiendlmeyer E et al. Beta-catenin up-regulates the expression of the urokinase plasminogen activator in human colorectal tumors. Cancer Res. 2004;64(4): 1209–14.

64. Gallagher SJ et al. Beta-catenin inhibits melanocyte migration but induces melanoma metastasis. Oncogene. 2013;32(17):2230–8.

65. Meyer S et al. A seven-marker signature and clinical outcome in malignant melanoma: a large-scale tissue-microarray study with two independent patient cohorts. PLoS One. 2012;7(6):e38222.

66. Soong SJ et al. Predicting survival outcome of localized melanoma: an electronic prediction tool based on the AJCC Melanoma Database. Ann Surg Oncol. 2010;17(8):2006–14.

67. Balch CM et al. The prognostic significance of ulceration of cutaneous melanoma. Cancer. 1980; 45(12):3012–7.

68. van Kilsdonk JW et al. Modulation of activated leukocyte cell adhesion molecule-mediated invasion triggers an innate immune gene response in melanoma. J Invest Dermatol. 2012;132(5):1462–70.

69. Florenes VA et al. Expression of activated TrkA protein in melanocytic tumors: relationship to cell proliferation and clinical outcome. Am J Clin Pathol. 2004;122(3):412–20.

70. Nishizawa A et al. Clinicopathologic significance of dysadherin expression in cutaneous malignant melanoma: immunohistochemical analysis of 115 patients. Cancer. 2005;103(8):1693–700.

71. Ruiter D et al. Melanoma-stroma interactions: structural and functional aspects. Lancet Oncol. 2002;3(1): 35–43.

72. Bakhshayesh M et al. Effects of TGF-beta and b-FGF on the potential of peripheral blood-borne stem cells and bone marrow-derived stem cells in wound healing in a murine model. Inflammation. 2012;35(1):138–42.

73. Hung CF et al. E-cadherin and its downstream catenins are proteolytically cleaved in human HaCaT keratinocytes exposed to UVB. Exp Dermatol. 2006;15(4):315–21.

74. Li G, Fukunaga M, Herlyn M. Reversal of melanocytic malignancy by keratinocytes is an E-cadherin-mediated process overriding beta-catenin signaling. Exp Cell Res. 2004;297(1):142–51.

75. McGary EC, Lev DC, Bar-Eli M. Cellular adhesion pathways and metastatic potential of human melanoma. Cancer Biol Ther. 2002;1(5):459–65.

76. Sanders DS et al. Alterations in cadherin and catenin expression during the biological progression of melanocytic tumours. Mol Pathol. 1999;52(3): 151–7.

77. Silye R et al. E-cadherin/catenin complex in benign and malignant melanocytic lesions. J Pathol. 1998; 186(4):350–5.

78. Rakosy Z et al. Integrative genomics identifies gene signature associated with melanoma ulceration. PLoS One. 2013;8(1):e54958.

79. Simka M. Cellular and molecular mechanisms of venous leg ulcers development—the "puzzle" theory. Int Angiol. 2010;29(1):1–19.

80. Elliott B et al. Long-term protective effect of mature DC-LAMP+ dendritic cell accumulation in sentinel lymph nodes containing micrometastatic melanoma. Clin Cancer Res. 2007;13(13):3825–30.

81. Eggermont AM et al. Long-term results of the randomized phase III trial EORTC 18991 of adjuvant therapy with pegylated interferon alfa-2b versus observation in resected stage III melanoma. J Clin Oncol. 2012;30(31):3810–8.

82. Eggermont AM et al. Is ulceration in cutaneous melanoma just a prognostic and predictive factor or is ulcerated melanoma a distinct biologic entity? Curr Opin Oncol. 2012;24(2):137–40.

83. Eggermont AM et al. Ulceration and stage are predictive of interferon efficacy in melanoma: results of

the phase III adjuvant trials EORTC 18952 and EORTC 18991. Eur J Cancer. 2012;48(2):218–25.

84. Eggermont AM et al. Adjuvant therapy with pegylated interferon alfa-2b versus observation alone in resected stage III melanoma: final results of EORTC 18991, a randomised phase III trial. Lancet. 2008;372(9633):117–26.

85. Thompson JF et al. Prognostic significance of mitotic rate in localized primary cutaneous melanoma: an analysis of patients in the multi-institutional American Joint Committee on Cancer melanoma staging database. J Clin Oncol. 2011;29(16):2199–205.

86. Harbst K et al. Molecular profiling reveals low- and high-grade forms of primary melanoma. Clin Cancer Res. 2012;18(15):4026–36.

87. Blow JJ, Dutta A. Preventing re-replication of chromosomal DNA. Nat Rev Mol Cell Biol. 2005;6(6):476–86.

88. Kundu LR et al. Deregulated Cdc6 inhibits DNA replication and suppresses Cdc7-mediated phosphorylation of Mcm2-7 complex. Nucleic Acids Res. 2010;38(16):5409–18.

89. Wheeler LW, Lents NH, Baldassare JJ. Cyclin A-CDK activity during G1 phase impairs MCM chromatin loading and inhibits DNA synthesis in mammalian cells. Cell Cycle. 2008;7(14):2179–88.

90. Schramm SJ et al. Review and cross-validation of gene expression signatures and melanoma prognosis. J Invest Dermatol. 2012;132(2):274–83.

91. Kauffmann A et al. High expression of DNA repair pathways is associated with metastasis in melanoma patients. Oncogene. 2008;27(5):565–73.

92. Song L et al. DNA repair and replication proteins as prognostic markers in melanoma. Histopathology. 2013;62(2):343–50.

93. Joosse A et al. Superior outcome of women with stage I/II cutaneous melanoma: pooled analysis of four European Organisation for Research and Treatment of Cancer phase III trials. J Clin Oncol. 2012;30(18):2240–7.

94. Thorn M et al. Long-term survival in malignant melanoma with special reference to age and sex as prognostic factors. J Natl Cancer Inst. 1987;79(5):969–74.

95. Joosse A et al. Gender differences in melanoma survival: female patients have a decreased risk of metastasis. J Invest Dermatol. 2011;131(3):719–26.

96. de Vries E et al. Superior survival of females among 10,538 Dutch melanoma patients is independent of Breslow thickness, histologic type and tumor site. Ann Oncol. 2008;19(3):583–9.

97. Joosse A et al. Sex is an independent prognostic indicator for survival and relapse/progression-free survival in metastasized stage III to IV melanoma: a pooled analysis of five European organisation for research and treatment of cancer randomized controlled trials. J Clin Oncol. 2013;31(18):2337–46.

98. Spatz A, Borg C, Feunteun J. X-chromosome genetics and human cancer. Nat Rev Cancer. 2004;4(8):617–29.

99. Agger K et al. UTX and JMJD3 are histone H3K27 demethylases involved in HOX gene regulation and development. Nature. 2007;449(7163):731–4.

100. Rivera MN et al. An X chromosome gene, WTX, is commonly inactivated in Wilms tumor. Science. 2007;315(5812):642–5.

101. Bauer J et al. BRAF mutations in cutaneous melanoma are independently associated with age, anatomic site of the primary tumor, and the degree of solar elastosis at the primary tumor site. Pigment Cell Melanoma Res. 2011;24(2):345–51.

102. Karram S et al. Predictors of BRAF mutation in melanocytic nevi: analysis across regions with different UV radiation exposure. Am J Dermatopathol. 2013;35(4):412–8.

103. Mar VJ et al. BRAF/NRAS wild-type melanomas have a high mutation load correlating with histologic and molecular signatures of UV damage. Clin Cancer Res. 2013;19(17):4589–98.

104. Scolyer RA, Long GV, Thompson JF. Evolving concepts in melanoma classification and their relevance to multidisciplinary melanoma patient care. Mol Oncol. 2011;5(2):124–36.

105. Broekaert SM et al. Genetic and morphologic features for melanoma classification. Pigment Cell Melanoma Res. 2010;23(6):763–70.

106. Udayakumar D et al. Genetic determinants of cutaneous melanoma predisposition. Semin Cutan Med Surg. 2010;29(3):190–5.

107. Freedberg DE et al. Frequent p16-independent inactivation of p14ARF in human melanoma. J Natl Cancer Inst. 2008;100(11):784–95.

108. Jones R et al. A CDKN2A mutation in familial melanoma that abrogates binding of p16INK4a to CDK4 but not CDK6. Cancer Res. 2007;67(19):9134–41.

109. Lewis JM, Truong TN, Schwartz MA. Integrins regulate the apoptotic response to DNA damage through modulation of p53. Proc Natl Acad Sci U S A. 2002;99(6):3627–32.

110. Karim RZ et al. Reduced p16 and increased cyclin D1 and pRb expression are correlated with progression in cutaneous melanocytic tumors. Int J Surg Pathol. 2009;17(5):361–7.

111. Soto JL et al. Mutation analysis of genes that control the G1/S cell cycle in melanoma: TP53, CDKN1A, CDKN2A, and CDKN2B. BMC Cancer. 2005;5:36.

112. Haferkamp S et al. p16INK4a-induced senescence is disabled by melanoma-associated mutations. Aging Cell. 2008;7(5):733–45.

113. Dahl C, Guldberg P. The genome and epigenome of malignant melanoma. APMIS. 2007;115(10):1161–76.

114. Bachmann IM, Straume O, Akslen LA. Altered expression of cell cycle regulators Cyclin D1, p14, p16, CDK4 and Rb in nodular melanomas. Int J Oncol. 2004;25(6):1559–65.

115. Nelson AA, Tsao H. Melanoma and genetics. Clin Dermatol. 2009;27(1):46–52.

116. Haluska FG, Hodi FS. Molecular genetics of familial cutaneous melanoma. J Clin Oncol. 1998;16(2): 670–82.

117. Sturm RA, et al. Phenotypic characterization of nevus and tumor PATTERNS in MITF E318K mutation carrier melanoma patients. J Invest Dermatol. 2014;134(1):141–9.

118. Davies JR et al. Inherited variants in the MC1R gene and survival from cutaneous melanoma: a BioGenoMEL study. Pigment Cell Melanoma Res. 2012;25(3):384–94.

119. Yokoyama S et al. A novel recurrent mutation in MITF predisposes to familial and sporadic melanoma. Nature. 2011;480(7375):99–103.

120. Bertolotto C et al. A SUMOylation-defective MITF germline mutation predisposes to melanoma and renal carcinoma. Nature. 2011;480(7375):94–8.

121. Eggermont A, Spatz A, Robert C. Cutaneous melanoma; an update. Lancet. 2014. In Press.

122. Bogenrieder T, Herlyn M. The molecular pathology of cutaneous melanoma. Cancer Biomark. 2010; 9(1–6):267–86.

123. Cooper C, Sorrell J, Gerami P. Update in molecular diagnostics in melanocytic neoplasms. Adv Anat Pathol. 2012;19(6):410–6.

124. Mehnert JM, Kluger HM. Driver mutations in melanoma: lessons learned from bench-to-bedside studies. Curr Oncol Rep. 2012;14(5):449–57.

125. Tremante E et al. Melanoma molecular classes and prognosis in the postgenomic era. Lancet Oncol. 2012;13(5):e205–11.

126. Walia V et al. Delving into somatic variation in sporadic melanoma. Pigment Cell Melanoma Res. 2012;25(2):155–70.

127. Woodman SE et al. New strategies in melanoma: molecular testing in advanced disease. Clin Cancer Res. 2012;18(5):1195–200.

128. Fedorenko IV, Gibney GT, Smalley KS. NRAS mutant melanoma: biological behavior and future strategies for therapeutic management. Oncogene. 2013;32(25):3009–18.

129. Kelleher FC, McArthur GA. Targeting NRAS in melanoma. Cancer J. 2012;18(2):132–6.

130. Tschandl P et al. NRAS and BRAF mutations in melanoma-associated nevi and uninvolved nevi. PLoS One. 2013;8(7):e69639.

131. Nikolaev SI et al. Exome sequencing identifies recurrent somatic MAP2K1 and MAP2K2 mutations in melanoma. Nat Genet. 2012;44(2):133–9.

132. Shull AY et al. Novel somatic mutations to PI3K pathway genes in metastatic melanoma. PLoS One. 2012;7(8):e43369.

133. Yajima I et al. RAS/RAF/MEK/ERK and PI3K/PTEN/AKT signaling in malignant melanoma progression and therapy. Dermatol Res Pract. 2012; 2012:354191.

134. Brose MS et al. BRAF and RAS mutations in human lung cancer and melanoma. Cancer Res. 2002;62(23): 6997–7000.

135. Davies H et al. Mutations of the BRAF gene in human cancer. Nature. 2002;417(6892):949–54.

136. Hodis E et al. A landscape of driver mutations in melanoma. Cell. 2012;150(2):251–63.

137. Colombino M et al. BRAF/NRAS mutation frequencies among primary tumors and metastases in patients with melanoma. J Clin Oncol. 2012; 30(20):2522–9.

138. Ekedahl H, et al. The clinical significance of BRAF and NRAS mutations in a clinic-based metastatic melanoma cohort. Br J Dermatol. 2013;169(5): 1049–55.

139. Richtig E et al. BRAF mutation analysis of only one metastatic lesion can restrict the treatment of melanoma: a case report. Br J Dermatol. 2013;168(2): 428–30.

140. Yancovitz M et al. Intra- and inter-tumor heterogeneity of BRAF(V600E) mutations in primary and metastatic melanoma. PLoS One. 2012;7(1): e29336.

141. Menzies AM et al. Distinguishing clinicopathologic features of patients with V600E and V600K BRAF-mutant metastatic melanoma. Clin Cancer Res. 2012;18(12):3242–9.

142. Amanuel B et al. Incidence of BRAF p.Val600Glu and p.Val600Lys mutations in a consecutive series of 183 metastatic melanoma patients from a high incidence region. Pathology. 2012;44(4):357–9.

143. Halait H et al. Analytical performance of a real-time PCR-based assay for V600 mutations in the BRAF gene, used as the companion diagnostic test for the novel BRAF inhibitor vemurafenib in metastatic melanoma. Diagn Mol Pathol. 2012; 21(1):1–8.

144. Marin C, et al. Detection of BRAF p.V600E mutations in melanoma by immunohistochemistry has a good interobserver reproducibility. Arch Pathol Lab Med. 2014 (In Press).

145. Wilmott JS et al. BRAF(V600E) protein expression and outcome from BRAF inhibitor treatment in BRAF(V600E) metastatic melanoma. Br J Cancer. 2013;108(4):924–31.

146. Busam KJ et al. Immunohistochemical analysis of BRAF(V600E) expression of primary and metastatic melanoma and comparison with mutation status and melanocyte differentiation antigens of metastatic lesions. Am J Surg Pathol. 2013;37(3):413–20.

147. Long GV et al. Immunohistochemistry is highly sensitive and specific for the detection of V600E BRAF mutation in melanoma. Am J Surg Pathol. 2013; 37(1):61–5.

148. Skorokhod A et al. Detection of BRAF V600E mutations in skin metastases of malignant melanoma by monoclonal antibody VE1. J Am Acad Dermatol. 2012;67(3):488–91.

149. Capper D et al. Assessment of BRAF V600E mutation status by immunohistochemistry with a mutation-specific monoclonal antibody. Acta Neuropathol. 2011;122(1):11–9.

150. Chapman PB et al. Improved survival with vemu-rafenib in melanoma with BRAF V600E mutation. N Engl J Med. 2011;364(26):2507–16.

151. Hauschild A et al. Dabrafenib in BRAF-mutated metastatic melanoma: a multicentre, open-label, phase 3 randomised controlled trial. Lancet. 2012; 380(9839):358–65.

152. Flaherty KT et al. Combined BRAF and MEK inhi-bition in melanoma with BRAF V600 mutations. N Engl J Med. 2012;367(18):1694–703.

153. Beadling C et al. KIT gene mutations and copy num-ber in melanoma subtypes. Clin Cancer Res. 2008;14(21):6821–8.

154. Carvajal RD et al. KIT as a therapeutic target in meta-static melanoma. JAMA. 2011;305(22):2327–34.

155. Zebary A et al. KIT, NRAS and BRAF mutations in sinonasal mucosal melanoma: a study of 56 cases. Br J Cancer. 2013;109(3):559–64.

156. Zebary A, et al. KIT, NRAS, BRAF and PTEN muta-tions in a sample of Swedish patients with acral lentigi-nous melanoma. J Dermatol Sci. 2013;72(3):284–9.

157. Guo J et al. Phase II, open-label, single-arm trial of imatinib mesylate in patients with metastatic mela-noma harboring c-Kit mutation or amplification. J Clin Oncol. 2011;29(21):2904–9.

158. Handolias D et al. Clinical responses observed with imatinib or sorafenib in melanoma patients express-ing mutations in KIT. Br J Cancer. 2010;102(8): 1219–23.

159. Hodi FS, et al. Imatinib for melanomas harboring mutationally activated or amplified KIT arising on mucosal, acral, and chronically sun-damaged skin. J Clin Oncol. 2013;31(26):3182–90.

160. Van Raamsdonk CD et al. Frequent somatic muta-tions of GNAQ in uveal melanoma and blue naevi. Nature. 2009;457(7229):599–602.

161. Van Raamsdonk CD et al. Mutations in GNA11 in uveal melanoma. N Engl J Med. 2010;363(23): 2191–9.

162. Derry JM et al. Developing predictive molecular maps of human disease through community-based modeling. Nat Genet. 2012;44(2):127–30.

Molecular Testing in Paediatric Tumours

23

Gino R. Somers and Paul S. Thorner

Introduction

Paediatric molecular diagnostics has revolutionized the diagnosis and prognosis of specific tumour types. This chapter will focus on two tumour types—paediatric sarcomas (specifically Ewing family of tumours, primitive round cell sarcomas (PRCS), infantile fibrosarcoma and embryonal rhabdomyosarcoma (ERMS)) and neuroblastoma. Each subtype benefits from the incorporation of molecular diagnostic techniques into the diagnostic regimen for diagnosis and/or prognosis. A summary of the more common and recurrent rearrangements in paediatric tumours and the role they play in diagnosis will be presented. In addition, the tools and techniques used to detect such abnormalities will be discussed, together with a summary of more advanced techniques making their way into the paediatric molecular diagnostic laboratory.

G.R. Somers, M.D., Ph.D. (✉) • P.S. Thorner, M.D., Ph.D.
Department of Paediatric Laboratory Medicine, Hospital for Sick Children, University of Toronto, Toronto, ON, Canada M5G 1X8

Department of Laboratory Medicine and Pathobiology, University of Toronto, Toronto, ON, Canada
e-mail: gino.somers@sickkids.ca; paul.thorner@sickkids.ca

Paediatric Sarcomas

Background

Up to 20 % of childhood solid malignancies are sarcomas [1]. Most sarcomas occur in the soft tissues and are presumed to have a mesenchymal origin. Such soft tissue sarcomas can occur in any region of the body and are generally divided into two major categories: rhabdomyosarcomas (RMS), which are the most common, and non-rhabdomyomatous sarcomas [2]. Examples of the latter category include Ewing sarcoma/peripheral neuroectodermal tumour (ES/PNET), synovial sarcoma (SS), malignant peripheral nerve sheath tumour (MPNST) and infantile fibrosarcoma. Accurate subclassification of sarcomas has important therapeutic implications [3, 4] and can be achieved by a variety of diagnostic methods including light microscopy and immunohistochemical analysis for particular cell antigens (e.g. CD99 in ES/PNET [5]). Molecular cytogenetic and genetic analyses have recently allowed the detection of certain chromosomal abnormalities associated with specific soft tissue sarcomas including the t(11;22) and t(21;22) associated with ES/PNET [6, 7] and the t(12;15) associated with infantile fibrosarcoma [8].

Chromosomal Abnormalities in Paediatric Sarcomas

Paediatric sarcomas fall into two major cytogenetic categories: those characterized by relatively simple, near diploid karyotypes with a small number of consistently rearranged chromosomal loci and those with complex karyotypes without recurrent abnormalities, suggestive of widespread genomic instability [9]. Tumours belonging to the former group include ES/PNET, alveolar RMS (ARMS) and SS [9–12], each of which have recurrent consistent translocations [6, 13–19]. The oncogenic mechanism of such fusion transcripts remains unclear; however, the prevailing view is that expression of aberrant transcripts leads to dysregulation of gene expression and transformation, possibly at the mesenchymal stem cell level [9]. The second group of tumours include ERMS, MPNST and osteosarcoma [9, 20]. Such complex karyotypes are indicative of chromosomal instability; subsequent gain-of-function mutations in oncogenes and loss-of-function mutations in tumour suppressor genes lead to tumour progression [9, 21, 22]. One change noted in a significant proportion of sarcomas with both simple and complex karyotypes is gain of chromosome 8 material, either as whole chromosomes or as amplification of specific regions [23–25]. Trisomy 8 has also been reported as the sole abnormality in extraskeletal mesenchymal chondrosarcoma and paediatric undifferentiated sarcomas [23, 26], suggesting a critical role for gain of chromosome 8 in tumour initiation, possibly through increased *MYC* gene dosage [23].

Sarcomas with Recurrent Rearrangements

Ewing Family of Tumours

The Ewing family of tumours (EFT) is a group of tumours with rearrangement of the *EWSR1* gene on 22q12. Such tumours include Ewing sarcoma (ES), angiomatoid fibrous histiocytoma (AFH), desmoplastic small round cell tumour (DSRCT), clear cell sarcoma (CCS), extraskeletal myxoid chondrosarcoma, myxoid/round cell liposarcoma and myoepithelial tumours ([27]; see Table 23.1).

Ewing sarcoma is the archetypal EFT, and much of the discussion will focus on this tumour. Previously divided into ES and primitive neuroectodermal tumour (pNET) depending on the amount of neuroectodermal differentiation (more in the latter), both subtypes are now considered one and the same tumour, and the World Health Organization has labelled them as ES/pNET. The diagnosis of ES rests upon a combination of histomorphological, immunohistochemical and molecular genetic features. The clinical and histological features have been extensively reviewed elsewhere [27]. Briefly, ES occurs more commonly in males and the incidence peaks in the second decade of life [6, 27]. The majority are primary bone tumours, with some 20–40 % being extraskeletal [27]. The tumour comprises sheets of small round cells with a high nuclear: cytoplasmic ratio; Homer–Wright rosettes and some spindling of the cells may be present. The cells have clear to vacuolated cytoplasm and round, hyperchromatic nuclei with inconspicuous nucleoli. Both lighter staining and darker staining cells can be discerned in the majority of ES using routine haematoxylin and eosin stains (Fig. 23.1). Cytoplasmic glycogen is prominent in many tumours [6, 27–29]. Immunohistochemistry shows evidence for neural differentiation (CD56, CD57, NSE). CD99, a transmembrane glycoprotein and the product of the *MIC2* gene [30, 31], is a more sensitive and specific immunostain [6, 28, 32]. The vast majority of ES show strong, diffuse membranous positivity; however, CD99 staining has also been reported in lymphoblastic lymphoma [33], mesenchymal chondrosarcoma [34] and poorly differentiated synovial sarcoma [35]. In such difficult cases, molecular testing is necessary for definitive diagnosis.

Up to 98 % of ES harbour diagnostic rearrangements of the *EWSR1* gene [36], with up to nine different partners described in a recent review [27]. In the vast majority of cases, *EWSR1* partners with a member of the *ETS* family of transcription factors [6, 13]. The most common partner is *FLI1* on 11q24 (85 % of ES) [6, 37], followed by *ERG* on 21q22 (10 % of ES) [6, 7]. Others include *ETV1* on 7p22 [38], *ETV4* on 17q22 [39] and *FEV* on 2q33 [40]. The *EWS/FLI1* fusion gene is the most extensively studied of the

Table 23.1 Ewing Family of Tumours

Tumour	Translocation	Fusion transcript	IHC	Age affected
Ewing sarcoma[a]	t(11;22)(q24;q12)	*EWSR1/FLI1*	CD99; FLI1; NSE	Peak in second decade
	t(21;22)(q22;q12)	*EWSR1/ERG*		
	t(7;22)(p22;q12)	*EWSR1/ETV1*		
	t(2;22)(q33;q12)	*EWSR1/FEV*		
	t(17;22)(q12;q12)	*EWSR1/ETV4*		
	t(16;21)(p11;q22)	*FUS/ERG*		
	t(2;16)(q35;p11)	*FUS/FEV*		
Angiomatoid fibrous histiocytoma	t(2;22)(q33;q12)	*EWSR1/CREB1*	Desmin; CD99; CD68; EMA	Mean age 20 years
	t(12;22)(q13;q12)	*EWSR1/ATF1*		
	t(12;16)(q13;p11)	*FUS/ATF1*		
Desmoplastic small round cell sarcoma	t(11;22)(p13;q12)	*EWSR1/WT1*	Keratin; EMA; desmin; NSE; WT1 (nuclear)	Peak in third decade
Clear cell sarcoma	t(12;22)(q13;q12)	*EWSR1/ATF1*	S100; HMB45; MART1	Peak in second and third decade
Extraskeletal myxoid chondrosarcoma	t(9;22)(q22;q12)	*EWSR1/NR4A3*	Vimentin	Median age in sixth decade
	t(9;17)(q22;q11)	*RBP56/NR4A3*		
Myoepithelial carcinoma	t(19;22)(q13;q12)	*EWSR1/ZNF444*	EMA, S100, SMA	Older adults, average age 55 years
	t(12;22)(q13;q12)	*EWSR1/ATF1*		
	t(1;22)(q23;q12)	*EWSR1/PBX1*		
	t(6;22)(p21;q12)	*EWSR1/POU5F1*		
Myxoid/round cell liposarcoma	t(12;22)(q13;q12)	*EWSR1/DDIT3*	S100	Peak incidence in fourth and fifth decade

[a]Only the more classical fusion transcripts are included

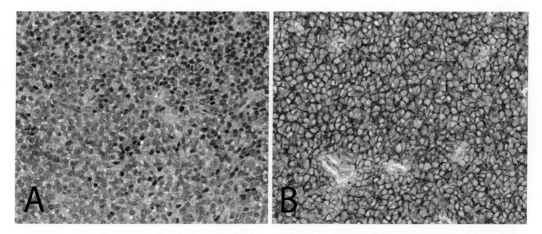

Fig. 23.1 Microscopic appearance and immunohistochemistry in Ewing sarcoma. (**a**) Ewing sarcoma is composed of sheets of polygonal cells with high nuclear:cytoplasmic ratios. Both light and dark cells are present, the latter appearing at *upper right*; (**b**) CD99 positivity highlighting the membranous pattern of staining ((**a**) hematoxylin and eosin; (**b**) immunoperoxidase; original magnification (**a**) and (**b**) ×400)

translocations. Structurally, the amino terminal of *EWS* fuses in frame to the carboxy terminal of *FLI1* and acts as an aberrant transcription factor [41, 42]. The fusion transcript has several reported breakpoints, but all contain the amino-terminal transactivation domain of *EWSR1* and the carboxy-terminal DNA-binding domain of *FLI1* [43]. No difference in biological activity between the different breakpoints has been reported [44]. *EWSR1/FLI1* has potent transforming activities [41] and is essential for maintenance of the transformed state in ES [45–47]. Expression of the *EWSR1/FLI1* fusion protein in vitro results in disrupted expression of a large number of target genes, including genes involved in oncogenic transformation, genes responsible for the maintenance of tumourigenesis and genes involved in the maintenance of the undifferentiated state (reviewed in [27, 44]). One study has shown a better prognosis associated with one specific type of *EWSR1/FLI1* fusion transcript ('type 1') [48], but more recent data suggest that current treatment protocols have eradicated this association [49].

It is worthy to note that a very small percentage of ES (<1 %) harbour rearrangements involving fusion of the *EWSR1* gene with non-ETS family members, including *NFAT2c*, *POU5F1*, *SMARCA5*, *ZSG* and *SP3* (reviewed in [44]). The presence of such rearrangements in ES tumours raises the intriguing question of what constitutes the definition of ES. Are such tumours ES, or do they represent another tumour type, albeit ES-like? Future studies are required to answer this question, but are limited by the rarity of such tumours.

Other EFT harbouring *EWSR1* gene rearrangements include AFH, DSCRT and CCS. CCS is discussed in Chap. 11. AFH is a tumour of borderline malignancy with an excellent prognosis [32]. The tumour generally occurs in children and young adults, with most cases being diagnosed under the age of 40 [32, 50]. The tumour usually presents as an asymptomatic, slow-growing subcutaneous mass; on occasion, systemic symptoms such as pyrexia and weight loss have been reported [32, 50]. Gross examination usually reveals a firm nodule a few centimetres in diameter with a cystic and haemorrhagic cut surface, occasionally mimicking a haematoma or haemangioma [29, 32, 50]. Histological features are characterized by a fibrous and chronically inflamed pseudocapsule, aggregates of lesional cells and interspersed blood-filled spaces. Lesional cells appear uniform and histiocyte-like, with pale cytoplasm and round to oval nuclei. Intracytoplasmic material, including hemosiderin and lipid, may be present, reinforcing the histiocyte-like appearance.

Cellular atypia is uncommon [29, 32, 50, 51] (Fig. 23.2).

The immunohistochemical staining pattern seen in AFH is helpful in coming to a diagnosis; CD68, desmin and CD99 are positive in approximately 50 % of cases, and EMA in approximately 40 % of cases. Vascular markers, other histiocytic markers and keratins are uniformly negative [32, 50, 51]. Electron microscopic analysis of AFH has been inconclusive, with several papers reporting either endothelial, histiocytic or myoid features of lesional cells [51–53].

Molecular genetic analysis of AFH has revealed three distinct fusion events. The most frequent is the t(2;22)(q33;q12) *EWSR1/CREB* rearrangement, followed by the t(12;22)(q13;q12) *EWSR1/ATF1* and the t(12;16)(q13;p11) *FUS/ATF1* rearrangements [50, 51, 54]. Both *EWSR1* and *FUS* are members of the TET family of genes and share structural and functional similarities [55]. Intriguingly, both *EWSR1*-containing fusion genes are identical to those found in CCS (see Chap. 11). The difference in clinical behaviour and phenotype in the presence of the same molecular abnormality is thought to relate to either a different cell of origin, the presence of additional molecular abnormalities or a combination of both [28, 56].

DSCRT is a rare, extremely aggressive EFT occurring in older children and young adults, usually presenting as a diffuse retroperitoneal mass encasing several organs [57]. Other sites of involvement include the lung [58], gonads [59, 60] and bone [61, 62]. It comprises trabeculae, sheets and islands of malignant round cells with Ewing-like features [63]. The cells are distributed within a dense, desmoplastic stroma, and there is often some compression and crushing of the constituent cells, leading to diagnostic difficulties on small biopsies. The cells are polyphenotypic, with variable positivity for desmin, CD99, keratins, EMA and neural markers [27, 57, 63]. The diagnostic molecular abnormality comprises a t(11;22)(p13;q12) rearrangement [64] leading to an *EWSR1/WT1* fusion transcript [28, 65]. The fusion transcript incorporates the carboxy portion of *WT1*, with subsequent expression

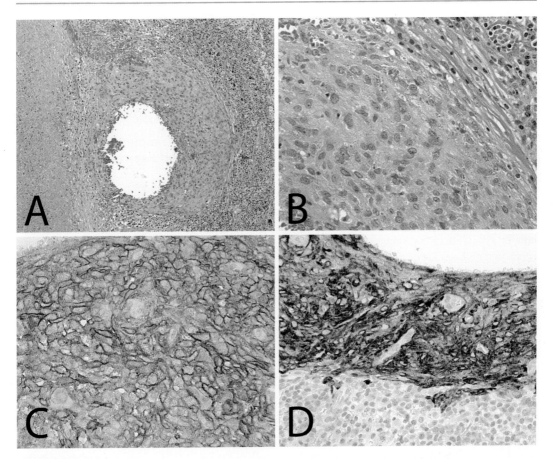

Fig. 23.2 Microscopic appearance and immunohisto-chemistry of angiomatoid fibrous histiocytoma. (**a**) Medium power view showing blood-filled spaces lined partly by histiocytoid cells with surrounding chronic inflammation. Hemosiderin can be seen at *upper right*; (**b**) high-power micrograph showing histiocytoid cells with minimal atypia and intracytoplasmic hemosiderin; (**c**) immunohistochemistry showing membranous positivity for CD99; (**d**) immunohistochemistry showing cytoplasmic positivity for desmin ((**a**, **b**) hematoxylin and eosin, original magnification (**a**) ×100, (**b**) ×400, (**c**, **d**) immunoperoxidase, original magnification ×400)

of only the carboxy terminal of the WT1 protein, a fact that can be utilized for immunohistochemical diagnosis of DSCRT [66]. Expression of the fusion gene is associated with overexpression of *PDGFA*, which is thought to play a central role in the development of DSRCT [67, 68].

Lesser known tumours harbouring *EWSR1* rearrangements include myxoid/round cell liposarcoma t(12;22)(q13;q12), resulting in a *EWSR1/DDIT3* fusion gene [69]; extraskeletal myxoid chondrosarcoma t(9;22)(q22;q12), resulting in *EWSR1/NR4A3* fusion transcript [70]; and myoepithelial tumours, including both myoepitheliomas and myoepithelial carcinomas [71].

The latter group of tumours are intriguing, with several different *EWSR1* partners reported including *POU5F1* [72], *PBX1* [73] and *ATF1* [74].

Congenital Infantile Fibrosarcoma

Congenital infantile fibrosarcoma usually occurs in infancy or early childhood; the majority of cases are diagnosed under the age of 2 years [8]. The tumour presents as a rapidly growing mass in the extremities or the head and neck [8]. Histologically, it comprises sheets of intersecting fascicles with a prominent 'herringbone' pattern of growth and foci of haemangiopericytoma-like vasculature [29, 75]. The immunohistochemical staining pattern is non-specific, with diffuse positivity for vimentin and, in a subset of cases, focal positivity for muscle markers [75].

Molecular genetics demonstrates the presence of a distinct rearrangement involving the transcription factor *ETV6* on 12p13 with the receptor tyrosine kinase *NTRK3* on 15q25 [76–78]. The resultant *ETV6/NTRK3* fusion gene has constitutively active tyrosine kinase activity encoded in the *NTRK3* domain, driving downstream activation of Ras–MAPK and PI3K–AKT pathways (reviewed in [79]). Interestingly, the same rearrangement is shared among several divergent tumour types, including congenital mesoblastic nephroma of the kidney [76, 80], secretory breast carcinoma [81] and acute myeloid leukaemia [82]. The findings suggest a common mechanism of tumourigenesis via tyrosine kinase activation in tumours of mesenchymal, epithelial and haematopoietic origin, and casts further doubt upon the canonical view that specific fusion genes are associated with specific tumours [78, 79].

Primitive Round Cell Sarcoma

PRCS have recently been recognized as a distinct subgroup of paediatric Ewing-like sarcomas [83–87]. Such sarcomas share several morphological and immunohistochemical features with ES, including variable and sometimes patchy CD99 positivity, but do not harbour *EWSR1* rearrangements. Up to 25 % of PRCS harbour a specific translocation involving chromosomes 4 and 19 [84, 87], resulting in fusion of most of the *CIC* gene (19q13) with the C-terminal portion of the *DUX4* gene (4q35). Limited information is known about the function of either gene. However, the *CIC* gene is the human homologue of the Drosophila gene *capicua* and encodes a high-mobility group box transcription factor [88]. The *DUX4* gene is a double homeobox gene whose normal function is poorly understood [89]. One recent study showed that overexpression of the *CIC–DUX4* fusion transcript in vitro induced increased anchorage-independent colony formation in murine NIH3T3 fibroblasts and induced overexpression of *ETS* family transcription factors [85]. However, the functional significance of *CIC–DUX4* in human mesenchymal progenitor

cells, and its role in the maintenance of the undifferentiated state, has not been clearly defined. Further work needs to be done in order to better understand the role of the fusion transcript in sarcomagenesis.

Sarcomas with Complex Karyotypes and No Recurrent Rearrangements

Several paediatric sarcomas have no diagnostic recurrent rearrangements and show complex, variable genetic aberrations. One such tumour, ERMS is described below. Others in this category include paediatric undifferentiated sarcoma of the soft tissues [23], liposarcoma, leiomyosarcoma, angiosarcoma and MPNST. The latter four tumours are discussed in Chap. 11.

Embryonal Rhabdomyosarcoma

ERMS is a tumour that occurs most frequently in children under the age of 10 years [90]. Common sites of involvement include the head and neck and genitourinary system, including the urinary bladder and prostate [90, 91]. Grossly, ERMS are infiltrative tumours that vary from solid, firm and fleshy to soft and myxoid [92]. A specific variant, sarcoma botryoides, has the appearance of a 'bunch of grapes', with multiple small sessile nodules; this variant has a predilection for mucosal sites. Microscopically, ERMS varies from a cellular tumour composed of round, slightly stellate cells with a small amount of cytoplasm to a myxoid tumour with larger spindle-shaped cells containing moderate amounts of eosinophilic cytoplasm [90, 92] (Fig. 23.3). The sarcoma botryoides variant has a cambium layer of condensed malignant cells directly beneath the epithelial layer [92] and is prognostically superior to the classical form [93]. Other variants include anaplastic [94], sclerotic [95, 96] and spindle cell [97], with the anaplastic variant having a worse prognosis when compared to the classical form [98]. Immunohistochemical analysis shows variable nuclear positivity for myogenin, and positivity can be rare; desmin shows more robust positivity [92].

The majority of ERMS show numerous chromosomal abnormalities, including gains of 2,

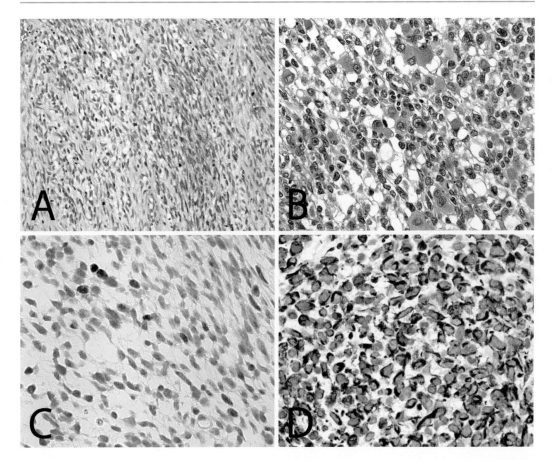

Fig. 23.3 Microscopic appearance and immunohisto-chemistry of embryonal rhabdomyosarcoma. (**a**) Medium power micrograph showing spindle-shaped cells with varying degrees of cellularity and myxoid stroma; (**b**) higher power view showing a posttreatment tumour with extensive cytodifferentiation; (**c**) immunohistochemical staining showing nuclear positivity for myogenin in the minority of cells; (**d**) immunohistochemical staining showing cytoplasmic positivity for desmin in the majority of cells ((**a**, **b**) haematoxylin and eosin, original magnification (**a**) ×200, (**b**) ×400; (**c**, **d**) immunoperoxidase original magnification (**c**, **d**) ×600)

5q35.2–35.3, 7, 8, 11, 12, 13q14 and 20 and losses of 1p36, 3p14–21, 9p21.3, 9q21–22, 10q22-qter, 16q, 17p, 17q11.2 and 22 [99, 100]. Interestingly, one study showed no significant difference in genomic imbalances between ARMS and ERMS [99]. A more specific abnormality is loss of heterozygosity (LOH) at 11p15, which is seen in the majority of ERMS [101, 102]. 11p15 is a highly imprinted chromosomal region implicated in Beckwith–Wiedemann syndrome, providing a link between 11p15, overgrowth syndrome and multiple embryonic tumours including ERMS, Wilms' tumour and hepatoblastoma (reviewed in [103]). Genes within this region include *IGF2* and *CDKN1C*. IGF2 is a pro-proliferative ligand acting via the IGF1 receptor and is implicated in many cancers (see [104] for review). IGF2 expression is upregulated in ERMS [105] and can be detected immunohistochemically in transloca-tion-negative RMS [106]. The tumour suppressor gene p53 also plays an important role in ERMS, and ERMS is associated with Li–Fraumeni syndrome in 1–10 % of patients with the tumour (reviewed in [107]). A recent study using high-resolution array comparative genomic hybridization (CGH) has identified numerous single-gene and gene-signalling abnormalities in ERMS, including loss of *CDKN2A/B*, a master regulator of p53 and Rb, as well as gain of function of *FGFR4*, *Ras* and *GLI1* [100].

Tools for the Diagnosis of Sarcomas

The diagnosis of paediatric sarcomas rests upon a combination of morphological, immunohisto-chemical and molecular genetic studies. Recurrent rearrangements can be detected using a variety of molecular genetic techniques, including traditional karyotypic analysis, spectral karyotyping (SKY), RT-PCR and fluorescence in situ hybridization (FISH).

Traditional karyotypic analysis and SKY require culture and growth of tumour cells. Both techniques have limitations, including failure of tumour cells to grow and a relatively labour- and time-intensive interpretation [108, 109]. Further, they are considered low resolution techniques, with an overall resolution of 3–5 Mb for conventional cytogenetics and 1–2 Mb for SKY [110, 111]. However, the advantages of karyotypic analysis include the ability to provide global information in a single assay [109] and the possibility of detecting novel or variant abnormalities associated with a specific tumour [84, 108].

RT-PCR can detect specific transcripts and has the advantage of being highly sensitive, rapid and requiring only small amounts of tumour RNA [109]. However, RT-PCR is limited by the fact that each primer set detects specific single fusion genes, and to test for multiple translocations requires multiple primer sets and polymerase chain reaction (PCR) reactions [108]. Further, it is not a screening test, and unusual or variant translocations will not be detected. FISH is also relatively rapid and has the advantage of detecting all rearrangements for a given probe, for example, an *EWSR1* break apart probe will detect rearrangement of *EWSR1*, regardless of the partner [108]. However, its strength is also its weakness, as the partner gene is not identified. This can be problematic when the tumour has overlapping features of several EFT tumour types.

Neuroblastoma

Clinical Features of Neuroblastoma

Neuroblastoma is an embryonic tumour derived from primitive neural crest cells of the sympathetic nervous system and can develop anywhere from the neck to the pelvis. It is the most common extracranial solid tumour of childhood affecting approximately 1 in 7,000 children [112], accounting for 15 % of cancer-related deaths in childhood and is the most common cause of death in children aged one to four years [113, 114]. The tumour occurs most frequently in children less than 5 years of age, with a median age at presentation of 18 months [115]. Neuroblastoma is characterized by a remarkable heterogeneity of histology and molecular biology, with a clinical outcome ranging from spontaneous regression to lethal metastatic disease [114, 116].

Risk Stratification

In an attempt to tailor therapy to the individual patient, children undergo risk stratification based on clinical and pathologic parameters and molecular genetic testing. Risk categorization schemes are continually undergoing refinement. The scheme that has been in use for some time by the Children's Oncology Group is based on stage, age, histology category, *MYCN* status and ploidy and divides patients into low, intermediate and high-risk disease (see [114] for details). Treatment for low-risk patients is usually resection or even just observation. Intermediate-risk tumours are usually treated with chemotherapy followed by resection. High-risk patients are given maximal therapy involving combinations of chemotherapy, surgery, radiation, autologous stem cell transplantation and immunotherapy. The overall survival for these groups is >98 %, 90–95 % and 40–50 %, respectively [117]. A more recent modification of this scheme adds also the parameters of tumour differentiation and 11q LOH, resulting in 16 categories associated with very low, low, intermediate and high-risk disease (see [118] for details). For institutions using this type of patient management, pathologists play a critical role in determining risk category and patient treatment. It is therefore important to obtain sufficient tumour for histological assessment as well as *MYCN*, 11q status and ploidy. This necessitates performing either open biopsies or multiple needle core biopsies.

Age

Patient age is one of the oldest prognostic indicators for neuroblastoma. Tumours in patients under 1 year of age tend to show a better outcome and are more likely to spontaneously regress or differentiate. Overall, 5-year survival for patients <1 year old is 94 %; for 1–4 years old, 60 %; and for 5–9 years old, 55 % [119]. Using 1 year of age as the cutoff value for favourable prognosis was convenient for clinical care but arbitrary, and more recent analyses on patients 12–18 months of age have resulted in the cutoff value for favourable prognosis being increased to 18 months of age [115, 120]. This brings the clinical parameter of age in line with the pathology classification system that started to be used almost 30 years ago (see below).

Staging of Neuroblastoma

Tumour stage is another long established prognostic marker for neuroblastoma. While different systems have been employed at various times and places, the one in use for over 20 years by the Children's Oncology Group is the International Neuroblastoma Staging System [121]. In this system, stage 1 is used for localized tumours that are grossly completely resected, with or without residual microscopic disease; stage 2, localized tumours not completely resected with (stage 2B) or without (stage 2A) ipsilateral lymph node involvement; stage 3, unresectable tumours that cross the midline (vertebral column) or located midline with bilateral extension; and stage 4 for disseminated tumours with metastatic involvement including bone, bone marrow, liver, skin and/or distant lymph nodes. Stage 4S is a special category for metastatic tumours in infants less than 18 months of age with a localized primary tumour (stage 1, 2A or 2B) and metastatic disease confined to liver, skin and/or bone marrow infiltration of <10 %.

Low stage neuroblastoma (stages 1 and 2) constitute only about 25 % of cases, but with overall survivals of 95–100 % [122, 123]. Survival for stage 3 disease ranges from 50 to 70 % and is dependent on patient age, tumour histology and tumour biology [124, 125]. Stage 4 patients have a survival of only about 40 % [126, 127]. Stage 4S tumours usually spontaneously resolve with no or minimal treatment, but some behave as high-risk tumours, and prognosis (and treatment planning) for individual patients can be better determined by other factors such as histology and tumour biology [128] (see below).

As part of the new risk classification system (see above), the staging of neuroblastoma is evolving to a more simplified system, but one that is highly dependent on pretreatment imaging [118, 129]. Stage L1 refers to a localized tumour, confined to one body compartment, and not involving vital structures according to a list of image-defined risk factors [130]. Stage L2 then refers to a localized tumour with one or more image-defined risk factors. Stages M and MS replace stages 4 and 4S in the International Neuroblastoma Staging System mentioned above. Using this staging system, stage L1 tumours have a survival of 90 % and stage L2, 78 % [129].

Pathology

Neuroblastoma shows a variable microscopic appearance, ranging from primitive neuroblastic cells to fully differentiated ganglion cells and Schwann cells, and all appearances in between. At the more primitive end of the spectrum, the tumour cells (i.e. neuroblasts) are relatively small cells (about twice the diameter of small lymphocytes) with no discernible cytoplasmic borders (Fig. 23.4). Nuclear chromatin patterns are coarse and small nucleoli are usually present (in contrast to some other small round cell tumours). The neuroblasts tend to form nests of cells separated by fibrovascular septa, and foci of calcification are a common finding. The neuroblasts may be tightly packed appearing as sheets of nuclei, or separated by varying amounts of eosinophilic fibrillary material, or neuropil, which is actually the cytoplasmic extensions of the neuroblasts, and not extracellular matrix. In some tumours, the neuroblasts organize in rosettes around a central core of neuropil, forming a Homer–Wright rosette. This is a helpful diagnostic clue to the diagnosis, but many cases

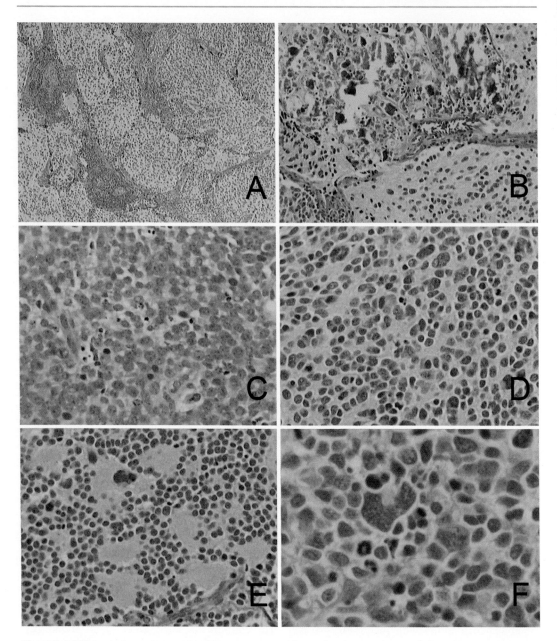

Fig. 23.4 Microscopic appearance of stroma-poor neuroblastoma. (**a**) Neuroblastoma typically forms nests of tumour cells separated by fibrovascular septa, often containing lymphocytes; (**b**) dystrophic calcification is a common histologic finding; (**c**) undifferentiated neuroblastoma consists of crowded primitive cells with no evidence of differentiation; (**d**) poorly differentiated neuroblastoma with primitive neuroblasts showing moderate nuclear pleomorphism and irregular chromatin patterns, separated by eosinophilic neurofibrillary material; (**e**) with better differentiation, neurofibrillary rosettes can be found; (**f**) neuroblastomas may contain anaplastic cells but this finding is not used to derive a histologic prognosis (haematoxylin and eosin, original magnifications: (**a**) ×40, (**b**) ×100, (**c–e**) ×200, (**f**) ×400)

lack this finding. Neuroblasts may also show anaplastic features. Better differentiated neuroblasts show ganglionic differentiation, recognizable as defined cytoplasmic borders and nuclear features that resemble mature ganglion cells. Better differentiated ganglion cells are seen in the most mature types of neuroblastoma. These cells acquire increased amounts of cytoplasm

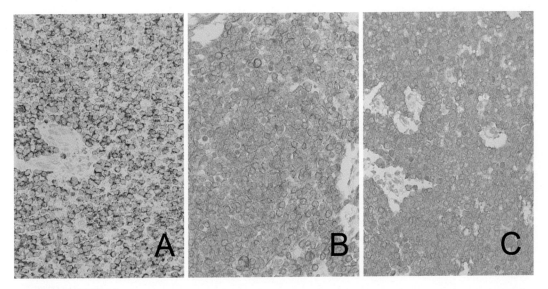

Fig. 23.5 Immunohistochemistry of neuroblastoma. Neuroblasts are diffusely positive for (**a**) NB84, (**b**) MAP2 and (**c**) tyrosine hydroxylase (immunoperoxidase, original magnifications: (**a–c**) ×200)

and more typical ganglion cell type nuclei with a prominent nucleolus, and the most mature forms cannot be distinguished from normal ganglion cells. Also with differentiation, the neuropil material becomes replaced by mature appearing Schwann cells arranged in interlacing fascicles. In most instances, the diagnosis of neuroblastoma can be made by routine light microscopy. However, tumours at the most primitive end of the differentiation spectrum will need immunohistochemistry and/or electron microscopy to confirm the diagnosis. Neuroblastoma is variably positive for neuron-specific enolase, chromogranin, synaptophysin and tyrosine hydroxylase. The two best markers for neuroblasts are NB84 and MAP-2 [131] (Fig. 23.5).

As a general rule, the more primitive neuroblastomas behave in a more aggressive fashion. In an attempt to deal with the different histological appearances and relate these more reliably to clinical behaviour, a classification system was created that standardizes the terminology for pathology reporting and assigns a prognostic value to each histological category as to 'favourable' or 'unfavourable'. The system was devised by Dr. Shimada and has been periodically updated and revised and is now referred to as the International Neuroblastoma Pathology Committee classification [132–135].

The features used for tumour categorization include the degree of differentiation (in terms of the neuroblasts and the Schwannian component), the number of cells in mitosis and/or undergoing karyorrhexis and the patient's age. The formal scheme is complicated at first glance and for details, the original references should be consulted [132–135]. A simplified working version is presented in Table 23.2. Tumours are first divided into stroma-poor and stroma-rich categories, based on the amount of Schwannian tissue or 'stroma', with <50 % considered to be 'stroma-poor'. Stroma-poor tumours constitute 80 % of neuroblastoma overall. For stroma-poor tumours, the patient's age can be used as the next parameter, with the older patients more likely in the unfavourable group, and always if the patient is older than 5 years of age. The degree of differentiation is based on the neuroblasts and to what extent they are becoming ganglionic in appearance. If ≥5 %, the tumour is referred to as 'differentiated'. If the tumour is so primitive, it cannot be diagnosed as neuroblastoma by light microscopy alone, it is referred to 'undifferentiated' and all others are 'poorly differentiated'. Any tumour with neuropil is at least poorly differentiated. Anaplastic cells are not part of the classification system, although this feature has been associated with a worse prognosis [132].

Table 23.2 Scheme for histological classification of neuroblastoma

Stroma-poor neuroblastoma			
>5 years old			Unfavourable
1.5–5 years old	Differentiated	MKI > 100/5,000	Unfavourable
		MKI < 100/5,000	Favourable
	Poorly differentiated		Unfavourable
	Undifferentiated		Unfavourable
<1.5 years old	Differentiated	MKI > 200/5,000	Unfavourable
		MKI < 200/5,000	Favourable
	Poorly differentiated	MKI > 200/5,000	Unfavourable
		MKI < 200/5,000	Favourable
	Undifferentiated		Unfavourable
Stroma-rich neuroblastoma (ganglioneuroblastoma)			
	Maturing		Favourable
	Intermixed		Favourable
	Nodular		Follow stroma-poor system

The last parameter to assess is the mitotic–karyorrhectic index. This refers to the combined number of cells in mitosis OR undergoing karyorrhexis, and the standard is to evaluate 5,000 cells for this count. It is not required to report an absolute value, only the category of low (<100/5,000 cells), intermediate (100–200/5,000 cells) or high (>200/5,000 cells). Fortunately, only about half of the categories in the classification are actually influenced by the MKI (see Table 23.2), and it need not be done in the other categories in order to assign prognosis. Histology is a strong prognostic indicator: favourable stroma-poor tumours have an overall survival of 84 % compared to 4.5 % for unfavourable ones [134, 135].

For the stroma-rich neuroblastoma (also referred to as ganglioneuroblastoma), the system is simpler. Two categories are favourable and are distinguished by the remaining neuroblastoma component, with greater numbers of neuroblasts in nests in the intermixed category, compared to the fewer isolated ones in the well-differentiated ganglioneuroblastoma (also known as maturing ganglioneuroma). Overall survival for these subtypes is 92 % for the intermixed and 100 % for the well-differentiated [134, 135]. The one unfavourable type of ganglioneuroblastoma is the relatively infrequent nodular subtype, which most commonly refers to a composite tumour showing a predominance of differentiated Schwannian stroma associated with one or more macroscopically visible nodules of neuroblastoma. Recently, it was determined that nodular ganglioneuroblastoma can be subcategorized as favourable or unfavourable according to the histopathology of the stroma-poor component, using the same criteria as for other stroma-poor neuroblastomas [136, 137]. Following this approach, unfavourable nodular ganglioneuroblastoma has an overall survival of 40 % compared to 95 % for favourable nodular ganglioneuroblastoma [136, 137].

Immunohistochemistry has generally not been found to be prognostic, although it often reflects differentiation. One exception is the neurotrophin genes *trkA*, *trkB* and *trkC* that encode the TrkA, TrkB and TrkC receptors, respectively. Trk genes encode receptor proteins for nerve growth factors and are important in differentiation and apoptosis of neural crest cells. High expression of TrkA is associated with a more favourable prognosis and high expression of TrkB with an unfavourable prognosis [138–140]. Expression of these proteins can be readily detected by immunohistochemistry, but this information is generally not in use to stratify patients and plan therapy. Nevertheless, TrkB inhibitors such as Lestaurtinib are being investigated as possible therapeutic agents in neuroblastoma [141].

Genetic Features of Neuroblastoma: Introduction

As with histology and clinical behaviour, there is great variability in the genetic changes that can occur in neuroblastoma. Although genetic changes are used in the vast majority of paediatric tumours to aid in diagnosis, this is not the case for neuroblastoma. Many genetic changes are strong prognostic markers and have been used to determine therapy for more than 20 years. Only some are currently included in risk stratification (see above). Genetic changes fall into two broad genetic categories: whole chromosome gains and segmental alterations (gains, losses, gene amplifications). Generally speaking, tumours with whole chromosome gains tend to occur in younger patients, have a lower stage, are more likely to differentiate and have a more favourable prognosis. The opposite tends to be the case for tumours with segmental alterations that tend to show involvement of chromosomes 1p, 11q, 17q and/or the *MYCN* oncogene [142, 143].

Genetic changes in neuroblastoma are detected using a variety of techniques including flow cytometry, in situ hybridization by fluorescence (FISH) or light microscopy chromogens (CISH), PCR and DNA arrays, based on either CGH or single nucleotide polymorphisms (SNPs). Excellent reviews are available on the advantages and disadvantages of these various techniques [144, 145].

DNA Content

DNA content or ploidy is one of the oldest genetic prognostic markers for neuroblastoma [146, 147] and is usually assessed by flow cytometry. While fresh tumour tissue is optimal, this parameter can be determined from paraffin-embedded tissue if necessary. Contrary to what might be predicted, diploid (DNA index of 1) tumours are unfavourable while aneuploid or triploid tumours (DNA index >1) are favourable [146–149]. This phenomenon reflects the finding that diploid tumours usually have prognostically unfavourable segmental changes in chromosomes, changes that are insufficient to alter the overall DNA content by much, and therefore such tumours appear diploid by flow cytometry. The prognostic value of DNA content is more significant in patients <12 months of age, and after 2 years becomes not significant. Ploidy is one of the genetic variables currently used in risk stratification (see above).

MYCN Oncogene

The *MYCN* gene is located on chromosome 2p24, and increased copies of this gene (amplification) are seen in 16–25 % of neuroblastoma tumours but in 40–50 % of high stage tumours (stages 3 and 4) and uncommonly (5–10 %) in low stage tumours (stage 1, 2 or 4S) [114, 150–153]. The *MYCN* gene is rarely mutated in neuroblastoma (1.7 % of cases) [154]. Amplification of *MYCN* has been known for about 30 years to be associated with a poor outcome in neuroblastoma [150, 151, 155]. For any stage, the prognosis is worsened if the tumour is *MYCN* amplified, and for stage 4/M disease, the overall 5-year survival drops to 25 % [153, 155]. *MYCN* copy number is one of the markers used in risk stratification (see above), and patients with amplification are considered to be high risk in the most recent system [118], regardless of other prognostic factors.

Copy number used to be determined from extracted DNA using Southern blotting [150] or quantitative PCR [156], techniques that gave an average result for a patient's tumour. These techniques have been replaced by FISH or CISH performed either on dispersed nuclei or intact tissue sections. Amplification is detected usually as extrachromosomal paired chromatin bodies (referred to as double minute chromosomes) (Fig. 23.6) and less commonly as multiple copies of the *MYCN* gene integrated as tandem repeats into one chromosome forming a homogeneously staining region (HSR). It is generally believed that HSRs develop from double minute chromosomes [157, 158]. The genetic form of amplification (double minute chromosomes vs. HSRs) has no prognostic significance [159].

ISH approaches have shown there is considerable heterogeneity in the number of double minute

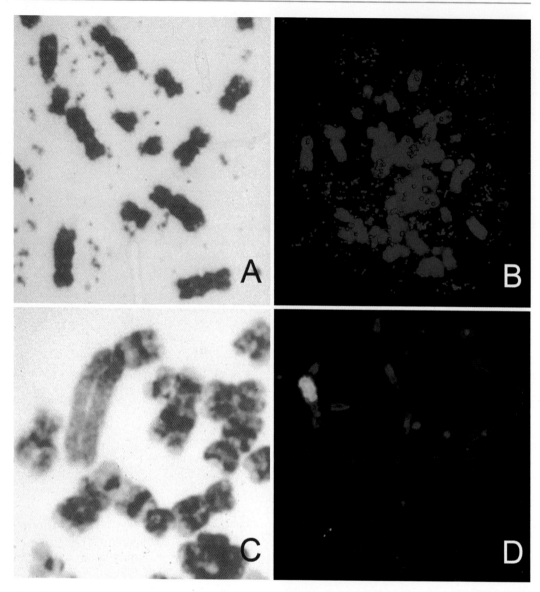

Fig. 23.6 *MYCN* amplification in neuroblastoma. (**a**) Metaphase spread showing numerous double minute chromosomes as paired extrachromosomal bodies; (**b**) FISH probe for *MYCN* tagged with Spectrum orange (*red*) showing the double minute chromosomes represent multiple copies of the *MYCN* gene (i.e. amplification); (**c**) metaphase spread showing a homogeneously staining region integrated into one chromosomes, lacking the normal banding pattern seen in the other chromosomes; (**d**) FISH probe for *MYCN* tagged with Spectrum green (*green*) showing the homogeneously staining region is a tandem series of copies of the *MYCN* gene

chromosomes observed per cell by FISH and CISH [160–165]. This is the result of unequal segregation of double minute chromosomes between daughter cells at mitosis, since double minute chromosomes lack centromeres and cannot be faithfully guided by the mitotic spindle. To deal with this, amplification is defined as >10 gene copies per diploid cell [148]. Values of 3–10 are referred to as *MYCN-gained* and often reflect increased copies of chromosome 2, where the *MYCN* gene resides. *MYCN* gain does not imply an unfavourable prognosis and is not used in risk stratification. Since 50 % of cases of metastatic neuroblastoma do not have *MYCN* amplification, it follows that the lack of amplification is not necessarily a favourable prognostic indicator. Levels of *MYCN* mRNA and MYCN protein have not been found to be prognostically useful [166]. However, recent studies have shown that some tumours have an unfavourable course due to elevated MYCN protein levels in the absence of *MYCN* amplification [167].

When comparing expression profiles in *MYCN*-amplified and non-amplified neuroblastomas, over 200 genes are associated with increased *MYCN* expression [168–172] and many of these genes are targets of MYCN. Upregulated genes include other transcription factors, genes related to proliferation, drug resistance and angiogenesis. Downregulated genes include those related to cell cycle regulation, apoptosis, signal transduction and neural differentiation. All of these changes would be permissive to tumour development and survival.

Chromosomal Changes in Neuroblastoma

Alterations of Chromosome 1p

Deletion of chromosome 1p occurs in 25–35 % of neuroblastoma overall, but LOH for this region occurs in up to 90 % of high stage cases [148, 173, 174]. The minimal common region of deletion has been narrowed to 1p36.2–1p36.3, but in many cases, the deletion is much larger [175]. Deletion is usually detected by FISH (Fig. 23.7), whereas detection of LOH requires other techniques such as PCR or SNP arrays, which are not generally in use in most diagnostic laboratories. Deletion of 1p or LOH of 1p is associated with a poor prognosis, but this genetic change is usually associated with *MYCN* amplification, as well as other unfavourable markers such as stage 4 disease, diploid chromosomal content and 17q gain [148, 173, 174, 176]. However, some tumours show 1p LOH without these other changes, supporting 1p LOH to be an independent marker for poor prognosis [177]. Despite this evidence, 1p status is not currently used for risk stratification.

The region 1p36.2–1p36.3 is believed to be the site of one or more tumour suppressor genes. Expression studies comparing neuroblastomas with and without 1p deletion identified ~25 known genes in this region including ones involved in neural differentiation, signal transduction in neural cells and cell cycle regulation [178]. However, complete loss of expression was *not* consistently found for any single gene. Another expression study concluded that the unfavourable prognosis from 1p deletion/LOH results from reduced expression of a combination of genes, rather than a single tumour suppressor gene [179]. Sequencing the entire region of minimal deletion on chromosome 1p identified 15 known genes, 9 unknown genes and 6 predicted genes [180]. Of these only *CDH5* (chromatin helicase-binding domain 5) showed high expression in neural tissue *and* no expression in neuroblastoma. This gene encodes VE-cadherin (CD144) and is involved in chromatin remodelling. CHD5 is an attractive candidate tumour suppressor gene for neuroblastoma: *CHD5* expression is lost in neuroblastoma cell lines and restoration leads to loss of tumourigenicity. The first allele is lost by deletion and the second is inactivated by promoter methylation. High *CDH5* expression correlates with other favourable parameters (age, stage, histology, ploidy, *MYCN* status, 1p status) and a favourable outcome [180–182].

Alterations of Chromosome 11q

11q deletion or LOH occurs in 21 % of cases of neuroblastoma [148]. The changes are centred on region 11q23, which is believed to be the site of one or more important tumour suppressor genes that to date have not been identified. As with 1p alterations, changes at 11q can be detected by FISH, PCR or DNA arrays. 11q deletion/LOH is associated with a poor outcome, with an overall survival rate of 45 % [183]. 11q23 changes are associated with gain at chromosome 17q, but are inversely associated with *MYCN* amplification and alterations at 1p [184]. This makes 11q status a powerful prognostic marker for cases that are not *MYCN* amplified and can be used to define a distinct biological group of neuroblastoma with a

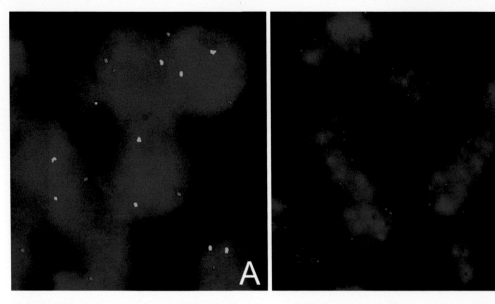

Fig. 23.7 Chromosomal gains and losses in neuroblastoma. (a) FISH probe for the 1p region tagged with Spectrum orange (*red*) showing one copy per interphase nucleus, whereas a centromere probe for chromosome 1 tagged with Spectrum green (*green*) shows two copies of chromosome 1 are present, indicating a deletion of 1p; (b) FISH probe for the 17q region tagged with Spectrum orange (*red*) showing 3–4 copies per interphase nucleus, indicating 17q gain

poor prognosis. Alterations of 11q are one of the parameters used in the latest risk stratification system [118].

Alterations of Chromosome 17q

In contrast to 1p and 11q that can be deleted in neuroblastoma, the region of 17q is often gained in neuroblastoma (48 % of cases), making this change the most common genetic change seen in neuroblastoma [148, 185]. It is most easily detected by FISH (Fig. 23.7). This region is sometimes involved in an unbalanced translocation, but the breakpoint is not consistent, other than occurring proximal to 17q22 [186]. This suggests the clinical effects of 17q gain are related to dosage effects of one or more genes in the distal portion of 17q acting as oncogenes, rather than disruption of a specific gene [186]. Genes that reside in this region that have been shown to be overexpressed in neuroblastoma include *NGFR*, *nm23-H1*, *nm23-H2* [187], *BiCR5* [188] and *PMM1D* [189]. *BiCR5* and *PMM1D* are related to cell proliferation and inhibition of apoptosis, changes that would promote a malignant phenotype. Of interest, *nm23-H1* and *nm23-H2* are both targets of the MYCN protein, but their exact role in neuroblastoma is not known. 17q gain is associated with a poor outcome, with an overall survival of 31 % [185]. This change, however, is associated with 1p deletion and *MYCN* amplification in two-thirds of patients. This genetic finding is not currently used for risk stratification in neuroblastoma.

Specific Genes Altered in Neuroblastoma

ALK Gene

The *ALK* gene is normally expressed in the developing nervous system (central and peripheral) and is involved in neuronal differentiation during embryogenesis and activation of cell proliferation, migration and survival (reviewed in [190]). Multiple malignancies harbour *ALK* alterations, including anaplastic large cell lymphoma and inflammatory myofibroblastic tumour, which are both encountered in the paediatric age group.

Germline mutations in *ALK* occur in ~50 % of cases of hereditary neuroblastoma [191, 192] and some of these pedigrees also have congenital anomalies of the central nervous system [193]. *ALK* alterations are not limited to familial neuroblastoma; *ALK* gain (from trisomy 2p) is seen in 23 % cases and *ALK* amplification in 2 % cases.

ALK mutations are equally distributed over all stages of neuroblastoma, and an association between most *ALK* mutations and reduced survival has not yet been established [190]. However, the prognostic significance may be mutation-specific; the F1174L mutation when associated with *MYCN* amplification correlates with a very poor outcome, worse than *MYCN* amplification alone [194]. This suggests a synergism between the *ALK* and *MYCN* genes in neuroblastoma, a concept supported by work in transgenic animal models. Transgenic animal models that overexpress human *MYCN* and the *ALK* F1174 mutation show increased tumour incidence and earlier tumour onset [195–197]. In this setting, the mutant ALK protein results in increased functional MYCN protein, in part through activation of the mTOR pathway [195]. *ALK* point mutations can occur in human neuroblastoma in the absence of *MYCN* amplification, suggesting the *ALK* mutation may be oncogenic in itself. This concept is also supported by animal studies; a transgenic mouse model that overexpresses the *ALK* F1174 mutation develops neuroblastoma with *MYCN* amplification and 17q loss [196]. Activation of *ALK* regulates cellular proliferation, differentiation and apoptosis via a number of different signalling pathways. The specific proteins and pathways involved in *ALK* mutations leading to neuroblastoma are still being worked out (reviewed in [190]).

ALK mutations are associated with high *ALK* expression but, paradoxically, high *ALK* expression can also be seen in tumours that lack *ALK* mutations [198, 199]. The ALK protein can be detected by immunohistochemistry. Greater than 50 % tumour cells positive by immunohistochemistry has been associated with a poor outcome [198]. Immunostaining would be simpler and cheaper than gene sequencing, but the prognostic significance of this remains unestablished. The importance of determining the *ALK* status for neuroblastoma patients lies mainly in the clin-ical potential. ALK inhibitors exist, and studies are ongoing to explore these as a therapeutic option in neuroblastoma. Knowledge of the specific mutation may be needed since some mutations are more resistant to certain ALK inhibitors than others [190]. mTOR inhibitors may be useful in overcoming resistance to ALK inhibitors [195]. It is unclear whether to treat only patients with *ALK* mutations or also those in whom the tumour is ALK positive by immunohistochemistry, but not *ALK* mutated. The decision will determine how the pathology laboratory assesses *ALK* gene status for neuroblastoma patients.

Other Genes

Phox2B: Germline mutations in the *Phox2B* gene have been reported in familial neuroblastoma [200–202]. Such patients may have other abnormalities, such as Hirschsprung disease and congenital hypoventilation syndrome (Ondine's curse). Only rarely are *Phox2b* mutations detected in sporadic neuroblastoma [203].

PTPN11: Germline mutations in the *PTPN11* gene are associated with Noonan syndrome, in which there is a predisposition to malignant tumours, in particular brain tumours, RMS and leukaemia, and rarely neuroblastoma [204, 205]. The overall mutation frequency in sporadic neuroblastoma is only 2.9 % [154, 204].

ATRX: The *ATRX* gene is involved in chromatin remodelling, nucleosome assembly and telomere maintenance [206]. Through whole genome sequencing, mutations were found in the *ATRX* gene in patients with stage 4 neuroblastoma that were strongly age-dependent: 44 % of cases in patients >12 years of age, 17 % of cases in patients 18 months to <12 years and 0 % of cases in patients <18 months [206]. Overall, the frequency of mutation is 9–10 % [154]. *ATRX* mutations were mutually exclusive of *MYCN* amplification, and patients with *ATRX* mutations had a more chronic and progressive course of disease.

LIN28b: Overexpression of *LIN28b* is a frequent finding in high-risk neuroblastoma (both *MYCN* amplified and non-amplified), but only a small proportion of cases are associated with amplification of the *LIN28b* gene on 6q21 [207]. High expression is a poor prognostic marker that is independent of *MYCN* amplification.

ARID1A/ARID1: Mutations have recently been detected in the genes *ARID1A* and *ARID1B* in 11 % of patients with neuroblastoma, with roughly equal involvement of both genes [208]. These mutations were associated with a poor outcome. The mutations lead to loss of function of the proteins, which normally are involved in chromatin remodelling as part of the SWI/SNF complex that is essential for the self-renewal of multipotent neural stem cells.

TP53: The tumour suppressor gene *TP53* is rarely mutated in neuroblastoma, although this can occur following cytotoxic therapy [209, 210]. However, disturbances in the p53 pathway in neuroblastoma may come via other routes. The *MDM2* gene normally inhibits p53 activity by degradation of p53. Amplification of *MDM2* is seen in sarcomas, gliomas and leukaemias [211] but not in neuroblastoma [212]. Instead, the *MDM2* gene is a target gene for MYCN, and neuroblastomas with *MYCN* amplification have high levels of MDM2 expression [212]. In turn, this leads to inhibition of p53 pathways.

Screening Technologies for Neuroblastoma

Expression Profiling

cDNA microarray studies have been widely used to study neuroblastoma [168–170, 172, 178, 213–226]. Some studies have examined neuroblastomas in general, and others have compared specific subgroups (e.g. tumours with and without 1p deletion, with and without *MYCN* amplification, low vs high telomerase expression, low vs. high stage). The goal has been to identify specific genes that play critical roles in determining the biology of neuroblastoma. Most studies have generated sets of 15–80 genes that are overexpressed in unfavourable tumours and another similar set overexpressed in favourable tumours.

Genes that are expressed in favourable type neuroblastomas include ones involved in neuronal differentiation, catecholamine metabolism, neuropeptide hormone activity, cell cycle regulation, apoptosis, signal transduction, cell adhesion and cell-to-cell signalling. Genes that are expressed in unfavourable type tumours include telomerase, transcription factors, DNA helicases, RNA binding proteins and genes involved in apoptosis escape. Overexpression of these would then lead to chromosomal instability, malignant transformation, invasiveness and metastatic spread.

As might be expected with a tumour of such complicated biology as neuroblastoma, no single marker has emerged as a strong predictor of outcome, but several studies have generated sets of genes, the expression profiles of which were useful for predicting prognosis. While these may be more accurate than the current risk stratification systems [220, 221], the need for high-quality RNA samples, expensive microarray technology and detailed computer-based analysis of the results makes this type of testing impractical for everyday clinical use. Nevertheless, specific genes of interest for prognosis or treatment purposes may be culled from such studies in the future.

miRNAs in Neuroblastoma

microRNAs (miRNAs) are small noncoding RNAs that generally act as negative regulators of gene expression by inhibiting translation or promoting RNA degradation [227, 228]. The primary miRNA is processed into its final form by the endonucleases DROSHA and DICER. Global downregulation of miRNAs has been reported in high-risk neuroblastoma associated with low expression of DICER and DROSHA [229].

Some miRNAs are targets of *MYCN* [230, 231]. By comparing *MYCN*-amplified and non-amplified tumours, at least 50 miRNAs are differentially regulated by *MYCN*. The majority are repressed including miRNAs involved in controlling cell cycle, apoptosis, differentiation and signal transduction (e.g. miR-184 and miR-542-5p). Some miRNAs show increased expression, and these normally promote cell proliferation, cell migration and inhibition of apoptosis (e.g. miR-9 and the miR-17-92 cluster). Such alterations would favour a malignant phenotype and metastatic spread. The expression of a small number (<35) of specific miRNAs has been reported to be useful in separating neuroblastoma patients into low-risk and high-risk groups [229, 232, 233]. This type of testing generally requires both high-quality RNA samples and array technology and is beyond the capabilities of most paediatric laboratories.

Whole Genomic Profiling in Neuroblastoma

High throughput sequencing technologies have found few recurrently mutated genes in neuroblastoma, largely limited to *ALK*, *PTPN11*, *ATRX*, *ARID1A* and *ARID1B* (see above) [154, 208]. Perhaps a more exciting result from this type of technology is the identification of specific alleles/variants in the *host* genome that are associated with not only susceptibility to develop neuroblastoma but also the clinical behaviour of the neuroblastoma. Such risk alleles can be identified by genome-wide association screening (GWAS), an approach that compares the genomes of a very large numbers of patients to an even larger number of controls to obtain statistical verification. From this type of work, it has been shown that specific SNPs in *BARD1*, *CHEK2*, *LMO1*, *LINC00340* and *PINK1* are associated with high-risk disease, whereas specific SNPs in *DUSP12*, *DDX4*, *IL31RA* and *HSD17B12* are associated with low-risk disease ([154, 234–238]). Moreover, children carrying 6–8 risk alleles have a threefold increased risk of developing high-risk neuroblastoma compared with those who carried 0–3 risk alleles [236]. The mechanisms on how the polymorphisms in these genes affect neuroblastoma tumour biology are just beginning to be worked out. As an example, *BARD1* is related to *BRCA1* that plays a role in breast cancer. One variant, *BARD1β*, is preferentially expressed in neuroblastoma and stabilizes the Aurora family of kinases in neuroblastoma cells [239]. The clinical relevance to this understanding is that Aurora kinase inhibitors exist and

these might offer a therapeutic option for neuroblastoma treatment.

There is also evidence that high-risk behaviour in neuroblastoma may be influenced by epigenetic modifications during tumour evolution, such as methylation. Since methylation generally results in gene silencing, this has a similar result to a loss of function mutation. Methylation can be detected using methylation-specific PCR [240]. In neuroblastoma, methylation of specific genes, such as *CASP8*, *DCR2*, *HIN-1*, *HIST1H3C*, *PRPH* and *ACSS3*, has been shown to be associated with a poor prognosis [240–242]. Caspase 8 function is involved in apoptosis and HIN1 in controlling cell migration, and *PRPH* encodes the cytoskeletal protein peripherin that is associated with maturation of a neuronal phenotype. Hence, loss of these functions would support a malignant phenotype.

Emergent Technologies

Several relatively recent techniques have the potential to be utilized in the diagnostic laboratory, namely, array technologies, NanoString RNA technology and whole genome sequencing.

Microarray CGH

Microarray CGH (mCGH) uses a DNA chip to detect copy number changes in tumour DNA [145, 243]. Multiple regions of genomic gain/amplification or deletion can be detected by one test using array technology versus multiple labour-intensive tests using the current, most commonly used technique of interphase fluorescence in situ hybridization (iFISH). mCGH has been recently applied to neuroblastoma, a tumour where certain DNA copy number changes are associated with prognosis (see previous neuroblastoma section). In addition to providing such clinical information, mCGH has also provided a large number of discovery-based findings that may form the basis of future prognostic targets [169, 244–247].

Expression Arrays

The use of expression arrays as routine diagnostic tools in the clinical laboratory has not been realized. It requires significant technical and financial resources, high-quality and demanding tissue handling protocols and results in a large amount of data requiring sophisticated computational algorithms for meaningful analysis [22, 248]. Further, reproducibility between studies has been variable. For these reasons, expression array studies have not been incorporated into the clinical laboratory.

Nevertheless, expression array technology has been extensively applied to neuroblastomas (see previous neuroblastoma section) and sarcomas in research settings. Studies analysing sarcomas have attempted to identify gene expression patterns associated with specific tumour subtypes, with the aim being to translate expression array data into clinically useful antibody markers for diagnosis, classification and prognosis (reviewed in [22, 248]). An example is the discovery of TLE1 as a specific marker for SS [249, 250] and the finding of cKIT expression associated with gastrointestinal stromal tumour [251]. More recent work has found specific markers distinguishing subtypes of osteosarcoma [252] and synovial sarcoma [253], enabling more accurate subclassification. Further, therapeutically relevant discoveries have been made, particularly with relation to the use of IGF pathway inhibition in the treatment of ES [254, 255] and HER2 in SS [249].

NanoString Technology

NanoString technology is a barcode-based system [256] that uses two types of probes: reporter probes and capture probes. Each probe has sequence-specific region that binds to the target sequence (either mRNA or DNA). Reporter probes are labelled with colour-coded bar tags, with each specific reporter probe having a unique colour code identifier. The capture probe then hybridizes with the target transcript–reporter pair and immobilizes the complex onto the surface of the chip.

Excess probe and nucleic acid are then washed away and the signal is read and decoded [256]. The methodology avoids the necessity of reverse transcription or amplification of the target genes. The system is extremely sensitive (500 attomolar quantities), and the hybridization-based technique minimizes background. Further, NanoString uses minimal amounts of DNA or RNA (50–100 ng) and can use up to 800 probes in a single reaction [257].

NanoString technology has been recently applied to paediatric sarcomas [258], as well as fusion transcript detection in adult cancers [259]. NanoString technology is ideally placed to detect fusion transcripts [258, 259]. Furthermore, the assay has the ability to test for multiple different fusion transcripts in a single reaction, avoiding the need for multiple different assays [256]. Some laboratories are currently exploring the utility of such a technique for the detection of diagnostically specific translocations in paediatric sarcomas.

Whole Genome and Whole Exome Sequencing

WG/WE sequencing has had limited use in the diagnostic oncology laboratory; however, there have been several discovery-related findings using such techniques. The general concepts of using this technology in paediatric neoplasia have been discussed under neuroblastoma.

Conclusion

The current state of molecular diagnostics for cancer in paediatrics is one of rapid change. With newer techniques comes additional molecular information that impacts diagnosis, prognosis and therapeutic options for individual tumours. Techniques such as NanoString and microarray CGH are making their way into diagnostic oncology laboratories, and whole genome sequencing is already being used for the detection of constitutional aberrations. The era of personalized medicine is upon us, and the pathologist will play a central role as we move forward to more accurate diagnoses and specific targeted therapies.

References

1. Mackall CL, Meltzer PS, Helman LJ. Focus on sarcomas. Cancer Cell. 2002;2(3):175–8.
2. Meyer WH, Spunt SL. Soft tissue sarcomas of childhood. Cancer Treat Rev. 2004;30(3):269–80.
3. Coffin CM, Dehner LP, O'Shea PA. Pediatric soft tissue sarcomas: a clinical, pathological and therapeutic approach. Baltimore, MD: Williams & Wilkins; 1997.
4. Rubin BP. Recent progress in the classification of soft tissue tumors: role of genetics and clinical implications. Curr Opin Oncol. 2001;13(4):256–60.
5. Coindre JM. Immunohistochemistry in the diagnosis of soft tissue tumours. Histopathology. 2003;43(1):1–16.
6. Ushigome S, Machinami R, Sorensen PH. Ewing sarcoma/primitive neuroectodermal tumour (PNET). In: Fletcher CDM, Unni KK, Mertens F, editors. World Health Organization classification of tumours: tumours of soft tissue and bone. Lyon: IARC Press; 2002. p. 297–300.
7. Sorensen PH, Lessnick SL, Lopez-Terrada D, Liu XF, Triche TJ, Denny CT. A second Ewing's sarcoma translocation, t(21;22), fuses the EWS gene to another ETS-family transcription factor, ERG. Nat Genet. 1994;6(2):146–51.
8. Coffin CM, Fletcher JA. Infantile fibrosarcoma. In: Fletcher CD, Unni KK, Mertens F, editors. World Health Organization classification of tumours: tumours of soft tissue and bone. Lyon: World Health Organization; 2002. p. 98–100.
9. Helman LJ, Meltzer P. Mechanisms of sarcoma development. Nat Rev Cancer. 2003;3(9):685–94.
10. Sandberg AA, Bridge JA. Updates on cytogenetics and molecular genetics of bone and soft tissue tumors: Ewing sarcoma and peripheral primitive neuroectodermal tumors. Cancer Genet Cytogenet. 2000;123(1):1–26.
11. Sandberg AA, Bridge JA. Updates on the cytogenetics and molecular genetics of bone and soft tissue tumors. Synovial sarcoma. Cancer Genet Cytogenet. 2002;133(1):1–23.
12. Sandberg AA, Bridge JA. Updates on the cytogenetics and molecular genetics of bone and soft tissue tumors. Desmoplastic small round-cell tumors. Cancer Genet Cytogenet. 2002;138(1):1–10.
13. Delattre O, Zucman J, Melot T, et al. The Ewing family of tumors—a subgroup of small-round-cell tumors defined by specific chimeric transcripts. N Engl J Med. 1994;331(5):294–9.
14. Delattre O, Zucman J, Plougastel B, et al. Gene fusion with an ETS DNA-binding domain caused by chromosome translocation in human tumours. Nature. 1992;359(6391):162–5.
15. Zucman J, Delattre O, Desmaze C, et al. Cloning and characterization of the Ewing's sarcoma and peripheral neuroepithelioma t(11;22) translocation breakpoints. Genes Chromosomes Cancer. 1992;5(4):271–7.
16. Galili N, Davis RJ, Fredericks WJ, et al. Fusion of a fork head domain gene to PAX3 in the solid tumour alveolar rhabdomyosarcoma. Nat Genet. 1993;5(3):230–5.
17. Davis RJ, D'Cruz CM, Lovell MA, Biegel JA, Barr FG. Fusion of PAX7 to FKHR by the variant t(1;13)(p36;q14) translocation in alveolar rhabdomyosarcoma. Cancer Res. 1994;54(11):2869–72.
18. Barr FG, Galili N, Holick J, Biegel JA, Rovera G, Emanuel BS. Rearrangement of the PAX3 paired box gene in the paediatric solid tumour alveolar rhabdomyosarcoma. Nat Genet. 1993;3(2):113–7.
19. Parham DM, Barr FG. Alveolar rhabdomyosarcoma. In: Fletcher CD, Unni KK, Mertens F, editors. World Health Organization classification of tumours: tumours of soft tissue and bone. Lyon: IARC Press; 2002. p. 150–2.
20. Squire JA, Pei J, Marrano P, et al. High-resolution mapping of amplifications and deletions in pediatric osteosarcoma by use of CGH analysis of cDNA microarrays. Genes Chromosomes Cancer. 2003; 38(3):215–25.
21. Mintz MB, Sowers R, Brown KM, et al. An expression signature classifies chemotherapy-resistant pediatric osteosarcoma. Cancer Res. 2005;65(5):1748–54.
22. Nielsen TO. Microarray analysis of sarcomas. Adv Anat Pathol. 2006;13(4):166–73.
23. Selvarajah S, Yoshimoto M, Prasad M, et al. Characterization of trisomy 8 in pediatric undifferentiated sarcomas using advanced molecular cytogenetic techniques. Cancer Genet Cytogenet. 2007;174(1):35–41.
24. Tarkkanen M, Larramendy ML, Bohling T, et al. Malignant fibrous histiocytoma of bone: analysis of genomic imbalances by comparative genomic hybridisation and C-MYC expression by immunohistochemistry. Eur J Cancer. 2006;42(8):1172–80.
25. Morrison C, Radmacher M, Mohammed N, et al. MYC amplification and polysomy 8 in chondrosarcoma: array comparative genomic hybridization, fluorescent in situ hybridization, and association with outcome. J Clin Oncol. 2005;23(36):9369–76.
26. Gatter KM, Olson S, Lawce H, Rader AE. Trisomy 8 as the sole cytogenetic abnormality in a case of extraskeletal mesenchymal chondrosarcoma. Cancer Genet Cytogenet. 2005;159(2):151–4.
27. Tsokos M, Alaggio RD, Dehner LP, Dickman PS. Ewing sarcoma/peripheral primitive neuroectodermal tumor and related tumors. Pediatr Dev Pathol. 2012;15(1 Suppl):108–26.
28. Romeo S, Dei Tos AP. Soft tissue tumors associated with EWSR1 translocation. Virchows Arch. 2010; 456(2):219–34.
29. Kempson RL, Fletcher CDM, Evans HL, Hendrickson MR, Sibley RK. Tumors of the soft tissues. 3rd ed. Washington, DC: Armed Forces Institute of Pathology; 2001.

30. Goodfellow PN, Pym B, Pritchard C, et al. MIC2: a human pseudoautosomal gene. Philos Trans R Soc Lond B Biol Sci. 1988;322(1208):145–54.

31. Fellinger EJ, Garin-Chesa P, Triche TJ, Huvos AG, Rettig WJ. Immunohistochemical analysis of Ewing's sarcoma cell surface antigen p30/32MIC2. Am J Pathol. 1991;139(2):317–25.

32. Weiss SW, Goldblum JR. Enzinger and Weiss's soft tissue tumors. 4th ed. St. Louis, MO: Mosby; 2001.

33. Ozdemirli M, Fanburg-Smith JC, Hartmann DP, et al. Precursor B-lymphoblastic lymphoma presenting as a solitary bone tumor and mimicking Ewing's sarcoma: a report of four cases and review of the literature. Am J Surg Pathol. 1998;22(7):795–804.

34. Granter SR, Renshaw AA, Fletcher CD, Bhan AK, Rosenberg AE. CD99 reactivity in mesenchymal chondrosarcoma. Hum Pathol. 1996;27(12):1273–6.

35. Pelmus M, Guillou L, Hostein I, Sierankowski G, Lussan C, Coindre JM. Monophasic fibrous and poorly differentiated synovial sarcoma: immunohistochemical reassessment of 60 t(X;18)(SYT-SSX)-positive cases. Am J Surg Pathol. 2002;26(11):1434–40.

36. Mackintosh C, Madoz-Gurpide J, Ordonez JL, Osuna D, Herrero-Martin D. The molecular pathogenesis of Ewing's sarcoma. Cancer Biol Ther. 2010;9(9):655–67.

37. Aurias A, Rimbaut C, Buffe D, Dubousset J, Mazabraud A. Chromosomal translocations in Ewing's sarcoma. N Engl J Med. 1983;309(8):496–8.

38. Jeon IS, Davis JN, Braun BS, et al. A variant Ewing's sarcoma translocation (7;22) fuses the EWS gene to the ETS gene ETV1. Oncogene. 1995;10(6):1229–34.

39. Kaneko Y, Yoshida K, Handa M, et al. Fusion of an ETS-family gene, EIAF, to EWS by t(17;22)(q12;q12) chromosome translocation in an undifferentiated sarcoma of infancy. Genes Chromosomes Cancer. 1996;15(2):115–21.

40. Peter M, Couturier J, Pacquement H, et al. A new member of the ETS family fused to EWS in Ewing tumors. Oncogene. 1997;14(10):1159–64.

41. May WA, Gishizky ML, Lessnick SL, et al. Ewing sarcoma 11;22 translocation produces a chimeric transcription factor that requires the DNA-binding domain encoded by FLI1 for transformation. Proc Natl Acad Sci U S A. 1993;90(12):5752–6.

42. May WA, Lessnick SL, Braun BS, et al. The Ewing's sarcoma EWS/FLI-1 fusion gene encodes a more potent transcriptional activator and is a more powerful transforming gene than FLI-1. Mol Cell Biol. 1993;13(12):7393–8.

43. Zucman J, Melot T, Desmaze C, et al. Combinatorial generation of variable fusion proteins in the Ewing family of tumours. EMBO J. 1993;12(12):4481–7.

44. Sankar S, Lessnick SL. Promiscuous partnerships in Ewing's sarcoma. Cancer Genet. 2011;204(7):351–65.

45. Tanaka K, Iwakuma T, Harimaya K, Sato H, Iwamoto Y. EWS-Fli1 antisense oligodeoxynucleotide inhibits proliferation of human Ewing's sarcoma

and primitive neuroectodermal tumor cells. J Clin Invest. 1997;99(2):239–47.

46. Lambert G, Bertrand JR, Fattal E, et al. EWS fli-1 antisense nanocapsules inhibits Ewing sarcoma-related tumor in mice. Biochem Biophys Res Commun. 2000;279(2):401–6.

47. Hu-Lieskovan S, Heidel JD, Bartlett DW, Davis ME, Triche TJ. Sequence-specific knockdown of EWS-FLI1 by targeted, nonviral delivery of small interfering RNA inhibits tumor growth in a murine model of metastatic Ewing's sarcoma. Cancer Res. 2005;65(19):8984–92.

48. de Alava E, Kawai A, Healey JH, et al. EWS-Fli-1 fusion transcript structure is an independent determinant of prognosis in Ewing's sarcoma. J Clin Oncol. 1998;16(4):1248–55.

49. van Doorninck JA, Ji L, Schaub B, et al. Current treatment protocols have eliminated the prognostic advantage of type 1 fusions in Ewing sarcoma: a report from the Children's Oncology Group. J Clin Oncol. 2010;28(12):1989–94.

50. Fanburg-Smith JC, Dal CP. Angiomatoid fibrous histiocytoma. In: Fletcher CD, Unni KK, Mertens F, editors. World Health Organization classification of tumours: tumours of soft tissue and bone. Lyon: IARC Press; 2002. p. 194–5.

51. Thway K. Angiomatoid fibrous histiocytoma: a review with recent genetic findings. Arch Pathol Lab Med. 2008;132(2):273–7.

52. Kay S. Angiomatoid malignant fibrous histiocytoma. Report of two cases with ultrastructural observations of one case. Arch Pathol Lab Med. 1985;109(10):934–7.

53. Wegmann W, Heitz PU. Angiomatoid malignant fibrous histiocytoma. Evidence for the histiocytic origin of tumor cells. Virchows Arch A Pathol Anat Histopathol. 1985;406(1):59–66.

54. Shao L, Singh V, Cooley L. Angiomatoid fibrous histiocytoma with t(2;22)(q33;q12.2) and EWSR1 gene rearrangement. Pediatr Dev Pathol. 2009;12(2):143–6.

55. Law WJ, Cann KL, Hicks GG. TLS, EWS and TAF15: a model for transcriptional integration of gene expression. Brief Funct Genomic Proteomic. 2006;5(1):8–14.

56. Rossi S, Szuhai K, Ijszenga M, et al. EWSR1-CREB1 and EWSR1-ATF1 fusion genes in angiomatoid fibrous histiocytoma. Clin Cancer Res. 2007;13(24):7322–8.

57. Antonescu CR, Gerald W. Desmoplastic small round cell tumour. In: Fletcher CD, Unni KK, Mertens F, editors. Pathology and genetics: tumours of soft tissue and bone. Lyon: IARC Press; 2002. p. 216–8.

58. Syed S, Haque AK, Hawkins HK, Sorensen PH, Cowan DF. Desmoplastic small round cell tumor of the lung. Arch Pathol Lab Med. 2002;126(10):1226–8.

59. Cummings OW, Ulbright TM, Young RH, Dei Tos AP, Fletcher CD, Hull MT. Desmoplastic small

round cell tumors of the paratesticular region. A report of six cases. Am J Surg Pathol. 1997;21(2): 219–25.

60. Young RH, Eichhorn JH, Dickersin GR, Scully RE. Ovarian involvement by the intra-abdominal desmoplastic small round cell tumor with divergent differentiation: a report of three cases. Hum Pathol. 1992;23(4):454–64.

61. Adsay V, Cheng J, Athanasian E, Gerald W, Rosai J. Primary desmoplastic small cell tumor of soft tissues and bone of the hand. Am J Surg Pathol. 1999;23(11):1408–13.

62. Murphy A, Stallings RL, Howard J, et al. Primary desmoplastic small round cell tumor of bone: report of a case with cytogenetic confirmation. Cancer Genet Cytogenet. 2005;156(2):167–71.

63. Chang F. Desmoplastic small round cell tumors: cytologic, histologic, and immunohistochemical features. Arch Pathol Lab Med. 2006;130(5):728–32.

64. Sawyer JR, Tryka AF, Lewis JM. A novel reciprocal chromosome translocation t(11;22)(p13;q12) in an intraabdominal desmoplastic small round-cell tumor. Am J Surg Pathol. 1992;16(4):411–6.

65. Ladanyi M, Gerald W. Fusion of the EWS and WT1 genes in the desmoplastic small round cell tumor. Cancer Res. 1994;54(11):2837–40.

66. Murphy AJ, Bishop K, Pereira C, et al. A new molecular variant of desmoplastic small round cell tumor: significance of WT1 immunostaining in this entity. Hum Pathol. 2008;39(12):1763–70.

67. Lee SB, Kolquist KA, Nichols K, et al. The EWS-WT1 translocation product induces PDGFA in desmoplastic small round-cell tumour. Nat Genet. 1997;17(3):309–13.

68. Gerald WL, Haber DA. The EWS-WT1 gene fusion in desmoplastic small round cell tumor. Semin Cancer Biol. 2005;15(3):197–205.

69. Panagopoulos I, Hoglund M, Mertens F, Mandahl N, Mitelman F, Aman P. Fusion of the EWS and CHOP genes in myxoid liposarcoma. Oncogene. 1996; 12(3):489–94.

70. Panagopoulos I, Mertens F, Isaksson M, et al. Molecular genetic characterization of the EWS/CHN and RBP56/CHN fusion genes in extraskeletal myxoid chondrosarcoma. Genes Chromosomes Cancer. 2002;35(4):340–52.

71. Rekhi B, Sable M, Jambhekar NA. Histopathological, immunohistochemical and molecular spectrum of myoepithelial tumours of soft tissues. Virchows Arch. 2012;461(6):687–97.

72. Antonescu CR, Zhang L, Chang NE, et al. EWSR1-POU5F1 fusion in soft tissue myoepithelial tumors. A molecular analysis of sixty-six cases, including soft tissue, bone, and visceral lesions, showing common involvement of the EWSR1 gene. Genes Chromosomes Cancer. 2010;49(12):1114–24.

73. Brandal P, Panagopoulos I, Bjerkehagen B, et al. Detection of a t(1;22)(q23;q12) translocation leading to an EWSR1-PBX1 fusion gene in a myoepithelioma. Genes Chromosomes Cancer. 2008;47(7):558–64.

74. Flucke U, Mentzel T, Verdijk MA, et al. EWSR1-ATF1 chimeric transcript in a myoepithelial tumor of soft tissue: a case report. Hum Pathol. 2012; 43(5):764–8.

75. Coffin CM, Alaggio R. Fibroblastic and myofibroblastic tumors in children and adolescents. Pediatr Dev Pathol. 2012;15(1 Suppl):127–80.

76. Knezevich SR, Garnett MJ, Pysher TJ, Beckwith JB, Grundy PE, Sorensen PH. ETV6-NTRK3 gene fusions and trisomy 11 establish a histogenetic link between mesoblastic nephroma and congenital fibrosarcoma. Cancer Res. 1998;58(22):5046–8.

77. Knezevich SR, McFadden DE, Tao W, Lim JF, Sorensen PH. A novel ETV6-NTRK3 gene fusion in congenital fibrosarcoma. Nat Genet. 1998;18(2): 184–7.

78. Fisher C. Soft tissue sarcomas with non-EWS translocations: molecular genetic features and pathologic and clinical correlations. Virchows Arch. 2010;456(2):153–66.

79. Lannon CL, Sorensen PH. ETV6-NTRK3: a chimeric protein tyrosine kinase with transformation activity in multiple cell lineages. Semin Cancer Biol. 2005;15(3):215–23.

80. Rubin BP, Chen CJ, Morgan TW, et al. Congenital mesoblastic nephroma t(12;15) is associated with ETV6-NTRK3 gene fusion: cytogenetic and molecular relationship to congenital (infantile) fibrosarcoma. Am J Pathol. 1998;153(5):1451–8.

81. Tognon C, Knezevich SR, Huntsman D, et al. Expression of the ETV6-NTRK3 gene fusion as a primary event in human secretory breast carcinoma. Cancer Cell. 2002;2(5):367–76.

82. Eguchi M, Eguchi-Ishimae M, Tojo A, et al. Fusion of ETV6 to neurotrophin-3 receptor TRKC in acute myeloid leukemia with t(12;15)(p13;q25). Blood. 1999;93(4):1355–63.

83. Somers GR, Shago M, Zielenska M, Chan HS, Ngan BY. Primary subcutaneous primitive neuroectodermal tumor with aggressive behavior and an unusual karyotype: case report. Pediatr Dev Pathol. 2004; 7(5):538–45.

84. Yoshimoto M, Graham C, Chilton-MacNeill S, et al. Detailed cytogenetic and array analysis of pediatric primitive sarcomas reveals a recurrent CIC-DUX4 fusion gene event. Cancer Genet Cytogenet. 2009; 195(1):1–11.

85. Kawamura-Saito M, Yamazaki Y, Kaneko K, et al. Fusion between CIC and DUX4 up-regulates PEA3 family genes in Ewing-like sarcomas with t(4;19) (q35;q13) translocation. Hum Mol Genet. 2006; 15(13):2125–37.

86. Italiano A, Sung YS, Zhang L, et al. High prevalence of CIC fusion with double-homeobox (DUX4) transcription factors in EWSR1-negative undifferentiated small blue round cell sarcomas. Genes Chromosomes Cancer. 2012;51(3):207–18.

87. Graham C, Chilton-MacNeill S, Zielenska M, Somers GR. The CIC-DUX4 fusion transcript is present in a subgroup of pediatric primitive round cell sarcomas. Hum Pathol. 2012;43(2):180–9.

88. Lee CJ, Chan WI, Cheung M, et al. CIC, a member of a novel subfamily of the HMG-box superfamily, is transiently expressed in developing granule neurons. Brain Res Mol Brain Res. 2002;106(1–2): 151–6.

89. Gabriels J, Beckers MC, Ding H, et al. Nucleotide sequence of the partially deleted D4Z4 locus in a patient with FSHD identifies a putative gene within each 3.3 kb element. Gene. 1999;236(1):25–32.

90. Parham DM, Barr FG. Embryonal rhabdomyosarcoma. In: Fletcher CDM, Unni KK, Mertens F, editors. World health classification of tumours: tumours of soft tissue and bone. Lyon: IARC Press; 2002. p. 146–9.

91. Newton Jr WA, Soule EH, Hamoudi AB, et al. Histopathology of childhood sarcomas, Intergroup Rhabdomyosarcoma Studies I and II: clinicopathologic correlation. J Clin Oncol. 1988;6(1):67–75.

92. Parham DM, Alaggio R, Coffin CM. Myogenic tumors in children and adolescents. Pediatr Dev Pathol. 2012;15(1 Suppl):211–38.

93. Qualman SJ, Coffin CM, Newton WA, et al. Intergroup Rhabdomyosarcoma Study: update for pathologists. Pediatr Dev Pathol. 1998;1(6):550–61.

94. Kodet R, Newton Jr WA, Hamoudi AB, Asmar L, Jacobs DL, Maurer HM. Childhood rhabdomyosarcoma with anaplastic (pleomorphic) features. A report of the Intergroup Rhabdomyosarcoma Study. Am J Surg Pathol. 1993;17(5):443–53.

95. Mentzel T, Katenkamp D. Sclerosing, pseudovascular rhabdomyosarcoma in adults. Clinicopathological and immunohistochemical analysis of three cases. Virchows Arch. 2000;436(4):305–11.

96. Croes R, Debiec-Rychter M, Cokelaere K, De Vos R, Hagemeijer A, Sciot R. Adult sclerosing rhabdomyosarcoma: cytogenetic link with embryonal rhabdomyosarcoma. Virchows Arch. 2005; 446(1):64–7.

97. Cavazzana AO, Schmidt D, Ninfo V, et al. Spindle cell rhabdomyosarcoma. A prognostically favorable variant of rhabdomyosarcoma. Am J Surg Pathol. 1992;16(3):229–35.

98. Qualman S, Lynch J, Bridge J, et al. Prevalence and clinical impact of anaplasia in childhood rhabdomyosarcoma: a report from the Soft Tissue Sarcoma Committee of the Children's Oncology Group. Cancer. 2008;113(11):3242–7.

99. Bridge JA, Liu J, Qualman SJ, et al. Genomic gains and losses are similar in genetic and histologic subsets of rhabdomyosarcoma, whereas amplification predominates in embryonal with anaplasia and alveolar subtypes. Genes Chromosomes Cancer. 2002; 33(3):310–21.

100. Paulson V, Chandler G, Rakheja D, et al. High-resolution array CGH identifies common mechanisms that drive embryonal rhabdomyosarcoma pathogenesis. Genes Chromosomes Cancer. 2011; 50(6):397–408.

101. Koufos A, Hansen MF, Copeland NG, Jenkins NA, Lampkin BC, Cavenee WK. Loss of heterozygosity in three embryonal tumours suggests a common pathogenetic mechanism. Nature. 1985;316(6026):330–4.

102. Scrable HJ, Witte DP, Lampkin BC, Cavenee WK. Chromosomal localization of the human rhabdomyosarcoma locus by mitotic recombination mapping. Nature. 1987;329(6140):645–7.

103. Choufani S, Shuman C, Weksberg R. Beckwith-Wiedemann syndrome. Am J Med Genet C Semin Med Genet. 2010;154C(3):343–54.

104. Samani AA, Yakar S, LeRoith D, Brodt P. The role of the IGF system in cancer growth and metastasis: overview and recent insights. Endocr Rev. 2007; 28(1):20–47.

105. El-Badry OM, Minniti C, Kohn EC, Houghton PJ, Daughaday WH, Helman LJ. Insulin-like growth factor II acts as an autocrine growth and motility factor in human rhabdomyosarcoma tumors. Cell Growth Differ. 1990;1(7):325–31.

106. Makawita S, Ho M, Durbin AD, Thorner PS, Malkin D, Somers GR. Expression of insulin-like growth factor pathway proteins in rhabdomyosarcoma: IGF-2 expression is associated with translocation-negative tumors. Pediatr Dev Pathol. 2009;12(2): 127–35.

107. Xia SJ, Pressey JG, Barr FG. Molecular pathogenesis of rhabdomyosarcoma. Cancer Biol Ther. 2002;1(2):97–104.

108. Bridge JA, Cushman-Vokoun AM. Molecular diagnostics of soft tissue tumors. Arch Pathol Lab Med. 2011;135(5):588–601.

109. Igbokwe A, Lopez-Terrada DH. Molecular testing of solid tumors. Arch Pathol Lab Med. 2011;135(1): 67–82.

110. Shaffer LG, Bejjani BA. A cytogeneticist's perspective on genomic microarrays. Hum Reprod Update. 2004;10(3):221–6.

111. Imataka G, Arisaka O. Chromosome analysis using spectral karyotyping (SKY). Cell Biochem Biophys. 2012;62(1):13–7.

112. Ross J, Davies S. Screening for neuroblastoma: progress and pitfalls. Cancer Epidemiol Biomarkers Prev. 1999;8:189–94.

113. Maris J, Matthay K. Molecular biology of neuroblastoma. J Clin Oncol. 1999;17:2264–79.

114. Maris J, Hogarty M, Bagatell R, Cohn S. Neuroblastoma. Lancet. 2007;369:2106–20.

115. London WB, Castleberry RP, Matthay KK, et al. Evidence for an age cutoff greater than 365 days for neuroblastoma risk group stratification in the Children's Oncology Group. J Clin Oncol. 2005; 23(27):6459–65.

116. Riley R, Heney D, Jones D, et al. A systematic review of molecular and biological tumor markers in neuroblastoma. Clin Cancer Res. 2004;10:4–12.

117. Maris JM. Recent advances in neuroblastoma. N Engl J Med. 2010;362(23):2202–11.

118. Cohn SL, Pearson AD, London WB, et al. The International Neuroblastoma Risk Group (INRG) classification system: an INRG Task Force report. J Clin Oncol. 2009;27(2):289–97.

119. Moroz V, Machin D, Faldum A, et al. Changes over three decades in outcome and the prognostic influence of age-at-diagnosis in young patients with neuroblastoma: a report from the International Neuroblastoma Risk Group Project. Eur J Cancer. 2011;47(4):561–71.

120. Schmidt ML, Lal A, Seeger RC, et al. Favorable prognosis for patients 12 to 18 months of age with stage 4 nonamplified MYCN neuroblastoma: a Children's Cancer Group Study. J Clin Oncol. 2005;23(27):6474–80.

121. Brodeur G, Pritchard J, Berthold F, et al. Revisions of the international criteria for neuroblastoma diagnosis, staging, and response to treatment. J Clin Oncol. 1993;11:1466–77.

122. Evans AE, Silber JH, Shpilsky A, D'Angio GJ. Successful management of low-stage neuroblastoma without adjuvant therapies: a comparison of two decades, 1972 through 1981 and 1982 through 1992, in a single institution. J Clin Oncol. 1996;14(9): 2504–10.

123. Matthay KK, Sather HN, Seeger RC, Haase GM, Hammond GD. Excellent outcome of stage II neuroblastoma is independent of residual disease and radiation therapy. J Clin Oncol. 1989;7(2):236–44.

124. Matthay KK, Perez C, Seeger RC, et al. Successful treatment of stage III neuroblastoma based on prospective biologic staging: a Children's Cancer Group study. J Clin Oncol. 1998;16(4):1256–64.

125. West DC, Shamberger RC, Macklis RM, et al. Stage III neuroblastoma over 1 year of age at diagnosis: improved survival with intensive multimodality therapy including multiple alkylating agents. J Clin Oncol. 1993;11(1):84–90.

126. Matthay K, Villablanca J, Seeger R, et al. Treatment of high-risk neuroblastoma with intensive chemotherapy, radiotherapy, autologous bone marrow transplantation, and 13-cis-retinoic acid. Children's Cancer Group. N Engl J Med. 1999;341:1165–73.

127. Zage PE, Kletzel M, Murray K, et al. Outcomes of the POG 9340/9341/9342 trials for children with high-risk neuroblastoma: a report from the Children's Oncology Group. Pediatr Blood Cancer. 2008;51(6):747–53.

128. Taggart DR, London WB, Schmidt ML, et al. Prognostic value of the stage 4S metastatic pattern and tumor biology in patients with metastatic neuroblastoma diagnosed between birth and 18 months of age. J Clin Oncol. 2011;29(33):4358–64.

129. Monclair T, Brodeur GM, Ambros PF, et al. The International Neuroblastoma Risk Group (INRG) staging system: an INRG Task Force report. J Clin Oncol. 2009;27(2):298–303.

130. Simon T, Hero B, Benz-Bohm G, von Schweinitz D, Berthold F. Review of image defined risk factors in localized neuroblastoma patients: results of the GPOH NB97 trial. Pediatr Blood Cancer. 2008; 50(5):965–9.

131. Krishnan C, Higgins JP, West RB, Natkunam Y, Heerema-McKenney A, Arber DA. Microtubule-associated protein-2 is a sensitive marker of primary and metastatic neuroblastoma. Am J Surg Pathol. 2009;33(11):1695–704.

132. Joshi V. Peripheral neuroblastic tumors: pathologic classification based on recommendations of international neuroblastoma pathology committee (modification of Shimada classification). Pediatr Dev Pathol. 2000;3:184–99.

133. Shimada H, Chatten J, Newton WJ, et al. Histopathologic prognostic factors in neuroblastic tumors: definition of subtypes of ganglioneuroblastoma and an age-linked classification of neuroblastomas. J Natl Cancer Inst. 1984;73:405–16.

134. Shimada H, Ambros IM, Dehner LP, et al. The International Neuroblastoma Pathology Classification (the Shimada system). Cancer. 1999;86(2):364–72.

135. Shimada H, Umehara S, Monobe Y, et al. International neuroblastoma pathology classification for prognostic evaluation of patients with peripheral neuroblastic tumors: a report from the Children's Cancer Group. Cancer. 2001;92(9):2451–61.

136. Peuchmaur M, d'Amore ES, Joshi VV, et al. Revision of the International Neuroblastoma Pathology Classification: confirmation of favorable and unfavorable prognostic subsets in ganglioneuroblastoma, nodular. Cancer. 2003;98(10):2274–81.

137. Umehara S, Nakagawa A, Matthay KK, et al. Histopathology defines prognostic subsets of ganglioneuroblastoma, nodular. Cancer. 2000;89(5):1150–61.

138. Brodeur GM, Minturn JE, Ho R, et al. Trk receptor expression and inhibition in neuroblastomas. Clin Cancer Res. 2009;15(10):3244–50.

139. Light JE, Koyama H, Minturn JE, et al. Clinical significance of NTRK family gene expression in neuroblastomas. Pediatr Blood Cancer. 2012;59(2):226–32.

140. Nakagawara A, Arima-Nakagawara M, Scavarda N, Azar C, Canter A, Brodeur G. Association between high levels of expression of the TRK gene and favorable outcome in human neuroblastoma. N Engl J Med. 1993;328:847–54.

141. Minturn JE, Evans AE, Villablanca JG, et al. Phase I trial of lestaurtinib for children with refractory neuroblastoma: a new approaches to neuroblastoma therapy consortium study. Cancer Chemother Pharmacol. 2011;68(4):1057–65.

142. Mosse YP, Diskin SJ, Wasserman N, et al. Neuroblastomas have distinct genomic DNA profiles that predict clinical phenotype and regional gene expression. Genes Chromosomes Cancer. 2007; 46(10):936–49.

143. Schleiermacher G, Janoueix-Lerosey I, Ribeiro A, et al. Accumulation of segmental alterations determines progression in neuroblastoma. J Clin Oncol. 2010;28(19):3122–30.

144. Li MM, Andersson HC. Clinical application of microarray-based molecular cytogenetics: an emerging new

era of genomic medicine. J Pediatr. 2009;155(3): 311–7.

145. Maciejewski JP, Tiu RV, O'Keefe C. Application of array-based whole genome scanning technologies as a cytogenetic tool in haematological malignancies. Br J Haematol. 2009;146(5):479–88.

146. Look A, Hayes F, Nitschke R, McWilliams N, Green A. Cellular DNA content as a predictor of response to chemotherapy in infants with unresectable neuroblastoma. N Engl J Med. 1984;311:231–5.

147. Look A, Hayes F, Shuster J, et al. Clinical relevance of tumor cell ploidy and N-myc gene amplification in childhood neuroblastoma: a Pediatric Oncology Group study. J Clin Oncol. 1991;9:581–91.

148. Ambros PF, Ambros IM, Brodeur GM, et al. International consensus for neuroblastoma molecular diagnostics: report from the International Neuroblastoma Risk Group (INRG) Biology Committee. Br J Cancer. 2009;100(9):1471–82.

149. Schneiderman J, London W, Brodeur G, Castleberry R, Look A, Cohn S. Clinical significance of MYCN amplification and ploidy in favorable-stage neuroblastoma: a report from the Children's Oncology Group. J Clin Oncol. 2008;26:913–8.

150. Seeger R, Brodeur G, Sather H, et al. Association of multiple copies of the N-myc oncogene with rapid progression of neuroblastomas. N Engl J Med. 1985;313:1111–6.

151. Brodeur G, Seeger R, Schwab M, Varmus H, Bishop J. Amplification of N-myc in untreated human neuroblastomas correlates with advanced disease stage. Science. 1984;224:1121–4.

152. Katzenstein H, Bowman L, Brodeur G, et al. The prognostic significance of age, MYCN oncogene amplification, tumor cell ploidy, and histology in 110 infants with stage D(S) neuroblastoma: The Pediatric Oncology Group experience. J Clin Oncol. 1998;16:2007–17.

153. Bagatell R, Beck-Popovic M, London WB, et al. Significance of MYCN amplification in international neuroblastoma staging system stage 1 and 2 neuroblastoma: a report from the International Neuroblastoma Risk Group database. J Clin Oncol. 2009;27(3):365–70.

154. Pugh TJ, Morozova O, Attiyeh EF, et al. The genetic landscape of high-risk neuroblastoma. Nat Genet. 2013;45(3):279–84.

155. Rubie H, Hartmann O, Michon J, et al. N-Myc gene amplification is a major prognostic factor in localized neuroblastoma: results of the French NBL 90 study. J Clin Oncol. 1997;15:1171–82.

156. Boerner S, Squire J, Thorner P, McKenna G, Zielenska M. Assessment of MYCN amplification in neuroblastoma biopsies by differential polymerase chain reaction. Pediatr Pathol. 1994;14:823–32.

157. Amler L, Schwab M. Amplified N-Myc in human neuroblastoma cells is often arranged as clustered tandem repeats of differently recombined DNA. Mol Cell Biol. 1989;9:4903–13.

158. Shimizu N, Shingaki K, Kaneko-Sasaguri Y, Hashizume T, Kanda T. When, where and how the bridge breaks: anaphase bridge breakage plays a crucial role in gene amplification and HSR generation. Exp Cell Res. 2005;302(2):233–43.

159. Moreau LA, McGrady P, London WB, et al. Does MYCN amplification manifested as homogeneously staining regions at diagnosis predict a worse outcome in children with neuroblastoma? A Children's Oncology Group study. Clin Cancer Res. 2006; 12(19):5693–7.

160. Shapiro D, Valentine M, Rowe S, et al. Detection of MYCN gene amplification by fluorescence in situ hybridization. Diagnostic utility for neuroblastoma. Am J Pathol. 1993;142:1339–46.

161. Cohen P, Seeger R, Triche T, Israel M. Detection of MYCN gene expression in neuroblastoma tumours by in situ hybridization. Am J Pathol. 1988;131: 391–7.

162. Taylor C, McGuckin A, Bown N, et al. Rapid detection of prognostic genetic factors in neuroblastoma using fluorescence in situ hybridisation on tumour imprints and bone marrow smears. Br J Cancer. 1994;69:445–51.

163. Misra D, Dickman P, Yunis E. Fluorescence in situ hybridization (FISH) detection of MYCN oncogene amplification in neuroblastoma using paraffin-embedded tissues. Diagn Mol Pathol. 1995;4:128–35.

164. Theissen J, Boensch M, Spitz R, et al. Heterogeneity of the MYCN oncogene in neuroblastoma. Clin Cancer Res. 2009;15(6):2085–90.

165. Thorner P, Ho M, Chilton-MacNeill S, Zielenska M. Use of chromogenic in situ hybridization to identify MYCN gene copy number in neuroblastoma using routine tissue sections. Am J Surg Pathol. 2006; 30:635–42.

166. Cohn S, London W, Huang D, et al. MYCN expression is not prognostic of adverse outcome in advanced-stage neuroblastoma with nonamplified MYCN. J Clin Oncol. 2001;18:3604–13.

167. Valentijn LJ, Koster J, Haneveld F, et al. Functional MYCN signature predicts outcome of neuroblastoma irrespective of MYCN amplification. Proc Natl Acad Sci U S A. 2012;109(47):19190–5.

168. Alaminos M, Mora J, Cheung N-K, et al. Genome-wide analysis of gene expression associated with MYCN in human neuroblastoma. Cancer Res. 2003;63:4538–46.

169. Chen Q, Bilke S, Wei J, et al. CDNA array-CGH profiling identifies genomic alterations specific to stage and MYCN-amplification in neuroblastoma. BMC Genomics. 2004;5:70.

170. Hiyama E, Hiyama K, Yamaoka H, Sueda T, Reynolds C, Yokoyama T. Expression profiling of favorable and unfavorable neuroblastomas. Pediatr Surg Int. 2004;20:33–8.

171. Krasnoselsky A, Whiteford C, Wei J, et al. Altered expression of cell cycle genes distinguishes aggressive neuroblastoma. Oncogene. 2005;24:1533–41.

172. Ohira M, Oba S, Nakamura Y, Hirata T, Ishii S, Nakagawara A. A review of DNA microarray analysis of human neuroblastomas. Cancer Lett. 2005;228:5–11.

173. Caron H, van Sluis P, van Hoeve M, et al. Allelic loss of chromosome 1p36 in neuroblastoma is of preferential maternal origin and correlates with *N-MYC* amplification. Nat Genet. 1993;4:187–90.

174. White P, Maris J, Beltinger C, et al. A region of consistent deletion in neuroblastoma maps to within 1p36.2-3. Proc Natl Acad Sci U S A. 1995;92:5520–4.

175. Caron H, Peter M, van Sluis P, et al. Evidence for two tumor suppressor loci on chromosomal bands 1p35-1p36 involved in neuroblastoma: one probably imprinted, another associated with N-myc amplification. Hum Mol Genet. 1995;4:535–9.

176. Fong C, Dracopoli N, White P, et al. Loss of heterozygosity for the short arm of chromosome 1 in human neuroblastomas: correlation with *N-myc* amplification. Proc Natl Acad Sci U S A. 1989;86:3753–7.

177. Maris J, Weiss M, Guo C, et al. Loss of heterozygosity at 1p36 independently predicts for disease progression but not decreased overall survival probability in neuroblastoma patients: A Children's Cancer Group study. J Clin Oncol. 2000;18:1888–99.

178. Janoueix-Lerosey I, Novikov E, Monteiro M, et al. Gene expression profiling of 1p35–36 genes in neuroblastoma. Oncogene. 2004;23:5912–22.

179. Fransson S, Martinsson T, Ejeskär K. Neuroblastoma tumors with favorable and unfavorable outcomes: significant differences in mRNA expression of genes mapped at 1p36.2. Genes Chromosomes Cancer. 2007;46:45–52.

180. Okawa ER, Gotoh T, Manne J, et al. Expression and sequence analysis of candidates for the 1p36.31 tumor suppressor gene deleted in neuroblastomas. Oncogene. 2008;27(6):803–10.

181. Fujita T, Igarashi J, Okawa E, et al. *CHD5*, a tumor suppressor gene deleted from 1p36.31 in neuroblastomas. J Natl Cancer Inst. 2008;100:940–9.

182. Garcia I, Mayol G, Rodriguez E, et al. Expression of the neuron-specific protein CHD5 is an independent marker of outcome in neuroblastoma. Mol Cancer. 2010;9:277.

183. Luttikhuis M, Powell J, Rees S, et al. Neuroblastomas with chromosome 11q loss and single copy MYCN comprise a biologically distinct group of tumours with adverse prognosis. Br J Cancer. 2001;17:531–7.

184. Guo C, White P, Weiss M, et al. Allelic deletion at 11q23 is common in *MYCN* single copy neuroblastomas. Oncogene. 1999;18:4948–57.

185. Bown N, Cotterill S, Lastowksa M, et al. Gain of chromosome arm 17q and adverse outcome in patients with neuroblastoma. N Engl J Med. 1999;340:1954–61.

186. Lastowska M, Roberts P, Pearson A, Lewis I, Wolstenholme J, Bown N. Promiscuous translocations of chromosome arm 17q in human neuroblastomas. Genes Chromosomes Cancer. 1997;19:143–9.

187. Godfried MB, Veenstra M, v Sluis P, et al. The N-myc and c-myc downstream pathways include the chromosome 17q genes nm23-H1 and nm23-H2. Oncogene. 2002;21(13):2097–101.

188. Islam A, Kageyama H, Takada N, et al. High expression of *Survivin*, mapped to 17q25, is significantly associated with poor prognostic factors and promotes cell survival in human neuroblastoma. Oncogene. 2000;19:617–23.

189. Saito-Ohara F, Imoto I, Inoue J, et al. PPM1D is a potential target for 17q gain in neuroblastoma. Cancer Res. 2003;63:1876–83.

190. Azarova AM, Gautam G, George RE. Emerging importance of ALK in neuroblastoma. Semin Cancer Biol. 2011;21(4):267–75.

191. Janoueix-Lerosey I, Lequin D, Brugieres L, et al. Somatic and germline activating mutations of the ALK kinase receptor in neuroblastoma. Nature. 2008;455(7215):967–70.

192. Mosse YP, Laudenslager M, Longo L, et al. Identification of ALK as a major familial neuroblastoma predisposition gene. Nature. 2008;455(7215): 930–5.

193. de Pontual L, Kettaneh D, Gordon CT, et al. Germline gain-of-function mutations of ALK disrupt central nervous system development. Hum Mutat. 2011;32(3):272–6.

194. Martinsson T, Eriksson T, Abrahamsson J, et al. Appearance of the novel activating F1174S ALK mutation in neuroblastoma correlates with aggressive tumor progression and unresponsiveness to therapy. Cancer Res. 2011;71(1):98–105.

195. Berry T, Luther W, Bhatnagar N, et al. The ALK(F1174L) mutation potentiates the oncogenic activity of MYCN in neuroblastoma. Cancer Cell. 2012;22(1):117–30.

196. Heukamp LC, Thor T, Schramm A, et al. Targeted expression of mutated ALK induces neuroblastoma in transgenic mice. Sci Transl Med. 2012;4(141): 141ra91.

197. Zhu S, Lee JS, Guo F, et al. Activated ALK collaborates with MYCN in neuroblastoma pathogenesis. Cancer Cell. 2012;21(3):362–73.

198. Duijkers FA, Gaal J, Meijerink JP, et al. High anaplastic lymphoma kinase immunohistochemical staining in neuroblastoma and ganglioneuroblastoma is an independent predictor of poor outcome. Am J Pathol. 2012;180(3):1223–31.

199. Schulte JH, Bachmann HS, Brockmeyer B, et al. High ALK receptor tyrosine kinase expression supersedes ALK mutation as a determining factor of an unfavorable phenotype in primary neuroblastoma. Clin Cancer Res. 2011;17(15): 5082–92.

200. Mosse YP, Laudenslager M, Khazi D, et al. Germline PHOX2B mutation in hereditary neuroblastoma. Am J Hum Genet. 2004;75(4):727–30.

201. Raabe EH, Laudenslager M, Winter C, et al. Prevalence and functional consequence of PHOX2B

mutations in neuroblastoma. Oncogene. 2008;27(4): 469–76.

202. Trochet D, Bourdeaut F, Janoueix-Lerosey I, et al. Germline mutations of the paired-like homeobox 2B (*PHOX2B*) gene in neuroblastoma. Am J Hum Genet. 2004;74:761–4.

203. Serra A, Haberle B, Konig IR, et al. Rare occurrence of PHOX2b mutations in sporadic neuroblastomas. J Pediatr Hematol Oncol. 2008;30(10):728–32.

204. Bentires-Alj M, Paez JG, David FS, et al. Activating mutations of the Noonan syndrome-associated SHP2/PTPN11 gene in human solid tumors and adult acute myelogenous leukemia. Cancer Res. 2004;64(24):8816–20.

205. Mutesa L, Pierquin G, Janin N, et al. Germline PTPN11 missense mutation in a case of Noonan syndrome associated with mediastinal and retroperitoneal neuroblastic tumors. Cancer Genet Cytogenet. 2008;182(1):40–2.

206. Cheung NK, Zhang J, Lu C, et al. Association of age at diagnosis and genetic mutations in patients with neuroblastoma. JAMA. 2012;307(10):1062–71.

207. Molenaar JJ, Domingo-Fernandez R, Ebus ME, et al. LIN28B induces neuroblastoma and enhances MYCN levels via let-7 suppression. Nat Genet. 2012;44(11):1199–206.

208. Sausen M, Leary RJ, Jones S, et al. Integrated genomic analyses identify ARID1A and ARID1B alterations in the childhood cancer neuroblastoma. Nat Genet. 2013;45(1):12–7.

209. Carr-Wilkinson J, O'Toole K, Wood KM, et al. High frequency of p53/MDM2/p14ARF pathway abnormalities in relapsed neuroblastoma. Clin Cancer Res. 2010;16(4):1108–18.

210. Tweddle DA, Malcolm AJ, Bown N, Pearson AD, Lunec J. Evidence for the development of p53 mutations after cytotoxic therapy in a neuroblastoma cell line. Cancer Res. 2001;61(1):8–13.

211. Onel K, Cordon-Cardo C. MDM2 and prognosis. Mol Cancer Res. 2004;2(1):1–8.

212. Slack A, Chen Z, Tonelli R, et al. The p53 regulatory gene *MDM2* is a direct transcriptional target of MYCN in neuroblastoma. Proc Natl Acad Sci. 2005;102:731–6.

213. Asgharzadeh S, Pique-Regi R, Sposto R, et al. Prognostic significance of gene expression profiles of metastatic neuroblastomas lacking MYCN gene amplification. J Natl Cancer Inst. 2006;98:1193–203.

214. Chen QR, Song YK, Yu LR, et al. Global genomic and proteomic analysis identifies biological pathways related to high-risk neuroblastoma. J Proteome Res. 2010;9(1):373–82.

215. Hiyama E, Hiyama K, Nishiyama M, Reynolds C, Shay J, Yokoyama T. Differential gene expression profiles between neuroblastomas with high telomerase activity and low telomerase activity. J Pediatr Surg. 2003;38:1730–4.

216. Krause A, Combaret V, Iacono I, et al. Genome-wide analysis of gene expression in neuroblastomas detected by mass screening. Cancer Lett. 2005;225: 111–20.

217. Lastowska M, Viprey V, Santibanez-Koref M, et al. Identification of candidate genes involved in neuroblastoma progression by combining genomic and expression microarrays with survival data. Oncogene. 2007;26(53):7432–44.

218. McArdle L, McDermott M, Purcell R, et al. Oligonucleotide microarray analysis of gene expression in neuroblastoma displaying loss of chromosome 11q. Carcinogenesis. 2004;25:1599–609.

219. Nevo I, Oberthuer A, Botzer E, et al. Gene-expression-based analysis of local and metastatic neuroblastoma variants reveals a set of genes associated with tumor progression in neuroblastoma patients. Int J Cancer. 2009;126(7):1570–81.

220. Oberthuer A, Berthold F, Warnat P, et al. Customized oligonucleotide microarray gene expression-based classification of neuroblastoma patients outperforms current clinical risk stratification. J Clin Oncol. 2006;24(31):5070–8.

221. Oberthuer A, Hero B, Berthold F, et al. Prognostic impact of gene expression-based classification for neuroblastoma. J Clin Oncol. 2010;28(21): 3506–15.

222. Ohira M, Morohashi A, Inuzuka H, et al. Expression profiling and characterization of 4200 genes cloned from primary neuroblastomas: identification of 305 genes differentially expressed between favorable and unfavorable subsets. Oncogene. 2003;22:5525–36.

223. Ohira M, Oba S, Nakamura Y, et al. Expression profiling using a tumor-specific cDNA microarray predicts the prognosis of intermediate risk neuroblastomas. Cancer Cell. 2005;7:337–50.

224. Schramm A, Schulte JH, Klein-Hitpass L, et al. Prediction of clinical outcome and biological characterization of neuroblastoma by expression profiling. Oncogene. 2005;24:7902–12.

225. Takita J, Ishii M, Tsutsumi S, et al. Gene expression profiling and identification of novel prognostic marker genes in neuroblastoma. Genes Chromosomes Cancer. 2004;40:120–32.

226. Wei J, Greer B, Westermann F, et al. Prediction of clinical outcome using gene expression profiling and artificial neural networks for patients with neuroblastoma. Cancer Res. 2004;64:6883–91.

227. Bartel DP. MicroRNAs: target recognition and regulatory functions. Cell. 2009;136(2):215–33.

228. Kim VN, Han J, Siomi MC. Biogenesis of small RNAs in animals. Nat Rev Mol Cell Biol. 2009;10(2):126–39.

229. Lin RJ, Lin YC, Chen J, et al. MicroRNA signature and expression of Dicer and Drosha can predict prognosis and delineate risk groups in neuroblastoma. Cancer Res. 2010;70(20):7841–50.

230. Bray I, Bryan K, Prenter S, et al. Widespread dysregulation of MiRNAs by MYCN amplification and chromosomal imbalances in neuroblastoma: association of miRNA expression with survival. PLoS One. 2009;4(11):e7850.

231. Buechner J, Einvik C. N-myc and noncoding RNAs in neuroblastoma. Mol Cancer Res. 2012; 10(10):1243–53.

232. Chen Y, Stallings RL. Differential patterns of microRNA expression in neuroblastoma are correlated with prognosis, differentiation, and apoptosis. Cancer Res. 2007;67(3):976–83.

233. De Preter K, Mestdagh P, Vermeulen J, et al. miRNA expression profiling enables risk stratification in archived and fresh neuroblastoma tumor samples. Clin Cancer Res. 2011;17(24):7684–92.

234. Maris JM, Mosse YP, Bradfield JP, et al. Chromosome 6p22 locus associated with clinically aggressive neuroblastoma. N Engl J Med. 2008;358(24):2585–93.

235. Capasso M, Devoto M, Hou C, et al. Common variations in BARD1 influence susceptibility to high-risk neuroblastoma. Nat Genet. 2009;41(6):718–23.

236. Capasso M, Diskin SJ, Totaro F, et al. Replication of GWAS-identified neuroblastoma risk loci strengthens the role of BARD1 and affirms the cumulative effect of genetic variations on disease susceptibility. Carcinogenesis. 2012;34(3):605–11.

237. Nguyen le B, Diskin SJ, Capasso M et al. Phenotype restricted genome-wide association study using a gene-centric approach identifies three low-risk neuroblastoma susceptibility loci. PLoS Genet. 2011;7:e1002026.

238. Wang K, Diskin SJ, Zhang H, et al. Integrative genomics identifies LMO1 as a neuroblastoma oncogene. Nature. 2011;469(7329):216–20.

239. Bosse KR, Diskin SJ, Cole KA, et al. Common variation at BARD1 results in the expression of an oncogenic isoform that influences neuroblastoma susceptibility and oncogenicity. Cancer Res. 2012;72(8):2068–78.

240. Yang Q, Kiernan CM, Tian Y, et al. Methylation of CASP8, DCR2, and HIN-1 in neuroblastoma is associated with poor outcome. Clin Cancer Res. 2007;13(11):3191–7.

241. Abe M, Watanabe N, McDonell N, et al. Identification of genes targeted by CpG island methylator phenotype in neuroblastomas, and their possible integrative involvement in poor prognosis. Oncology. 2008;74(1–2):50–60.

242. Decock A, Ongenaert M, Hoebeeck J, et al. Genome-wide promoter methylation analysis in neuroblastoma identifies prognostic methylation biomarkers. Genome Biol. 2012;13(10):R95.

243. Gondek LP, Haddad AS, O'Keefe CL, et al. Detection of cryptic chromosomal lesions including acquired segmental uniparental disomy in advanced and low-risk myelodysplastic syndromes. Exp Hematol. 2007;35(11):1728–38.

244. Wolf M, Korja M, Karhu R, et al. Array-based gene expression, CGH and tissue data defines a 12q24 gain in neuroblastic tumors with prognostic implication. BMC Cancer. 2010;10:181.

245. Mosse YP, Greshock J, Weber BL, Maris JM. Measurement and relevance of neuroblastoma DNA copy number changes in the post-genome era. Cancer Lett. 2005;228(1–2):83–90.

246. Scaruffi P, Coco S, Cifuentes F, et al. Identification and characterization of DNA imbalances in neuroblastoma by high-resolution oligonucleotide array comparative genomic hybridization. Cancer Genet Cytogenet. 2007;177(1):20–9.

247. Chen QR, Bilke S, Khan J. High-resolution cDNA microarray-based comparative genomic hybridization analysis in neuroblastoma. Cancer Lett. 2005;228(1–2):71–81.

248. West RB. Expression profiling in soft tissue sarcomas with emphasis on synovial sarcoma, gastrointestinal stromal tumor, and leiomyosarcoma. Adv Anat Pathol. 2010;17(5):366–73.

249. Allander SV, Illei PB, Chen Y, et al. Expression profiling of synovial sarcoma by cDNA microarrays: association of ERBB2, IGFBP2, and ELF3 with epithelial differentiation. Am J Pathol. 2002;161(5):1587–95.

250. Terry J, Saito T, Subramanian S, et al. TLE1 as a diagnostic immunohistochemical marker for synovial sarcoma emerging from gene expression profiling studies. Am J Surg Pathol. 2007;31(2):240–6.

251. Nielsen TO, West RB, Linn SC, et al. Molecular characterisation of soft tissue tumours: a gene expression study. Lancet. 2002;359(9314):1301–7.

252. Kubista B, Klinglmueller F, Bilban M, et al. Microarray analysis identifies distinct gene expression profiles associated with histological subtype in human osteosarcoma. Int Orthop. 2011;35(3):401–11.

253. Nakayama R, Mitani S, Nakagawa T, et al. Gene expression profiling of synovial sarcoma: distinct signature of poorly differentiated type. Am J Surg Pathol. 2010;34(11):1599–607.

254. McKinsey EL, Parrish JK, Irwin AE, et al. A novel oncogenic mechanism in Ewing sarcoma involving IGF pathway targeting by EWS/Fli1-regulated microRNAs. Oncogene. 2011;30(49):4910–20.

255. Prieur A, Tirode F, Cohen P, Delattre O. EWS/FLI-1 silencing and gene profiling of Ewing cells reveal downstream oncogenic pathways and a crucial role for repression of insulin-like growth factor binding protein 3. Mol Cell Biol. 2004;24(16):7275–83.

256. Geiss GK, Bumgarner RE, Birditt B, et al. Direct multiplexed measurement of gene expression with color-coded probe pairs. Nat Biotechnol. 2008;26(3):317–25.

257. Fortina P, Surrey S. Digital mRNA profiling. Nat Biotechnol. 2008;26(3):293–4.

258. Luina-Contreras A, Jackson S, Ladanyi M. Highly multiplexed detection of translocation fusion transcripts without amplification using the NanoString platform. In: [1901] United States and Canadian Association of Pathologists, 2010, Washington, DC; 2010.

259. Lira ME, Kim TM, Huang D, et al. Multiplexed gene expression and fusion transcript analysis to detect ALK fusions in lung cancer. J Mol Diagn. 2013;15(1):51–61.

Pharmacogenomics in Molecular Oncology

Soya S. Sam and Gregory J. Tsongalis

Introduction

During the last decade, the field of pharmacogenomics (PGx) has revolutionized our approach to prognosis, screening, diagnosis, and targeting therapies by means of personalized and predictive medicine with the rapid evolution of genetic and genomic technologies. These have not only defined the way the clinical practice is evolving today but also indicate how it will be practiced in the future.

While pharmacogenetics involves the relationship between response to drugs and single genes, PGx comprises influence of different genes that determine drug behavior or the whole genome including germline variation (single-nucleotide polymorphisms [SNPs], gene copy number alterations) and acquired changes (tumor mutations) that relate to drug response, adverse drug reactions (ADRs), or toxicity [1, 2]. In contrast to disease genetics, PGx focuses specifically on personalized or predictive medicine involving genetic biomarkers of outcome from pharmacologic interventions based on both drug efficacy and ADRs. However, sometimes both pharmacogenetics and pharmacogenomics are used interchangeably in terms to characterize and understand drug-genome relation.

The term "pharmacogenetics" was first coined by Friedrich Vogel in 1959, to describe the study of genetically inherited conditions which alters pharmacokinetics and pharmacodynamics mechanisms, while the term "pharmacogenomics" has been introduced during the 1990s to transmit the idea that variability in drug response may reflect sets of variants within an individual or across a population using the broadened pharmacogenetic approaches with the advent of novel genomic techniques [3]. P4 medicine is a term coined by biologist Leroy Hood more recently and is short for "predictive, preventive, personalized, and participatory medicine" to denote an ongoing revolution in medicine, moving from a reactive to a proactive discipline that envisions to maximize wellness for each patient rather than to treat the patient [4, 5].

Pharmacogenomics in Oncology

The field of oncology is being revolutionized by incorporating many of the strategies of personalized medicine, especially within the realm of PGx. It particularly has a significant role in the pharmacotherapy of cancer, because most clinically used anticancer drugs have narrow therapeutic indices, variable response rates, rapid and severe systemic toxicity, and unpredictable efficacy which are the hallmarks of cancer therapies and ultimately exhibit a large interindividual

S.S. Sam, Ph.D.
Dartmouth Hitchcock Medical Center, One Medical Center Drive, Lebanon, NH 03756, USA

G.J. Tsongalis, Ph.D. (✉)
Department of Pathology, Geisel School of Medicine at Dartmouth and the Dartmouth Hitchcock Medical Center, One Medical Center Drive, Lebanon, NH, USA
e-mail: Gregory.J.Tsongalis@Hitchcock.org

G.M. Yousef and S. Jothy (eds.), *Molecular Testing in Cancer*,
DOI 10.1007/978-1-4899-8050-2_24, © Springer Science+Business Media New York 2014

Table 24.1 Pharmacogenomics biomarkers and targeted therapeutics for common cancers

Tumor type	Molecular biomarker	Frequency (%)	Clinical utility
Breast cancer	ER/PR	55–75	Sensitivity to hormonal therapy
	ERBB2 (*HER2*)	20–30	Sensitivity to trastuzumab, pertuzumab
Colorectal	KRAS	35–40	Sensitivity to cetuximab and panitumumab
	MSI	15	Resistance to 5-fluorouracil
	UGT1A1*28	39	Adverse reaction to irinotecan
Gastrointestinal stromal tumors	KIT	~85	Sensitivity to imatinib, sunitinib
Leukemia (chronic myelogenous leukemia)	BCR-ABL	>95	Sensitivity to imatinib, dasatinib, nilotinib, bosutinib, ponatinib
Leukemia (acute promyelocytic leukemia)	PML-RAR-alpha translocation	100	Sensitivity to all-trans retinoic acid and arsenic trioxide
Leukemia (acute myeloid leukemia)	FLT3	40	Prognostic relevance
	NPM1	55	
	CEBPA	17	
Leukemia (acute lymphoblastic leukemia)	TPMT	10	Increased risk of 6-mercaptopurine-induced neutropenia
Melanoma	*BRAF* V600E	40–60	Sensitivity to vemurafenib
NSCLC	EML4-ALK	5–7	Sensitivity to crizotinib
	EGFR	15	Sensitivity to erlotinib, gefitinib

pharmacokinetic and pharmacodynamics variability [6]. The implementation of PGx in cancer treatment offers the potential for clinicians to better predict the differences in drug response, resistance, efficacy, and toxicity among chemotherapy and targeted therapy patients and to optimize the treatment regimens based on these differences.

Oncologists have long recognized that there exists a considerable variation among the cancer patients in their response to a drug and to the toxic effects of the drug. Through individualized medicine a realistic goal can be attained by profiling the patients' genetic framework using the molecular biology concepts of PGx which has the potential to revolutionize the cancer therapy. PGx is especially important for oncology as it focuses on severe systemic toxicity and unpredictable efficacies that are hallmarks of cancer therapies [6, 7]. In the practice of oncology medicine, ADRs in cancer therapy have become almost synonymous with the therapy themselves. ADRs are a significant health burden worldwide.

It is ranked as the fifth leading cause of death in the United States and causes over two million severe reactions and claims 100,000–218,000 lives annually and costs over $100 billion dollars annually [8]. It is also an important source of morbidity and mortality among cancer patients.

PGx has been shown to be a powerful predictor of ADRs and has the potential to prevent patients who are predisposed to ADRs from potentially iatrogenic adverse outcomes.

Although many factors influence the effect of medications, genetic factors often account for a significant proportion of interindividual drug response variability [9]. In cancer medicine, clinical molecular diagnostics and biomarker discoveries are constantly advancing as the molecular mechanisms involved in neoplastic cell transformation are increasingly understood. Ultimately, these have the potential to make therapy safer and more effective by determining selection and dosing of drugs for an individual patient.

The cancer biomarkers can be classified as prognostic and predictive biomarkers. Prognostic biomarkers are associated with clinical outcome, such as overall survival or recurrence-free survival, independent of therapy, whereas predictive biomarkers are associated with drug response and utilized for predicting clinical decisions [10]. Rapid developments in new molecular technologies for genomic analysis now provide the means to perform comprehensive analyses of cancer genome mutations. In this review, we discuss the commonly used prognostic and predictive biomarkers in clinical molecular oncology testing (Table 24.1).

Breast Cancer

Breast cancer is the most common cancer in women worldwide. It is the second leading cause of cancer-related mortality among women and accounts for 14 % of cancer deaths [10]. According to the National Cancer Institute, an estimated 232,340 women will be diagnosed with the disease, and 39,620 will die from it in 2013 in the United States [11]. Approximately 5–10 % of breast cancers are reported to be hereditary [12]. Inherited loss-of-function mutations in the tumor suppressor genes *BRCA1*, *BRCA2*, and multiple other genes such as *TP53*, *PTEN*, *CHEK2*, *MLH1*, and *MSH2* predispose to high risks of breast and/or ovarian cancer. *BRCA1* and *BRCA2* mutations account for 5–10 % of breast cancers in Caucasian women in the United States [10].

Approximately 55–75 % of breast cancers are estrogen receptor (ER)-positive, and the hormone receptor status of the cancer can predict the outcome to suppression therapy with tamoxifen or raloxifene [13, 14]. Among the breast cancers that express ER, more than half of these tumors also express progesterone receptor (PR). Tamoxifen is an antagonist of the estrogen receptor and hence competes with estrogen from binding to the ER via its active metabolite, hydroxytamoxifen, and has been used as a first-line therapy for many years. In premenopausal women, tamoxifen is usually administered for hormone receptor-positive breast cancer and also as a standard in postmenopausal women though aromatase inhibitors are used more frequently in this group [15]. If the tumor is hormone receptor-negative, the v-erb-b2 erythroblastic leukemia viral oncogene homolog 2 and neuro-/glioblastoma-derived oncogene homolog (*c-ERBB2* or *HER2/neu*) receptor 2 status will predict the efficacy of trastuzumab [16]. Amplification or overexpression of the *HER2* gene occurs in approximately 20–30 % of breast cancers. Trastuzumab (Herceptin; Genentech, South San Francisco) is a recombinant, humanized anti-HER2 monoclonal antibody and the first clinically active anti-HER2 therapy to be developed for targeting *HER2* overexpressed tumors. Trastuzumab consists of two antigen-specific sites that bind to the extracellular juxtamembrane portion of the HER2 receptor and that prevent the activation of its intracellular tyrosine kinase. Other possible mechanisms by which trastuzumab decreases signaling include prevention of HER2 receptor dimerization, increased endocytotic destruction of the receptor, inhibition of shedding of the extracellular domain, and immune activation [16]. Pertuzumab, another monoclonal antibody, which inhibits dimerization of HER2 receptor which is hypothesized to result in delayed tumor growth, was approved by the FDA for use in combination with trastuzumab in June 2012. Ado-trastuzumab emtansine (Kadcyla) was approved in February 2013 by the FDA, which is the first antibody-drug conjugate for treating HER2-positive metastatic breast cancer [17]. An accurate determination of HER2 status is critically important for clinical decision-making. While there are several methods available to detect *HER2* status, fluorescence in situ hybridization (FISH) and immunohistochemistry (IHC) are the two most commonly employed methods.

Colorectal Cancer

Colorectal cancer is one of the leading causes of cancer-related mortality worldwide. It is estimated that about 102,480 colon and 40,000 rectal cancers will be diagnosed in the United States in 2013 [18]. Colorectal cancer develops through a series of events that lead to the transformation of normal mucosa to adenoma and then to carcinoma where genomic instability plays an integral part in the transformation process. The three distinct molecular pathways identified in colorectal cancer are the chromosomal instability pathway, microsatellite instability pathway, and the CpG island methylator phenotype pathway [19].

Mutations in the KRAS proto-oncogene are overexpressed in colorectal cancer but are common in many other types of cancers, including pancreatic, lung, and ovarian cancer [20]. KRAS is a signaling molecule downstream of the epidermal growth factor receptor (EGFR), a transmembrane receptor for extracellular signaling, and upstream of RAF in the RAS/RAF/MAPKs signaling pathway. The wild-type KRAS mediates signal transduction through its GTPase activity by switching the GDP bound inactive form to the GTP bound active form [20, 21].

Mutations in *KRAS* are reported in 35–40 % of colorectal tumors [22]. Activating mutations in *KRAS* are among the most common mutations in human cancers [23]. The most common *KRAS* mutations are missense mutations leading to amino acid substitutions at codons 12 and 13 of exon 2 that account for about 95 % of all mutation types with mutation at codon 12 being most prevalent and tumorigenic, with approximately 80 % occurring in this codon [24–26]. The common amino acid substitution at both codons 12 and 13 is a glycine to an aspartate residue. In addition, mutations in codons 61, 146, and 154 have been documented but are rare [24]. The KRAS is a membrane-anchored guanosine triphosphate-/guanosine diphosphate (GTP/GDP)-binding protein and is widely expressed in most human cells. All of the *KRAS* mutations enhance the oncogenic potential of *KRAS* by disabling the intrinsic GTPase activity of *KRAS* and preventing GTPase-activating proteins (GAP) from associating with *KRAS* [27]. During normal physiological conditions, upstream signals activate wild-type *KRAS* by promoting the exchange of bound GDP for GTP, and this process is transient because of GAP-mediated GTP hydrolysis. However, when the *KRAS* gene is mutated, this process becomes transformed [28].

As *KRAS* is the most frequently mutated factor downstream of the EGFR signaling pathway, it was considered a candidate molecular biomarker for anti-EGFR therapy. Target-specific treatments, such as cetuximab and panitumumab, monoclonal antibodies directed against EGFR, improved progression-free survival in patients with colorectal cancer that have not responded to traditional chemotherapies [21]. Nevertheless, metastatic colorectal cancer patients whose tumors harbor mutations in *KRAS* do not benefit from anti-EGFR therapies [29]. Therefore, screening of patients who are candidates for these therapies for KRAS mutations has been recommended. Molecular testing for these mutations can be performed by various techniques including real-time PCR, Sanger sequencing, pyrosequencing, and microbead arrays.

The discovery of the microsatellite instability (MSI), the molecular fingerprint of a defective mismatch repair system, is an important feature in about 15 % of colorectal tumors. These tumors with MSI have distinctive features, including a tendency to arise in the proximal colon, lymphocytic infiltrate, and a poorly differentiated, mucinous, or signet ring appearance [30]. While MSI tumors have a better prognosis than microsatellite stable colorectal tumors, MSI cancers mostly do not have the same response to the chemotherapeutics used to treat microsatellite stable tumors. MSI tumors might not benefit from 5-fluorouracil-based adjuvant chemotherapy regimens especially in stage II MSI tumors [30]. MSI testing is conducted using a PCR-based assay and/or immunohistochemical staining for MMR protein expression.

Irinotecan is a topoisomerase I inhibitor approved worldwide for the treatment of metastatic colorectal cancer. A genetic variation in *UGT1A1* increases the risk of irinotecan-induced toxicity. It is responsible for conjugating activated irinotecan, SN-38, to a glucuronide inactive metabolite, SN-38G, through glucuronidation. Mutations in *UGT1A1* can result in significant reduction in glucuronidation, leading to increased exposure of SN-38 and an increased risk of severe neutropenia [31]. Patients who are homozygous for the *UGT1A1*28* allele are at the highest risk of developing severe toxicity, whereas heterozygous patients seem at intermediate risk. The *UGT1A1*28* allele seems to confer reduced gene expression compared with the wild-type allele, *UGT1A1*1*, leading to increased exposure of patients to the cytotoxic metabolite SN-38. The accumulated evidence prompted the US FDA and the pharmaceutical sponsor to revise the irinotecan label in June 2005. The label includes homozygosity for the *UGT1A1*28* genotype as one of the risk factors for severe neutropenia [32, 33]. A US FDA-approved *UGT1A1*28* genotyping method is also commercially available [34].

Gastrointestinal Stromal Tumors

Gastrointestinal stromal tumor (GIST) is one of the most common mesenchymal tumors of the gastrointestinal tract. It is estimated that there are 3,300–6,000 new cases of GIST that occur yearly in the United States, mostly in adults [35]. The pathologic characterization of GIST was first described in 1983, and it was later demonstrated that mutational activation of a proto-oncogene, *KIT*, stimulated the growth of the cancer cells and represents the molecular hallmark of GIST [36]. In healthy individuals, the role of *KIT* usually is to signal cells to grow and divide, a signal which limits cell division and growth. However, in patients with GIST, a malfunctioning of KIT signals the cells to constantly grow and divide out of control becoming cancerous [37].

Targeted agents were developed in the form of small molecule tyrosine kinase inhibitors, such as imatinib and sunitinib, where they block signaling via *KIT* by binding to the adenosine triphosphate-binding pocket required for phosphorylation and activation of the receptor resulting in inhibition of tumor proliferation [38]. Those GIST patients carrying *KIT* exon 11 mutations (deletions or substitutions) tend to have a relatively higher response rate, reduced risk of progression, and long median survival, compared with those carrying wild-type or exon 9 mutations [39]. IHC staining for *KIT* identifies most GISTs. The US FDA approved the use of regorafenib (Stivarga) in February 2013, for locally advanced, unresectable GISTs that no longer respond to imatinib or sunitinib. In a pivotal phase III GRID, trial of 199 patients with metastatic or unresectable GIST demonstrated that regorafenib along with best supportive care (BSC) significantly improved progression-free survival compared to placebo with BSC [40].

Chronic Myelogenous Leukemia

Chronic myelogenous leukemia (CML) or chronic granulocytic leukemia is a myeloproliferative disorder characterized by the proliferation of myeloid cells in the bone marrow [41]. It accounts for about 20 % of all leukemias affecting adults especially middle-aged individuals and it is uncommon in children. According to the cancer statistics data of 2013, an annual decline in mortality rate of 8.4 % was reported for CML when data were analyzed from 2000 to 2009 [18].

The myeloproliferative disease is relatively easy to diagnose because the leukemic cells of more than 95 % of patients have a distinctive cytogenetic abnormality, the Philadelphia chromosome (Ph1) [42, 43]. The Ph1 results from a reciprocal translocation between the long arms of chromosomes 9 and 22. The translocation involves the transfer of the *Abelson* (*ABL*) gene on chromosome 9 oncogene area to the *breakpoint cluster region* (*BCR*) of chromosome 22, resulting in a fused *BCR-ABL* gene [44] (Fig. 24.1). The fusion gene produces a protein, p210 (b2a2 (e13a2) and b3a2 (e14a2)), an abnormal tyrosine kinase that plays a key role in the development of CML [45]. It results in deregulated proliferation and reduced adherence to the bone marrow stroma and impaired apoptotic response to mutagenic stimuli [46]. CML with p190 BCR-ABL and p230 BCR-ABL is less frequent [45].

Usually, CML presents in a chronic phase but progresses to an accelerated phase and a terminal blast crisis [47]. The understanding of the abnormal signaling in CML cells led to the design and development of small molecules that target the tyrosine kinase activity of BCR-ABL, of which imatinib mesylate (Gleevec) was first to be used, which significantly improved outcomes for Ph1-positive CML patients [48]. Tyrosine kinase inhibitor imatinib competes with ATP for binding to the BCR-ABL kinase domain, thus preventing phosphorylation of tyrosine residues. Disruption of this oncogenic signal is critical for disease control, especially when used in initial chronic phase of the disease. Nevertheless, the emergence of subclones of leukemic progenitor cells with point mutation in the coding sequence of the ABL kinase domain of BCR-ABL prevents the binding of the inhibitor to the kinase domain that can lead to imatinib resistance [49]. The more potent second-generation BCR-ABL inhibitors

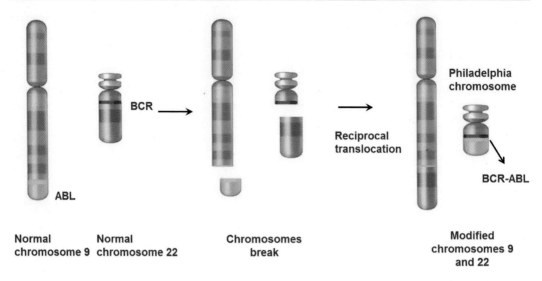

Fig. 24.1 The translocated *abl* gene inserts to the *bcr* gene forming Philadelphia chromosome [http://www.cancer.gov/cancertopics/pdq/treatment/CML/Patient/page1]

dasatinib (Sprycel) and nilotinib (Tasigna), with bosutinib (Bosulif) and ponatinib (Iclusig), having been recently approved for market inclusion could circumvent this form of drug failure in the case of most kinase domain mutations associated with imatinib resistance [49, 50]. Resistance has been associated with more than 50 different amino acid residues within BCR–ABL [51]. In vitro, dasatinib and nilotinib are effective against all imatinib-resistant *BCR–ABL* mutants tested except T315I. However, each inhibitor has reduced potency toward specific mutants compared with unmutated *BCR–ABL*: F317L and E255V for dasatinib, and Y253F/H, E255K/V, and F359V for nilotinib whereas bosutinib is less active in V299L and E255K/V mutant carriers and inactive against T315I [52, 53]. Dasatinib, nilotinib, and bosutinib have a 325-fold, 10–50-fold, and 25-fold increased potency, respectively, over imatinib against *BCR-ABL1* kinase activity [54]. Therefore, in addition to monitoring *BCR-ABL1* levels, it has become important to screen imatinib-resistant CML cases for mutations in the fusion gene.

The important prognostic indicator is the response to therapy at the hematologic, cytogenetic, and molecular level [55, 56]. Imatinib currently has a complete cytogenetic response rate

of 70–90 %, with a 5-year progression-free survival and overall survival between 80 and 95 % [57]. In most patients, following the imatinib therapy, transcripts of *BCR-ABL* remain detectable by quantitative RT-PCR [58]. Therefore, patients need to be continually monitored in order to detect the level of *BCR-ABL* transcripts. Measurement of minimum residual disease using molecular analysis (real-time quantitative PCR) has become the gold standard of measuring response to therapy, considering its higher sensitivity compared with other cytogenetic or FISH testing [59].

Acute Promyelocytic Leukemia

Acute promyelocytic leukemia (APL), a distinctive subtype of AML, comprises about 5–8 % of AML cases [60], with an abnormal accumulation of immature granulocytes called promyelocytes in the blood and bone marrow. Early diagnosis in APL is essential because it is associated with life-threatening disseminated intravascular coagulation [61]. The disease is characterized by a chromosomal translocation involving the (15;17) (q22;q12) leading to fusion of the promyelocytic gene (PML) on chromosome 15 with the *retinoic* acid receptor (*RARα*) gene on chromosome 17, a diagnostic hallmark of APL. This translocation produces a chimeric protein that blocks the myeloid differentiation at the promyelocytic stage leading to increased proliferation of promyelocytes [62].

The blasts are highly sensitive to the anthracycline-based chemotherapy in APL patients. During the past decades, two therapeutic drugs have been introduced that have dramatically improved the treatment outcome of this disease. The all-trans retinoic acid (ATRA), a vitamin A derivative that targets the RARa domain of the fusion protein, is the first drug discovered. This significantly increased clinical remission and improved the 5-year disease-free survival rates from below 40 % to more than 80 % [63]. The second drug is arsenic trioxide (ATO), a component that targets PML and was discovered to be very effective in treating APL as a single agent [64]. Currently, ATRA in combination with chemotherapy is employed as the frontline therapy, while ATO is being used for refractory or relapsed patients. Studies have revealed a positive synergistic effect of these drugs, suggesting that future therapy of newly diagnosed patients may involve a combination of the two reagents [65–68].

Various diagnostic tools such as cytogenetics, FISH, monoclonal anti-PML antibodies, or RT-PCR are necessary for genetic confirmation of the aberrant *PML–RARa* fusion oncogene. The only technique that can identify the *PML–RARa* isoform useful for the monitoring of MRD is RT-PCR [69, 70] whereas quantitative RT-PCR improves the predictive value of MRD monitoring. By employing quantitative RT-PCR, it evaluates response to treatment and assess prognosis of disease and therefore guides therapy in order to reduce the rate of relapse [71]. Once, APL was considered the most malignant human leukemia associated with the worst prognosis, and this has been transformed in the past few decades into the most frequently curable, with advancement in diagnostic molecular testing, sensitive MRD monitoring by PCR techniques, predicting relapse-risk categories, and adoption of risk-adapted strategies [72].

Acute Myeloid Leukemia

It has long been appreciated that acute myeloid leukemia (AML) belongs to a heterogeneous group of neoplastic disorders with marked variability in both response to therapy and overall survival. It is heterogeneous regarding clinical feature, morphological and immunophenotypic features, and karyotypic and genetic abnormalities, as well as in the genetic and molecular basis of pathology.

In the AML, accumulation of acquired genetic variations in the myeloid progenitor cell transforms normal growth, proliferation, and cell differentiation. Nevertheless, only 55 % of the patients with AML have chromosomal abnormalities detectable by standard cytogenetic analyses [73, 74]. Cytogenetically normal (CN) group of these neoplasms that account for about 45 % belongs to molecularly heterogeneous disease entity in which mutations in certain genes have been linked to prognostic significance. Mutant variations in the internal tandem duplications (ITD) of the *fms-like tyrosine kinase 3* (*FLT3*) gene and mutations in *NPM1* and *CEBPA* genes are the most common prognostic markers [75, 76] (Fig. 24.2).

Nucleophosmin (*NPM1*) gene also known as nucleolar phosphoprotein B23 or numatrin located at 5q35.1 is a ubiquitously expressed phosphoprotein that belongs to the nucleoplasmin family of nuclear chaperones. The gene continuously shuttles between the nucleus and cytoplasm with predominant nucleolar localization, a significant characteristic feature of patients with AML who have a normal karyotype [77]. It is involved in critical cell functions such as control of ribosome formation and export, stabilization of the oncosuppressor p14^{Arf} protein in the nucleolus, and regulation of centrosome duplication [78]. Among the AML mutations, *NPM1* gene mutations represent the single most common genetic alteration in adult de novo AML. These gene mutations account for about 35 % of all cases with 50–60 % cases having cytogenetically normal karyotype [79]. *NPM1* mutations occur in exon 12 and are most frequently characterized by a 4-bp insertion, leading to frameshift

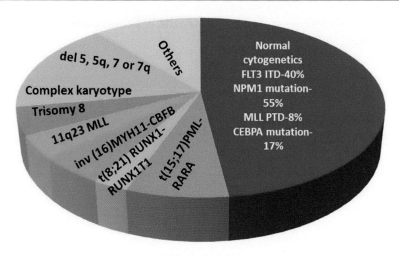

Fig. 24.2 Relative frequencies of common recurrent genetic abnormalities in AML [76]

and an elongated protein, which is retained in the cytoplasm. Mutation A accounts for about 70–80 % of all adult cases due to a TCTG duplication at position 960 whereas mutation B and D together account for 15–20 % of all cases. There are about 50 other mutations that have been identified till date [80]. Therefore, a reliable molecular method is necessary for accurate identification of the NPM1 mutations. Simultaneous detection of the most common *NPM1* mutations in exon 12 (A, B, D, and J) is employed by multiplex RT-PCR followed by multiplex detection on the Luminex® 100 IS™ or 200™ System. In addition, fragment analysis is yet another molecular diagnostic assay for detection of these mutations.

Activating mutations in the *FLT3* gene are the most common mutations in AML and are associated with a higher risk of relapse and indicate poor prognosis [81]. The *FLT3* gene is located on 13q12 and encodes a membrane-bound receptor tyrosine kinase (RTK) that belongs to the RTK subclass III family, characterized by five immunoglobulin-like extracellular domains, a single transmembrane domain, a juxtamembrane domain (JMD), and an intracellular domain consisting of two protein tyrosine kinase (PTK) domains linked by a kinase-insert domain [81].

Mutations of the *FLT3* are of major clinical relevance in AML because they guide treatment decisions as independent indicators of poor prognosis [75, 82]. The most common mutation

of *FLT3* in AML is the internal tandem duplication (*FLT3-ITD*). *FLT3-ITD* results from a duplication of a fragment within the juxtamembrane domain coding region (encoded by exons 14 and 15) of *FLT3*. It is found in 15–35 % of AML patients [83], and this is first described by Nakao et al. in a high proportion of patients with AML [83]. The mutation is rare in infant AML but increases to 5–10 % in age 5–10 years, 20 % in young adults, and >35 % in AML patients older than 55 years [84]. This mutation enhances autodimerization and autophosphorylation of the receptor, which turns it constitutively phosphorylated and activating AKT, a key serine-threonine kinase within the phosphatidylinositol 3-kinase pathway [85–87].

The second most common type of *FLT3* mutations is the *FLT3-TKD* found in 5–10 % of AML, and they rarely coexist with *FLT3-ITD*. The mutation occurs in codon 835 with a change of an aspartic acid to tyrosine (D835Y or Asp835Tyr). *FLT3-TKD* promotes ligand-independent proliferation through autophosphorylation and constitutive receptor activation, similar to that of *FLT3-ITD*. They promote activation of different downstream effectors and trigger different biological responses [88, 89]. The presence of *FLT3-ITD* is an independent prognostic factor for poor outcome in AML. Sorafenib, an inhibitor of multiple kinases including FLT3, has demonstrated promising effect in *FLT3-ITD*-positive AML [90].

Transcription activation   DNA binding and dimerization

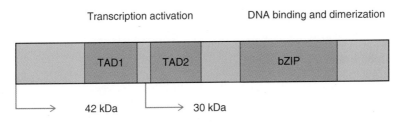

Fig. 24.3 Schematic of transactivation and basic region leucine zipper domains

However, the drug is not effective in the treatment of *FLT3-ITD*-positive AML relapsing after allogeneic hematopoietic stem cell transplantation [90]. Detection of activating mutations in the receptor tyrosine kinase FLT3 can be conducted by fluorescence-based multiplex PCR fragment analysis. The testing would help selecting AML cases that are appropriate for targeted therapy.

The *CEBPA* gene located on chromosome 19q13.1 encodes a member of the basic leucine zipper (bZIP) domain transcription factor family and is a critical regulator of granulopoiesis [91]. The CEBPA mutations can be classified broadly into two groups: N-terminal frameshift mutations and C-terminal in-frame mutations in a basic leucine zipper (bZIP) domain. Mutation in the N-terminal specifically abolishes the translation of the full length (42-kDa) CEBPA protein, leading to the overexpression of a shorter, dominant-negative 30-kDa isoform of CEBPA (Fig. 24.3). Mutations in the C-terminal lead to proteins with disrupted homo- and hetero-dimerization domains and ultimately result in impaired DNA binding activities [92, 93]. The majority of AML patients with *CEBPA* mutations harbor a mutation at both domains (CEBPA double mutants), and these are located on different alleles, resulting in the lack of wild-type C/EBPα p42 expression in these patients. However, both types can occur as single *CEBPA* mutations, in which expression of the wild-type product is retained at lower levels [94, 95]. A fluorescence-based multiplex PCR fragment analysis and a direct sequencing method are commonly employed for detecting *CEBPA* mutations in patients with acute myeloid leukemia.

Acute Lymphoblastic Leukemia

Acute lymphoblastic leukemia, also known as acute lymphocytic leukemia (ALL), is the most common cancer diagnosed in children and represents 23 % of cancer diagnoses among children younger than 15 years. This represents 12 % of all leukemia cases, with a worldwide incidence projected to be 1–4.75 per 100,000 people [96]. It occurs at an annual rate of about 30–40 cases per million people in the United States [97]. Thiopurine S-methyltransferase (TPMT) is a cytosolic enzyme ubiquitously expressed in the human body and catalyzes the S-methylation of thiopurines such as 6-mercaptopurine (6-MP) which is a standard drug therapy in ALL. The *TPMT* heterozygous individuals (6–11 % of white individuals) have intermediate TPMT activity, and homozygous mutant individuals (0.2–0.6 % of white individuals) have very low TPMT activity. About 20 variant alleles (*TPMT*2-*18*) have been identified, which are associated with decreased activity compared with the *TPMT*1 wild-type allele. Through molecular profiling, more than 95 % of defective TPMT activity can be addressed by the most frequent mutant alleles, TPMT*2 and TPMT*3(A-D) [98–101]. Genetic variation in *TPMT* is associated with myelosuppression after treatment with 6-MP. Patients may experience moderate to severe myelosuppression such that drug dose reduction may be warranted. Low TPMT activity levels could put a patient at risk for developing toxicity, since too much drug would be converted to 6-thioguanine nucleotides (6-TGNs), the cytotoxic active metabolite incorporated into DNA.

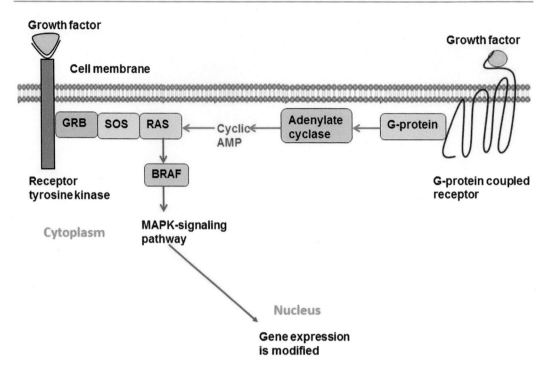

Fig. 24.4 The *BRAF* and signal transduction: The RAS-RAF-MAPK (mitogen-activated protein kinase) signaling pathway is a pivotal molecular cascade through which extracellular signal can be transmitted into the nucleus, to control cell proliferation or differentiation by changes in gene expression. Extracellular signals (growth factors) that activate one of two types of receptor, receptor tyrosine kinases and G-protein-coupled receptors, can result in the activation of RAS, leading to activation of BRAF and the downstream cascade [104]

However, patients with high TPMT activity levels would need higher than standard doses of a thiopurine drug to respond well to the therapy, since a large amount of the drug is being inactivated before it can be converted to 6-TGNs. Additionally, genetic testing of TPMT may be important not only for determining TPMT-related 6-MP toxicity but also for determining response to 6-MP, measured by minimal residual disease (MRD), in the early course of childhood ALL. Therefore, dose modifications based on TPMT genetic testing are now recommended by the FDA [98, 99]. Real-time PCR method is one of the techniques routinely employed for the molecular detection

Melanoma

Melanoma is the leading cause of death from skin disease that accounts for 4 % of incident cancers, and its mortality rate is increasing [102]. Although the prognosis is better in early-stage cases upon surgical excision and adjuvant therapy, many will develop disseminated disease [103]. Melanoma is a complex genetic disease, and multiple genetic variations have been reported to play a role in pathogenesis of disease progression. More recently, preclinical discoveries have led to the understanding of molecular pathogenesis of melanoma and the key molecular signaling events underlying the disease. Approximately 40–60 % of melanomas harbor activating mutations in the BRAF, a serine/threonine protein kinase that leads to constitutive activation of downstream signaling in the MAP kinase/ERK pathway (Fig. 24.4) [104]. In 80–90 % of the cases, the activating mutation consists of a single-base missense transversion (T to A at nucleotide 1,799) resulting in substitution of glutamic acid for valine at amino acid 600 (V600E) in exon 15. The effects of other less frequent observed BRAF mutations have also been reported. Among melanomas with mutated

BRAF, about 5–12 % are V600K (valine to lysine) and 5 % or less are V600R (valine to arginine) or V600D (valine to aspartic acid) [105]. These less frequent mutations, similar to BRAFV600E, result in an increase in BRAF kinase activity and increased MEK and ERK phosphorylation [106].

The *BRAFV600E* mutation became a popular target in drug development due to the high prevalence in melanoma. Sorafenib was one of the first multi-kinase inhibitors which targeted BRAF but lacked selectivity and potency. Additionally, it is a highly potent inhibitor of VEGFR2, VEGFR3, and several other kinases critical in cancerous processes [107, 108]. Later, vemurafenib, a novel BRAF inhibitor with greater specificity to mutant *BRAFV600E* than the wild-type protein, has been developed. This orally available selective BRAF inhibitor, vemurafenib, has potent cytotoxicity against melanoma cells in vitro and in vivo and clinically has improved survival of melanoma patients [109, 110]. Vemurafenib also asserts its inhibitory action on other BRAF mutations such as *BRAFV600D*, *BRAFV600K*, and *BRAFV600R* in preclinical trials [111, 112]. *BRAFV600K* and *BRAFV600E* both show better responses to the MEK inhibitor, trametinib (GSK1120212), compared to patients with wild-type BRAF melanomas [113, 114].

Non-small Cell Lung Cancer

Non-small cell lung cancer (NSCLC) is the most common type of lung cancer and accounts for approximately 85 % of all lung cancers [115]. The introduction of genome-wide analyses has dramatically broadened our view on the molecular landscape of NSCLC. A number of molecular variations have been identified in NSCLC which include *EML4-ALK* translocation fusions, *EGFR* mutations and amplifications, *KRAS* mutations, *PIK3CA* mutations, *MET* mutations, alternative splicing, amplification, and overexpression [116].

Among the three common types of NSCLC, adenocarcinoma is the most common type of lung cancer seen in the United States that accounts for about 50 % of the cases whereas squamous cell carcinoma in 30 % of the cases and large cell cancers in 10 % of the cases [117]. Adenocarcinoma

is also the most frequently occurring cell type in nonsmokers. Gene expression profiling using DNA microarrays has identified subtypes of lung adenocarcinomas (e.g., bronchioid, squamoid, magnoid) which correlate with stage-specific survival and metastatic pattern. Importantly, bronchioid tumors were associated with increased survival in early-stage disease, whereas squamoid tumors were associated with increased survival in advanced disease [118].

In patients with NSCLC, mutations in epidermal growth factor receptor (*EGFR*) and anaplastic lymphoma kinase (*ALK*) are mutually exclusive, and the presence of one mutation in lieu of another can influence response to targeted therapy. Therefore, molecular testing for these mutations and tailoring therapy accordingly is widely accepted as standard practice.

A significant development in molecular diagnostic and clinical oncology is the discovery of the *EML-ALK* fusion oncogene which was first identified in 2007 in a small proportion of patients with NSCLC. This fusion oncogene arises from an inversion on the short arm of chromosome 2, inv(2) (p21p23), that joins exons 1–13 of EML4 to exons 20–29 of ALK [119, 120]. The resulting fusion protein, EML4-ALK, contains an N-terminus derived from EML4 and a C-terminus containing the entire intracellular tyrosine kinase domain of ALK. Multiple variants of *EML-ALK* have been reported, all of which encode the same cytoplasmic portion of ALK but contain different truncations of EML4. The fusion protein is expressed aberrantly and activates canonical signaling pathways, including Ras/Mek/Erk and PI3K/Akt cascades (Fig. 24.5). In addition, combinations of *ALK* with other partners including TRK-fused gene *TFG* and *KIF5B* have also been described in lung cancer patients but appear to be much less common than *EML4-ALK* [121]. Crizotinib is an oral tyrosine kinase inhibitor, which silences the protein product of the *ALK* fusion gene and has been approved in 2011 for the treatment of NSCLC [122]. The *ALK* gene rearrangements or the resulting fusion proteins may be detected using FISH, IHC, and reverse transcription polymerase chain reaction. The gold standard tool for diagnosing *ALK*-positive NSCLC is FISH.

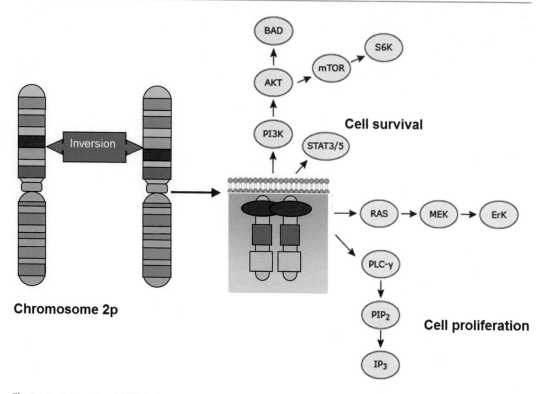

Fig. 24.5 Schematic of ALK fusion oncogene and important downstream signaling pathways [121]

In the FISH analysis, the break-apart probes include two differently colored (red and green) probes that flank the highly conserved translocation breakpoint within ALK. In the setting of an ALK rearrangement, red and green probes are separated and splitting of the red and green signals is observed; while in the non-rearranged cells or wild-type cells, the overlying red and green probes result in a yellow (fused) signal. Atypical patterns of cell rearrangement have also been detected, and these are also responsive to ALK inhibition with crizotinib (Fig. 24.6).

In the United States, mutations in the EGFR tyrosine kinase are observed in approximately 15 % of NSCLC adenocarcinoma and occur more frequently in nonsmokers [123]. The most commonly found *EGFR* mutations in patients with NSCLC are deletions in exon 19 (E19del in 45 % of patients) and a mutation in exon 21 (L858R in 40 % of patients). In advanced NSCLC, the presence of an *EGFR* mutation confers a more favorable prognosis and strongly predicts sensitivity to EGFR tyrosine kinase inhibitors such as erlotinib and gefitinib [117].

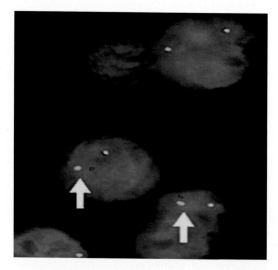

Fig. 24.6 Fluorescence microscopy image using ALK break-apart probes of cells from a NSCLC tumor, demonstrating an ALK gene rearrangement. The red and green probes hybridize to regions that flank the highly conserved translocation breakpoint within the ALK gene. *Arrow*: in the setting of an ALK rearrangement, these probes are separated, and splitting of the red and green signals is observed. In the wild-type intact ALK gene, the closely apposed red and green probes result in a yellow signal (adapted from UpToDate)

Conclusion

Achieving personalized care is increasingly important among cancer patients as they often require complex and coordinated ongoing medical attention and require multiple long-term medications to prevent disease recurrence, manage disease-related symptoms, or treat long-term therapy-induced toxicities. Rapid developments in new molecular technologies for genomic analysis now provide the means to perform comprehensive analyses of cancer genome mutations. As our knowledge of tumor heterogeneity and tumor resistance mechanisms evolves, more rational therapies and combinations of therapies can be expected. Pharmacogenomics provides a unique approach toward investigating and therapeutically serving the individual cancer patient through personalized medicine. By using the information gleaned from pharmacogenomics and molecular testing, it is anticipated that cancer chemotherapy can be tailored to the individual patient or tumor phenotype, making therapy safer and more effective for cancer patients.

References

1. Wang L, McLeod HL, Weinshilboum RM. Genomics and drug response. N Engl J Med. 2011;364:1144–53.
2. Watson RG, McLeod HL. Pharmacogenomic contribution to drug response. Cancer J. 2011;17:80–8.
3. Motulsky A. From pharmacogenetics and ecogenetics to pharmacogenomics. Med Secoli. 2002;14:683–705.
4. Hood L, Balling R, Auffray C. Revolutionizing medicine in the 21st century through systems approaches. Biotechnol J. 2012;7:92–1001.
5. Hood L, Friend SH. Predictive, personalized, preventive, participatory (P4) cancer medicine. Nat Rev Clin Oncol. 2011;8:184–7.
6. Feng X, Brazill B, Pearson D. Therapeutic application of pharmacogenomics in oncology: selective biomarkers for cancer treatment. US Pharm. 2011;36(Oncology Suppl):5–12.
7. Wheeler HE, Maitland ML, Dolan ME, Cox NJ, Ratain MJ. Cancer pharmacogenomics: strategies and challenges. Nat Rev Genet. 2013;14:23–34.
8. Ross CJ, Visscher H, Rassekh SR, Castro-Pastrana LI, Shereck E, Carleton B, et al. Pharmacogenomics of serious adverse drug reactions in pediatric oncology. J Popul Ther Clin Pharmacol. 2011;18:e134–51.
9. Kalow W, Tang BK, Endrenyi L. Hypothesis: comparisons of inter- and intra-individual variations can substitute for twin studies in drug research. Pharmacogenetics. 1998;8:283–9.
10. Ong FS, Das K, Wang J, Vakil H, Kuo JZ, Blackwell WL, et al. Personalized medicine and pharmacogenetic biomarkers: progress in molecular oncology testing. Expert Rev Mol Diagn. 2012;12:593–602.
11. http://www.cancer.gov/cancertopics/types/breast
12. http://www.breastcancer.org/risk/factors/genetics
13. Barnadas A, Estévez LG, Lluch-Hernández A, Rodriguez-Lescure A, Rodriguez-Sanchez C, Sanchez-Rovira P. An overview of letrozole in postmenopausal women with hormone-responsive breast cancer. Adv Ther. 2011;28:1045–58.
14. Tiwary R, Yu W, de Graffenried LA, Sanders BG, Kline K. Targeting cholesterol-rich microdomains to circumvent tamoxifen-resistant breast cancer. Breast Cancer Res. 2011;13:R120.
15. BIG 1–98 Collaborative Group, Mouridsen H, Giobbie-Hurder A, Goldhirsch A, Thürlimann B, Paridaens R, et al. Letrozole therapy alone or in sequence with tamoxifen in women with breast cancer. N Engl J Med. 2009;361:766–76.
16. Hortobagyi GN. Trastuzumab in the treatment of breast cancer. N Engl J Med. 2005;353:1734–6.
17. Traynor K. Ado-trastuzumab emtansine approved for advanced breast cancer. Am J Health Syst Pharm. 2013;70:562.
18. Siegel R, Naishadham D, Jemal A. Cancer statistics, 2013. CA Cancer J Clin. 2013;63:11.
19. Goel A, Arnold CN, Niedzwiecki D, Chang DK, Ricciardiello L, Carethers JM, et al. Characterization of sporadic colon cancer by patterns of genomic instability. CancerRes. 2003;63:1608–14.
20. Jančík S, Drábek J, Radzioch D, Hajdúch M. Clinical relevance of KRAS in human cancers. J Biomed Biotechnol. 2010;2010. Article ID 150960. doi:10.1155/2010/150960.ci
21. El Zouhairi M, Charabaty A, Pishvaian MJ. Molecularly targeted therapy for metastatic colon cancer: proven treatments and promising new agents. Gastrointest Cancer Res. 2011;4:15–21.
22. Phipps AI, Buchanan DD, Makar KW, Win AK, Baron JA, Lindor NM, Potter JD, Newcomb PA. Br J Cancer. 2013;108(8):1757–64.
23. Ikediobi ON, Davies H, Bignell G, Edkins S, Stevens C, O'Meara S, et al. Mutation analysis of 24 known cancer genes in the NCI-60 cell line set. Mol Cancer Ther. 2006;5:2606–12.
24. Normanno N, Tejpar S, Morgillo F, De Luca A, Van Cutsem E, Ciardiello F. Implications for KRAS status and EGFR-targeted therapies in metastatic CRC. Nat Rev Clin Oncol. 2009;6:519–27.
25. Guerrero S, Casanova I, Farré L, Mazo A, Capellà G, Mangues R. K-ras codon 12 mutation induces higher level of resistance to apoptosis and predisposition to anchorage-independent growth than codon 13 mutation or proto-oncogene overexpression. Cancer Res. 2000;60:6750–6.

26. Forbes S, Clements J, Dawson E, Bamford S, Webb T, Dogan A, et al. COSMIC 2005. Br J Cancer. 2006;94:318–22.

27. Di Fiore F, Sesboüé R, Michel P, Sabourin JC, Frebourg T. Molecular determinants of anti-EGFR sensitivity and resistance in metastatic colorectal cancer. Br J Cancer. 2010;103:1765–72.

28. Tan C, Du X. KRAS mutation testing in metastatic colorectal cancer. World J Gastroenterol. 2012;18: 5171–80.

29. Behl AS, Goddard KA, Flottemesch TJ, Veenstra D, Meenan RT, Lin JS, et al. Cost-effectiveness analysis of screening for KRAS and BRAF mutations in metastatic colorectal cancer. J Natl Cancer Inst. 2012; 104:1785–95.

30. Boland CR, Goel A. Microsatellite instability in colorectal cancer. Gastroenterology. 2010;138: 2073–87.

31. Innocenti F, Kroetz DL, Schuetz E, Dolan ME, Ramírez J, Relling M, et al. Comprehensive pharmacogenetic analysis of irinotecan neutropenia and pharmacokinetics. J Clin Oncol. 2009;27: 2604–14.

32. O'Dwyer PJ, Catalano RB. Uridine diphosphate glucuronosyltransferase (UGT) 1A1 and irinotecan: practical pharmacogenomics arrives in cancer therapy. J Clin Oncol. 2006;24:4534–8.

33. Innocenti F, Ratain MJ. Pharmacogenetics of irinotecan: clinical perspectives on the utility of genotyping. Pharmacogenomics. 2006;7:1211–21.

34. US Food and Drug Administration. FDA clears genetic test that advances personalized medicine test helps determine safety of drug therapy. http://www.fda.gov/bbs/topics/NEWS/2005/NEW01220.htm

35. Corless CL, Heinrich MC. Molecular pathobiology of gastrointestinal stromal sarcomas. Annu Rev Pathol. 2008;3:557–86.

36. Siehl J, Thiel E. C-kit, GIST, and imatinib. Recent Results Cancer Res. 2007;176:145–51.

37. Licence for imatinib in UK for patients with GIST. Oncology Times UK: June 2009;6:18.

38. Blanke CD, Demetri GD, von Mehren M, Heinrich MC, Eisenberg B, Fletcher JA, et al. Long-term results from a randomized phase II trial of standard-versus higher-dose imatinib mesylate for patients with unresectable or metastatic gastrointestinal stromal tumors expressing KIT. J Clin Oncol. 2008; 26:620–5.

39. Quek R, George S. Gastrointestinal stromal tumor: a clinical overview. Hematol Oncol Clin North Am. 2009;23:69–78.

40. http://www.fda.gov/NewsEvents/Newsroom/Press Announcements/ucm340958.htm

41. Kantarjian HM, Deisseroth A, Kurzrock R, Estrov Z, Talpaz M. Chronic myelogenous leukemia: a concise update. Blood. 1993;82:691–703.

42. Kurzrock R, Kantarjian HM, Druker BJ, Talpaz M. Philadelphia chromosome-positive leukemias: from basic mechanisms to molecular therapeutics. Ann Intern Med. 2003;138:819–30.

43. Goldman JM, Melo JV. Chronic myeloid leukemia—advances in biology and new approaches to treatment. N Engl J Med. 2003;349:1451–64.

44. Faderl S, Talpaz M, Estrov Z, Kantarjian HM. Chronic myelogenous leukemia: biology and therapy. Ann Intern Med. 1999;131:207–19.

45. Ritchie DS, McBean M, Westerman DA, Kovalenko S, Seymour JF, Dobrovic A. Complete molecular response of e6a2 BCR-ABL-positive acute myeloid leukemia to imatinib then Dasatinib. Blood. 2008; 111:2896–8.

46. Deininger MW, Goldman JM, Melo JV. The molecular biology of chronic myeloid leukemia. Blood. 2000;96:3343–56.

47. Sawyers CL. Chronic myeloid leukemia. N Engl J Med. 1999;340:1330–40.

48. Kantarjian H, Sawyers C, Hochhaus A, Guilhot F, Schiffer C, Gambacorti-Passerini C, et al. Hematologic and cytogenetic responses to imatinib mesylate in chronic myelogenous leukemia. N Engl J Med. 2002;346:645–52.

49. Guilhot F, Roy L, Tomowiak C. Current treatment strategies in chronic myeloid leukemia. Curr Opin Hematol. 2012;19:102–9.

50. Simoneau CA. Treating chronic myeloid leukemia: improving management through understanding of the patient experience. Clin J Oncol Nurs. 2013;17: E13–20.

51. Apperley JF. Part I: mechanisms of resistance to imatinib in chronic myeloid leukaemia. Lancet Oncol. 2007;8:1018–29.

52. O'Hare T, Walters DK, Stoffregen EP, Jia T, Manley PW, Mestan J, et al. In vitro activity of Bcr-Abl inhibitors AMN107 and BMS-354825 against clinically relevant imatinib-resistant Abl kinase domain mutants. Cancer Res. 2005;65:4500–5.

53. Redaelli S, Piazza R, Rostagno R, Magistroni V, Perini P, Marega M, et al. Activity of bosutinib, dasatinib, and nilotinib against 18 imatinib-resistant BCR/ABL mutants. J Clin Oncol. 2009;27:469–71.

54. Shami PJ, Deininger M. Evolving treatment strategies for patients newly diagnosed with chronic myeloid leukemia: the role of second-generation BCR-ABL inhibitors as first-line therapy. Leukemia. 2012;26:214–24.

55. Marin D, Ibrahim AR, Lucas C, Gerrard G, Wang L, Szydlo RM, et al. Assessment of BCR-ABL1 transcript levels at 3 months is the only requirement for predicting outcome for patients with chronic myeloid leukemia treated with tyrosine kinase inhibitors. J Clin Oncol. 2012;30:232–8.

56. Baccarani M, Saglio G, Goldman J, Hochhaus A, Simonsson B, Appelbaum F, et al. Evolving concepts in the management of chronic myeloid leukemia: recommendations from an expert panel on behalf of the European LeukemiaNet. Blood. 2006; 108:1809–20.

57. Swerdlow SH. WHO classification of tumours of haematopoietic and lymphoid tissues. Lyon, France: International Agency for Research on Cancer; 2008.

58. Quintás-Cardama A, Kantarjian HM, Cortes JE. Mechanisms of primary and secondary resistance to imatinib in chronic myeloid leukemia. Cancer Control. 2009;16(2):122–31.

59. Foroni L, Gerrard G, Nna E, Khorashad JS, Stevens D, Swale B, et al. Technical aspects and clinical applications of measuring BCR-ABL1 transcripts number in chronic myeloid leukemia. Am J Hematol. 2009;84:517–22.

60. Jing Y. The PML-RARalpha fusion protein and targeted therapy for acute promyelocytic leukemia. Leuk Lymphoma. 2004;45:639–48.

61. Miller Jr WH, Kakizuka A, Frankel SR, Warrell Jr RP, DeBlasio A, Levine K, et al. Reverse transcription polymerase chain reaction for the rearranged retinoic acid receptor alpha clarifies diagnosis and detects minimal residual disease in acute promyelocytic leukemia. Proc Natl Acad Sci U S A. 1992; 89:2694–8.

62. Wang ZY, Chen Z. Acute promyelocytic leukemia: from highly fatal to highly curable. Blood. 2008;111:2505–15.

63. Huang ME, Ye YC, Chen SR, Chai JR, Lu JX, Zhoa L, et al. Use of all-trans retinoic acid in the treatment of acute promyelocytic leukemia. Blood. 1988;72: 567–72.

64. Sun HD, Ma L, Hu XC, Zhang TD. Ai-Lin 1 treated 32 cases of acute promyelocytic leukemia. Chin J Integrat Chin West Med. 1992;12:170–2.

65. Estey E, Garcia-Manero G, Ferrajoli A, Faderl S, Verstovsek S, Jones D, et al. Use of all-trans retinoic acid plus arsenic trioxide as an alternative to chemotherapy in untreated acute promyelocytic leukemia. Blood. 2006;107:3469–73.

66. Hu J, Liu YF, Wu CF, Xu F, Shen ZX, Zhu YM, et al. Long-term efficacy and safety of all-trans retinoic acid/arsenic trioxide-based therapy in newly diagnosed acute promyelocytic leukemia. Proc Natl Acad Sci U S A. 2009;106:3342–7.

67. Shen ZX, Shi ZZ, Fang J, Gu BW, Li JM, Zhu YM, et al. All-trans retinoic acid/As2O3 combination yields a high quality remission and survival in newly diagnosed acute promyelocytic leukemia. Proc Natl Acad Sci U S A. 2004;101:5328–35.

68. Wang G, Li W, Cui J, Gao S, Yao C, Jiang Z, et al. An efficient therapeutic approach to patients with acute promyelocytic leukemia using a combination of arsenic trioxide with low-dose all-trans retinoic acid. J Hematol Oncol. 2004;22:63–71.

69. Grimwade D, Jovanovic JV, Hills RK, Nugent EA, Patel Y, Flora R, et al. Prospective minimal residual disease monitoring to predict relapse of acute promyelocytic leukemia and to direct pre-emptive arsenic trioxide therapy. J Clin Oncol. 2009;27:3650–8.

70. Lewis C, Patel V, Abhyankar S, Zhang D, Ketterling RP, McClure RF, et al. Microgranular variant of acute promyelocytic leukemia with normal conventional cytogenetics, negative PML/RARA FISH and positive PML/RARA transcripts by RT-PCR. Cancer Genet. 2011;204:522–3.

71. Reiter A, Lengfelder E, Grimwade D. Pathogenesis, diagnosis and monitoring of residual disease in acute promyelocytic leukaemia. Acta Haematol. 2004;112: 55–67.

72. Lo-Coco F, Cicconi L. History of acute promyelocytic leukemia: a tale of endless revolution. Mediterr J Hematol Infect Dis. 2011;3:e2011067.

73. Grimwade D, Walker H, Harrison G, Oliver F, Chatters S, Harrison CJ, et al. The predictive value of hierarchical cytogenetic classification in older adults with acute myeloid leukemia (AML): analysis of 1065 patients entered into the United Kingdom Medical Research Council AML11 trial. Blood. 2001;98:1312–20.

74. Slovak ML, Kopecky KJ, Cassileth PA, Harrington DH, Theil KS, Mohamed A, et al. Karyotypic analysis predicts outcome of preremission and postremission therapy in adult acute myeloid leukemia: a Southwest Oncology Group/Eastern Cooperative Oncology Group Study. Blood. 2000; 96:4075–83.

75. Schlenk RF, Döhner K, Krauter J, Fröhling S, Corbacioglu A, Bullinger L, et al. Mutations and treatment outcome in cytogenetically normal acute myeloid leukemia. N Engl J Med. 2008;358:1909–18.

76. Gulley ML, Shea TC, Fedoriw Y. Genetic tests to evaluate prognosis and predict therapeutic response in acute myeloid leukemia. J Mol Diagn. 2010;12: 3–16.

77. Borer RA, Lehner CF, Eppenberger HM, Nigg EA. Major nucleolar proteins shuttle between nucleus and cytoplasm. Cell. 1989;56:379–90.

78. Grisendi S, Mecucci C, Falini B, Pandolfi PP. Nucleophosmin and cancer. Nat Rev Cancer. 2006;6: 493–505.

79. Dohner K, Döhner H. Molecular characterization of acute myeloid leukemia. Haematologica. 2008;93: 976–82.

80. Falini B, Nicoletti I, Martelli MF, Mecucci C. Acute myeloid leukemia carrying cytoplasmic/mutated nucleophosmin (NPMc+AML): biologic and clinical features. Blood. 2007;109:874–85.

81. Gregory TK, Wald D, Chen Y, Vermaat JM, Xiong Y, Tse W. Molecular prognostic markers for adult acute myeloid leukemia with normal cytogenetics. J Hematol Oncol. 2009;2:23.

82. Patel JP, Gönen M, Figueroa ME, Fernandez H, Sun Z, Racevskis J, et al. Prognostic relevance of integrated genetic profiling in acute myeloid leukemia. N Engl J Med. 2012;366:1079–89.

83. Nakao M, Yokota S, Iwai T, Kaneko H, Horiike S, Kashima K, et al. Internal tandem duplication of the flt3 gene found in acute myeloid leukemia. Leukemia. 1996;10:1911–8.

84. Meshinchi S, Alonzo TA, Stirewalt DL, Zwaan M, Zimmerman M, Reinhardt D, et al. Clinical implications of FLT3 mutations in pediatric AML. Blood. 2006;108:3654–61.

85. Kiyoi H, Ohno R, Ueda R, Saito H, Naoe T. Mechanism of constitutive activation of FLT3 with

internal tandem duplication in the juxtamembrane domain. Oncogene. 2002;21:2555–63.

86. Griffith J, Black J, Faerman C, Swenson L, Wynn M, Lu F, et al. The structural basis for autoinhibition of FLT3 by the juxtamembrane domain. Mol Cell. 2004;13:169–78.

87. Brandts CH, Sargin B, Rode M, Biermann C, Lindtner B, Schwäble J, et al. Constitutive activation of Akt by Flt3 internal tandem duplications is necessary for increased survival, proliferation, and myeloid transformation. Cancer Res. 2005;65:9643–50.

88. Schnittger S, Schoch C, Dugas M, Kern W, Staib P, Wuchter C, et al. Analysis of FLT3 length mutations in 1003 patients with acute myeloid leukemia: correlation to cytogenetics, FAB subtype, and prognosis in the AMLCG study and usefulness as a marker for the detection of minimal residual disease. Blood. 2002;100:59–66.

89. Grundler R, Miething C, Thiede C, Peschel C, Duyster J. FLT3-ITD and tyrosine kinase domain mutants induce 2 distinct phenotypes in a murine bone marrow transplantation model. Blood. 2005;105:4792–9.

90. Sharma M, Ravandi F, Bayraktar UD, Chiattone A, Bashir Q, Giralt S, et al. Treatment of FLT3-ITD-positive acute myeloid leukemia relapsing after allogeneic stem cell transplantation with sorafenib. Biol Blood Marrow Transplant. 2011;17:1874–7.

91. Antonson P, Xanthopoulos KG. Molecular cloning, sequence, and expression patterns of the human gene encoding CCAAT/enhancer binding protein alpha (C/EBP alpha). Biochem Biophys Res Commun. 1995;215:106–13.

92. Gombart AF, Hofmann WK, Kawano S, Takeuchi S, Krug U, Kwok SH, et al. Mutations in the gene encoding the transcription factor CCAAT/enhancer binding protein alpha in myelodysplastic syndromes and acute myeloid leukemias. Blood. 2002;99:1332–40.

93. Asou H, Gombart AF, Takeuchi S, Tanaka H, Tanioka M, Matsui H, et al. Establishment of the acute myeloid leukemia cell line Kasumi-6 from a patient with a dominant-negative mutation in the DNA-binding region of the C/EBPalpha gene. Genes Chromosom Cancer. 2003;36:167–74.

94. Lin LI, Chen CY, Lin DT, Tsay W, Tang JL, Yeh YC, et al. Characterization of CEBPA mutations in acute myeloid leukemia: most patients with CEBPA mutations have biallelic mutations and show a distinct immunophenotype of the leukemic cells. Clin Cancer Res. 2005;11:1372–9.

95. Barjesteh van Waalwijk van Doorn-Khosrovani S, Erpelinck C, Meijer J, van Oosterhoud S, van Putten WL, Valk PJ, Berna Beverloo H, et al. Biallelic mutations in the CEBPA gene and low CEBPA expression levels as prognostic markers in intermediate-risk AML. Hematol J. 2003;4:31–40.

96. Redaelli A, Laskin BL, Stephens JM, Botteman MF, Pashos CL. A systematic literature review of the clinical and epidemiological burden of acute lymphoblastic leukaemia (ALL). Eur J Cancer Care (Engl). 2005;14:53–62.

97. http://www.cancer.gov/cancertopics/pdq/treatment/childALL/HealthProfessional/page1

98. McLeod HL, Krynetski EY, Relling MV, Evans WE. Genetic polymorphism of thiopurine methyltransferase and its clinical relevance for childhood acute lymphoblastic leukemia. Leukemia. 2000;14:567–72.

99. Schaeffeler E, Fischer C, Brockmeier D, Wernet D, Moerike K, Eichelbaum M, et al. Comprehensive analysis of thiopurine S-methyltransferase phenotype-genotype correlation in a large population of German-Caucasians and identification of novel TPMT variants. Pharmacogenetics. 2004;14:407–17.

100. Indjova D, Atanasova S, Shipkova M, Armstrong VW, Oellerich M, Svinarov D. Phenotypic and genotypic analysis of thiopurine s-methyltransferase polymorphism in the Bulgarian population. Ther Drug Monit. 2003;25:631–6.

101. Ganiere-Monteil C, Medard Y, Lejus C, Bruneau B, Pineau A, Fenneteau O, et al. Phenotype and genotype for thiopurine methyltransferase activity in the French Caucasian population: impact of age. Eur J Clin Pharmacol. 2004;60:89–96.

102. Jemal A, Siegel R, Xu J, Ward E. Cancer statistics, 2010. CA Cancer J Clin. 2010;60:277–300.

103. Sullivan RJ, Flaherty KT. BRAF in melanoma: pathogenesis, diagnosis, inhibition, and resistance. J Skin Cancer. 2011;2011. Article ID 423239. doi:10.1155/2011/423239.

104. Pollock PM, Meltzer PS. Lucky draw in the gene raffle. Nature. 2002;417:906–7.

105. Lovly CM, Dahlman KB, Fohn LE, Su Z, Dias-Santagata D, Hicks DJ, et al. Routine multiplex mutational profiling of melanomas enables enrollment in genotype-driven therapeutic trials. PLoS One. 2012;7:e35309.

106. Wan PT, Garnett MJ, Roe SM, Lee S, Niculescu-Duvaz D, Good VM, et al. Cancer genome project. Mechanism of activation of the RAF-ERK signaling pathway by oncogenic mutations of B-RAF. Cell. 2004;116:855–67.

107. Wilhelm SM, Carter C, Tang L, Wilkie D, McNabola A, Rong H, et al. BAY 43–9006 exhibits broad spectrum oral antitumor activity and targets the RAF/MEK/ERK pathway and receptor tyrosine kinases involved in tumor progression and angiogenesis. Cancer Res. 2004;64:7099–109.

108. Chang YS, Adnane J, Trail PA, Levy J, Henderson A, Xue D, et al. Sorafenib (BAY 43–9006) inhibits tumor growth and vascularization and induces tumor apoptosis and hypoxia in RCC xenograft models. Cancer Chemother Pharmacol. 2007;59:561–74.

109. Chapman PB, Hauschild A, Robert C, Haanen JB, Ascierto P, Larkin J, et al. BRIM-3 Study Group. Improved survival with vemurafenib in melanoma with BRAF V600E mutation. N Engl J Med. 2011;364:2507–16.

110. Young K, Minchom A, Larkin J. BRIM-1, -2 and -3 trials: improved survival with vemurafenib in metastatic melanoma patients with a BRAF(V600E) mutation. Future Oncol. 2012;8:499–507.

111. Rubinstein JC, Sznol M, Pavlick AC, Ariyan S, Cheng E, Bacchiocchi A, et al. Incidence of the V600K mutation among melanoma patients with BRAF mutations, and potential therapeutic response to the specific BRAF inhibitor PLX4032. J Transl Med. 2010;8:67.

112. Yang H, Higgins B, Kolinsky K, Packman K, Go Z, Iyer R, et al. RG7204 (PLX4032), a selective BRAFV600E inhibitor, displays potent antitumor activity in preclinical melanoma models. Cancer Res. 2010;70:5518–27.

113. Flaherty KT, Robert C, Hersey P, Nathan P, Garbe C, Milhem M, et al. Improved survival with MEK inhibition in BRAF-mutated melanoma. N Engl J Med. 2012;367:107–14.

114. Salama AK, Kim KB. Trametinib (GSK1120212) in the treatment of melanoma. Expert Opin Pharmacother. 2013;14:619–27.

115. Molina JR, Yang P, Cassivi SD, Schild SE, Adjei AA. Non-small cell lung cancer: epidemiology, risk factors, treatment, and survivorship. Mayo Clin Proc. 2008;83:584–94.

116. Ma PC. Personalized targeted therapy in advanced non–small cell lung cancer. Cleve Clin J Med. 2012;79:e-S56–60.

117. Ettinger DS, Akerley W, Borghaei H, Chang AC, Cheney RT, Chiriac LR, et al. J Natl Compr Canc Netw. 2012;10:1236–71.

118. Hayes DN, Monti S, Parmigiani G, Gilks CB, Naoki K, Bhattacharjee A, et al. Gene expression profiling reveals reproducible human lung adenocarcinoma subtypes in multiple independent patient cohorts. J Clin Oncol. 2006;24:5079–90.

119. Soda M, Choi YL, Enomoto M, Takada S, Yamashita Y, Ishikawa S, et al. Identification of the transforming EML4-ALK fusion gene in non-small-cell lung cancer. Nature. 2007;448:561–6.

120. Sasaki T, Rodig SJ, Chirieac LR, Jänne PA. The biology and treatment of EML4-ALK non-small cell lung cancer. Eur J Cancer. 2010;46:1773–80.

121. Shaw AT, Solomon B. Targeting anaplastic lymphoma kinase in lung cancer. Clin Cancer Res. 2011;17:2081–6.

122. Ou SH. Crizotinib: a novel and first-in-class multi-targeted tyrosine kinase inhibitor for the treatment of anaplastic lymphoma kinase rearranged non-small cell lung cancer and beyond. Drug Des Devel Ther. 2011;5:471–85.

123. Zhang Z, Stiegler AL, Boggon TJ, Kobayashi S, Halmos B. EGFR-mutated lung cancer: a paradigm of molecular oncology. Oncotarget. 2010;1:497–514.

Quality Assurance in Molecular Testing of Cancer

25

Sylviane Olschwang, Simon Patton,
Etienne Rouleau, and Elisabeth Dequeker

Introduction

In the past 20 years, the demand for molecular genetic testing has increased enormously. Clinical laboratory science has been transformed by generic molecular genetic technologies crossing traditional boundaries between diverse laboratory disciplines, including genetics, haematology, clinical chemistry and microbiology. Also, many of the laboratories offering diagnostic molecular genetic testing on a routine basis originated from a research-based setting. In bringing these new technologies into diagnostic practice, issues of quality have not been given adequate attention.

The exponential growth of the clinical diagnostic molecular genetic laboratories together with improving technical approaches has forced these laboratories to reorganise and standardise their methods and procedures and to manage their increasing dataflow more efficiently that is important for confirmation of a clinical diagnosis. The results of DNA diagnostic tests are of major importance in clinical decision-making, and therefore, the quality of the whole laboratory process, from sample reception to reporting of the results, from calibration of equipment to training of personnel and from documentation to method validation, should be managed systematically. Laboratories need to ensure that all the process is well controlled in terms of quality, using reference materials. External quality assessment (EQA) schemes are one of the ways to validate and improve this quality. Several have been established to help laboratories measure their performance against other centres and against fixed standards.

Cancer is now known to be a heterogeneous disease at the molecular level, with genetic and genomic factors underlying its aetiology. Understanding how these factors contribute to the development and treatment of both sporadic and hereditary cancers is important in cancer risk assessment, prevention, diagnosis, treatment and long-term management and surveillance. Now, a set of molecular analyses is well implemented in routine laboratories and covers these different aspects. The molecular results can now be integrated early in the decision process for the management of both patient and cancer.

S. Olschwang, Ph.D. (✉)
UMR_S910, INSERM, Marseille, France

Department of Gastroenterology, Ambroise Paré
Hospital, Marseille, France
e-mail: sylviane.olschwang@inserm.fr

S. Patton, Ph.D.
European Molecular Genetics Quality Network
(EMQN) Genetic Medicine, St. Mary's Hospital,
Manchester, UK

E. Rouleau, Ph.D.
Department of Genetics, Institut Curie, Paris, France

E. Dequeker, Ph.D.
Department of Public Health, Research Unit,
University of Leuven, Leuven, Belgium

G.M. Yousef and S. Jothy (eds.), *Molecular Testing in Cancer*,
DOI 10.1007/978-1-4899-8050-2_25, © Springer Science+Business Media New York 2014

In medical genetics, it is used to assess the exact nature of a cancer predisposition and to further establish the risk of asymptomatic relatives for developing cancer. Mutation carriers then enter specific early detection programmes and prophylactic recommendations referred to as personalised follow-up.

Recent advances in pharmacogenetics and pharmacogenomics have gradually unveiled the genetic basis of individual differences in drug responses. Molecular tests are used to characterise or classify tumours, detect specific alterations that relate to prognosis or define targets that predict therapy response or adverse effects. The results of these tests directly influence the clinical management of individual patients and participate to the so-called personalised therapy. Given the complexity of this genetic information (tumour mutation, gene overexpression, chromosomal translocation and germ line variations), as well as the variable level of scientific evidence, a subtle and moving classification of the tests has been proposed as a standard, optional or recommended complement to the therapeutic or diagnostic evaluation. That is why the quality of the result produces a very crucial point as any false positive or negative will bias the decision and reduce the chance to be correctly managed or treated for a patient.

In the following sections, we address the best practice recommendations for genetic testing through examples taken within one of the most frequent pathologies in oncology that is colorectal cancer. Colorectal cancer management indeed takes advantage of all the approaches mentioned above. Major genetic predispositions encounter for about 10 % of colorectal cancer and are genetically identified as polyposis syndromes and Lynch syndrome linked to germ line mutations in the APC, MYH, SMAD4, BMPR1A and STK11 genes and mismatch repair (MMR, i.e. MSH2, MLH1, MSH6, PMS2) genes, respectively. Recently developed drugs, which target molecular pathways altered in cancer cells, are only effective in the subset of patients that carries a molecular alteration that is targeted by a particular drug. For the identification of such molecular alterations, the term "predictive molecular

pathology" has become popular. An example of a personalised therapy is the use of KRAS gene mutation analysis constraining the prescription of EGFR-targeting drugs in patients with metastatic colorectal adenocarcinoma [1]. Microsatellite instability (MSI) in patients with stage II colorectal cancer is also a strong predictive factor for deciding on adjuvant treatment, and systematic testing has been retained as a standard but is not limiting test prior to therapeutic decision. On the contrary, although the ColoPrint(®) and Oncotype Dx(®) gene expression signatures have been shown to have prognostic value, no consensus yet exists concerning their use in clinical practice [2, 3]. Overall response rates after adjuvant chemotherapy remain low, with high rates of toxicity and pharmacogenetics aims at predicting adverse effects in individual patients [4, 5]. As an example, UGT1A1*28 leads to reduced conjugation of the active metabolite of irinotecan, resulting in an increased rate of adverse effects, especially neutropenia. Several other polymorphisms are known to influence drug efficacy, but the interpretation of pharmacogenetic tests is complicated, although results imply a promising way of pretreatment evaluation.

Quality Management

Models for integrated quality care have been progressively developed, based on the circle initially proposed by Demming that shows the constant process of quality care divided into four important phases: Plan—Do—Check—Act. Together, these models lifted the concept of quality from the primary process of producing high-quality goods to a higher level in an organisation, including its management [6].

First of all, developing a quality policy is the responsibility of management, but the attainment of quality requires the participation of all the members of an organisation, as defined in the rules of the International Standards Organisation's (ISO) standard ISO 9000. As the organisation implementing a quality management process can be held legally responsible, it is therefore important to chart an outline of the hierarchic and organisational structure of the laboratory. The managerial and technical personnel of the organisation must have the authority and resources needed to carry out their duties correctly. Job descriptions have to be updated regularly to clarify and reinforce the staff's duties and responsibilities within the laboratory, and documented training procedures have to be in place. A molecular genetic laboratory produces a lot of test data, and the scientist or technician performing the test is often the first person to interpret the results. It is common practice in many laboratories that the results and their interpretation are authorised by a second suitably qualified person, independent from the scientist or technician performing the test. A fully interpretative report on the results is normally forwarded to the referring clinician by the scientific staff. The workload of such laboratory is gradually increasing in line with new advances in technologies and research, and consequently, there is a continual need for additional extra well-trained personnel. Laboratory management also needs to ensure that there are clear criteria defining who is able to perform the second independent check of data. To ensure that the quality management system is implemented and adhered to, laboratory management should appoint a laboratory quality manager with a defined role and responsibilities and the authority to implement them.

Second, standards are an important part of quality management. The process by which a laboratory gains recognition from an external agency that its activities and products have a guaranteed high quality and meet the set standards is accreditation. Accreditation involves an external audit of the ability of the laboratory to provide a service of high quality. By declaring a defined standard of practice and having this independently confirmed, accredited laboratories attain a hallmark of performance and offer reassurance to users of their service. Over the world, there is a growing trend towards complying with the international standards ISO 15189 for medical laboratories and ISO 17025 for testing and calibration laboratories. In parallel to quality management, those standards stress technical expertise in the process. Any method needs to have a validation process before

any implementation. Performance needs the use of internal and external quality controls. All people involved in the process have to be empowered regularly. The molecular genetic test reports have to be "fit for purpose" and responsive to the needs of the user (http://www.eurogentest.org/laboratories/).

In daily practice, it is of most importance to guarantee reproducibility (same method on identical sample materials under different circumstances, i.e. technician, equipment, time) and repeatability (same method on identical sample materials under the same circumstances) of results. Three lines of controls have to be set up to secure these goals.

The first line controls: To daily validate assays. PCR blanks (no DNA template added to the PCR reaction) to check for contaminations, size markers to check for correct length of the PCR products, visual checks (e.g. equal reaction volumes in 96 well plates) and normal controls (DNA samples with no mutation in the genes being tested) to check the quality of the method. Repeated testing of positive control samples (DNA samples with a known mutation in the gene being tested). Reference material is an issue in molecular testing in cancer.

In order to demonstrate the efficacy of the test, laboratories should, where possible, include at least one positive control for every region scanned. However, laboratories cannot be expected to have positive control samples for every region scanned. Now, collection of mutated biological samples and banking of corresponding lymphoblastoid cell lines have been set up by European agencies, which provide relevant DNAs to the medical laboratories for their quality controls.

The second line controls: To validate the internal coherence of the results. Analysis of two DNA extracts from the same blood sample isolated in two separate rounds (this is a check of the reproducibility of the DNA isolation method and on sample swaps). In predisposition, the coherence can also be checked with clinical information as correct segregation of haplotypes in a family. In molecular pathology, some co-occurrences are very rare as BRAF and KRAS activating mutations in colorectal cancer or EGFR and KRAS activating mutations in lung cancer. All this information is important to consider in a daily practice as they warrant the coherence of the results.

The use of these two line controls may vary depending on the reason of referral. For example, mutation analysis in a family with a known mutation should always include a positive and a normal control. The approach used to detect the mutation should be a direct technique such as sequence analysis or mutation-specific PCR. However, several choices are possible for requests for mutation analysis in a family with an as yet undetermined mutation, so-called mutation-scanning analysis. Whole gene scans are preferably done in large batches with many samples. For gene scans using direct sequencing in genes without mutational hotspots, a minimum of two samples in a scanning series will suffice to obtain a normal pattern enabling the detection of a variant pattern. There is therefore no need for a separate normal control sample that reduces the costs of testing.

The third line controls: Laboratories can check the performance and spread of their results, quality controls and procedures by participating in organised external quality assessment (EQA) schemes for molecular genetics. Examples of such schemes include those organised by the European Molecular Genetics Quality Network (EMQN) and the United Kingdom National External Quality Assessment Scheme (UKNEQAS) for molecular cancer genetics or other national organisms in Italy and France. The performance of the laboratory is assessed on the basis of its ability to correctly genotype DNA samples in the context of a mock clinical question and to give a full interpretation of the test results. EQA schemes also assess the clerical accuracy of reports. Assessment of the results of EQA schemes is often guided by best practice guidelines that are a consensus statement by the diagnostic molecular genetics community on the best approaches to take in the molecular diagnosis of a disease [7, 8].

In summary, the implementation of a quality management system in a laboratory is a time of major disruption and can have a significant impact on the job of the referring clinicians, i.e. the pre-analytical steps. For example, the criteria for accepting a blood sample are often narrowed, and laboratories tend to stick more consistently to these criteria. The implementation of a quality system is often the beginning of a stricter, more formal sample acceptance policy. The referring clinician will be asked to fill out the forms completely and label sample tubes correctly. Best practice guidelines for laboratory internal quality control have been produced by the EMQN (http://www.emqn.org/emqn/Best+Practice). Incomplete forms and incorrectly labelled tubes often result in a sample not being accepted for testing.

Cancer Genetics: Germ Line Variations in Cancer

Hereditary predispositions to cancer are genetic prone diseases that highly increase the risk of individuals that bear germ line mutations for developing various types of cancers. Specific syndromes are defined on the basis of tumours spectra, but phenotypes often remain complex to recognise at the clinical level. As an example, BRCA1/2 mutation carriers are at high risk for breast and ovarian adenocarcinomas but also pancreas, prostate and at lower level colorectal cancers. Lynch syndrome is mainly characterised by colorectal and endometrial adenocarcinomas, but the tumour spectrum is much larger, including cancers from stomach, ovary, biliary tract, urinary tract and small intestine. Glioblastoma (i.e. Turcot syndrome) or skin cancers (i.e. Muir-Torre syndrome) are also part of Lynch syndrome. Pancreatic cancer increased risk is still debated. A common trait of these cancer predispositions is however an early-age at cancer development compared with general population.

As people carrying a mutation are often asymptomatic at time of genetic diagnosis, i.e. ask for predictive diagnosis, they thus enter specific and sometimes complex surveillance programmes. These consensus programmes guarantee the detection of tumours at early stages allowing to cure them in almost all cases. They have to be started at an early age, usually between 20 and 30 years depending on the mutated gene, sometimes in the childhood, and then have to be maintained the entire life. People not carrying the mutation segregating in their family are not at increased risk for cancer and do not enter specific surveillance protocols. Unclear or misinformed laboratory reports have major clinical implications since the presence or absence of a pathogenic mutation is often instrumental to decisions made about patient management. It is thus of most importance to characterise rigorously all genomic variations found during screening procedures of index cases to identify exactly that responsible for the predisposing disease.

External quality assessment is yearly provided for all frequent and several rare cancer predispositions by accredited organisms like EMQN or UKNEQAS since more than 10 years. We experienced laboratory performances in some diseases including Lynch syndrome, one of the most frequent cancer predispositions [9]. Since the first pilot scheme in 2003, annual EQAs have enabled the identification of the most frequent difficulties encountered by the participating labs, addressing disease-/gene-specific points to improve the standard of testing strategies. Globally, the performance of laboratories increased each year as well as the number of participants, and a high technical standard of genotyping has been reached with the decreasing use of home-made reagents and manual procedures. This result is very encouraging for labs, which aim to become referent with long-term agreements. The feedback to the labs integrated the genotyping assessment and keypoints to get the quality of the reports themselves better. For example in 2009, two separate reports were requested in one of the mock clinical questions—one for the index case (confirmation of the screening analysis) and one for a predictive test: 11 labs did not re-analyse the index case and 16 labs mixed the information from both cases in a single report, i.e. 25 % of the participants failed

to write a reliable report. Best practice guidelines on reporting are available which give clear guidance on the appropriate reporting procedures (http://www.sgmg.ch/view_page_professional.php?view=page&page_id=19). Specifically to the cancer predisposition studied, the conclusion should have restated the genetic status in the clinical context with discussion on the patient's main risks (related cancers, mode of inheritance) and the suitable prospective analyses when needed. At the end of the report, the reader should be convinced of the biological consequences of the genotype. In the 2008 scheme, 80 % of participants provided consistent information since no case referred to missense variants. In contrast, the 2005 and 2009 schemes included such a situation, and only 25 % of them reached the maximum score. This observation points out the difficulty linked to the interpretation of missense mutations itself rather than the lack of experience in quality controls. In complex diseases approached through the EMQN schemes, results emphasise that it is very important to have good background knowledge of the genes being tested to guarantee the reliability of genetic testing as part of the medical evaluation, especially as relevant and validated information is now available on free access international and national mutation databases.

Molecular Pathology: Somatic Variations in Cancer

The requirements for the reliability of molecular pathology are high since the results, which generally extend beyond histologically recognisable subtypes, are used to determine the eligibility of a patient for treatment using a specific class of drug and unreliable results might lead to over- or undertreatment of patients. Since these drugs are expensive, the availability of reliable tests will also significantly improve the cost-effectiveness of these new treatment modalities. In view of their widespread use in clinical practice, molecular tests need to be both accurate and readily available. Contrary to the USA, where

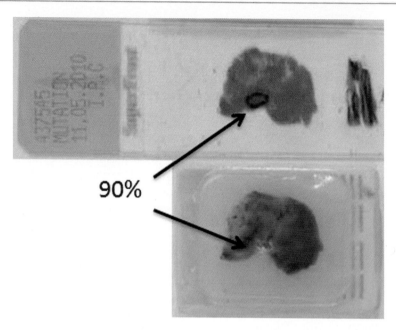

90%

Fig. 25.1 Histological control of a tumour sample. Before tumour DNA analysis, selection of the most accurate part of the sample is performed by the pathologist on a coloured slide, and the proportion of neoplastic cells is indicated for the selected region and the entire slide. In case of very small fragments, it is possible to use them without dissection when tumour cell compound is over 50 %. Dissection can be done by biopsies directly on the paraffin-embedded block as shown at the bottom of the figure

in vitro diagnostic (IVD) product regulation has been developed and directly related to drugs, in Europe no regulatory framework exists on which assay(s) is eligible as drug response marker: personalised drugs are related to a biomarker in Europe, whereas in the USA, they are related to a specific in vitro diagnostic product. However, as molecular testing allows getting a unique result using several different technical approaches, which under appropriate laboratory and expertise conditions might provide reliable results. However, the equivalence of the results can be only established through inter-laboratory comparison. To attain this goal, EQA programmes are essential.

The large majority of molecular tests in pathology are performed on formalin-fixed, paraffin-embedded tumour tissue. Considering the diversity and heterogeneity of tumour tissue, pathology review and assessment of section quality is mandatory. For instance, due to the limitations of most routinely utilised techniques, it is important to determine the percentage of neoplastic cell content in the material to be analysed.

The molecular test itself then includes DNA extraction, validation of the methods used for the test and accuracy of the result. Finally, reporting has to reflect the reliability of all different aspects: identification of the sample analysed, information on the type of assay used, adequacy of the sample relative to the underlying request and the test used, and accurate assessment of the clinical implications of the result.

The best practice is to assess the pathology review, the molecular analysis as well as reporting of the results, suggesting that reports should be divided into separate sections [10].

The "pre-analytical" phase includes examination of the sample by a pathologist, assessment of the adequacy of the test sample, evaluation of the percentage of neoplastic cells and whether or not the sample needs to be dissected (Fig. 25.1). This evaluation will have an impact on the performance of the method. This phase can also include other parameters related to the histological evaluation of the sample. However, quality assurance of pathological diagnosis of the specimens does not fall within this scope.

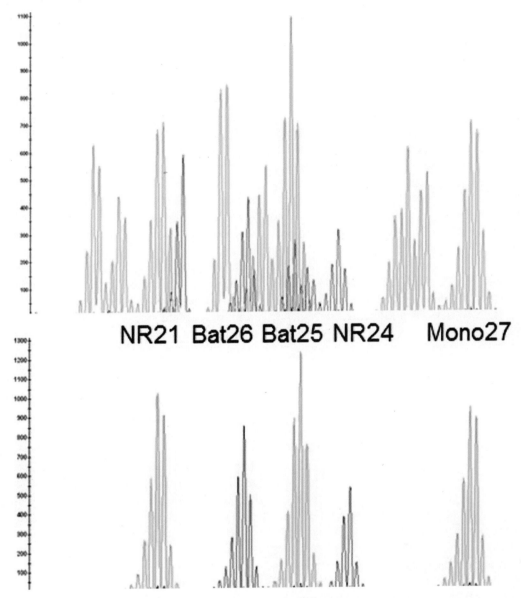

NR21 Bat26 Bat25 NR24   Mono27

Fig. 25.2 Characterisation of the MMR function in tumour cells by genotyping. A multiplex PCR is performed using the MSI Analysis System v1.2 (Promega, Charbonnières, France). The five loci are unambiguously detected after electrophoresis as shown on the normal profile presented on the top. Below, abnormal PCR products are observed at all five loci, indicating a tumour DNA of MSI genotype. The result is easy to obtain, but, depending on the indication of the analysis, the conclusion might be completely different: in a context of locally advanced colorectal cancer with bad-prognosis factors, the decision of 5-FU-based adjuvant treatment depends on the MMR function of cancer cells. In a context of early-onset colorectal cancer or family history suggesting a Lynch syndrome, this analysis is helpful to manage further germ line analyses

The "analytical" phase corresponds to DNA isolation and genotyping. Genotyping is the core of most currently practised tests in molecular genetics (Fig. 25.2). There is no specificity for molecular pathology towards any genetic testing. Some real-time PCR-based methods do not distinguish between different mutations in the same codon. Likewise, for some commercially available kits, the validation studies limit the result to whether a sample is mutant or not. Such methods are not to be preferred as only the genotype will certify the full quality of the process and avoid any false positive. Nevertheless, some screening approaches are not able to detect some mutations as the p.Val600Lys in the BRAF gene, for example.

The "post-analytical" phase includes interpretation and reporting of the results of the analysis, replaced in its clinical context. As the report will be sent to the clinicians and participate directly to the decision process, it is highly important to have standardisation and minimum items to be easily interpreted. This report is also the external reflect of the quality in a laboratory. Finally, interpretation becomes a major point with the increase of data produced per tumour sample. Databases and guidelines are very useful to help the biologist to explain the impact of variants, specifically outside the well-known hotspots.

Further Developments

In a clinical setting, next-generation sequencing (NGS) approaches for the enrichment and re-sequencing of DNA targets will progressively replace the current molecular techniques in oncology. In cancer predispositions, the NGS workflow targeted on BRCA1/2 genes for mutation detection was recently evaluated and has been reported as accurate and easy to incorporate into conventional workflow [11, 12]. If dedicated NGS projects might have similar performance in routine testing, the implementation of multi-targets will change the way for integrating and handling the results. In tumour analysis, despite the complexity revealed by a detailed analysis of many tumours, sequencing seems to find its place today. Set up a list of all the alterations present in the DNA of a tumour cell is an interesting way for research laboratories, but focus on a set of 100–200 genes whose involvement in the process of oncogenesis is known and for which a specific therapy is already effective (or will likely be) will play an important role in clinical practice. Contrary to targeted testing, this approach is interesting because it does not require the use of

specialised panels for each tumour type. Two tests are currently being validated that examine 176 and 128 genes, respectively [13, 14]. Sequencing can be done either on a high-end machine (Illumina HiSeq) by multiplexing the samples or, in urgent cases, on new clinical systems (Ion Torrent from Life Technologies or MiSeq from Illumina) that produce results faster, but at a higher cost. The pilot study results are encouraging, with a response time of less than 1 month, the frequent detection of mutations already known and the possibility to offer targeted therapy in all cases. Things are quite advanced, and indeed in the UK, the National Health Service has launched an appeal for such tests, with a maximum cost of 350 euros each. For those applications that are already part of the clinical management, laboratories have to follow identical standard rules for molecular testing, from DNA extraction to reporting. Quality management of those new techniques has no specificity. The use of internal controls will help to correctly follow any change in the process and the potential impact for the result. In the external quality assessment, one is just shifting from locus-specific EQA to genome-specific EQA. Three important aspects have to be mentioned at this stage: the quality criteria to be met by a sequence for clinical use, the question of the interpretation of the sequence and, finally, the ethical issues about informed consent in this context.

Conclusions

In summary, molecular testing of cancer needs to implement several quality controls in the testing process. EQA has demonstrated to be one of the major tools to alert laboratories to problems and shortcomings and, in time, will improve laboratory services, in general. Regular participation in EQA will help labs in achieving and maintaining proficient testing. In addition, the issue is to produce a certified reference material for internal and external quality follow-up. The shortcoming challenge will be the implementation in a routine process of the NextGen sequencing technology.

The quality management of a new technique should be hindered by those new approaches but implies a specific issue. For this purpose, a scheme is proposed in collaboration between EMQN and the UKNEQAS for molecular genetics. The scheme will be platform-independent and designed so that labs can "plug in" the EQA sample to their normal lab testing process without too much additional work.

References

1. García-Alfonso P, Salazar R, García-Foncillas J, Musulén E, García-Carbonero R, Payá A, et al.; Spanish Society of Medical Oncology (SEOM); Spanish Society of Pathology (SEAP). Guidelines for biomarker testing in colorectal carcinoma (CRC): a national consensus of the Spanish Society of Pathology (SEAP) and the Spanish Society of Medical Oncology (SEOM). Clin Transl Oncol. 2012;14:726–39.
2. Maak M, Simon I, Nitsche U, Roepman P, Snel M, Glas AM, et al. Independent validation of a prognostic genomic signature (ColoPrint) for patients with stage II colon cancer. Ann Surg. 2013;257:1053–8.
3. Kelley RK, Venook AP. Prognostic and predictive markers in stage II colon cancer: is there a role for gene expression profiling? Clin Colorectal Cancer. 2011;10:73–80.
4. Aiello M, Vella N, Cannavò C, Scalisi A, Spandidos DA, Toffoli G, et al. Role of genetic polymorphisms and mutations in colorectal cancer therapy. Mol Med Rep. 2011;4:203–8.
5. Henriette Tanja L, Guchelaar HJ, Gelderblom H. Pharmacogenetics in chemotherapy of colorectal cancer. Best Pract Res Clin Gastroenterol. 2009;23:257–73.
6. Voorhoeve E, Kneppers AL, Patton S. Quality management in molecular genetics molecular diagnosis of genetic diseases. Methods Mol Med. 2004;92:359–68.
7. Hastings RJ, Howell RT. The importance and value of EQA for diagnostic genetic laboratories. J Community Genet. 2010;1:11–7.
8. Losekoot M, van Belzen MJ, Seneca S, Bauer P, Stenhouse SA, Barton DE. EMQN/CMGS best practice guidelines for the molecular genetic testing of Huntington disease. Eur J Hum Genet. 2013;21:480–6.
9. Qiu J, Hutter P, Rahner N, Patton S, Olschwang S. The educational role of external quality assessment in genetic testing: a 7-year experience of the European Molecular Genetics Quality Network (EMQN) in Lynch syndrome. Hum Mutat. 2011;32:696–7.
10. van Krieken JH, Normanno N, Blackhall F, Boone E, Botti G, Carneiro F, et al. Guideline on the requirements of external quality assessment programs in molecular pathology. Virchows Arch. 2013;462:27–37.
11. Feliubadaló L, Lopez-Doriga A, Castellsagué E, Del Valle J, Menéndez M, Tornero E, et al. Next-generation sequencing meets genetic diagnostics: development of a comprehensive workflow for the analysis of BRCA1 and BRCA2 genes. Eur J Hum Genet. 2012;19. doi:10.1038/ejhg.2012.270.
12. Chan M, Ji SM, Yeo ZX, Gan L, Yap E, Yap YS, et al. Development of a next-generation sequencing method for BRCA mutation screening: a comparison between a high-throughput and a benchtop platform. J Mol Diagn. 2012;14:602–12.
13. Ross J, Lipson D, Yelensky R, et al. Comprehensive next-generation sequencing for clinically actionable mutations from formalin-fixed cancer tissues. Chicago: ASCO; June 2011. http://www.foundationmedicine.com/pdf/posters-abstracts/2011-06_ASCO_Poster.pdf.
14. Wagle N, Berger MF, Davis MJ, Blumenstiel B, Defelice M, Pochanard P, et al. High-throughput detection of actionable genomic alterations in clinical tumor samples by targeted, massively parallel sequencing. Cancer Discov. 2012;2:82–93.

Index

Printed by Printforce, the Netherlands